DESIGNING AND CONDUCTING HEALTH SURVEYS

DESIGNING AND CONDUCTING HEALTH SURVEYS

A Comprehensive Guide

SECOND EDITION

LU ANN ADAY

Foreword by Ronald M. Andersen

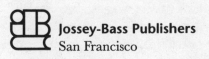

Jossey-Bass Publishers
San Francisco

Substantial discounts on bulk quantities of Jossey-Bass books are available to corporations, professional associations, and other organizations. For details and discount information, contact the
special sales department at Jossey-Bass Inc., Publishers (415) 433–1740; Fax (800) 605–2665.

For sales outside the United States, please contact your local Simon & Schuster International Office.

 Manufactured in the United States of America on Lyons Falls Pathfinder Tradebook. This paper
is acid-free and 100 percent totally chlorine-free.

Library of Congress Cataloging-in-Publication Data

Aday, Lu Ann.
    Designing and conducting health surveys : a comprehensive guide /
Lu Ann Aday; foreword by Ronald M. Andersen. — 2nd ed.
        p.   cm.
    Includes bibliographical references and index.
    ISBN 0-7879-0294-2
    1. Health surveys.   2. Health surveys—Statistical methods.
    I. Title.
    RA40.5.A33   1996
    614.4'2—dc20   96-18108

SECOND EDITION
HB Printing   10 9 8 7 6 5 4 3 2 1

CONTENTS

List of Figures, Tables, and Exhibits   ix

Foreword by *Ronald M. Andersen*   xiii

Preface   xv

Acknowledgments   xxi

The Author   xxiii

1 Thinking About Topics for Health Surveys   1

2 Matching the Survey Design to Survey Objectives   25

3 Defining and Clarifying the Survey Variables   44

4 Thinking Through the Relationships Between Variables   75

5 Choosing the Methods of Data Collection   91

6 Deciding Who Will Be in the Sample   112

7 Deciding How Many Will Be in the Sample   143

8 General Principles for Formulating Questions   177

9 Formulating Questions About Health   200

10 Formulating Questions About Demographics and Behavior   222

11 Formulating Questions About Knowledge and Attitudes   243

12 Guidelines for Formatting the Questionnaire   261

13 Monitoring and Carrying Out the Survey   281

14 Preparing the Data for Analysis   305

15 Planning and Implementing the Analysis of the Data   322

16 Writing the Research Report   350

Resource A   Personal Interview Survey: National Center for
                Health Statistics Health Interview Survey, 1995   359

Resource B   Telephone Interview Survey: Chicago
                Area General Population Survey on AIDS   399

Resource C   Mail Questionnaire Survey:
                Washington State Study of Dentists'
                Preferences in Prescribing Dental Therapy   442

Resource D   Selected Sources on Health Surveys   461

Resource E   Selected Examples of Health Surveys   467

References   481

Name Index   523

Subject Index   529

LIST OF FIGURES, TABLES, AND EXHIBITS

Figures

1.1 Framework for Classifying Topics in Health Surveys 11

1.2 Steps in Designing and Conducting a Survey 19

2.1 Stating the Study Objectives and Hypotheses for Different Study Designs 36

3.1 Evaluating the Reliability of Study Variables 52

3.2 Evaluating the Validity of Study Variables 59

3.3 Constructing Typologies and Indexes to Summarize Study Variables 64

4.1 Testing the Main Study Hypothesis 78

4.2 Elaborating the Main Study Hypothesis—Explanation 81

4.3 Elaborating the Main Study Hypothesis—Interpretation 83

4.4 Elaborating the Main Study Hypothesis—Interaction 85

4.5 Elaborating the Main Study Hypothesis—Replication 87

6.1 Types of Probability Sample Designs—Random Samples 117

6.2 Types of Probability Sample Designs—Complex Samples 119

6.3 Procedures for Selecting the Respondent—Selection Tables 130

6.4 Probability Sample Designs for Sampling Rare Populations 134

7.1 Normal Sampling Distribution 145

7.2 Selected Resources for Power Analysis 158

8.1 Basic Elements and Criteria in Designing Survey Questionnaires 192

9.1 Selected Utility-Related Scales 205

15.1 Using Nonparametric Bivariate Statistics to Test for Relationships Between Variables 335

15.2 Using Parametric Bivariate Statistics to Test for Relationships Between Variables 338

15.3 Using Nonparametric Multivariate Statistics to Explain Relationships Between Variables 340

Tables

1.1 Types of Errors in Designing and Conducting Surveys 21

2.1 Types of Study Designs 27

2.2 Stating the Research Question for Different Study Designs 33

2.3 Selected Examples of Research Questions, Objectives, Hypotheses, and Study Designs 40

3.1 Applying Different Levels of Measurement to Define Study Variables 48

3.2 Methods of Computing Reliability 54

3.3 Methods of Computing Validity 62

3.4 Constructing Scales to Summarize Study Variables 66

5.1 Comparison of Personal Interviews, Telephone Interviews, and Self-Administered Questionnaires 96

6.1 Advantages and Disadvantages of Different Probability Sample Designs 122

6.2 Sampling with Probability Proportionate to Size (PPS) 125

6.3 Procedures for Selecting the Respondent—Respondent Characteristics 132

6.4 Selected Examples of Probability Sample Designs 140

7.1a Sample Size Estimation—Descriptive Studies: Selected Examples 148

7.1b Sample Size Estimation—Descriptive Studies: Selected Examples 150

7.2 Type I and Type II Errors 153

7.3 Sample Size Estimation—Analytical and Experimental Studies: Selected Examples 156

7.4 Additional Adjustments in Computing the Sample Size 163

7.5 Calculation of Response Rate 166

7.6 Weighting the Sample Data to Reflect the Population 170

9.1 Selected General Health Status Measures 206

11.1 Selected Patient Satisfaction Measures 258

13.1 Schedule for Chicago AIDS Survey 299

13.2 Budget for Chicago AIDS Survey 300

15.1   Measurement Matrix Based on Dental Clinical Decision-Making
       Study   324
15.2   Using Univariate Statistics to Describe the Sample   330
15.3   Using Parametric Multivariate Statistics to Explain Relationships
       Between Variables   342
15.4   Mapping Out the Analysis Plan   344
16.1   Outline of the Research Report   352
 E.1   Selected Examples of Health Surveys   474

Exhibits

1.1   A Typical Survey Research Project   18
 4.1   Setting Up Mock Tables for the Analysis   88
 7.1   Criteria for Estimating the Sample Size Based on the Study Design   147
12.1   Do's and Don'ts of Questionnaire Design   264

FOREWORD

Ronald M. Andersen

In the foreword to the first edition of *Designing and Conducting Health Surveys* I wrote, "There is nothing like Aday's book currently available. I use it, assign it to my students and recommend it to my colleagues. I expect it to be the basic reference for health survey work for years to come." All that remains true and now will be true for even more years to come with the publication of this second edition.

Although everything valuable from the first edition is still here, additional guides and illustrations further assist the person interested in designing and conducting health surveys. In addition, this volume is substantially updated to emphasize the concept of total survey error to guide survey design; describe the rapidly expanding use of computers to access information as well as to conduct health surveys and process and analyze health survey data; and summarize new thinking about health questionnaire development based on research from multiple disciplines, including cognitive psychology and utility theory from economics.

Aday's success with this volume continues to be based on her clarity of purpose and a good plan meticulously carried out. She provides a comprehensive description of the process of doing a survey—from conceptualizing the problem to writing up the results. She covers all the key processes—variable development, planning and analysis, sampling, formulating questions, constructing the questionnaire, and collecting and analyzing the data. She provides principles pertaining to each part of the survey process, operational guides for applying the principles, and concrete examples of their implementation. Based on her own extensive experience and exceptional command of the literature she is able to impart successfully to the reader a sense of "how to," that is, how each step is carried out, why each step is important, and how the various processes are interrelated.

This volume provides both a road map for conducting health surveys and guidelines for orderly processes applicable to all social surveys. The bonuses for health survey students are the excellent discussion of formulating specific questions about health and the examples throughout the book drawn from health surveys conducted by mail or telephone or through face-to-face interviews.

Novices to health survey research will surely have an increased appreciation for the complexity of good survey research after reading *Designing and Conducting Health Surveys* and they will be in a better position to evaluate the use of survey research. Students learning to do survey research will also find the book very useful. It can serve as a fine textbook. And, somehow, Aday has also managed to include plenty of "grist for the mill" of the health survey researchers and practitioners. They will want to read the book and keep it handy as a reference guide.

July 1996   Ronald M. Andersen
                                                     Wasserman Professor and Chair
                                                     Department of Health Services
                                                     School of Public Health
                                                     University of California, Los Angeles

PREFACE

Designing and Conducting Health Surveys provides a guide for institutions and individuals interested in conducting or using health surveys. Drawing on methodological work on surveys in general and health surveys in particular, the book presents principles and approaches that should be applied in developing high-quality surveys.

The first edition of the book, published in 1989, identified a number of trends in the design and conduct of health surveys that continue to unfold today: the topics addressed remain sensitive and complex; the populations that are the focus of health surveys are hard to reach; computerized data gathering technologies present new possibilities, as well as problems, in gathering high-quality survey data; and a richer theoretical understanding of how respondents go about *answering* survey questions can help provide practical guidance to survey developers regarding how best to *ask* them.

This second edition of the book is intended to strengthen the preparedness of survey developers in taking on these and other challenges in designing high-quality health surveys. This edition draws heavily on the most recent methodological research in survey design in general and the rich storehouse of insights and implications provided by cognitive research on question and questionnaire design in particular. A total survey error framework is presented as a useful compass for charting the dangerous waters between the Scylla and Charybdis of systematic and random errors that inevitably accompany the survey design enterprise.

Each chapter ends with guidelines for minimizing errors in the aspect of designing a study that is the focus of that chapter. In addition, the three studies for which questionnaires were included in the first edition of the book—the National Center for Health Statistics National Health Interview Survey, the Chicago AIDS survey, and the Washington State Dentists Clinical Decision-Making Study—are used to illustrate the range of design alternatives available at each stage of a survey's development and to suggest a sound basis for choosing among them. Special populations get special attention as well in surfacing, at the end of each chapter, instructive perspectives and approaches for assuring that we have a better sense of the size and shape of their moccasins before insisting they try on ours in posing survey questions.

For those who would like to explore in greater depth any aspect of survey design discussed in the book, an extensive set of references is provided. In addition, selected sources most relevant to the topics addressed in the respective chapters are highlighted at the end of each.

The number, complexity, and scope of both privately and governmentally funded health care surveys—on the institutional, local, state, national, and international levels—have increased dramatically in recent years in response to the growing need for information about the sources, magnitude, and impact of health problems as well as about the roles of the programs and providers delivering services to address these problems. Many hospitals, health maintenance organizations (HMOs), and other health care businesses are struggling for their share of the consumer market. AIDS and new morbidities such as stress-related illness are placing increasing strain on the health care system as a whole. The issue of how to provide reasonable access to quality medical care in cost-effective ways with limited resources is a major problem in the United States and in other countries. Health surveys have been and will continue to be important sources of information about the impact of these dynamic and complex changes taking place in the health care marketplace. The purpose of this book is to provide a state-of-the-art resource for individuals and institutions charged with designing and conducting such surveys.

Audience

This book is intended to be a reference for health care marketing personnel, strategic planners, program designers, agency administrators, and health professionals charged with conducting or contracting for health studies. It will also serve as a resource for academics and researchers who are interested in collecting, analyzing, and evaluating health survey data and as a text for teaching students in public health, medical sociology, health administration, health education, medicine, nursing, dentistry, allied health, health program evaluation, and related fields how to design and conduct good surveys.

The issues involved in designing high-quality surveys parallel those to be considered in evaluating the quality of medical or nursing care. Certain norms of practice are taught during clinical training, based on research and experience in the profession. The precise relationship of these norms to whether the patient lives, or at least improves, is not always clear or systematically documented. What clinical researchers discover in the laboratory and what works for practitioners on the wards do provide the practical basis for training new professionals in sound medical practice. Doing good surveys is, similarly, a combination of science and practical experience.

Overview of the Contents

Chapter One lays the groundwork for thinking about what topics could be the focus of a health survey and what related studies to review before beginning one's own study. The chapter also looks ahead to the topics, technologies, and methodological and ethical challenges that are likely to affect the way health surveys are designed and conducted in the future and it introduces the total survey error framework as a foundation for identifying and mitigating the systematic and random errors that accompany any survey.

The fundamental starting point for a study is the definition of survey objectives. The process begins with the specification of the health topic or topics to be addressed in the survey. Deciding on the basic research questions to be addressed requires determining when, where, who, and what the focus of the study will be. Chapter Two describes major survey designs for addressing different research questions and presents guidelines for formulating detailed study objectives or hypotheses based on those questions.

The research questions and study hypotheses and objectives are usually phrased in general—or conceptual—terms. For example, "Are patients of higher socioeconomic status more likely to engage in preventive self-care practices?" During survey preparation, these concepts are translated into more directly measurable indicators such as, "Are patients with more education and higher family incomes more likely to exercise regularly?" Chapter Three reviews the techniques for developing working definitions of the topics or issues addressed in health surveys. It also provides two important criteria to use in evaluating just how useful these working definitions are: (1) Do they seem to mean the same thing all the time and/or to different people? (In other words, are they reliable?) and (2) Are they accurate translations of what the investigators originally had in mind? (That is, are they valid?) Techniques are also discussed for reducing the number of variables produced by many different survey questions to a more economical set of indicators through the use of summary typologies, indexes, and scales.

Chapter Four reviews the logic and methods to use in formulating the analysis plan for a survey. Analyzing the data is one of the last steps in the survey process. Having some idea of the analysis plan for the study can, however, help guide decisions made at every subsequent stage of the survey. Survey researchers should, like good scouts, be prepared and know before setting out what they want to accomplish.

Chapter Five explains the advantages and disadvantages of different ways of collecting data in general and data on health topics in particular. Methods of data collection considered here include face-to-face interviews, telephone interviews, and self-administered questionnaires. Any of these can be either recorded on paper copy questionnaires or input directly into a computer. Combinations of these various data gathering approaches can be used depending on the funding and technical capabilities at the researcher's disposal.

All the decisions made up to this point, especially those relating to the method of data collection, influence the process of sampling or selecting the people or organizations to be included in the study. Chapter Six reviews the basic types of sample designs used in surveys and presents examples of each from major health studies. Chapter Seven introduces an approach to estimating the sample size required for a given study. It also discusses the problems or errors that can arise in the sampling process and ways to deal with these, both in the course of the study and later, in data analysis using a particular sample design.

The heart of the survey is generally a questionnaire containing questions designed to elicit the information the investigator wants from study participants. Although rules for asking these questions are not always clear-cut, in recent years methodological research has yielded some useful guidelines for composing valid and reliable questions. Chapter Eight provides a general overview, based on the emerging research, of some of the issues to consider in formulating questions in general regarding both the form of the question itself and the possible response categories to use with it. Similarly, Chapters Nine, Ten, and Eleven present guidelines for developing particular types of questions—objective questions about respondents' characteristics or behavior, subjective questions about their attitudes toward or knowledge about certain health issues, and questions about their perceived or clinically evaluated health status. Examples of each type of question, drawn from health surveys, are also presented.

Individual questions are simply the building blocks of the survey questionnaire itself. The order or context in which questions are placed in the questionnaire and the form and clarity of the questionnaire have been found to influence the quality of data obtained in surveys. The type of data collection method chosen (face-to-face, telephone, or self-administered) can also significantly influence

the phrasing of individual questions and the form and format of the questionnaire itself. Chapter Twelve presents general rules of thumb to consider in designing questionnaires and the adaptations required for different modes of data
collection.

The issue of quality control during data collection is discussed in Chapter
Thirteen. The way the survey is actually conducted is shaped by all the prior decisions about study design and by the dress rehearsals (pilot studies or pretests)
done to see how well the questionnaires and procedures are performing, by the
training and experience of the data collection staff, and through the management
and monitoring of the data gathering process.

Coding the data entails assigning numbers to answers so that they can be
processed by computers. Before the data can be analyzed, adjustments may have
to be made to correct for missing or incomplete data from certain types of respondents on certain questions. The method of data collection—especially if computerized—can directly affect the ways the data are subsequently coded, processed,
and cleaned. (Cleaning refers to the process of identifying and correcting errors.) Chapter Fourteen discusses these preparations.

Chapter Fifteen reviews the major univariate, bivariate, and multivariate
methods for analyzing survey data. The methods the researcher uses will depend on the analysis plan chosen for the study (Chapter Four), the research question being addressed, the design of the study, and the measurement of the survey
variables to be used in the analysis.

The final step in designing and carrying out a survey is writing up what has
been learned in a report to interested audiences. Such a report may be addressed
to the funder as evidence of fulfillment of grant or contract objectives; to an op-
erating agency's administration or board of directors as input to their strategic
planning process; or to legislative committees, task forces, or staff as background
research on a particular piece of pending legislation. The survey may also be
the basis for a thesis, book, or journal article. This final chapter describes what the
form and content of a basic research report based on the survey might be.

The resources at the end of the book include questionnaires used in face-to-
face, telephone, and mail surveys. The most important sources of information on
health surveys and an inventory of health survey archives are also provided. Many
specific examples of health surveys at the international, national, state, and local
levels are presented.

In summary, this book provides an overview of the basic tenets of good health
survey design for those who have a role in gathering, analyzing, or interpreting
health survey data.

July 1996   Lu Ann Aday
Houston, Texas

ACKNOWLEDGMENTS

I gratefully acknowledge the contributions of many people to this book. I would like to thank the mentors and colleagues who first contributed to my understanding of how to design and conduct high-quality health surveys: Ronald M. Andersen (University of California, Los Angeles), Odin W. Anderson (University of Wisconsin), and Robert L. Eichhorn (Purdue University).

Numerous colleagues across the country provided comments on the first edition of the book and information on their experiences (or those of their institution) in designing and carrying out health surveys. I extend a special thanks to Norman Bradburn (National Opinion Research Center), Marcie Cynamon (National Center for Health Statistics), and Renee Slobasky (Westat, Inc.) for helping to coordinate visits to their institutions.

Particular thanks go to those colleagues who read all or part of the working manuscript for the book and provided invaluable comments, all of which I took seriously in making the final revisions to the book: Gary Albrecht, Ronald M. Andersen, Charles Begley, Steven Botman, Marcie Cynamon, David Grembowski, Asha Kapadia, David Lairson, Diane O'Rourke, Beatrice Selwyn, Carl Slater, and Richard Warnecke. The anonymous Jossey-Bass reviewers also provided very helpful feedback on the first edition of the book to consider in writing the second.

I also wish to express my thanks to the head librarians and their staff who facilitated my access to state-of-the-art sources both on-line and in the stacks—Stephanie Normann, University of Texas School of Public Health, and Pat Bova,

National Opinion Research Center—as well as Cassandra Perkins, Information Services Librarian, at the Texas Medical Center Library.

Special thanks go also to the graduate assistants who helped locate and copy many of the sources on which the revisions were based (Contessa Fincher, Jeannette Goode, and Wally Thomas) and to Lynn D. Binnicker in particular who created and compiled the bibliographic database for the extensive set of references cited in the book.

I gratefully acknowledge the patience and expertise of my secretary, Regina Fisher, in assisting with the preparation of the manuscript.

I am grateful for the supportive environment at the University of Texas School of Public Health (UTSPH), which allowed me the flexibility to write this book, and to the students in my Health Survey Research Design course throughout the years, who facilitated my thinking through how best to teach others about surveys.

Finally, my thanks go to my friend Katherine V. Wilcox, who read the draft of the manuscript with a teacher's eye for clarity. Her suggestions were extremely helpful in ensuring that the manuscript would make sense to someone besides the author. She also helped copy and assemble the extensive set of sources referenced in the book.

I enjoyed and learned from writing this book. My hope is that others will learn from and enjoy reading it.

—L.A.A.

THE AUTHOR

LU ANN ADAY is professor of behavioral sciences and management and policy sciences at the University of Texas School of Public Health. She received her B.S. degree (1968) in economics from Texas Tech University and her M.S. (1970) and Ph.D. (1973) degrees in sociology from Purdue University.

Aday's principal research interests have focused on the conceptual, empirical, and policy dimensions of equity of access to care for vulnerable populations. She has conducted major national and community surveys and evaluations of national demonstrations and has published extensively in this area. She is the principal author of eight books:

The Utilization of Health Services: Indices and Correlates—A Research Bibliography (1972)

Development of Indices of Access to Medical Care (1975)

Health Care in the United States: Equitable for Whom? (1980)

Access to Medical Care in the U.S.: Who Has It, Who Doesn't (1984)

Hospital-Physician Sponsored Primary Care: Marketing and Impact (1985)

Pediatric Home Care: Results of a National Evaluation of Programs for Ventilator-Assisted Children (1988)

At Risk in America: The Health and Health Care Needs of Vulnerable Populations in the United States (1993)

Evaluating the Medical Care System: Effectiveness, Efficiency, and Equity (1993)

Aday is also coauthor of *Ambulatory Care and Insurance Coverage in an Era of Constraint* (1987) with R. M. Andersen, C. S. Lyttle, L. J. Cornelius, and M. Chen.

CHAPTER ONE

THINKING ABOUT TOPICS
FOR HEALTH SURVEYS

Chapter Highlights

1. Surveys systematically collect information on a topic by asking individuals questions to generate statistics on the group or groups that those individuals represent.
2. Health surveys ask questions about a variety of factors that influence, measure, or are affected by people's health.
3. Health survey researchers should review the major international, national, state, and local health surveys relevant to their interests before undertaking their own study.
4. Good survey design is basically a matter of good planning.
5. The total survey error framework alerts researchers to ways to identify and mitigate both bias and variable errors in surveys.

This book provides guidance for designing and conducting health surveys. These surveys systematically collect information on a topic of interest (such as state abortion rights legislation) by asking individuals questions (about their attitudes toward the legislation) to generate statistics (percent who favor and percent who oppose it) for the group or groups those individuals represent (registered voters in the state).

This chapter addresses (1) the topics, techniques, and ethical issues that will characterize the design and conduct of health surveys in the future; (2) the defining features of surveys compared with other data collection methods; and (3) the reasons for studying health surveys. It also provides (4) a framework for classifying the topics addressed in health-related surveys, (5) illustrative examples of health surveys to be used in this book, and (6) an overview of the total survey design approach to designing and conducting health surveys.

Future Health Surveys

Health surveys have been and will continue to be important sources of information for health care policymakers, public health professionals, private providers, insurers, and health care consumers concerned with the planning, implementation, and evaluation of health-related programs and policies. The design and conduct of health surveys in the future will, however, be shaped by changes in the diversity, complexity, and sensitivity of the topics addressed in these studies, the innovative techniques and technologies that are being developed for carrying them out, and the new or intensified ethical dilemmas that are a result of these changes.

Topics

The topics addressed in future health surveys will be sensitive and complex ones. Such sociomedical morbidities as AIDS, child abuse, sexual dysfunction, drug and alcohol addiction, and family violence, among others, are now encompassed in definitions of public health and medical problems. The issue of access to medical care focuses on vulnerable and hard-to-locate populations differentially experiencing these new morbidities—homosexual males and bisexual males and females, drug abusers, the homeless, medically fragile children and the elderly, and undocumented migrant and refugee populations. Health care program designers are concerned with the number of people in these vulnerable groups, the particular health problems they experience, the barriers to care they confront, the ways in which their knowledge, attitudes, and behaviors exacerbate the risk of their contracting serious illnesses, and the resources they have to deal with these problems.

These trends in asking tough questions of hard-to-locate respondents in order to gain information for the design of cost-effective public and private health programs to address the needs of these respondents are likely to continue.

Techniques and Technologies

The topics to be addressed in health surveys present new and intensified challenges at each stage of the design and conduct of a study. Corresponding to these developments, however, is the emergence of new technologies for assisting with these tasks.

Rapid growth in the number and diversity of journals and specialized publications dealing with health topics has made the job of identifying the major research in any given area more difficult. It is challenging for most survey researchers to keep current with the literature in their own principal areas of interest, much less to master the literature in other fields. Computerized text search programs have greatly facilitated access to published research, but time is required to learn how to carry out these searches efficiently. Initially the databases used in these systems tended to focus on professional journals and related periodical literature, though increasingly computerized access to books, government publications, and unpublished research in progress relevant to the topic is being facilitated by online library and database systems. For those health topics for which little information is available because of the newness of the topic or the corollary lag in publication of research results, the survey designer will need to contact relevant public or private funding agencies and colleagues in the field who are known to have research in progress on the issue.

In the interest of learning about health and health-related attitudes, knowledge, and behaviors, survey researchers are attempting to penetrate more deeply into the traditionally best-kept family and personal secrets. The application of principles of cognitive psychology to the design and evaluation of such questions promises to challenge many of the standardized approaches to asking questions that have evolved since World War II. At a minimum, in the early stages of questionnaire development survey designers should ask respondents what went through their minds when they were asked sensitive questions about themselves or other members of their family. Moreover, prominent survey methodologists have called for the development of theories of surveys. These theories would focus on the decisions that could be made at each stage of designing and carrying out a survey to maximize quality and minimize costs (Groves, 1987, 1989; Sudman, Bradburn, & Schwarz, 1995).

The technology that has had the largest influence on the techniques used in the design and conduct of health surveys is computerized information processing. Survey designers should consider how these methods can be used to facilitate research on different survey techniques or methodologies (such as using different approaches to sampling respondents, phrasing questions, training interviewers, and so on). The rapid turnaround of information made possible by computerized methods should expedite choices among design alternatives of this kind. More attention needs to be given to evaluating the overall quality of the information obtained using computerized approaches, the impact on the interviewers and respondents of using computers to display the questions and enter respondents' answers, and the costs at each stage of the study compared with traditional paper-and-pencil surveys. Computerized survey technologies are wonderful innovations. As with any new invention, however, the most effective and efficient means of producing and using it needs to be explored and tested rather than simply assumed.

The topics and technologies evolving for health surveys present both challenges and opportunities in designing the samples for these studies. As mentioned earlier, health surveys have increasingly focused on rare or hard-to-locate populations. Innovative approaches are required to identify the universe or target population of interest, develop cost-effective methods for drawing the sample, and then find individuals to whom the questionnaire or interview should be administered. Survey designers must be aware of the methods that have been developed to identify and oversample rare populations and prepared to invest time and resources to come up with the best sample design for their study.

Ethics

Asking people questions in surveys about aspects of their personal or professional lives always involves a consideration of the ethical issues posed by this process. Are they fully informed about the study and do they voluntarily agree to participate? What benefits or harm may they experience if they participate? Will their right to remain anonymous and the confidentiality of the information they provide be maintained when the findings are reported? The evolution of the topics, techniques, and technologies just reviewed promises to heighten, rather than diminish, the importance of these ethical questions in the design and conduct of health surveys.

Informed Consent. The increasing use of cold contact (unannounced) calls in random digit dialing telephone surveys permits very little advance information to be provided to the respondent about the nature of the study and the ways in which the information will be used. Survey designers are reluctant to spend much time giving respondents details on the survey for fear they will hang up. There is also little opportunity to elicit the formal written consent of respondents for what might be particularly sensitive topics. Respondents with what are perceived to be socially undesirable diseases and little means to pay for health care also may feel obligated to participate in a study if their providers ask them to do so, fearing that they will subsequently be refused treatment if they do not.

Benefit Versus Harm. Rational and ethical survey design attempts to ensure that the benefits outweigh the costs of participating. Asking people sensitive questions about threatening or difficult topics may call forth memories or emotions that are hard for them to handle. Most survey designers do not explicitly consider such "costs" to the respondents.

Providing monetary incentives does increase people's willingness to participate in surveys. However, more research is needed to examine the effect of such incentives on the quality of the information provided. Do respondents feel more obligated, for example, to give answers they think the interviewer wants to hear?

Rights of Anonymity and Confidentiality. Finally, an issue that continues to be an important one in the design and conduct of surveys is guaranteeing the anonymity of survey respondents and the confidentiality of the information they provide. This issue is made more salient with the possibility of computerized linkages between sources, such as databases that link phone numbers to household addresses or between survey data and medical records or billing information from providers.

The United States has become an increasingly litigious society, as evidenced by the growing number of malpractice suits brought against health care providers. Survey designers can thus expect to confront more detailed and cumbersome review procedures for evaluating how the rights of study participants will be protected in carrying out the survey.

Defining Features of Surveys

Several key dimensions define the survey approach: (1) a research topic or problem of interest has been clearly delineated; (2) information on the issue is gathered by asking individuals questions; (3) the data collection process itself is systematic and well defined; (4) the purpose of the study is to generate group-level summary statistics; and (5) the results are generalizable to the groups represented by the individuals included in the study (American Statistical Association, 1995).

A number of these features are not unique to surveys, but taken together they tend to distinguish this data gathering method from such other approaches as using existing record data, conducting participant or nonparticipant observational studies, or carrying out case studies of one or a limited number of programs, institutions, or related units. Researchers should not necessarily assume that surveys are always the best approach to use in gathering data. That decision depends on what best enables investigators to address the research questions of interest to them. Further, survey developers are increasingly making use of qualitative research methods (such as focus groups, in-depth unstructured interviews, or ethnographies) to guide the development and interpretation of more structured surveys (Bauman & Adair, 1992; Mechanic, 1989; Stange & Zyzanski, 1989; Steckler, McLeroy,

Goodman, Bird, & McCormick, 1992; Sudman, 1989; Sudman, Bradburn, & Schwarz, 1995). The similarities and differences between these methods and surveys are reviewed in the following discussion.

Existing Record Sources

Health care investigators might decide that existing record data, such as the medical records available in hospitals or physicians' offices, claims data from private or public third-party insurers, or vital statistics records on births and causes of deaths are the most useful and relevant sources for the types of information they need to gather for their study. It will then not be necessary to ask people questions directly to get the information. This is particularly true for factual data on concrete events that are fully and completely documented in existing sources. If the investigator wishes to obtain more subjective, attitudinal data from individuals or to explore the probable accuracy or completeness of the information in the record sources, then designing a survey to ask people questions about the topic is warranted.

Participant or Nonparticipant Observation

In a second important method of data collection that differs from the survey approach, the investigator directly observes rather than asks individuals questions about particular situations or events. These observations may be relatively unstructured ones in which the researchers become, in effect, direct participants in the events. For example, this approach is used by medical anthropologists who live and work with members of a cultural subgroup (such as minority drug users or prostitutes) in order to establish the trust and rapport required to gain an understanding of certain health practices within that group.

Structured observational methods require that the investigator have clearly delineated guidelines that indicate what to look for while observing the behaviors of interest. For example, researchers might want to record systematically patterns of interaction among family members during counseling sessions dealing with the addictive behavior of one of them. To do this, they could call on the procedures that social psychologists have developed for systematically inventorying and classifying such interactions. These approaches are also used in coding interviewers' and respondents' behaviors for the purpose of identifying problem questions during the instrument development phase of the study or to improve interviewer performance.

The principal way in which observational methods differ from surveys is that individuals are not asked questions directly to obtain needed information. In addition, the purpose of such research may be exploratory, that is, the investigator may want to get a better idea of what relationships or behaviors should be examined before going on to develop a comprehensive, formalized approach to gathering data on the topic. The investigator is usually not so interested in generating aggregate summary statistics that can be generalized to a larger target population when these methods are used. Instead, the focus is on the microcosm of activity being observed in the particular situation and what the investigator can learn from it.

Case Studies

Case studies of particular institutions or agencies (such as hospitals, health maintenance organizations [HMOs], or neighborhood clinics) ask key informants questions about the organization, observe aspects of what is going on in the agency, or examine extant administrative or other record sources. The main difference between case studies and surveys, however, is that in case studies the investigators tend to focus on *a few elements to illustrate the type of unit* they are interested in learning about whereas in a survey they gather information *on a number of elements intended to represent a universe of units of that type.* Case studies take on more of the features of survey-based approaches to the extent that individuals are asked questions about themselves or their institutions; that a systematic, well-defined approach is used in deciding what questions to ask; and that the institutions or informants are selected with consideration given to the groups they represent.

If the investigators determine that a survey is the preferred method to elicit the information they need, they then have to decide whether they will try to do the study themselves, contract with a survey firm to carry it out, or make use of data that have already been gathered on the topic in other surveys.

Reasons for Studying Health Surveys

1. To design good surveys with small budgets. Most designers of health surveys do not have large grants or substantial institutional resources to support the conduct of large-scale studies. Students generally have a shoestring budget to carry out required thesis research. Academic researchers often use students in their classes or draw on limited faculty research funds to carry out surveys locally in their institutions or communities. State and community agency budgets are generally tight, and the boards of hospitals and health care organizations may encourage staff interested in conducting surveys to make use of institutional resources such as phone, mail, or computer services to keep survey costs down. And doing good surveys does not always require large budgets—either a Cadillac or a Ford will get you where you want to go; the same basic principles of sound engineering design apply to both. Survey developers should be aware of the fundamental principles behind the good design even of small surveys. It may be a matter of what you can afford. However, it is important to remember that the costs of poor survey design are also high.

2. To learn about and from well-designed, large-scale surveys with large budgets. Hundreds of millions of dollars have been spent in designing and executing large-scale national health surveys. The decennial census and Census Bureau-sponsored Current Population Surveys are useful sources of selected indicators of the health of the U.S. population. The National Center for Health Statistics routinely conducts surveys of the health of the U.S. population and the providers of health care. Since 1977 the Agency for Health Care Policy and Research (formerly the National Center for Health Services Research) and the National Center for Health Statistics have conducted several large-scale special surveys on the health practices of the U.S. population and their levels and patterns of expenditures for medical care. In addition, a variety of methodological studies have been conducted in conjunction with these and other large-scale health surveys to identify sources of errors in this type of study and the decisions that should be made to reduce or eliminate them (Berk, Wilensky, & Cohen, 1984; Cox & Cohen, 1985). The results of such studies are routinely published in the proceedings of conferences held by the American Statistical Association and the U.S. Bureau of the Census, as well as other governmental agencies (see Resource D).

Individuals interested in health surveys should be aware of these large-scale studies because they are a rich source of data on the nation's health and health care system. They also provide a gold mine of questions for inclusion in related studies, the answers to which can then be compared with national data. Finally, they have a great deal to teach us about how to do good surveys since resources are provided in the budgets of these surveys to assess the quality of the research itself.

3. To be aware of what to look for in conducting secondary analyses of existing health survey data sets. Many researchers do not have the time or resources to carry out their own surveys. In recent years extensive archives of national and local health survey data sets have been developed. Students, researchers, and program administrators and planners are being encouraged to make greater use of these secondary data sources, that is, data they were not involved in collecting (Connell, Diehr, & Hart, 1987; DeFriese, 1991; Hakim, 1982; Kiecolt & Nathan, 1985; Stewart, 1984). These analyses can involve efforts to use existing data sets—state or national data collected for other purposes—to address a particular research question, such as the influence of the types of food children consume on obesity, or to make estimates for specific local areas or populations, such as the percent of the population without insurance coverage. "Small area estimation" procedures have been developed to generate these latter estimates (Braden & Cohen, 1992; Johnson,

1993; Malec, 1995; Malec & Sedransk, 1993; Malec, Sedransk, & Tompkins, 1993; Marker, 1993; National Center for Health Statistics, 1977, 1979).

Users of secondary data sources should raise a number of questions, however, in considering the relevance of these data for their own research. How were people chosen for inclusion in the study? Were efforts made to evaluate the accuracy of the data obtained? How did researchers deal with people who refused to participate in the study or to answer certain questions? Are there particular features of how the sample was drawn that should be taken into account in analyzing the data? Awareness of these and other issues is essential to being an informed user of secondary health survey data sources.

4. *To know how to evaluate and choose firms to conduct health surveys.* Health survey research is big business. Nonprofit, university-based survey organizations as well as for-profit commercial firms compete to obtain contracts with government agencies, academic researchers, and provider institutions for conducting national, state, and local health surveys. Some university-based or affiliated survey research organizations that have conducted health surveys on a variety of topics include NORC (National Opinion Research Center, University of Chicago), Survey Research Center (University of California, Berkeley), Survey Research Center (University of Michigan), Survey Research Laboratory (University of Illinois), and the Wisconsin Survey Research Laboratory (University of Wisconsin). Other not-for-profit firms that have been engaged in conducting large-scale health surveys include the Research Triangle Institute (University of North Carolina) and the RAND Corporation (Santa Monica, Calif.). A number of commercial, for-profit firms have also carried out a range of health surveys under contract with public and private sponsoring agencies, including Chilton Research Services (Radnor, Penn.), Gallup (Princeton, N.J.), Louis Harris and Associates (New York), Mathematica Policy Research (Princeton, N.J.), and Westat (Rockville, Md.). *Survey Research,* a newsletter published quarterly by the Survey Research Laboratory at the University of Illinois, provides an overview of the studies currently being conducted by university-based and other nonprofit survey research firms.

These organizations emphasize different methods of data collection—in-person interviews, computer-assisted telephone interviews, or computer-assisted personal interviews—and different basic sample designs, and they use different types of data-editing and data-cleaning procedures. Researchers and agency and organizational representatives considering contracting with such organizations need to know their experience in doing health surveys and evaluate their capabilities for carrying out the proposed study.

5. *To become a better-informed consumer of health survey results.* Opinion polls that summarize the American public's attitudes toward issues, such as whether children with AIDS should be admitted to public schools, often report that estimates vary plus or minus 3 percent for the sample as a whole or as much as plus or minus

7 percent for certain subgroups (African Americans, Hispanics) because only a small sample of the American public was interviewed to make these estimates. How does one use this information to decide whether a difference of 10 percent reported between African Americans and whites in support of the issue is "real" then? An HMO administrator is interested in the results of a survey of plan members' satisfaction with services in which only 50 percent of the members returned the questionnaire. Should she be concerned about whether the survey accurately represents all enrollees' attitudes toward the plan? Students and faculty conduct literature reviews of studies relevant to concepts of interest prior to formulating their own research proposals. If a study reports that an indicator of patient functional ability had a reliability coefficient of .80 when administered at two different times in the course of a week to a group of elderly patients, does that mean it is a fairly good measure? These are examples of the types of questions that could occur to consumers of health survey findings. This book identifies the criteria that can be applied when one attempts to answer these and other questions about the quality of health survey data.

Framework for Classifying Topics in Health Surveys

Health surveys can cover a variety of topics, such as the ecology (distribution) and etiology (causes) of disease, the response to illness or maintenance of health on the part of the patient or the public, and the personnel and organizations in the health care professions (Aday, 1993a; Aday, Sellers, & Andersen, 1981; Cartwright, 1983; Suchman, 1967).

Health status is the explicit or implicit focus of health surveys, as defined here—studies that ask questions about factors that directly or indirectly influence, measure, or are affected by people's health. It is important to point out that health surveys may address more than one topic. A study may focus on one area of interest (out-of-pocket expenditures for care) but also include a range of related issues (health status, utilization of services) to examine their relationships to the major study variable. As will be discussed later, a survey may be principally concerned with describing a particular situation or with analyzing relationships between variables to explain why the situation is the way it is. The blocks outlined in Figure 1.1 reflect aspects that influence, measure, or are influenced by a person's health, and the arrows between them indicate relationships commonly hypothesized to exist between those elements. Health surveys can be used to examine the broader political, cultural, social, economic, and physical environment of a community, as well as the characteristics of the people who live there and the health care system that has evolved to serve them.

FIGURE 1.1. FRAMEWORK FOR
CLASSIFYING TOPICS IN HEALTH SURVEYS.

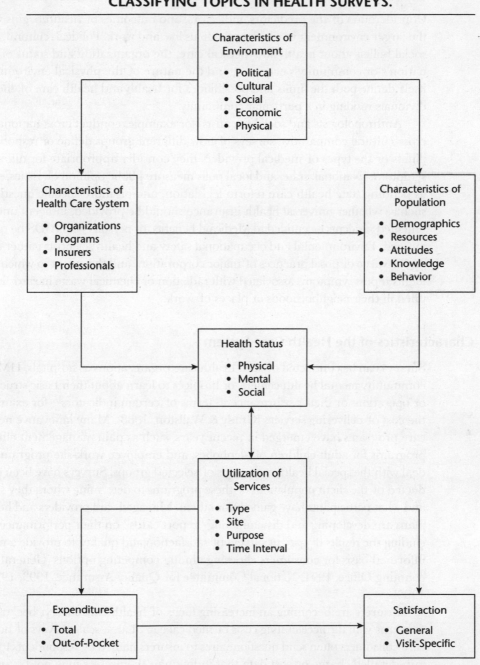

Characteristics of the Environment

Consideration of the predictors, indicators, and outcomes of health begins with the larger environment in which individuals live and work. Political, cultural, and social beliefs about health and medical care, the organization and status of the nation's or community's economy, and the nature of the physical environment itself define both the limits and possibilities for health and health care of the individuals residing in a particular community.

Anthropologists and social scientists, for example, conduct cross-national or cross-cultural comparative surveys of how different groups define or respond to illness or the types of medical providers they consider appropriate for different symptoms. National, state, and local polls measure public opinion on issues, such as pending state health care reform legislation, and on more specific questions, such as whether universal health insurance should be provided, indigent undocumented residents be entitled to Medicaid benefits, or persons with AIDS be quarantined. Environmental and occupational safety and health scientists gather data on the waste disposal practices of major corporations and the extent to which residents report symptoms associated with radiation or chemical waste hazards identified in their neighborhoods or places of work.

Characteristics of the Health Care System

Surveys can be conducted of such health care organizations as hospitals, HMOs, community mental health centers, or hospices to learn about their basic structure or operations or their performance in terms of certain indicators—for example, the cost of delivering services (Grady & Wallston, 1988). Many innovative health care programs have emerged in recent years, such as pain management clinics, programs for adult children of alcoholics, and employee work-site programs, to deal with the special health care needs of selected groups. Surveys have been conducted of the client populations of these programs to determine whom they serve and what participants have gained from them. Managed care providers and health plans are developing and disseminating "report cards" on their performance, including the results of patient surveys of satisfaction and quality, to provide a more informed basis for consumers choosing among competing options (General Accounting Office, 1994; National Committee for Quality Assurance, 1993, 1995a, 1995b).

Insurers are becoming an increasing focus of health care surveys because of concerns with the accelerating costs of medical care. Large-scale surveys of health care consumers often send questionnaires to insurers named by respondents to obtain detailed charge or cost data that individuals themselves may not be aware of when third parties pay their medical bills directly.

Health care professionals—physicians, dentists, nurses, allied health workers—have been a frequent focus of health care surveys. Surveys of health professionals have yielded information about the people who choose to go into the profession and why, the nature of the professional socialization experience and students' responses to it, factors that enter into the choice of specialty or practice location, the actual content and norms of care in professional practice, and the level of professional job or career satisfaction.

Characteristics of the Population

Surveys of the population at risk in a community have been widely used in needs assessment and strategic planning or marketing studies for new health care facilities or programs. Demographics, such as the age, sex, ethnic, and racial composition of a community, indicate the potential need and demand for certain medical services, such as prenatal care, preventive immunizations, hypertension screening, or elderly day care. Income levels and the type and extent of insurance coverage in a community reflect the resources available to individuals for purchasing medical care when they need it.

Responses to questionnaires about an individual's health and health care attitudes and knowledge may signal which groups are at particular risk of contracting certain illnesses (such as AIDS or cervical cancer) because of beliefs that demonstrate their ignorance of the disease or its causes or their unwillingness to seek appropriate screening or treatment services for it. There is increasing evidence that people who engage in certain personal health practices or behaviors, such as excessive smoking or alcohol consumption, and not others, such as exercising or eating breakfast regularly, experience higher morbidity (disease) and mortality (death) rates. With the promulgation by the U.S. Department of Health and Human Services of national objectives for promoting health and preventing disease, there has been a corresponding increase in national and local surveys that collect information on individual lifestyles and preventive self-care behaviors (National Center for Health Statistics, 1995).

Health Status. A tremendous amount of effort has gone into clarifying and defining what is meant by the term *health* and in trying to develop valid and reliable indicators of the concept. The World Health Organization (WHO) offers a comprehensive definition of health as a "state of complete physical, mental, and social well-being and not merely the absence of disease or infirmity" (World Health Organization, 1948, p. 1). The concept of health outlined in Figure 1.1 reflects this comprehensive WHO definition.

To determine health status, surveys can be based either on individuals' own reports of their health or on clinical judgments or exams conducted by health professionals. Further, reports by individuals can reflect simply their subjective perceptions of how healthy they are (is their health excellent, good, fair, or poor?) or describe the impact that being ill had on their ability to function in their daily lives (did they have to take time off from work because of illness?). Differing conclusions about "health" can thus result depending on the particular dimension examined and the specific indicators chosen to measure it. An increasing concern on the part of policymakers, consumers, insurers, and providers with measuring the outcomes of medical care has provided an added impetus to clarifying and refining both the predictors and indicators of health status (Patrick & Erickson, 1993).

Utilization of Services. The environment in which individuals find themselves, the health care system available to serve them, their own characteristics and resources, and their state of health and well-being all influence whether they seek medical care and with what frequency. Surveys of health care utilization could ask questions to determine the type of service used (hospital, physician, dentist), the site or location at which the services are received (inpatient ward, emergency room, doctor's office, public health clinic), the purpose of the visit (preventive, illness-related, or long-term custodial care), and the time interval of use (whether services were received or not, the volume of services received, or the continuity or pattern of visits during a given time period) (Aday, 1993b). Presumably, the use of health services also ultimately leads to improved health. This concept of health as both a predictor and an outcome of utilization is reflected in Figure 1.1 in the double-headed arrow between "health status" and "utilization of services." The growing focus on measuring the outcomes of medical care presents special challenges to survey researchers and others in developing or choosing the appropriate measures of health status and in designing studies that can accurately attribute observed outcomes to provider decision making. As when choosing health status measures in surveys, survey researchers should consider the particular dimensions they want to tap in their study and how precedents from other studies or methodological research on various ways of collecting health care utilization data inform those choices.

Expenditures. The cost of medical care has become a particular concern among consumers, policymakers, and health care providers. A number of large-scale national surveys and program demonstrations have examined patterns of expenditures for health care services for the U.S. population as a whole and for individuals in different types of health insurance plans (see Resource E).

Surveys are particularly useful for obtaining information on out-of-pocket expenditures for medical care and the private or public third-party payers, if any, that covered the bulk of the medical bills. As mentioned earlier, it is often necessary to go to insurers or providers directly to obtain information on the total charges for services individuals received. It may require even more effort and creativity on the part of the researcher to estimate the actual "costs" of the care, which may differ from the "charges" for it because of markups to cover other services or patients for whom no payment was received.

Satisfaction. The experience people have when they go for medical care and how much they have to pay for it out of pocket have been found to be important influences on their satisfaction with medical care in general or with a particular visit to a health provider. Because of an increased emphasis on patient-centered care, many hospitals and provider settings have assigned greater weight to developing and implementing surveys of patient satisfaction with the services received (Delbanco, 1992; Gerteis, Edgman-Levitan, Daley, & Delbanco, 1993). A number of different questions and attitude scales for measuring patient satisfaction with medical care have been developed and used in health surveys. (Specific examples are discussed in Chapter Eleven.) Designers of health surveys incorporating patient satisfaction measures should learn about these and other ways of asking satisfaction questions, how well they have worked in other studies, their relevance for the particular survey being considered, and how to modify them to increase their relevance or applicability to the population to be studied.

Examples of Health Surveys

Literally thousands of health surveys on a variety of topics have been conducted since the first studies were carried out in the early part of this century in the United States. It is not possible in the context of this book to provide a comprehensive inventory of the health surveys that have been conducted in the United States and other countries. However, Resource D offers a summary of sources of information on health surveys and Resource E provides selected examples of major surveys that have been conducted internationally, nationally, and at the state and local levels. For each survey, a profile of the topics addressed, the research design, the population or sample included, and the method of data collection used are provided. Health survey researchers should be aware of the analyses that these studies have yielded on the topics of interest to them as well as the questions or methods used in those studies that they might employ in designing their own surveys.

In addition to numerous other examples, three surveys in particular will be used to illustrate many of the aspects of survey and questionnaire design that will be discussed in the chapters that follow. These are the 1995 National Center for

Health Statistics–National Health Interview Survey (NCHS–NHIS), which included supplements to obtain detailed information on childhood immunizations, disability, family resources, behaviors related to the Year 2000 Public Health Objectives for the Nation, and knowledge and attitudes regarding AIDS; the Chicago Area General Population Survey on AIDS; and the Washington State Study of Dentists' Preferences in Prescribing Dental Therapy. The questionnaires for these studies are included in Resources A, B, and C, respectively.

These three studies were chosen principally because they provide examples of the range of design alternatives that are available in doing health surveys. First, each involved different methods of data collection. The NCHS–NHIS was conducted through personal interviews with family members in households selected for the study; the AIDS survey collected data through telephone interviews; and the dentists' preferences study sent a mail questionnaire to eligible providers. The NHIS is national in scope, the AIDS survey was a general population survey of people with telephones in a large urban area, and the dentists survey focused on practitioners in a four-county area in one state.

The basic research designs for the studies were also different. (The different types of research designs that can be chosen in developing health surveys are discussed in Chapter Two.) The National Health Interview Survey has been conducted annually since 1957. The 1995 study included items relating to the issues of health promotion and disease prevention in particular. A number of those items have also appeared in other NCHS–NHIS studies to facilitate monitoring changes over time in these particular indicators of the population's health and health practices. The 1994 and 1995 surveys also added extensive batteries of follow-up questions for adults, children, the elderly who reported experiencing disability, and polio survivors, who were identified in the core NHIS questionnaire and disability supplement in an effort to monitor the health and access impacts of the 1990 Americans with Disabilities Act (Hendershot, 1990; Verbrugge, 1994). The AIDS survey was undertaken prior to the introduction of a major AIDS education intervention in the Chicago area to provide baseline data on the general public's knowledge of AIDS, attitudes toward the disease, and lifestyle and health behaviors related to the risk of contracting the disease; it also sought to identify those groups or areas of the city in which the intervention might be most effectively targeted. The dentists survey was a one-time cross-sectional study that provided information on why dentists chose certain treatment alternatives over others. Its purpose was ultimately to relate dentists' expressed preferences for different types of treatment procedures to the volume and variations in the rates of utilization of these and related procedures in their practices.

The sample designs for the studies differed as well, with the NCHS–NHIS relying on an area probability method of sampling, the AIDS survey on random digit dialing, and the dentists survey on a list sample (these three designs are discussed in more detail in Chapter Six). The core NCHS–NHIS interview gathered information on everyone in the family, whereas the AIDS survey selected one random adult to be interviewed from each sampled household.

The survey questionnaires for the respective studies also reflect an array of health topics and different categories of questions relating to demographic characteristics, health behaviors, attitudes, knowledge, and need measured in a variety of ways. In the NCHS–NHIS, supplements addressing varying topics are added to the core interview each year. These three studies thus illustrate the range of choices that a researcher has in designing a survey.

Steps in Designing and Conducting a Survey

Good survey design is basically a matter of good planning. Exhibit 1.1 presents a picture of the survey research process experienced by investigators who fail to think about the steps involved in doing a study before they begin.

The principal steps in designing and conducting surveys and the chapters of this book in which they are discussed are displayed in Figure 1.2. A number of feedback loops appear in Figure 1.2 to reflect the fact that designing surveys is a dynamic, iterative, and interactive process. Many decisions have to be made in tandem; the advent of computerized systems that can be used to carry out many or all phases of the survey has made this even more true.

Previous experience and personal or professional interests can lead researchers to want more information about a particular issue. For academically oriented researchers, the problem could be stated in terms of study hypotheses about what they expect to find given their theoretical understanding of the topic. For business-oriented investigators, the problem could be stated in terms of precise questions that need to be answered to inform a firm's marketing, strategic planning, program development, or institutional evaluation decision-making activities.

The specification of the problem should be guided by what others have learned and written about it already. Reviewing the literature on related research, acquiring copies of questionnaires or descriptions of procedures used in studies on comparable topics, and consulting with experts knowledgeable in the field or associated with one's own institution can be extremely valuable in clarifying the focus of the survey.

The statement of the problem that emerges from this process should then serve as the reference point for all the steps that follow. This statement is the most visible marker on the landscape to guide the rest of the steps in the journey. These steps include defining the variables to be measured in the study, planning how the

EXHIBIT 1.1. A TYPICAL SURVEY RESEARCH PROJECT.

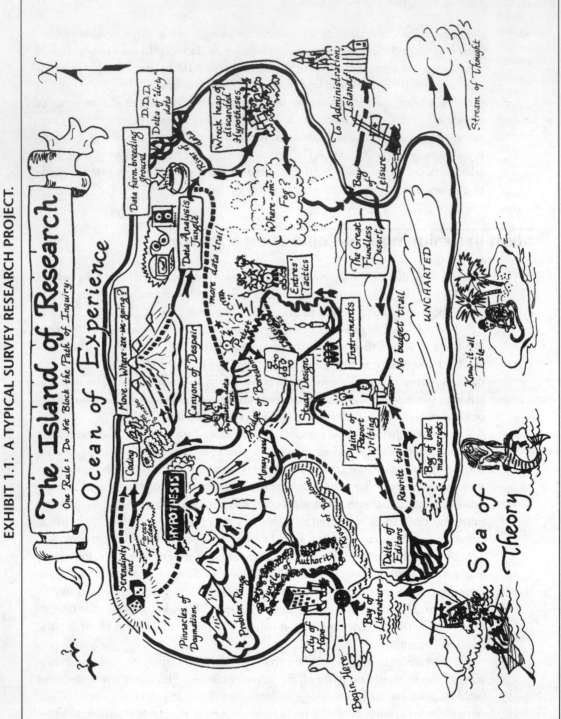

Note: Permission to reprint this figure granted by Ernest Harburg, University of Michigan, Ann Arbor.

FIGURE 1.2. STEPS IN DESIGNING AND CONDUCTING A SURVEY.

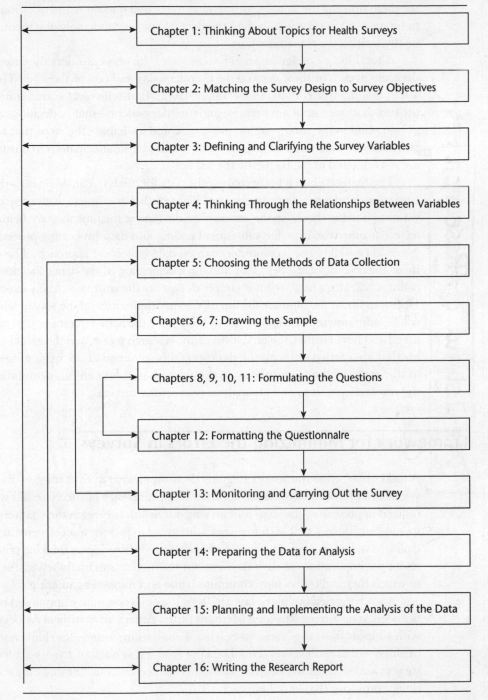

data will be used (or analyzed), choosing the methods for actually collecting the data, drawing the sample, formulating the actual questions and questionnaire to be used in the survey, collecting the data, preparing and analyzing them, and, finally, writing the research report.

A total survey design approach to planning surveys considers the impact of decisions at each of these steps on the overall quality and cost of the study (Groves, 1989; Schuman & Kalton, 1985; Tanur, 1982). It also involves consideration of the fact that these steps are iterative and interdependent—that is, decisions made at one point in the survey design process should anticipate the steps that follow and revisions to the original design will be required if unanticipated circumstances are encountered in the course of the study.

The method chosen for preparing the data for analysis can affect how the investigator decides to collect the data (see Figure 1.2). For example, if the researcher wants to build in checks on the accuracy of the data at the time they are being collected or otherwise expedite subsequent coding and data-processing procedures, it would be well to use a computer-assisted data collection approach. The quality of the training of the field staff and the specification of the data collection procedures will affect how well the sample design for the study is actually executed. Decisions about the ultimate format of the questionnaire and the way in which it will be administered to respondents will influence the actual questions that can be asked and how. Further, the final form of the research report and the actual analyses that are carried out with the data should be planned at the beginning—not at the end—of the study, and they should be based on careful formulation of the research questions and an analysis plan for the project.

Framework for Minimizing the Errors in Surveys

A total survey error framework to guide decision making at each stage of the survey design process to help ensure accuracy and consistency of survey results will be utilized in presenting the steps for carrying out health surveys in the chapters that follow. (See Table 1.1.) This framework is intended to provide a set of general principles, as well as specific guidelines, to facilitate survey developers thinking critically about the implications of their decisions for the quality and usefulness of the data to which they and others have committed time and resources gathering.

A study carried out in the late 1970s by a special committee appointed by the Subsection on Survey Research Methods of the American Statistical Association, with support from the National Science Foundation, found—perhaps not surprisingly—that most surveys could be improved. Fifteen out of twenty-six federal surveys and seven of ten nonfederal surveys studied had one or more major study design problems (Bailar & Lanphier, 1978).

TABLE 1.1. TYPES OF ERRORS IN DESIGNING AND CONDUCTING SURVEYS.

A. No Bias, Low Variable Error

```
                    x
                    x
                    x
                    x
              x     x     x
              x     x     x
        x     x     x     x     x
        x     x     x     x     x
        x     x     x     x     x
        x     x     x     x     x
```

B. High (–) Bias, Low Variable Error

```
        x
        x
        x
        x
  x     x     x
  x     x     x
x  x    x     x     x
x  x    x     x     x
x  x    x     x     x
x  x    x     x     x
```

C. No Bias, High Variable Error

```
                    x     x
              x     x     x     x
        x     x     x     x     x     x
     x     x     x     x     x     x     x
     x     x     x     x     x     x     x     x     x
```

D. High (–) Bias, High Variable Error

```
              x     x
        x     x     x     x
     x     x     x     x     x
  x     x     x     x     x     x
x     x     x     x     x     x     x     x
```

– Bias	$\overline{X}$ (True Value)	+ Bias

In 1979 Andersen and his colleagues at the University of Chicago used a total survey error framework for identifying all the possible sources of bias and variable errors associated with both the sampling and nonsampling steps in designing health surveys. They then applied this framework to measure directly the magnitude of certain of these errors in a 1970 national survey of health care utilization and expenditures. The authors found that the type and magnitude of errors varied for different types of health and health care variables (Andersen, Kasper, Frankel, & Associates, 1979).

Presentations at a series of conferences on health survey research methods and procedures sponsored by the Agency for Health Care Policy and Research (formerly the National Center for Health Services Research) and other public and private sources have argued for the utility of a total survey design and related total survey error framework in enhancing the quality and reducing the costs of health surveys (Fowler, 1989b; National Center for Health Services Research, 1977a, 1979, 1981a, 1984). Robert Groves (1989) and others (Biemer, Groves, Lyberg, Mathiowetz, & Sudman, 1991; Fienberg & Tanur, 1989; Lessler & Kalsbeek, 1992; Schwarz & Sudman, 1995; Sudman, Bradburn, & Schwarz, 1995; Tanur, 1992) have made significant theoretical and empirical contributions to identifying the major types and costs of errors associated with the sampling and nonsampling aspects of designing both health and other surveys. The total survey error framework has led to the practical application of the related principles of Continuous Quality Improvement (CQI) and Total Quality Management (TQM) in designing systems to enhance the quality of survey data collection and processing (Biemer & Caspar, 1994; Fecso, 1989; Groves, 1990a; McCall & Rogers, 1992; Smith & Vincent, 1990).

The errors frequently made in designing and conducting surveys can be classified as either systematic ("bias") or random ("variable") errors (see Table 1.1). A bias involves a fixed departure of a statistic (such as a mean or proportion) across samples (or replications) in a particular (positive or negative) direction from the underlying actual (or true) population value for the estimate. Thus, the sample values are consistently higher or lower than the real value. Variable errors involve varying departures of the statistic (sometimes in a positive, sometimes in a negative direction) from the true population value. This means that the sample values vary or are spread out around the true value across samples (Andersen, Kasper, Frankel, & Associates, 1979; Groves, 1987, 1989; Schuman & Kalton, 1985). The combined or total error may be expressed as the mean square error (MSE), or the sum of the variable error (variance) and bias squared:

$$MSE = VARIANCE + BIAS^2$$

The further the estimate for the sample (such as a mean) is from the true population value—whether higher (+) or lower (−)—and the wider the spread (or variation) in the values obtained for a given sample, the greater the total survey error.

Though rarely measured fully and directly in a survey, the reference point provided by the concept of these two types of errors considered separately and in combination is useful for identifying and mitigating their occurrence or magnitude through thoughtful survey design. These two types of total survey error are portrayed graphically in Table 1.1 and discussed in the following paragraphs.

A. No bias, low variable error. When survey procedures yield estimates that basically cluster around the true value—as with example A in Table 1.1—they are said to be both unbiased and consistent. These are surveys in which the questions are valid and reliable. No substantial noncoverage or nonresponse problems were encountered in designing and executing the sample. That is, everyone who should have been eligible for the study had an opportunity to be included in the sample, a high proportion of those who were selected actually responded, and the size of the sample was large enough to minimize the standard (sampling) errors of the estimates derived from it.

B. High bias, low variable error. If procedures yield consistently inaccurate estimates (as with example B in the table), then the degree of bias is very high. One could, for example, design a question to ask about average weekly alcohol consumption that would yield fairly similar results if asked of the same respondents six months apart but that would still underestimate the rates of use for alcoholics. The refusal of heavy drinkers to participate in the survey could also create problems in this kind of study. The resulting nonresponse bias would also contribute to the underestimation of alcohol use in the target population.

C. No bias, high variable error. Some measures or procedures may yield different results on different occasions or in different survey situations without any consistent pattern in one direction (higher or lower than the true value), as with example C in the table. These results could occur when questions with low reliability (stability) are used to measure the concept of interest (X) or when the sample size is too small to provide very precise estimates.

D. High bias, high variable error. If, in contrast, the researcher gets different answers each time the question is asked and these answers are consistently different (higher or lower, for example) from the right answer to the question, then the resulting estimate has a high degree of bias *and* variable error. Survey results are just the opposite of those described in example A. They are neither consistent nor accurate (as in example D in the table).

The total survey error summarized here and depicted in Table 1.1 will guide the presentation of both specific and general principles to apply in the aspects of designing a survey addressed in the chapters that follow.

No survey is ever error-free. However, this book is intended to increase the reader's awareness of standards to use in identifying the type and magnitude of the problems that can arise in designing and conducting surveys and the alternatives available to minimize them.

Supplementary Sources

For a history and general overview of academic, governmental, and market-oriented polling and survey research, see Bradburn and Sudman (1988), Converse (1987), and Fienberg and Tanur (1990). Consult Resources D and E for additional sources and examples of health surveys. For an overview of survey design in general, see Czaja and Blair (1996) and *The Survey Kit* (1995). The approach to total survey error is discussed more fully in Chapters Eight and Sixteen.

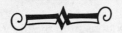

CHAPTER TWO

MATCHING THE SURVEY DESIGN TO SURVEY OBJECTIVES

Chapter Highlights

1. Study designs for health surveys differ principally in terms of the number of groups explicitly included in the study—based on the criteria for including them—and the number of points in time and reference periods for collecting the data.
2. The first step in choosing the appropriate design for a survey is to formulate the research question to be addressed in the study based on who and what the focus of the survey will be, when and where it will be conducted, and (if applicable) what the researcher expects to find and why.
3. Study objectives help clarify what the researcher needs to do to answer the research question, while study hypotheses are statements of the answers the researcher expects to find based on previous research or experience.

This chapter provides guidance for designing surveys to address different types of research questions. In particular, it presents the types of designs that can be used to address various questions (Table 2.1), shows how to state the questions themselves (Tables 2.2 and 2.3), and discusses related study objectives and hypotheses (Figure 2.1).

The discussion that follows draws upon contributions from the disciplines of epidemiology and sociology. Epidemiology is the study of the distribution and causes of disease and related medical conditions in populations. It addresses research questions such as, "Who gets sick in a community and why?" Susser (1985), in a review of the development and evolution of epidemiology in the United States since World War II, pointed out that since chronic, rather than infectious, diseases are now the leading cause of death, the discipline has turned to examining the total environment of an individual and the multitude of factors that can affect whether he or she develops a particular disease rather than focusing on a single causal agent of the condition. Corresponding to these developments, population-based health surveys are being increasingly used by epidemiologists to explore the person's environment as a whole (community, family, and work) and the variety of factors (diet, stress, smoking behavior) that could give rise to serious chronic illness.

Sociologists have also made major contributions to developing and refining the use of the survey method for gathering information from individuals representative of some population of interest (Babbie, 1990). They have, for example, developed broad conceptual frameworks to explain health care behavior that can be used to guide the development of study hypotheses and the selection of questions to include in the survey. Often, however, there is not an adequate translation of concepts and methods from either epidemiology or sociology in designing health surveys. This chapter draws upon contributions from both disciplines to provide guidance for what different types of health survey designs can accomplish.

Types of Study Designs

Epidemiologists usually identify two major types of epidemiological study designs—*experimental* and *observational* (Hennekens & Buring, 1987; Hulley & Cummings, 1988). The two are distinguished principally with respect to whether the treatment or intervention (or major factor of interest in the study) is under the control of the investigator or not. In experimental studies, the investigator actually introduces a factor or intervenes in the environment of the study subjects (such as introducing a mass immunization program for preschool children in a certain community) to see what impact the intervention has on the study subjects (incidence of measles) compared with a group of subjects (in another community) that did not have the intervention.

In observational studies, the investigators do not directly intervene but instead develop methods for describing events that occur naturally without their direct intervention (identifying which children have already been immunized and which have not) and the effect that this has on study subjects (incidence of measles for both groups).

Further, observational studies can be either descriptive or analytical in emphasis, depending on the types of research questions they address. *Descriptive surveys* provide a profile of the characteristics of a population or group of interest (proportion with measles). *Analytical studies* ask why the group has the characteristics (measles) it does (by examining the prior immunization status of study objects, for example). In general, the methods that have been increasingly used by epidemiologists over the last fifty years are much more analytical than descriptive in design (Susser, 1985).

There are three major types of observational study designs—*cross-sectional, group-comparison,* and *longitudinal.* The distinguishing features of these three designs, as well as of the experimental study design, are summarized in Table 2.1. The designs differ principally in two ways: (1) the number of groups explicitly included in the study and the criteria for choosing them and (2) the number of points in time and reference periods for gathering the data.

Cross-sectional designs generally focus on a single group representative of some population of interest. Data are gathered at a single point in time. The reference period for the characteristics that study subjects are asked to report may, however, be either for that point in time or for some reasonable period of time that they can recall in the past.

TABLE 2.1. TYPES OF STUDY DESIGNS.

| | Characteristics | | | |
| | Groups | | Time Periods | |
Types of Study Design	Number of Groups	Criteria for Selection of Groups	Number of Periods of Data Collection	Reference Periods for Data Collection
Observational Cross-sectional (One-group)	1	Population of interest	1	Present (and Recall of Past)
Group-comparison (Case-control)	2+	Population subgroups with and without characteristic of interest	1	Present and Recall of Past
Longitudinal (Prospective)	1 or 2+	Population or subgroups that are and are not likely to develop characteristic of interest	2+	Present and Future
Experimental "True" experiment	2+	Randomly determined subgroups of population	2+	Present and Future

Group-comparison designs explicitly focus on two or more groups chosen because one has a characteristic of interest and the other does not. Data are collected at one point in time, as is the case with the cross-sectional design. Similarly, the reference period for asking study subjects questions may be either the present or some period of time in the past. Analytical group-comparison designs (termed *case-control* or *retrospective* designs in epidemiological studies) make an explicit effort to look back in time at the factors that may have given rise to one group having the characteristic (a particular disease, for example) and the other not having it.

Longitudinal designs focus on a population or subgroups, some members of which will be exposed to or experience certain events over time while others will not. Data are collected at more than one point in time and the reference period is prospective, rather than retrospective—that is, the investigator looks to the future, rather than the past, in describing and explaining the occurrence of the characteristic of interest.

In contrast to observational studies, experimental designs involve directly testing whether a treatment or a program that is thought to produce certain outcomes actually does produce them by assigning the treatment to one group but not another and then comparing the changes that take place in the two groups over time. Experimental designs thus include elements of cross-sectional, group-comparison, and longitudinal research designs.

Most observational studies actually combine elements of these respective designs as well. The following discussion presents examples of each of the major types of observational and experimental designs to illuminate the distinctive features of each. Descriptive and analytical examples of each observational study design are also provided.

Observational Designs

As noted earlier, the three principal types of observational designs are cross-sectional, group-comparison, and longitudinal designs.

Cross-Sectional Designs. A researcher may decide to do a one-time survey to profile a population or group of interest; this would be a descriptive cross-sectional survey design. It provides a slice of life at a particular point in time. For example, epidemiological prevalence studies describe the prevailing rates of illness or related conditions in a population at a designated point in time (Hennekens & Buring, 1987; Hulley & Cummings, 1988; Last, 1988). Thus, a public health department might conduct a house-to-house survey in a neighborhood with high concentrations of Hispanics to estimate the proportion of preschool children who have not been immunized. Such a study would provide an assessment of the need for this service in the community at that particular time.

Analytical cross-sectional surveys search for explanations by examining the statistical association (or correlation) of variables gathered in a one-time survey. This type of survey addresses questions such as, Are homosexual males who say they practice "safe sex" less likely to have AIDS or HIV antibodies in their blood than are sexually active homosexual males who do not use these methods? Analytical designs generally assume that the investigator has a specific hypothesis in mind to test.

Many epidemiologists, as well as social scientists, do not draw sharp distinctions between descriptive and analytical cross-sectional surveys. Most investigators are interested in looking at the relationships of certain characteristics of the study subjects (such as their age, sex, race, and so on) to others (presence or absence of a disease) when doing cross-sectional surveys.

Designers of cross-sectional surveys should determine whether they simply want a snapshot of the population they will be surveying or if there are relationships between factors they will ultimately want to examine once the data are collected in order to be sure to ask questions about those factors in their survey. Even if the investigator simply wants to profile the population, thought should be given to what characteristics it is important to profile and why—*before* undertaking the study.

Group-Comparison Designs. In descriptive group-comparison designs, different groups are compared at approximately the same point in time. For example, a hospital administrator might be interested in the attitudes of physicians, nurses, and nonclinical staff toward a ban on smoking in the hospital. A survey could be administered to each of the groups and the results compared.

Analytical group-comparison designs are what epidemiologists call *case-control* or *retrospective* studies. In these studies the past history of groups with and without a disease are retraced and compared to address the question of why the one group contracted it and the other did not. They are called "case-control" studies because the cases (that have the disease) are compared with the control group (that does not). With retrospective designs, the groups being compared are identified after the fact—it is known that one group has the illness (or condition) and the other does not. This is in contrast to prospective designs that wait and see if the illness develops *over time* and for whom or to cross-sectional studies that take a look at who has the illness *now* and who does not and explore why statistically. (See Armenian [1994] for a review of applications of the case-control design.)

However, epidemiologists do not generally distinguish between cross-sectional and between-group retrospective designs since both could focus on the recall of factors in the past that help explain a current characteristic of the groups of interest.

Longitudinal Designs. Surveys may also be conducted at different points in time to describe how things change longitudinally or over time. These longitudinal survey designs differ primarily in terms of whether the sample or populations surveyed are the same or different at the successive time periods (Babbie, 1990; Kalton & Citro, 1993).

Trend studies may be viewed as a series of cross-sectional surveys. They basically involve different samples of comparable populations over time. The National Center for Health Statistics, for example, conducts a National Health Interview Survey of the U.S. population annually. The size and composition of this population change each year, as does the particular sample chosen for the survey itself. Nevertheless, the National Health Interview Survey provides a rich source of data over time on the health and health care of the American people. (See Resource A for the 1995 National Health Interview Survey questionnaire.)

Panel studies attempt to study the same sample of people at different times. The Medicare Current Beneficiary Survey, sponsored by the Health Care Financing Administration, is an example of a panel survey design. Respondents are interviewed three times each year over a three-year period. This panel design is intended to capture changes in health status, use, and coverage over time as well as to facilitate the quality and completeness of the complex utilization and expenditure data gathered in that study based on a shorter recall period (Edwards, Sperry, & Edwards, 1992).

Longitudinal designs are used in epidemiological studies of disease "incidence," that is, the rate of new occurrences (or incidents) of the disease over time (Last, 1988; Hennekens & Buring, 1987; Hulley & Cummings, 1988). Analytical longitudinal surveys refer to what epidemiologists term "prospective" or "cohort" studies. These involve studies of samples of populations over time to see whether people who are exposed at differing rates to factors (such as engaging in "unsafe" homosexual acts) thought likely to affect the occurrence of a disease (such as AIDS) do indeed ultimately contract the illness at correspondingly different rates. This type of design is termed *prospective* because it looks to the future "prospects" of the person's developing the illness, given the chances he takes over time in engaging in high-risk behavior. Studies of this kind provide a better opportunity than one-time cross-sectional studies to examine whether certain behaviors do in fact lead to (or cause) the disease.

Experimental Designs

The most powerful type of design to test what factors cause an illness or lead to certain outcomes are experiments in which the researcher directly controls who receives a certain type of treatment. Surveys can be used to collect both baseline (pretreatment) and follow-up (posttreatment) data on those who received the treatment (experimental group) and those who did not (control group). "True" experiments generally assume that individuals in the experimental and control groups are equivalent, so that the only reason they might differ on the outcomes of interest is the program or intervention itself. Randomly assigning a subject to either the experimental or control group is the means generally used to establish equivalence between the two groups. However, numerous ethical issues arise in implementing these kinds of studies. As a result, many social experiments or program evaluations are actually quasi-experiments in which some aspect of a true experiment has to be modified or dropped because of ethical or other real-world constraints (Campbell & Stanley, 1963; Kish, 1987).

Randomized trials have been a key component of clinical and pharmaceutical research to evaluate the efficacy of alternative therapeutic regimens and are being increasingly applied in health services research on the cost, quality, and effectiveness of medical care (Balas, Austin, Ewigman, Brown, & Mitchell, 1995). Epidemiologists have conducted community trials in which entire communities are exposed to certain public health interventions, such as a water fluoridation program or health education campaign, and indicators of health outcomes are compared over time or with communities that did not have such programs (Murray, et al., 1994). The RAND Health Insurance Experiment (described in Resource E) is an example of a large-scale social experiment to test the impact of varying the type and extent of insurance coverage on people's health, as well as on their utilization of and expenditures for health care. Surveys were a major part of that study.

Many things can go wrong in the data collection process with surveys that take on special importance in social survey-based experiments or quasi-experimental program evaluations (Burstein, Freeman, Sirotnik, Delandshere, & Hollis, 1985). In those studies, it is particularly important "to keep the noise down" so that one can detect whether the signals that the program worked are loud and clear. A variety of factors in the design of surveys administered at different points in time (such as minor revisions in question wording) or changes in the health care environment as a whole (improved medical diagnostic procedures, for example) that are not taken into account in designing longitudinal surveys can also directly affect interpretations of data collected to reflect changes in the nation's health over time (Wilson, 1981; Wilson & Drury, 1984).

This discussion of alternative designs for health surveys is intended to provide a framework to refine and clarify what a particular study might accomplish and at what level of effort and complexity.

Stating the Research Question for Different Study Designs

What are you interested in finding out? *Whom* do you want to study? *Where* are these people or organizations located? *When* do you want to do the survey? What do you expect to learn and *why?* These are the questions survey designers should ask themselves as guides to formulating the major research question or statement of the problem to be addressed by the study (see Table 2.2).

What investigators will be studying should be guided by the health topics they are interested in and what they would like to learn about them. A survey researcher might, for example, be interested in the topic of smoking. Is he or she interested in people's attitudes or knowledge about smoking, their actual smoking behavior, or all these aspects of the issue? Further, is the researcher interested in studying smoking in general or one particular type of smoking, such as cigarette smoking? Perhaps the investigator is concerned with smoking as an aspect of some broader concept, such as health habits or self-care behavior. The researcher should then have an idea of how a study of smoking fits into learning about these more general concepts of interest. In either case, the investigator should clearly and unambiguously state *what* he or she is interested in studying and have in mind specific questions that could be asked of real-world respondents to get at those issues. In determining what the focus of their study will be, researchers should be guided not only by their own interests but also by the previous research that has been conducted on the topic.

A review of the example provided in Table 2.2 suggests that the focus of a study may be different for different survey designs. Descriptive studies focus on the characteristics of interest for a group at a particular point in time (cross-sectional design) or over time (longitudinal design) or on the differences that exist between certain groups on the characteristics of interest (group-comparison design). Analytical designs speculate on the relationship of the characteristics of interest (cigarette smoking behavior, for example) with some other factors (friends' smoking behavior). Experimental designs directly test the impact of a program or intervention (antismoking seminars) on some outcome of interest (incidence of first-time smokers) in the experiment.

The principal distinguishing features of descriptive and analytical designs may be summarized as follows:

Descriptive	*Analytical*
Describes	Explains
Is more exploratory	Is more explanatory
Profiles characteristics of group	Analyzes why group has characteristics
Focuses on *what?*	Focuses on *why?*
Assumes no hypothesis	Assumes a hypothesis
Does not require comparisons (between groups or over time)	Requires comparisons (between groups or over time)

TABLE 2.2. STATING THE RESEARCH QUESTION FOR DIFFERENT STUDY DESIGNS.

| | Descriptive | | | Analytical | | | |
| | Cross-Sectional | Group-Comparison | Longitudinal | Cross-Sectional | Case-Control | Prospective | Experimental |
Elements of Research Question							
What?	What is the *prevalence* of cigarette smokers	Do the characteristics of those who are cigarette smokers and those who are not *differ*	What is the *incidence* of cigarette smokers	Are cigarette smokers *more likely* than nonsmokers	Are cigarette smokers *more likely* than nonsmokers	Is the *incidence* of cigarette smokers *greater*	Is the *incidence* of cigarette smokers *less*
Who?	among seniors	among seniors	among seniors	among seniors	among seniors	among seniors	among seniors
Where?	of a large urban high school	of a large urban high school	of a large urban high school	of a large urban high school	of a large urban high school	of a large urban high school	of a large urban high school
When?	in the last month of school?	in the last month of school?	between the first and the last month of school?	in the last month of school	in the last month of school	between the first and the last month of school	between the first and the last month of school
Why?	—	—	—	to have friends who smoke?	to have friends who have a history of smoking?	for those whose friends start to smoke?	for those randomly assigned to a teen peer antismoking program?

Study Designs

At the same time that the investigator decides what the primary focus of the study will be, he or she should consider *who* will be the focus of the survey. The choice should be a function of conceptual, cost, and convenience considerations. Conceptually, whom does it make the most sense to study, given the investigator's interests? For example, is there a concern with learning about smoking behavior in the general U.S. population, among pregnant women, among nurses or other health professionals, among patients in the oncology ward of a particular hospital, or among high school students? All are possibilities; the choice depends on the researcher's interests and the constraints imposed by the varying costs of the study with different groups.

Deciding who will be the focus of the study is critical for determining the ultimate sampling plan for the survey. A researcher, for example, might be interested in learning about high school students' smoking behaviors and the impact that peer pressure has on their propensity to smoke (Table 2.2), but because of time and resource constraints, the study will have to be limited to a single high school in a city rather than include all the high school students in the community or a sample of students throughout the state.

A related issue is *where* the study will take place. This decision, too, is subject to time and resource constraints. There are also such issues as whether clearance can be obtained for conducting the survey in certain institutional settings or with selected population groups.

When the data will be collected is also a function of what and whom the investigator is interested in studying and the research design chosen for the study, as well as practical problems related to gathering data at different times of the year. The *what* and the *who* may dictate the best time for data collection. It may make the most sense, for example, to gather information on students during the regular school year or on mothers of newborns just before discharge from the hospital or on recent HMO enrollees immediately following a company's open enrollment period.

As indicated in the example in Table 2.2, longitudinal and prospective as well as true experimental designs assume that data are collected at more than one point in time. The researcher will simultaneously need to consider whether there are seasonal differences that could show up on certain questions (incidence of upper respiratory illnesses, for example) depending on when the data are collected or if there might be problems with reaching prospective respondents at certain times of the year (such as during the Christmas holidays). Analytical and experimental designs attempt to explore *why* groups have certain characteristics in contrast to descriptive designs, which simply focus on *what* these characteristics are. The former types of designs assume that the researchers have some hypotheses in mind about what they expect to find and why. Here is where previous experience and an acquaintance with existing research can be particularly helpful in shaping the research question and the particular issues to be pursued in any given study.

Stating the Study Objectives and Hypotheses for Different Study Designs

The research question is the major question that the study designer wants to try to answer. The specification of the study objectives and hypotheses are the first steps toward formulating an approach to answering this question. Study objectives reflect what the researcher wants *to do* to try to answer the question. Study hypotheses are statements of the answers the researcher expects to find and why, based on previous research or experience. Figure 2.1 provides templates for formulating the study objectives and hypotheses for different types of survey designs.

Study objectives may be stated in a form parallel to that of the expression *to do* to reflect the actions that the researcher will undertake to carry out the study. As suggested in the figure, the principal objectives will differ depending on whether the study is primarily descriptive, analytical, or experimental in focus. Again, the objective of descriptive studies is *to describe,* of analytical studies *to explain,* and of experimental studies *to test the impact of* certain factors of interest to the investigator. Whether the focus of the study is on a certain group at a particular point in time, over time, between different groups, or some combination of these will depend on the specific research question chosen by the investigator.

It is possible to address more than one research question in a study. An investigator may, for example, be interested in describing the characteristics or behaviors of certain groups (such as women who begin prenatal care after the first trimester of their pregnancy), in determining whether there are changes in their behavior over time (do they come in regularly for prenatal care, once seen?), and in discovering how they differ from other groups (such as women who begin prenatal care earlier). However, the precise question or set of questions the investigator wants to answer and the corresponding design or combination of designs and accompanying study objectives must be specified before the survey begins. In addition, an investigator should not try to build too many objectives into a single study because the focus and nature of the study may become overly complex or ambiguous.

A clear statement of the study's objectives is essential to shaping the analyses that will be carried out to answer the major research question. Different data analysis plans and statistical methods are dictated by different survey designs. The three objectives—to describe, to explain, and to test the impact of—require different types of data analysis procedures. Having a clear idea of the study design

FIGURE 2.1. STATING THE STUDY OBJECTIVES AND HYPOTHESES FOR DIFFERENT STUDY DESIGNS.

Study Designs	Objectives	Hypotheses	
		Why?	What?
Descriptive	*To describe. . .*		
Cross-sectional	the characteristics (X, Y) of population.	—	
Group-comparison	whether the characteristics (X, Y) of subgroups A and B are different.	—	
Longitudinal	whether the characteristics (X, Y) of population or subgroups A and B change over time.	—	

(What? column diagram: box containing X over box containing Y)

Study Designs	Objectives	Why?	What?
Analytical	*To explain whether. . .*	*Predictor. . .is related to. . .outcome.*	
Cross-sectional	the characteristics Y of population are related to characteristics X.		
Case-control	differences in the characteristics Y of subgroups A and B are related to differences in characteristics X.		
Prospective	changes in the characteristics Y of population or subgroups A and B are related to changes or differences in characteristics X.		

(Diagram: Independent Variable X → [+ or – or 0] → Dependent Variable Y)

Study Designs	Objectives	
Experimental	*To test the impact of program (or treatment) X on Y for Group A that had it compared to Group B that did not.*	*Pretest. . .intervention. . .posttest.*

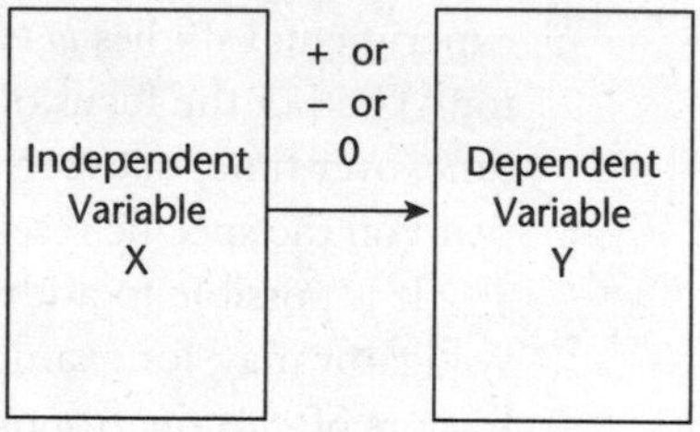

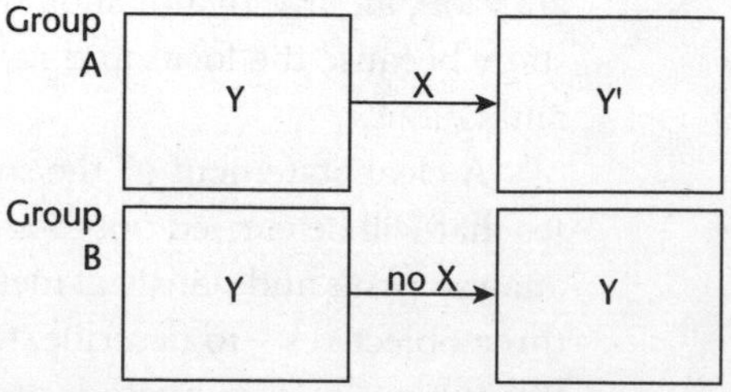

(Diagram:
Group A: Y —X→ Y'
Group B: Y —no X→ Y)

and accompanying study objectives needed to address the major research question will greatly facilitate the specification of the analyses most appropriate to that design.

Study hypotheses are statements about what the researcher expects to find in advance of carrying out the study and why. Hypotheses are used in the physical and social sciences to express propositions about why certain phenomena occur. A theory represents an integrated set of explanations for these occurrences— explanations based on logical reasoning, previous research, or some combination of the two. Hypotheses, which are assumptions or statements of fact that flow from these theories, must of course be measured and tested in the real world. If the hypotheses are supported (or, more appropriately, not rejected), this provides evidence that the theory may be a good one for explaining how the world works. Theories provide the ideas and hypotheses provide the empirical tests of these ideas; in other words, they guide real-world observations of whether the theory's predictions do or do not actually occur.

Theories or frameworks predicting health and health care behavior can be tested in health surveys by empirically examining hypotheses that are based on those theories (Grembowski, et al., 1993). Quite often, however, health surveys are applied rather than theoretical in focus. That is, they apply the theoretical perspectives to generate the questions that should be included in a study—to shed light on a health or health care problem and the best ways of dealing with that problem—rather than use the results to evaluate whether the theory itself is a good one. It was noted earlier that the science of epidemiology is concerned with studying the distribution and causes of disease in a community. Most often the data gathered in epidemiological surveys are used to design interventions to prevent or halt the spread of illness in a given community. In these applied surveys, theories about the spread of certain diseases can guide the selection of questions to be included in the study. But the survey results can also be examined to see whether they tend to support those theories per se, that is, do the findings agree with what the theory predicted?

In either case, researchers should begin with a review of the theoretical perspectives and previous research in an area before undertaking a study. They will then better understand what questions have and have not been answered already about the health topic that interests them, how their research can add to the current body of knowledge on the topic, and what the theories in the field suggest about the questions that should be included in studying it. They will also gain insights into ways in which their own research can serve to test the accuracy of prevailing theories in the field.

As stated earlier, hypotheses generally state what the investigator expects to find and why. In some instances, however, theories or previous research on a topic of interest will be limited. The researchers will then have to conduct exploratory studies to gather information on the issue or to generate hypotheses, using their own or others' practical experience in the area.

Descriptive studies are often exploratory in nature in that the investigator does not necessarily have well-developed assumptions about the characteristics or behaviors of the groups being studied. In these descriptive designs, there is no effort to address *why* certain findings are expected. The investigators may simply present what was found. Or, if they have some prior assumptions about what they expect to find, they may phrase a hypothesis about the magnitude of some characteristic of interest (such as the average number of visits to a physician in a year by HMO enrollees), noting whether they expect this to change over time or whether it might differ from comparable estimates for some other group (enrollees in a regular indemnity plan). They can then determine if these assumptions are borne out.

More traditionally, hypotheses refer to statements about *why* certain characteristics or behaviors are likely to be observed. These causal hypotheses are what guide the conduct of analytical or experimental survey designs. In these cases, the hypotheses go beyond simple descriptions of certain characteristics to statements about the relationships between these characteristics. The phenomena for which explanations or causes are being sought are termed *dependent variables*, while factors suggested as the explanations or causes of these phenomena are termed *independent variables*. The hypothesis states that some relationship exists between these (independent and dependent) variables. If the hypothesis suggests that as one variable changes, the other changes in the same direction, the variables are positively (+) associated. If they change in opposite directions, they are inversely or negatively (−) associated. A hypothesis may also theoretically state that there is no (0) relationship between the variables. (This null form of the hypothesis is also used in statistical tests of relationships that are hypothesized in theory to be either positive or negative.)

The hypothesis underlying the analytical study designs in Table 2.2 is, "The prevalence (or incidence) of smoking (dependent variable) will be higher (+ relationship) among high school seniors who have friends who smoke (or start to smoke) (independent variable)."

Analytical surveys focus on whether there are empirically observed relationships between certain characteristics of interest. Theories, previous research, or the investigators' own experiences can help suggest which should be considered the dependent and which the independent variable in the hypothesized or observed relationship. However, for the independent variable to be considered a "cause" of the dependent variable, (1) there has to be some theoretical, conceptual, or practical basis for the hypothesized relationship; (2) the variables have to be statistically associated (that is, as one changes, so does the other); (3) the occurrence of the independent variable has to precede the occurrence of the dependent variable in time; and (4) other explanations for what might "cause" the dependent variable have to be ruled out.

In the real world, however, and especially in the health and social sciences, there are very often a variety of explanations for some phenomenon of interest. In that case, the major study hypothesis will have to be elaborated (more variables will have to be considered) to test adequately whether the hypothesized predictor (independent) variable is the "cause" of the outcome (dependent) variable of interest. Most importantly, the researcher must think through the variables of interest before undertaking the study in order to reduce the chance that a critical variable for stating or elaborating the study objectives or hypotheses will be omitted.

Special Considerations for Special Populations

The underlying objectives and associated design for addressing them have direct implications regarding whom to include in the study. Both the complexity and costs of capturing the target population for a survey are increased if the groups of interest are rare, hard to locate, highly mobile, non-English speakers, or otherwise different from modal demographic or social-cultural groupings. These implications will be addressed more fully in Chapter Six, in discussing the design of the sampling plan for the survey. It is, however, none too soon to anticipate these parameters in the initial formulation of the study design on which it is based.

Selected Examples

The research questions, objectives, hypotheses and study designs for the surveys in Resources A, B, and C are summarized in Table 2.3.

The 1995 National Health Interview Survey is part of a continuing series of annual surveys carried out through the National Center for Health Statistics–National Health Interview Survey program to monitor trends in the health status and health care utilization of the civilian noninstitutionalized population. Supplements to the 1995 survey were intended to monitor progress toward the Year 2000 Health Promotion and Disease Prevention Objectives for the Nation's Health, which were developed by the Department of Health and Human Services, as well as the impact of the Americans with Disabilities Act of 1990 (Hendershot, 1990; Verbrugge, 1994). The formulation of questions to be included in

TABLE 2.3. SELECTED EXAMPLES OF RESEARCH QUESTIONS, OBJECTIVES, HYPOTHESES, AND STUDY DESIGNS.

Elements	Examples		
	NCHS–NHIS	Chicago Area Survey on AIDS	Washington Dentists Survey
Research Question			
What?	What are the health status, health care utilization, childhood immunization status, disability, family resources, health behaviors, and knowledge and attitudes related to AIDS	What are the knowledge, attitudes, and behaviors related to AIDS	Are the preferences for particular therapies
Who?	of the civilian noninstitutionalized population	of adults 18 and over	of general practice dentists who provide services to Washington Education Association members and their dependents
Where?	in the United States	in the Chicago metropolitan area	in a four-county area of Washington State
When?	in 1995	in 1987	during 1984 and 1985
Why?	in order to monitor changes in these characteristics over time?	prior to an AIDS health education program intervention?	due principally to technical, patient, cost, or other factors?
Objectives			
1. To describe	the health status, health care utilization, childhood immunization status, disability, family resources, health behaviors, and knowledge and attitudes related to AIDS	the knowledge, attitudes, and behaviors related to AIDS	the importance of technical, patient, and cost factors in influencing preferences for particular therapies
2. To compare	by demographic groups.	by racial/ethnic groups.	by dentists practicing in different countries.
3. To analyze	—	—	the relative importance of practice beliefs, practice characteristics and organization, and patient characteristics as predictors of the factors influencing dentists' preferences.
Hypothesis	—	—	Practice beliefs, practice characteristics and organization, and patient characteristics predict the major factors influencing dentists' preferences.
Design	Longitudinal Descriptive	Quasi-experimental	Cross-sectional Analytic

the surveys was guided by previous epidemiological research. Two examples include an Alameda County, California, study documenting the importance of seven health habits (having never smoked, drinking less than five drinks at one sitting, sleeping seven to eight hours a night, exercising, maintaining desirable weight for height, avoiding snacks, and eating breakfast regularly) for predicting good health and lower death rates over time (Berkman & Breslow, 1983) and health services research on the health and health care needs of persons with disabilities (Institute of Medicine, 1991).

The Chicago Area General Population Survey on AIDS (Resource B) was the baseline survey for a quasi-experimental study to investigate the impact of a major health education intervention in the Chicago metropolitan area on the general population's perceptions and behavior in response to the disease (Albrecht, 1989, 1993; Albrecht, Levy, Sugrue, Prohaska, & Ostrow, 1989; Albrecht & Zimmerman, 1993; Prohaska, Albrecht, Levy, Sugrue, & Kim, 1990). As is often the case with applied, real world research, funding for the planned postintervention, follow-up study to assess changes over time in many of the indicators for which data were gathered in the survey was not forthcoming. However, the descriptive data obtained in the survey did provide useful baseline information for the design of the AIDS education program itself. The conceptualization for the issues addressed in that study was based on the Health Belief Model. This is a social psychological model that examines the likelihood that the following elements will contribute to taking preventive action: individual perceptions (perceived susceptibility to and perceived seriousness of the disease); modifying factors (demographic, sociopsychological, and structural variables, as well as cues to action) that affect the perceived threat of the disease to the individual; and the perceived benefits and barriers to engaging in some health practice to prevent the disease (Becker, 1974).

The Washington State Study of Dentists' Preferences in Prescribing Dental Therapy (Resource C) is an example of an analytical cross-sectional survey concerned with examining the relative importance of patient, technical, and cost factors in explaining dentists' propensity to use certain clinical procedures rather than others. It was a part of a larger collaborative effort carried out by the University of Washington to examine the practice patterns of dentists in a homogeneous population of patients. The design of the study was based on a conceptual model developed by Barbara Starfield, in which both structural (personnel, facilities, organization, and financing) and functional (problem recognition, technical care issues) aspects of the practice interact with patient behavior to determine the nature of clinical decision making (Grembowski, Milgrom, & Fiset, 1988, 1989, 1990a, 1990b, 1991). The purpose of this study was to examine the relative importance of technical and patient factors (including preference and cost issues) in the dentists' choice of alternative therapies.

Guidelines for Minimizing Survey Errors

Two major types of errors are of primary concern in formulating analytical and experimental designs: *internal validity* and *external validity* (Campbell & Stanley, 1963; Cook & Campbell, 1979). Internal validity refers to whether the design adequately and accurately addresses the study's hypotheses, particularly with respect to demonstrating a causal relationship between the independent and dependent variables. External validity deals with how widely or universally the findings are likely to apply to related populations or subgroups. These types of validity can be affected by both the variable and systematic errors that plague a given design.

Internal Validity

Analytical cross-sectional designs have the least control over two major conditions in determining whether a hypothesized relationship between two variables (X, Y) is causal or not: the temporal priority of the independent variable in relationship to the dependent variable and the ability to rule out other explanations. Case-control designs try to rule out competing explanations about whether some factor X caused one group to have a condition Y and another group not to have that condition by matching the groups as nearly as possible on everything else that could "cause" Y. Prospective designs attempt to establish more clearly whether one factor (X) does indeed precede the other (Y) in time.

The true experimental design provides the most direct test of whether a certain outcome Y is "caused" by X. In this case, the hypothesis is that the experimental group (Group A) that receives the intervention or program (X) is more likely to have an outcome (Y') than the control group (Group B) that does not receive the intervention (no X). Data are collected over time for both groups before and after X is administered to Group A, to establish the temporal priority of X, and the groups are made as equivalent as possible through randomization to rule out any other possible explanations for differences observed between the groups except for X. However, much applied public health and health services research is based on quasi-experimental designs that do not entail the full randomization of individuals to experimental and control conditions. These types of designs present more threats to the internal validity of the study. (See Campbell and Stanley, 1963, and Cook and Campbell, 1979, for a discussion of these threats for different designs.)

External Validity

The major limitations with respect to the external validity of a design are directly linked to its spatial and temporal dimensions, that is, where and with whom, in addition to when, the study is done. The results of cross-sectional surveys, as well as those based on other designs, are generalizable only to those groups and time periods that were eligible to be represented in the study. Group-comparison designs place a special premium on who is included in the study and longitudinal designs on when it is conducted. A defining strength of experimental designs from the point of their internal validity (random assignment of participants to the experimental and control conditions) may, in contrast, introduce problems in terms of their external validity or generalizability (because of the artificiality of the experimental situation or who is willing to participate in such experiments).

The different types of study designs may be viewed as maps that are available to chart the spatial and temporal dimensions of the study—or where, with whom, and when the survey will be done. The research questions reflect the destination or what the investigator is interested in discovering. The specific itinerary is mapped out in the study objectives based on the guidance provided by an appropriately chosen research design. The hypotheses represent the points of interest the traveler (or researcher) expects to find once the undertaking is completed.

If survey researchers fail to articulate clearly the research questions, study design and objectives, and their interrelationship, they may not accomplish what they set out to do and may spend resources in gathering data that will ultimately be disappointingly irrelevant or imprecise.

Supplementary Sources

Sources to consult on alternative research designs for surveys from the point of view of different disciplines include the following: epidemiology (Abramson, 1990; Hennekens & Buring, 1987; Hulley & Cummings, 1988); sociology and the social sciences (Creswell, 1994; deVaus, 1991; Miller, 1991); and program evaluation (Campbell & Stanley, 1963; Cook & Campbell, 1979; Rossi & Freeman, 1993; Shortell & Richardson, 1978).

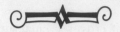

CHAPTER THREE

DEFINING AND CLARIFYING
THE SURVEY VARIABLES

Chapter Highlights

1. The researcher should first have a clear idea of the concept that he or she wants to measure to guide the choice of questions to ask about that concept.
2. The phrasing of the questions chosen to operationalize the concept of interest should reflect the level of measurement—nominal, ordinal, interval, or ratio—appropriate for the types of analysis that the researcher wants to carry out using those questions.
3. The reliability of survey questions can be evaluated in terms of the stability of responses to the same questions over time (test-retest reliability) and their equivalence between data gatherers or observers (inter-rater reliability). They can also be evaluated in terms of the consistency of different questions related to the same underlying concept (internal consistency reliability).
4. The validity or accuracy of survey measures can be evaluated in terms of how well they sample the content of the concept of interest (content validity) and how well they predict (predictive validity) or agree with (concurrent validity) some criterion. Their validity is also based on the extent to which empirically observed relationships between measures of the concepts agree with what theories hypothesize about the relationships between the concepts (construct

validity), that is, whether they are correlated (convergent validity) or not (discriminant validity).

5. Survey items that relate to the same topic can be summarized into typologies, indexes, or scales (such as Likert, Guttman, Thurstone, or Rasch scales), depending on the level of measurement desired.

Once they start looking at questionnaires used in other studies, researchers can identify literally dozens of questions they may wish to include in their survey. This chapter presents criteria to apply both in deciding the types of questions it would be appropriate to take from existing sources and in evaluating the soundness of items that researchers develop themselves. Researchers should, in particular, have a clear idea of (1) the precise concept they want to capture in asking the question; (2) how the question should be asked and how variables should be created from it to yield the type and amount of information required for analyzing the data in certain ways (Table 3.1); and (3) the methods and criteria to use in evaluating the reliability and validity of the question (Figures 3.1 and 3.2 and Tables 3.2 and 3.3).

The reliability of information obtained on a topic by asking a question about it in a survey refers to the extent of *random variation* in the answers to the question as a function of (1) when it is asked, (2) who asked it, and (3) that it is simply one of a number of questions that could have been asked to obtain the information.

The validity of a survey question about a concept of interest (such as health) refers to the extent to which there is a *systematic departure* in the answers given to the question from (1) the meaning of the concept itself, (2) answers to comparable questions about the same concept, and (3) hypothesized relationships with other concepts.

In the measurement of attitudes toward various health issues or practices, a variety of different questions are often asked to capture a respondent's opinion. Procedures have been developed to collapse responses to numerous items of this kind into single summary scores (or scales) that reflect how respondents feel about an issue. The procedures used to develop such scales and to integrate the answers from several different survey questions into one variable (or scale score) as well as the procedures for critically evaluating the potential sources of errors in these procedures will be presented in this chapter (Figure 3.3 and Table 3.4). An understanding of these data summary or reduction devices can facilitate the development of empirical definitions of complex concepts that are both parsimonious and meaningful, reduce the overall number of variables required to carry out the analyses of these concepts, and acquaint the researcher with criteria to use for determining whether the summary devices that other researchers have developed are valid and reliable—and, therefore, worth using in his or her own studies.

The criteria and procedures for developing a multidimensional approach to measuring health status in connection with the Medical Outcomes Study (MOS), a major health services research study that compared health outcomes for patients in health maintenance organizations (HMOs), multispecialty groups, and solo practices in three cities (Boston, Chicago, and Los Angeles), will be used to illustrate reliability and validity analyses and associated scale construction procedures (McHorney, Ware, Lu, & Sherbourne, 1994; McHorney, Ware, & Raczek, 1993; Stewart & Ware, 1992; Ware, Kosinski, Bayliss, et al., 1995; Ware, Kosinski, & Keller, 1994, 1995; Ware & Sherbourne, 1992; Ware, Snow, Kosinski, & Gandek, 1993).

Translating Concepts into Operational Definitions

Researchers often begin with a variety of concepts they would like to measure in a health survey. For example, they may be interested in finding out about levels of alcohol consumption or drug use of survey respondents and how these levels affect people's reported well-being as well as if the findings are different for people at different income levels, for men and women, for employed and unemployed persons, for individuals who are married and those who are not, and so on. The precise selection of topics and the relationships to be examined between them are dictated by the study's principal research question and associated study objectives and hypotheses.

The actual questions to be asked or the procedures to be used to gather information about the major concepts of interest in a study are called the *operational definitions* of the concepts. They specify the concrete operations that will be carried out to obtain answers to the overall research questions posed by the investigator. Other surveys that have dealt with comparable issues should be the starting point for the selection of the questions to be asked. In the absence of previous questions on a topic, the researcher will have to draft new questions based on an understanding of the concept of interest and the principles of good question design (detailed in Chapters Eight to Eleven). The answers to these survey questions will then be coded into the variables that will ultimately be used in analyzing the data.

It is imperative that the precise questions asked in the survey and the resulting variable definitions adequately and accurately capture the concepts that the investigator has in mind. Formal methods for testing the correspondence between these empirical measures and the original theoretical or hypothetical concepts will be presented later when various approaches to evaluating the validity of survey variables are discussed. In general, however, researchers should consider exactly what they want to capture in operationalizing the concept (such as "obesity") and how they expect to use the data gathered on that concept (for example, to construct an objective composite index of the relationship between the respondent's height and weight) in deciding how best to phrase a survey question about it.

The process for translating ideas or concepts into questions to be asked of study subjects in a survey is illustrated in Table 3.1. The particular questions used in the table represent modifications of related items used in the National Center for Health Statistics–National Health Interview Survey (NCHS–NHIS).

Applying Different Levels of Measurement to Define Study Variables

The form and meaning of the variables constructed from answers to survey questions have important implications for the types of analyses that can be carried out with the data (Khurshid & Sahai, 1993). As will be discussed in more detail in Chapter Fifteen, certain statistical techniques assume that the study variables are measured in certain ways. Table 3.1 summarizes examples of ways in which study concepts would be operationalized differently depending on the type or level of measurement used in gathering the data. The items from the NCHS–NHIS survey were modified, as appropriate, for the purpose of illustrating the different levels of measurement that can be used in developing survey questions. The respective measurement procedures—nominal, ordinal, and interval, or ratio— provide increasingly more quantitative detail about the study variable.

In general, constructing variables involves assigning numbers or other codes to represent some qualitative or quantitative aspect of the underlying concept being measured. The codes assigned should, however, be mutually exclusive in that a value should represent only one answer (not several). They should also be exhaustive, that is, the codes should encompass the range of possible answers to that question. For example, the use of only two income categories, such as 0–$25,000 and $25,000–$50,000, would reflect groupings that are neither exhaustive (some people may earn more than $50,000) nor mutually exclusive (persons with incomes of $25,000 could place themselves in either category).

Nominal Variables

Nominal variables reflect the names, nomenclature, or labels that can be used to classify respondents into one group or another, such as male or female; African American, white, or Hispanic; and employed, unemployed, or not in the labor force. Numerical values assigned to the categories of a nominal scale are simply codes used to differentiate the resulting categories of individuals.

TABLE 3.1. APPLYING DIFFERENT LEVELS OF MEASUREMENT TO DEFINE STUDY VARIABLES.

Definitions and Selected Examples	Levels of Measurement		
	Nominal	*Ordinal*	*Interval or Ratio*
Conceptual definition (concept or issue of interest) . . . family income from wages or salaries. . . . obesity.	*Classification* of study subjects by . . .	*Ranking* of study subjects according to . . .	*Quantifying* or comparing *levels* reported by study subjects on . . .
Operational Definition (questions asked to obtain information on concept or issue)	Did anyone in your family have income from wages or salaries in the past twelve months?	Which of the following categories (SHOW CARD) best describes your family's total income from wages and salaries in the past twelve months?	What was your family's total income from wages and salaries during the past twelve months?
	Do you consider yourself overweight, underweight, or just about right?	Would you say you are very overweight, somewhat overweight, or only a little overweight?	About how tall are you without shoes? *and* About how much do you weigh without shoes?
Variable Definition (variable constructed from questions to be used in the analysis of the data)	*Family Wages and Salaries* 1 = had wages or salaries 2 = did not have wages or salaries	*Family Wages and Salaries* 1 = income category 1 2 = income category 2 k = income category k	*Family Wages and Salaries* = \$_____ /year
	Obesity 1 = overweight 2 = underweight 3 = about right	*Obesity* 1 = very overweight 2 = somewhat overweight 3 = only a little overweight	*Obesity* *Construct* index of obesity, based on body mass index (BMI), calculated as weight divided by height, squared.

Nominal scales do not permit the following types of quantitative statements to be made about study respondents: "The first respondent is higher than the second on this indicator," or "The difference between respondents on the measure is X units." These more quantitative applications are possible only with the other (ordinal, interval, or ratio) measurement procedures.

Data for the concepts in Table 3.1—family income from wages and salaries and obesity—could be summarized in quantitative terms, depending on how the question is asked. The examples given of a nominal level of measurement for these concepts reflect questions primarily intended to classify a respondent into one group or another: (1) whether someone in the family had income from wages or salaries or not, and (2) whether the person considers himself or herself to be overweight, underweight, or just right. To obtain more detailed quantitative information on these concepts, different questions (such as those listed under the other levels of measurement in Table 3.1) would have to be asked.

Ordinal Variables

Ordinal variables are a step up on the measurement scale in that they permit some ranking or ordering of survey respondents on the study variable. Ordinal measures assume an underlying continuum along which respondents can be ranked on the characteristic of interest—from high to low, excellent to poor, and so on. In Table 3.1, for example, people who say they are overweight are asked to indicate the extent to which they think they are overweight—very, somewhat, or only a little. However, ordinal scales make no assumptions about the precise distances between the points along this continuum (that is, how much more obese a man who says he is "very" overweight is compared with another who says he is "only a little" overweight).

The Medical Outcomes Study developed a number of ordinal-level questions related to dimensions of physical, mental, and social role functioning and well-being. Among these, for example, was a question asking if the respondent's health limited his or her activities during a typical day (such as lifting or carrying groceries or climbing several flights of stairs) a lot, a little, or not at all (Stewart & Ware, 1992; Ware & Sherbourne, 1992).

Interval or Ratio Variables

Interval and ratio levels of measurement assume that the underlying quantitative continuum on which the study variable is based has intervals of equal length or distance, much as the inches of a ruler do. The main difference between interval scales and ratio scales is that the latter have an absolute zero point—meaning that the total absence of the attribute can be calibrated—while the former do not. Because of the anchor provided by this zero point, the ratio scale allows statements to be made about the ratio between these distances, that is, whether one score is X times higher or lower than another, as well as about the magnitude of these distances.

Examples of interval scales are measures of intelligence and temperature. Theoretically, there is never a total absence of these attributes and, therefore, no real zero point on the scales that measure them. On certain variables used in health surveys, such as measures of a person's height or weight or scores on interval-level attitude scales, a substantively meaningful zero point either does not exist or is hard to define. Scales used in measuring other variables in health surveys, including some of those in the National Center for Health Statistics–National Health Interview Survey—such as number of physician visits, nights spent in the hospital, number of cigarettes smoked per day, days of limited activity due to illness during the year, and so on—do have meaningful zero points. Interval-level measures are treated like ratio measures for most types of analysis procedures in the social sciences. Interval and ratio measures can be collapsed to create nominal variables (saw a doctor or not) or ordinal variables (0, 1–2, 3–4, 5 or more visits).

In summary, survey researchers should think through how much and what kind of qualitative and quantitative information they want to capture in asking a question about some concept of interest in their study. Knowing whether the resultant survey variable represents a nominal, ordinal, or interval or ratio level of measurement will help in deciding which way of asking the question is best given the objectives of the study.

Evaluating the Reliability of Study Variables

The reliability of a survey measure refers to the *stability* and *equivalence* (or reproducibility) of measures of the same concept over time or across methods of gathering the data. The stability of a measure refers to the consistency of the answers people give to the same question when they are asked it at different points in time, assuming no real changes have occurred that should cause them to answer differently. In contrast, the equivalence of different data gathering methods refers to the consistency of the answers when different data gatherers use the same questionnaire or instrument or when different but presumably equivalent (or parallel) instruments are used to measure the same individuals at the same point in time (Alwin, 1989; American Psychological Association, 1985; DeVellis, 1991; Nunnally & Bernstein, 1994; Traub, 1994).

Questions with low reliability are ones in which the answers respondents give vary widely as a function of when the questions are asked, who asks them, and the fact that the particular questions chosen from a set of items seem to be asking the same thing but are not.

The consistency of answers to the same questions over time may vary as a function of transient personal factors, such as a respondent's mental or physical state at the different time periods; situational factors (are other people present at the interview or not?); variations in the ways interviewers actually phrase the questions at the different time periods; and real changes that may have taken place between these periods.

Variations in the consistency of responses to what are thought to be equivalent ways of asking a question could be the result if different observers or interviewers elicit or record the data differently or if apparently equivalent items do not actually tap the same underlying concept.

Estimates derived from survey data always reflect something of the "true value" of the estimate as well as random errors that result from unreliability of the measure itself. Good survey design attempts to anticipate the sources of these variations and to the maximum extent possible control and minimize them in the development and administration of the study questionnaire.

The estimates of reliability to be examined reflect the extent to which (1) the same question yields consistent results at different points in time, (2) different people collecting or recording data on the same questions tend to get comparable answers, and (3) different questions that are assumed to tap the same underlying concept are correlated. These are termed *test-retest, inter-rater,* and *internal consistency reliability,* respectively (Carmines & Zeller, 1979; DeVellis, 1991).

Figure 3.1 summarizes the various procedures for evaluating the reliability of survey variables. Correlation coefficients are the statistics used most often in developing *quantitative measures* of reliability (these statistics will be discussed in more detail in Chapter Fifteen). Quantitative measures can also be readily computed using standard social science and biomedical computer software. In general, correlation coefficients reflect the degree to which the measures "correspond" or "co-relate." That is, if one tends to be high or low, to what extent is the other high or low as well? Correlation coefficients normally range from −1.00 to +1.00. The most reliable measures are ones for which the reliability (correlation) coefficient is closest to +1.00.

The precise coefficient (or formula) to use in estimating the reliability of an indicator differs for different approaches to measuring reliability (Carmines & Zeller, 1979; Crocker & Algina, 1986; Cronbach, 1951; DeVellis, 1991; Nunnally & Bernstein, 1994). The following sections discuss the appropriate coefficient to

FIGURE 3.1. EVALUATING THE RELIABILITY OF STUDY VARIABLES.

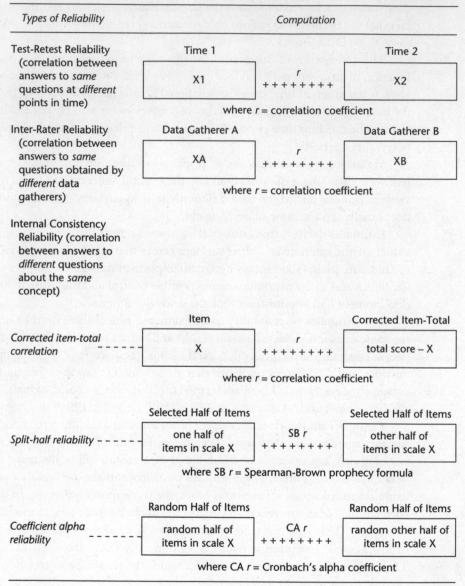

Types of Reliability	Computation

Test-Retest Reliability (correlation between answers to *same* questions at *different* points in time)

Time 1 r Time 2

X1   + + + + + + + +   X2

where r = correlation coefficient

Inter-Rater Reliability (correlation between answers to *same* questions obtained by *different* data gatherers)

Data Gatherer A r Data Gatherer B

XA   + + + + + + + +   XB

where r = correlation coefficient

Internal Consistency Reliability (correlation between answers to *different* questions about the *same* concept)

Corrected item-total correlation

Item r Corrected Item-Total

X   + + + + + + + +   total score – X

where r = correlation coefficient

Split-half reliability

Selected Half of Items   SB r Selected Half of Items

one half of items in scale X   + + + + + + + +   other half of items in scale X

where SB r = Spearman-Brown prophecy formula

Coefficient alpha reliability

Random Half of Items   CA r Random Half of Items

random half of items in scale X   + + + + + + + +   random other half of items in scale X

where CA r = Cronbach's alpha coefficient

use with particular approaches and the criteria that can be applied to evaluate the reliability of a given question based on the resulting value of the coefficient.

Test-Retest Reliability

The test-retest reliability coefficient reflects the degree of correspondence between answers to the same questions asked of the same respondents at different points in time. A survey designer might, for example, try out some questions on a test sample of respondents and then go back a month later to see if they give the same answers to the questions asked earlier, such as how many drinks of alcoholic beverages they have on average each week. There could be *real* changes in the behavior or situation about which the questions are asked to account for a less than perfect correspondence between the data gathered at different points in time. Changes that occur at random between the respective time periods could also give rise to any differences observed. The researcher needs to consider these possibilities in selecting the questions to include in a test-retest reliability analysis, in deciding how long to wait before going back, and in ultimately interpreting the coefficient obtained between the two time periods.

In the Medical Outcomes Study data were gathered on the same person for selected questions four months apart. Because real changes in health could occur over this time period, the correlation between answers at the two time periods was deemed to represent the "lower-bound estimate of reliability," that is, it was likely to represent the lowest reliability coefficient for a given question, especially compared to its likely performance in terms of internal consistency reliability (Stewart & Ware, 1992, p. 83). It would be desirable to have a much shorter period of time between the first and second measurements (perhaps two to four weeks), particularly if there is a possibility that real changes might take place in the underlying construct of interest (emotional well-being) within a short period of time.

Test-retest reliability can be computed using correlation coefficients such as the Pearson correlation coefficient for interval-level data, the Spearman rank order coefficient for ordinal-level variables, or nominal-based measures of association for categoric data to examine the association between the answers a respondent gave to the same question (or item) at two different points in time (Table 3.2). (See also Chapter Fifteen.) The closer the resulting value of the coefficient is to + 1.00, the more stable or consistent the indicator can be said to be at different points in time. In general, minimum test-retest reliabilities of .70 are satisfactory for studies focusing on group-level differences. Higher coefficients (.90 or above) are preferred when the emphasis is on changes in individuals over time, especially if the measure is to be used to make clinical judgments regarding treatment or outcomes on a case-by-case basis.

TABLE 3.2. METHODS OF COMPUTING RELIABILITY.

Types of Reliability	Data Records		Correlation Coefficients	
	Cases	Data/Answer		
Test-retest		Item Over Time		
	Respondent	Time 1	Time 2	Interval:	Pearson r
	1	X11	X12	Ordinal:	Spearman rho
	2	X21	X22	Nominal:	Chi-square-based
	3	X31	X32		
	4	X41	X42		
	5	X51	X52		
Inter-rater		Item Across Data Gatherers		where two data gatherers = A,B	
	Respondent	A	B	Interval:	Pearson r
	1	X1A	X1B	Ordinal:	Spearman rho
	2	X2A	X2B	Nominal:	Kappa
	3	X3A	X3B		
	4	X4A	X4B	where three+ data gatherers = A,B,C, etc.	
	5	X5A	X5B	Mixed:	Intra-class correlation (eta)
Internal Consistency	Respondent	Item 1	Item 2		
	1	X11	X12	Interval or Ordinal:	Corrected item total r
	2	X21	X22		Spearman-Brown
	3	X31	X32		Cronbach's alpha
	4	X41	X42	Dichotomy:	Kuder-Richardson
	5	X51	X52		

Formula: Cronbach's alpha = $kr/[1+(k-1)r]$

where,
k = number of items in the scale
r = average correlation between items

Example: Cronbach's alpha = $10(.32)/[1+(10-1)*.32]$
= 3.20/[1+(9)*.32]
= 3.20/3.88
= .825

where,
k = 10
r = [.185+.451+.048+...+.233 = 14.557]/45 = .32

Correlation Matrix (numbers in cells = correlation between items)

	1	2	3	4	5	6	7	8	9	10
1	–	.185	.451	.399	.413	.263	.394	.352	.361	.204
2		–	.048	.209	.248	.246	.230	.050	.277	.270
3			–	.350	.399	.209	.381	.427	.276	.332
4				–	.369	.415	.469	.280	.358	.221
5					–	.338	.446	.457	.317	.425
6						–	.474	.214	.502	.189
7							–	.315	.577	.311
8								–	.299	.374
9									–	.233
10										–

Inter-Rater Reliability

Inter-rater reliability examines the equivalence of the information obtained by different data gatherers or raters on the same (or comparable) groups of respondents.

We saw earlier, in the examples of possible sources of variation in survey questions, that different interviewers may ask the survey questions differently. Survey designers may also engage raters or observers to record and observe behaviors rather than to ask questions directly. For example, observers might report on study subjects' level of functioning on physical tasks or patterns of interaction with family members. Inter-rater reliability coefficients reflect the level of agreement between interviewers or observers in recording this information. As indicated in Table 3.2, a Pearson, Spearman rank order or a kappa coefficient can be used to measure the strength of agreement between *two* data gatherers (A and B) for interval, ordinal, or nominal-level variables. An intraclass correlation coefficient measures the agreement among *all* the data gatherers in the study (A, B, C, and so on) (Nunnally & Bernstein, 1994; Soeken & Prescott, 1986). In general, a correlation of the answers between or among raters of .80 or higher is desirable.

The inter-rater reliability between survey interviewers is rarely computed. Different interviewers do not usually go back to ask respondents the same questions and groups of respondents interviewed by different interviewers are not always comparable. Especially in personal interview surveys, interviewers may be assigned to different areas of a city or region that differ a great deal compositionally. Survey designers should, however, consider what might give rise to random variation in interviewers' performance before starting the study and standardize the training and field procedures to reduce these sources of variation as much as possible.

Internal Consistency Reliability

Whereas test-retest and inter-rater reliability analysis can be used to evaluate individual items or summary scales, internal consistency reliability analysis is used primarily in constructing and evaluating summary scales. The sources of variability examined with this type of reliability analysis include the inconsistency or nonequivalence of different questions intended to measure the same concept. If the questions are not really equivalent, then different conclusions about the concept will result depending on which questions are used in constructing the summary scale to measure it. The main procedures for estimating the internal consistency or intercorrelation among a number of different questions that are supposed to reflect the same concept are the *corrected item-total correlation* and *split-half* and *alpha reliability coefficients*. The procedures were originally developed in connection with multiple-item summary scores or scales of people's attitudes toward a particular topic. People's attitudes (toward persons with AIDS or banning smoking in public places, for example) are often complex and multidimensional and therefore difficult to tap with a single survey question.

As will be seen later in this chapter, the process of developing attitude scales begins with the identification of a large number of questions that seem to capture some aspect of how a respondent feels about an issue. The corrected item-total correlation, split-half and internal consistency reliability procedures are used to estimate the extent to which these items tap the same basic attitude (toward persons with AIDS, for example, rather than toward homosexuals, who are one of several risk groups for the disease; or toward policies about banning smoking in the workplace, rather than toward the practice of smoking in general). There could, of course, be a variety of dimensions that characterize the attitudes that individuals hold on certain topics. Attitude scaling and the reliability analyses required to construct those scales help identify what those dimensions are and which survey items best tap those dimensions.

A useful indicator for initially assessing whether all the items that are intended to measure a given concept do and therefore warrant being combined into a single scale is the correlation of the item with the sum of all the other items in the scale. This is sometimes referred to as the *corrected item-total correlation* since the item is not included in computing the total scale score. Doing this serves to remove the bias associated with correlating an item with itself. This correlation is available in the SPSS RELIABILITY procedure as well as in other software packages that compute the split-half and Cronbach's alpha reliability coefficients (Norusis, 1990, 1992). A correlation of .40 or higher was used as a cutoff for identifying candidate items in constructing a 36-item health status questionnaire in the Medical Outcomes Study. This was deemed to be a substantively meaningful and robust level of association between variables. All the items except one exceeded this criterion (McHorney, Ware, Lu, & Sherbourne, 1994).

Split-half reliability reflects the correspondence between answers to two subsets of questions when an original set of questions about a topic (such as patient satisfaction with various aspects of medical care) is split in half, and a correlation coefficient is computed between scores from the two halves. The correlation coefficient used to compute the correspondence between the scores for these two subsets of items is the Spearman-Brown prophecy formula (Carmines & Zeller, 1979; DeVellis, 1991; Nunnally & Bernstein, 1994). The reliability estimate based on this formula will be higher (1) the more questions asked about the topic and (2) the higher the correlation between the scores for the respective halves of the entire set of questions.

The process for computing *coefficient alpha reliability* is similar to that for the split-half approach except that it is based on all possible ways of splitting and comparing sets of questions used to tap a particular concept. Cronbach's alpha or coefficient alpha is the correlation coefficient used to estimate the degree of equivalence between answers to sets of questions constructed in this fashion (Cronbach, 1951). The Kuder-Richardson formula is a special case of the alpha coefficient that is used when the response categories for the questions are dichotomous rather than multilevel. In other words, they require a *yes* or *no* rather than a *strongly agree, agree, uncertain, disagree*, or *strongly disagree* response to a statement that reflects an attitude toward some topic (Carmines & Zeller, 1979; DeVellis, 1991; Nunnally & Bernstein, 1994).

The coefficient alpha (and associated Kuder-Richardson) formula is used more often than the split-half formula in most internal consistency analyses of multiple-item scales because it enables the correlations between scores on all possible halves of the items to be computed. The coefficient alpha will be higher (1) the more questions asked about the topic and (2) the higher the average correlation between the scores for all possible combinations of the entire set of questions.

In most applied studies, the lowest acceptable level of internal consistency reliability is .70 for group-level and .90 or higher for individual-level analysis (Nunnally & Bernstein, 1994). Values any lower than this mean that some items in the summary scale do not tap the attitude in the same way as the others. When a researcher evaluates scales that others have constructed, an alpha of less than .70 should be a red flag that the items used in the scale to tap a particular concept are not entirely consistent in what they reflect about the person's attitudes toward the issue. These internal consistency coefficients are then helpful in deciding whether different questions are yielding similar answers.

A formula based on the number of questions (or items) in a scale and the average correlation among the items, as well as an example of the computation of Cronbach's alpha using this formula, is provided in Table 3.2. The values in the correlation matrix reflect the correlations among items in a 10-item scale of self-esteem reported by Carmines and Zeller (1979, p. 64). The average correlation is a mean (.32) of all (forty-five) unduplicated correlations in the correlation matrix (which range from .048 to .577). The coefficient alpha resulting (.825) reflects an acceptable level of reliability. If the alpha for the scale as a whole increases when an item is removed, this suggests its correlation with the other items is low and should perhaps be deleted. If the alpha remains unchanged or decreases, then it should be retained.

Internal consistency reliability coefficients were computed for eight summary scales used to tap various dimensions of health status in the Medical Outcomes Study (McHorney, Ware, Lu, & Sherbourne, 1994). These coefficients ranged from a low of .78 to .93, well above the overall standards for reliability. However, the MOS investigators pointed out that if the principal analyses involve comparisons between groups (such as patients in different delivery settings), the minimum reliability standard could perhaps be somewhat lower (.50 to .70). But if the focus is on individuals (whether a particular patient experiences an improvement in health over time), then a more rigorous standard may be required (.90 to .95) to assure that sound decisions are made regarding the individuals' care.

Evaluating the Validity of Study Variables

The validity of survey questions refers to the degree to which there are systematic differences between the information obtained in response to the questions relative to (1) the full meaning of the concept they were intended to express, (2) related questions about the same concept, and (3) theories or hypotheses about their relationships to other concepts. Such differences generally reflect assessments of content validity, criterion validity, and construct validity, respectively. Figure 3.2 summarizes these three approaches to estimating the validity of survey measures and Table 3.3 highlights the principal methods used to evaluate each (American Psychological Association, 1985; Carmines & Zeller, 1979; Nunnally & Bernstein, 1994).

Content Validity

Content validity relies on judgments about whether the questions chosen are representative of the concepts they are intended to reflect. More precisely, content validity refers to how good a sample the empirical measures are of the theoretical domain they are presumed to represent. It is, therefore, important that there be some clear idea of the domain or universe of meaning implied in the concept being evaluated. One way to ensure that a series of questions have a fair amount of content validity is to begin with questions and variables on the same topic that have been used in other studies. The researcher could also ask expert consultants in the area whether, in their judgment, the questions being asked adequately represent the concept.

Investigators in the Medical Outcomes Study were interested in validating empirical measures of the dimensions of physical, mental, and social functioning and well-being as well as general health perceptions and satisfaction. The content validity analyses in that study involved thorough reviews of the literature on the concepts and measures within each dimension. The content of the items being considered for inclusion in the study was then compared with the universe of items distilled from this literature review to evaluate whether at least one item was included to represent each of the major dimensions of health and certain concepts within each dimension (such as depression and anxiety within the mental health dimension) and whether a sufficient number of items were included to represent adequately each dimension and concept (Stewart & Ware, 1992).

FIGURE 3.2. EVALUATING THE VALIDITY OF STUDY VARIABLES.

	Computation	
Types of Validity	Measure	"True Value"

Content Validity (extent to which measures adequately represent concept)	Variables		Concept

Content Validity (extent to which measures adequately represent concept)

Variables
```
x1
x2       =
x3    ========
x4
```
Concept
```
X1
X2
X3
X4
```

Criterion Validity (extent to which measure predicts or agrees with criterion indicator of concept)
—*Predictive*
—*Concurrent*

Variable
```
x1
```

r
+ + + + + + + +

where r = correlation coefficient

Criterion
```
x1'
```

Variable (x1)   Criterion (x1')

		+	−
	+	a = true +	b = false +
	−	c = false −	d = true −

Sensitivity =
$a \div (a + c)$

Specificity =
$d \div (b + d)$

Construct Validity (extent to which relationships between measures agree with relationships predicted by theories or hypotheses)
—*Convergent*
—*Discriminant*

Observed Relationships
```
        +
x1 + + + + + x1'
        0
x1 + + + + + x2
        0
x1 + + + + + x3
        +
x1 + + + + + x4
```

=
========

Theoretical Relationships
```
        +
X1 + + + + + X1'
        0
X1 + + + + + X2
        0
X1 + + + + + X3
        +
X1 + + + + + X4
```

Criterion Validity

Criterion validity refers to the extent to which the survey measure predicts or agrees with some criterion of the "true" value (or "gold standard") for the measure. The two major types of criterion-based validity are *predictive* and *concurrent validity*, depending on whether the criterion is one that can be predicted by or currently corresponds with the survey estimate.

Both types of criterion validity are generally quantified through correlation coefficients between the survey measure and the (future or concurrent) criterion source value. The higher the correlation, the greater the validity of the survey measure is said to be. The predictive validity of a survey-based measure of functional status, for example, could be based on the correlation of this measure with the ability of the respondent to carry out certain physical tasks in the future. This form of validity analysis is often used in designing tests to choose good candidates for certain programs (such as health promotion programs) based on the correlation of scores (of probable adherence) on screening tests with participants' later performance in the program (actual adherence to prescribed health promotion regimens). Concurrent validity, in contrast, reflects the correspondence between the survey measure and a criterion measure obtained at essentially the same point in time. For example, concurrent validity could be evaluated by correlating patient reports of the types of conditions for which they had seen their physicians during a year with the physicians' medical records for the same time period.

Another approach to quantifying both predictive and concurrent criterion validity is to use sensitivity and specificity analyses. The diagram in Figure 3.2 shows the outcomes that could result, for example, when patient and physician data are compared by means of this approach. The proportion represented by the number of times that the patient reports a condition that also appears in the physician records $[a/(a+c)]$ reflects the "sensitivity" of the survey question to picking up the condition in the survey when it is known, from the physician records, to have occurred. The extent to which patients do *not* report conditions that do *not* appear on the medical record $[d/(b+d)]$ reflects the "specificity" or accuracy of the aim of the measure in *not* netting something it should not. When a respondent reports an extra condition that is not found in the physician's record, it is said to be a "false positive" response. If, in contrast, the respondent fails to report a condition that is found in the medical record, it is said to be a "false negative" survey response. The higher the sensitivity and specificity of the survey measure, and correspondingly, the lower the false positive and false negative rates of the indicator when compared with the criterion source, the greater its criterion validity. Highly unreliable survey measures are likely to have low sensitivity and specificity as well (Hennekens & Buring, 1987; Kehoe, Wu, Leske, & Chylack, 1994).

Examples of concurrent validity analyses conducted in the Medical Outcomes Study included examining the correlation between a survey-based measure of depression and a gold standard measure derived from the Diagnostic Interview Schedule of the *Diagnostic and Statistical Manual of Mental Disorders* (American Psychiatric Association, 1995), as well as the correlation of a short-form measure of physical functioning with a validated longer form measure of the same concept. The predictive validity of a perceived health measure gathered at the time of enrollment in the study was assessed by examining its association with the use of health services in the following year (Stewart & Ware, 1992).

Construct Validity

Evaluations of the construct validity of a survey variable assume that there are well-developed theories or hypotheses about the relationships of that variable to others being measured in the study. Construct validity examines whether and how many of the relationships predicted by these theories or hypotheses are empirically borne out when the data are analyzed. The more often these hypothetical relationships are confirmed, the greater the construct validity of the survey variables is assumed to be.

The distinction between criterion and construct validity analysis is primarily a function of the purpose of the analysis and the assumptions underlying it. Criterion (particularly concurrent) validity principally examines the strength of the association of the survey measure with what is deemed to be an accurate measure of the same concept. Construct validity tests whether a hypothesized association between the survey measure and a measure of the same concept (convergent validity) or a different concept (discriminant validity) is confirmed.

Correlational analyses can be used to quantify construct validity as well. For example, in the Medical Outcomes Study, it was hypothesized that different indicators of physical health (such as physical functioning, mobility, and pain) would be correlated (as in the example of the positive correlation between x1 and x1' in Figure 3.2). Measures of physical health (x1) would not, however, be highly correlated with measures of mental or social health (x2 or x3, respectively). Further, measures of general health status and vitality (x4) would be correlated with the measures of physical health (x1) as well as with the mental and social health indicators. The construct validity analyses in that study did in fact confirm these hypothesized relationships for the health status variables (McHorney, Ware, & Raczek, 1993).

The more different measures meant to measure the same concept (such as physical health) agree (that is, have convergence) and the more they differ from those intended to tap other concepts (such as mental or social health), the greater the convergent and discriminant validity of the indicators, respectively, is said to be. Other approaches to examining convergent and discriminant construct validity, in addition to correlational analyses, include known-groups comparisons, factor analysis, and the multitrait multimethod approach (MTMM) (Table 3.3) (Streiner & Norman, 1991).

Known-groups validity analysis is based on comparing a given health survey measure of physical or cognitive functioning, for example, between groups with known clinically diagnosed (physical or mental) status. The hypothesis would be that the survey measures would clearly differ between the groups on those measures that were most reflective of the underlying clinical differences between them. The Medical Outcomes Study compared four different patient groups—those with (1) minor chronic medical conditions, (2) serious chronic medical conditions, (3) psychiatric conditions only, or (4) serious medical and psychiatric conditions—on both physical and mental health status measures. The results confirmed hypotheses regarding expected differences between the groups on the respective types of health status measures (McHorney, Ware, & Raczek, 1993).

Factor analysis basically uses the correlation matrix between variables as the basis for examining whether subsets of the variables are related in such a way (or form a factor) so as to suggest that they are measuring the same underlying concept. Factor loadings are used to express the correlation between each item and a given factor (DeVellis, 1991; Kim & Mueller, 1978; Nunnally & Bernstein, 1994).

The MOS conducted extensive factor analyses of the variety of scales developed to measure physical or mental health status or overall health status and vitality. A strong correlation (or factor loading) was defined to be greater than or equal to .70, moderate to substantial as .30 to .70, and weak as less than .30. The results strongly confirmed that the hypothesized associations among the respective dimensions of health status at a strong, moderate, or weak level were correlated as expected (McHorney, Ware, & Raczek, 1993).

TABLE 3.3. METHODS OF COMPUTING VALIDITY.

Methods	Types of Validity		
	Content	Criterion	Construct
Literature review	X		
Expert judgment	X		
Sensitivity-specificity analysis		X	
Correlation coefficients		X	X
Known-groups validity			X
Factor analysis			X
Multitrait multimethod			X

Psychologists have developed the multitrait multimethod (MTMM) approach to formally test the construct validity of measures of complex concepts. A matrix is constructed that displays the correlations between two or more health concepts (physical and cognitive functioning), for example, measured by two or more methods (health survey and clinical exam). With this approach, a measure is hypothesized to be more highly correlated with other measures of the same concept (physical or cognitive functioning) across methods (survey or clinical exam) than with a different concept measured using the same method. The matrix also provides a look at the underlying internal consistency reliability of the items intended to measure the same construct (Campbell & Fiske, 1959; Shortell & Richardson, 1978). The multitrait multimethod approach was not used in evaluating the MOS survey measures because the information used to measure the health status constructs were gathered through essentially the same data collection method (respondent self-reports) (Stewart & Ware, 1992).

It is important for the researcher to have a good idea of the soundness of the theory or hypotheses on which the predictions about the relationships between variables are based in order to make judgments about the construct validity of the measures.

Measures must be reliable to be valid. Empirically, the maximum observable correlation between two scales (used to measure the criterion or construct validity of one of them, for example) is defined by the theoretically maximum correlation multiplied (reduced) by the square root of the product of the respective scale's reliability coefficients (test-retest or coefficient alpha, for example). The maximum possible correlation between two scales with coefficient alphas of .60 and .80, even if the concepts they measure were theoretically perfectly correlated (1.00), would be only .69, that is, 1.00* (.60 * .80) (Carmines & Zeller, 1979).

Constructing Typologies, Indexes, and Scales to Summarize Study Variables

As indicated in the previous discussion, many different questions may be asked in a survey to obtain information about a concept of interest. Using several questions rather than only one or two to tap concepts that are particularly complex or have a number of different dimensions (such as health status or preventive care behavior) can result in more valid and reliable data. For example, if the researcher wants to operationalize adequately the comprehensive World Health Organization (WHO) definition of health, it will be necessary to ask questions about the physical, mental, and social well-being of the respondent. Sources and summary scales tapping a number of common social, psychological, and health status concepts are highlighted in Chapter Nine.

Figure 3.3 and Table 3.4 present different approaches for collapsing and summarizing a variety of questions about the same underlying concept into typologies, indexes, or scales that capture the overall meaning of a number of different measures of a concept. However, the choice of a method for summarizing the data is dependent on the level of measurement (nominal, ordinal, interval or ratio) of the variables to be included.

Typologies

An approach to combining one or more variables that are basically nominal scales, for example, might be a cross-classification of these variables to create a typology mirroring the concept of interest. Each cell of the cross-classification table results in identification of a type of respondent or study subject. For example, Shortell, Wickizer, and Wheeler (1984), in an analysis of the characteristics of community hospital–based group practices to improve the delivery of primary medical care in selected communities, created a typology of the groups based on whether their institutional and community environment was favorable or unfavorable to a group's development (*X1*) and the actual performance (high or low) of the group in meeting its goals (*X2*) (see Figure 3.3). The resulting classification of these

FIGURE 3.3. CONSTRUCTING TYPOLOGIES AND INDEXES TO SUMMARIZE STUDY VARIABLES.

Typologies and Indexes	Level of Measurement	Scoring Methods			
		Methods			Scoring
Typology (cross-classification of answers to questions)	Nominal	Variable X2	Variable X1 1 2		Codes
		1	1 = Type 11	2 = Type 21	1 = Type 11 2 = Type 21
		2	3 = Type 12	4 = Type 22	3 = Type 12 4 = Type 22
Index (accumulation of scores assigned to answers to questions)	Ordinal	*Variable*	*Answers*		*Scores*
		X1	1 = yes		1
		X2	2 = no		0
		X3	1 = yes		1
		X4	1 = yes		1
		X5	1 = yes		1
					―
					4

two variables yielded a profile of different *types* of programs. Those programs that were started in a favorable environment and did well were called "hotshots" (Type 11). "Overachievers" were initiated in unfavorable environments but did well anyway (Type 21). In contrast, "underachievers" began in favorable settings but did not really achieve what they set out to accomplish (Type 12). "Underdogs" did not have favorable environments and, in fact, did poorly (Type 22).

Indexes

Another approach to summarizing a number of survey questions about an issue is simply to add up the scores (or codes) of the variables related to the concept that the researcher wants to measure. The resulting total is a simple summary measure or index of the constituent items. This is a particularly useful approach for summing up the correct answers to questions that test the respondent's knowledge regarding a certain topic, such as the risk factors for AIDS or breast cancer.

Index scores do not, however, provide information on the patterns of the responses that were given. For example, do respondents seem to have more knowledge about certain diseases than others? Index construction per se does not assume a process for verifying that the individual items tap the same underlying concept: do they reflect knowledge about these conditions or some underlying attitude toward the scientific practice of medicine? Further, such summaries may make more sense for certain types of variables than others, depending on what the constituent numbers mean in terms of the respective levels of measurement. The sum of codes for *types* of the kind described earlier, for example, has no meaning in itself. The process of constructing scales to summarize questions presumed to tap the same underlying concept attempts to address these issues.

Scales

The construction of scales follows this pattern: (1) a large number of items or questions thought to reflect a concept are identified; (2) items that are poorly worded or seemingly less clear-cut indicators of the concept are eliminated; and (3) some process for deciding whether the items fit into the structure for the variables that are assumed by a particular scale is chosen (that is, are they "scalable" according to that scale's requirements?). The three major types of scales discussed here and presented in Table 3.4 are the Likert, Guttman, and Thurstone Equal-Appearing Interval Scales.

An implicit assumption in the construction of a summary scale is that the scale items are observable (empirical) expressions of an underlying, unobservable (latent) construct (attitude). Scale development methods such as internal consistency

TABLE 3.4. CONSTRUCTING SCALES TO SUMMARIZE STUDY VARIABLES.

Scales	Level of Measurement	Scaling and Scoring Methods

Likert Scale (sum of scores assigned to answers to questions in scale) — Level of Measurement: **Ordinal**

Methods

Variables	Response Categories					Scoring
	Strongly Agree	Agree	Uncertain	Disagree	Strongly Disagree	Scores
X1	1	2	3	(4)	5	4
X2	1	(2)	3	4	5	2
X3	1	2	3	4	(5)	5
X4	(1)	2	3	4	5	1
X5	1	2	(3)	4	5	3
						15

Guttman Scale (cumulative pattern of scores assigned to answers to questions in scale) — Level of Measurement: **Ordinal**

Responses	Variables					Scoring
	X1	X2	X3	X4	X5	Scores
+ + + + +	Agree	Agree	Agree	Agree	Agree	5
+ + + +	Agree	Agree	Agree	Agree	Disagree	4
+ + +	Agree	Agree	Agree	Disagree	Disagree	3
+ +	Agree	Agree	Disagree	Disagree	Disagree	2
+	Agree	Disagree	Disagree	Disagree	Disagree	1
−	Disagree	Disagree	Disagree	Disagree	Disagree	0

Thurstone Equal-Appearing Interval Scale (average of *scale interval* scores assigned to answers to questions in scale) — Level of Measurement: **Interval**

Variables	Response Categories		Scoring
	Agree	Disagree	Scores
X1	+		4
X2		+	0
X3	+		5
X4	+		3
X5	+		3
			$15 \div 4 = 3.8$

reliability and construct validity analyses serve to quantify the extent to which responses to the survey questions that are actually developed to measure this construct are correlated with or may be said to be "caused by" this underlying abstract but nonetheless real influence (Crocker & Algina, 1986; DeVellis, 1991; Jöreskog & Sörbom, 1979; Kim & Mueller, 1978; Nunnally & Bernstein, 1994).

As mentioned earlier, survey designers may want to use scales developed by other researchers. In that case, they should have some idea of how the respective scales are constructed, what they mean, whether the reliability and (when possible) the validity of the scales have been documented, and whether the findings for the populations included in those studies are relevant to the current population of interest. With the first two types of scaling procedures (the Likert and Guttman approaches), investigators can include items in the survey that they have developed on their own and that they think can be collapsed into these scales and then test the actual scalability of the data during analysis. Or, ideally, if the necessary time and resources are available at the front end of the study, the investigators can develop and test such scales on a set of subjects similar to those who will be in the survey and then incorporate only those items in the study questionnaire that turn out to be scalable.

The *Likert* approach to developing questions and summary scales is used with great frequency in surveys. It basically relies on an ordinal response scale in which the respondent indicates the level of his or her agreement with an attitudinal or other statement. This, of course, reflects a subjective rather than a factual response of the individual to an issue. Question 17 in the Dentists' Preferences study (Resource C), which asks about dentists' "practice beliefs," is an example of a Likert-type format for survey questions. Generally five categories—strongly agree, agree, disagree, strongly disagree, and uncertain (or neutral)—are used in such questions, although as few as three or as many as ten could be used. Questions 31 to 35 in the Chicago Area AIDS survey (Resource B) also reflect a Likert-type question response scale to measure the intensity of respondents' feelings about their fear of different illnesses, the likelihood of contracting them, their perceptions of the seriousness of the illnesses, and so on.

Scores can be assigned to each of the responses to reflect the strength and direction of the attitude expressed in a particular statement. For example, a code of 1 could be used to indicate that respondents strongly agree with a statement regarding their satisfaction with an aspect of medical care and 5 when they strongly disagree. The scores associated with the answers that respondents provide to each question (indicated in parentheses in Table 3.4) would then be added up to produce a total summary score of the strength and direction of a respondent's attitude on the subject (with a higher score meaning a more positive attitude, for example). Likert-type scales are referred to as *summative scales* because the scores on the constituent question are summed or added up to arrive at the total scale score.

A good scale should have a mix of positive and negative statements (about satisfaction with aspects of medical care, for example). Let us assume that the following codes are used to reflect responses to such statements: 1=strongly agree, 2=agree, 3=uncertain, 4=disagree, and 5=strongly disagree. A person who strongly disagrees (code of 5) with a negative statement ("I am sometimes ignored by the office staff in my doctor's office") or strongly agrees (code of 1) with a positive statement ("The office staff treats me with respect") would be deemed to have a positive attitude about their care (Weiss & Senf, 1990). When summing the answers to each question to create a summary score, if a higher score were intended to represent higher levels of satisfaction on this five-item scale, then a code of 1 assigned for strongly agreeing with a positive statement would need to be recoded to 5, for example. A formula for converting (reversing) the coding for this and other possible responses is as follows: $R=(H+L) - I$, where H is the highest possible value or response (5), L is the lowest possible value (1), and I is the actual response (or code) for a given item. For a five-item ordinal response scale that ranges from 1 to 5 the results would be: $(5+1) - 1 = 5$; $(5+1) - 2 = 4$; $(5+1) - 3 = 3$; $(5+1) - 4 = 2$; $(5+1) - 5 = 1$ (Spector, 1992, p. 22).

The reliability indicators reviewed earlier can then be used to determine just how stable and consistent these summary scores are over time, across interviewers, and among the array of items on which the summary scores are based. The alpha coefficient can be used to assess the feasibility of combining a variety of attitudinal items into a Likert-type scale. As mentioned earlier, a minimum coefficient of .70 is required to document that items included are fairly consistent in how they tap the underlying concept.

More sophisticated procedures, such as factor analysis, can also be carried out to determine whether different factors or subdimensions of the same concept are being tapped by different subgroups of questions.

The Medical Outcomes Study has made extensive use of many of the procedures outlined here in developing Likert-type summary scales of health status, including the MOS 36-Item Short-Form Health Survey (SF-36) and related forms of this scale (the SF-20 and SF-12, for example) (McHorney, Ware, Lu, & Sherbourne, 1994; McHorney, Ware, & Raczek, 1993; Stewart & Ware, 1992; Ware & Sherbourne, 1992; Ware, Kosinski, Bayliss, et al., 1995; Ware, Kosinski, & Keller, 1994, 1995; Ware, Snow, Kosinski, & Gandek, 1993).

Survey researchers need to consider whether they may be tapping a variety of different subdimensions of a concept when creating summary scores based on different questions; they should also be aware of formalized procedures for testing whether they are in fact doing so.

Unlike a Likert summary score, the *Guttman scale* reflects the patterns of answers to particular questions in the score itself (Crocker & Algina, 1986). This scale assumes that there is a gradient (or hierarchy) in the attitude that the items are intended to represent and that this gradient can be used as the basis for selecting and scoring those items. For example, an investigator might be interested in attitudes about the degree of intimacy people would be willing to have with persons with AIDS. The researcher could then ask respondents whether they agreed or disagreed with the following statements:

X5—I would be willing to have sex with someone who has AIDS.

X4—I would be willing to live in the same house with someone who has AIDS.

X3—I would be willing to occasionally visit someone who has AIDS.

X2—I would be willing to sit next to someone on a bus who has AIDS.

X1—I would be willing to talk on the phone to a person with AIDS.

These items imply a range in the extent of physical intimacy respondents would be willing to have with a person with AIDS, reflected in whether they agree or disagree with the respective items. As in the Guttman scale example in Table 3.4, a score of 5 would be assigned to someone who agreed with all the items and would, therefore, be presumed to be the most willing to have close contact with AIDS victims, a score of 4 would be assigned to those who agree to items X1, X2, X3, and X4 but not X5, 3 to those who agree to X1, X2, and X3 but not X4 and X5, and so on, to those who would be the least willing to have any personal contact with the person with AIDS (said no to all the items). Specific patterns of responses or "scale types" would then theoretically be reflected in each of these scores (+ + + + +, + + + +, + + +, + +, +, −). Guttman scales are referred to as *cumulative scales* because the total scale score reflects a cumulative pattern of answers to the individual questions included in the scale.

Some respondents, however, might not fit these (theoretical) cumulative patterns. For example, if someone disagreed only with item X3 (would not be willing to visit occasionally with someone with AIDS) then their actual pattern of response (++ − ++) would not correspond with the expected pattern (+ + + + −) for someone with a total score of 4 on the scale. These departures from the pattern of answers implied by a particular scale score are termed *scale errors*. To the extent that scale types can be verified and the errors of classifying respondents' answers into these types minimized, the questions can be considered scalable into a Guttman-type format.

The MOS study elected not to use Guttman scales principally because they require dichotomous response formats (agree or disagree) and tend to be limited to a few (five or six) items, which limits the amount of information that can be obtained. They also tend to be more cumbersome and ambiguous to construct and interpret (Stewart & Ware, 1992, p. 79).

A third method for scaling responses to a variety of questions on the same topic is the Thurstone Equal-Appearing Interval Scale (Nunnally & Bernstein, 1994). This scale has to be constructed in advance of selecting the items to include in the survey questionnaire. To that end, a panel of judges is given a large number of attitude statements (usually a hundred or more) about some issue of interest. The judges are asked to rate the statements according to whether they think a particular item reflects a generally favorable or unfavorable attitude toward the issue, using a scale with 11 points at equal-appearing intervals along the scale: the number 11 would be deemed the very favorable end of the scale, 1 the very unfavorable end, and 6 neutral. The judges are then asked to place the statements, as appropriate, at points spaced all along the 11 points on the scale.

The median (or middle) value among all the judges' ratings of a statement is taken to represent its overall degree of favorableness (on a scale from 1 to 11). The median value is the score that falls exactly in the middle of the judges' ratings for a given item, with half the judges giving a score below that value and half above it. The range or degree of variability in the judges' responses to any particular item is also computed. Items for which there seem to be the least agreement among the judges would be eliminated. Thurstone scales are generally limited to twenty to twenty-two items intended to represent each of the points along a scale that measures the degree of favorableness toward the topic.

After the items are selected, they can then be incorporated into a questionnaire and respondents can be asked to indicate whether they agree or disagree with the statements. The respondents are not aware of the scale scores for the items but the values for those with which they agree can be summed and an average value computed to assess the overall favorableness of the attitudes respondents are said to hold (on a scale from 1 to 11). In the example in Table 3.4, the scores for the items tend to reflect relatively unfavorable attitudes (have values less than 6). When added up and averaged, the scores for the specific questions with which the respondents agree (X1, X3, X4, X5) indicate a negative attitude toward some topic, such as the convenience and availability of health care services for residents of an inner-city neighborhood.

Hulka, Kupper, Daly, Cassel, and Schoen (1975) developed a scale of patient satisfaction based on a modified Thurstone-type technique. This type of scale requires a considerable amount of preliminary effort to develop the items and obtain and process the judges' ratings. Nevertheless, survey designers should be aware of this method and consider its utility for concepts they might want to address in their studies (Roberts & Tugwell, 1987).

Two other types of scaling that have been used in connection with health status index development in particular include Rasch item response theory (IRT) and utility scaling. IRT is utilized to guide the development of summary scales that are hierarchical (items progress from easy to difficult along a hypothesized continuum, such as indicators of physical functioning); unidimensional (represent a single dominant concept); and reproducible (the order and meaning of the points along the scale, such as degree of difficulty, are not highly variable across different groups and over time) (Andrich, 1988; Hambleton, Swaminathan, & Rogers, 1991). IRT assumes that each item has its own characteristic sensitivity to the underlying concept being measured that can be expressed as a logistic probability function (or the probability of answering the question in a certain way as a function of the magnitude of the underlying level of functioning). This approach can be particularly useful if one is interested in classifying scale items according to an underlying hierarchy (of task difficulty, for example) ranging from tasks that may be relatively easy (bathing and dressing) to relatively difficult (engaging in vigorous physical activity) to perform. An IRT analysis of the ten-item physical functioning scale (PF-10) from the MOS SF-36 confirmed that the items in this scale could be arrayed in this fashion (Haley, McHorney, & Ware, 1994). Utility-scaling approaches to health status scale development will be discussed in more detail in Chapter Nine.

Special Considerations for Special Populations

Other important criteria, in addition to those reviewed here, for evaluating items and summary measures used in surveys are practical ones related to their responsiveness, interpretability, burden, and cultural and language sensitivity. These are important criteria to consider in general but they take on particular importance in studies of special populations. *Responsiveness* refers to the tool's ability to detect changes (in health status, for example) that are deemed relevant by individuals (persons with HIV/AIDS) targeted for a particular intervention (a new drug). *Interpretability* means that the quantitative findings on the measure (scale scores) can be translated into qualitative meanings (health status) that can be understood by users or consumers (patients or providers). *Burden* refers to the time and effort in administering the instrument as well as responding to it. *Cultural and language sensitivity* is concerned with the assessment of conceptual and linguistic equivalence of other language versions of the instrument as well as whether their psychometric properties (reliability and validity) are comparable for different language or cultural groups. It may also be important to evaluate the reading level of the survey instrument in relationship to the likely literacy levels of the target population (Medical Outcomes Trust, Scientific Advisory Committee, 1995; Sullivan, et al., 1995).

Generalizability theory uses analysis of variance to explore formally the extent to which the measurement process is similar across different measurement situations (data gatherers or mode of administration), referred to as facets. This procedure may be particularly useful to employ in evaluating the equivalence of items using different data collection modes or language versions of an instrument (Crocker & Algina, 1986).

Selected Examples

The 1996 and subsequent NHIS surveys reflect a substantial redesign of the core survey questionnaire and data collection procedures in response to methodological research conducted by NCHS and academic researchers (Smith & Lancashire, 1995). A major criticism that has been made of the NCHS–NHIS is that while it provides a useful battery of an array of discrete questions on health status and related constructs, there has been insufficient attention to the development of indexes or summary scales from these items to measure the underlying constructs (Patrick & Erickson, 1993).

A Knowledge of AIDS Index was constructed from selected questions on the Chicago AIDS survey to provide an assessment of respondents' knowledge about the behavioral factors associated with HIV virus transmission (Prohaska, Albrecht, Levy, Sugrue, & Kim, 1990). The six items used in constructing the index (and scores for the correct answer) were as follows (see Resource B): Q. 10: Is the number of people with AIDS likely to increase or decrease over the next five years (increase = 1); Q. 13: Compared to catching a cold, is it easier, harder, or about the same to catch AIDS (harder = 1); Q. 14a,b,c: Is it possible for pregnant woman to pass to her child, . . . for a woman to get AIDS from having sex with a man with AIDS, . . . for a man to get AIDS from having sex with a woman with AIDS (possible = 1); and Q. 15: If a man uses a condom, does this make getting AIDS less likely or not (less likely = 1)? Total scores ranged from 0 to 6, with higher score indicating more knowledge.

In the dentists' preferences study several constructs reflective of the dentists' practice beliefs were derived based on a factor analysis of selected questionnaire items (see Resource C) (Grembowski, Milgrom, & Fiset, 1988, 1991). These beliefs and the items from which they were constructed are the following: the extent to which prevention and patient education are emphasized (Q. 17a, 17e); the role of the patient in influencing the type of treatment rendered (Q. 17c, 17f); and the extent to which the dentist should share information with the patient about treatment options (Q. 17b, 25). The response to each question was recoded to 1 or 0 as appropriate to provide a uniform basis for combining the items.

Guidelines for Minimizing Survey Errors

Reliability and validity analysis represent classic and important approaches to evaluating the magnitude of random and systematic error in survey data. A consideration of these norms may be applied at many stages of survey design: in identifying the relevant principles to apply in wording certain types of questions (threatening, nonthreatening, attitudinal, and so on) in order to ensure the accuracy and stability of people's answers; in evaluating the questions or scales developed in other studies; in designing a pretest or pilot study to evaluate the reliability and validity of the instrument before going into the field; and in constructing and validating summary scales based on the information gathered in the survey on a key study concept of interest.

High reliability and validity coefficients for a scale to measure a given concept do not in and of themselves assure that the scale is either meaningful or relevant. Theoretical knowledge and practical wisdom are both useful in informing the development of questionnaire items and summary scales to measure a concept of interest. Limiting the dimensions of consumer satisfaction considered to the experiences of those who regularly use medical care may fail to surface the considerable dissatisfaction of those who do not. And asking questions that make sense to people who stroll the main street in Peoria may not necessarily "play" to those who live out their days on the mean streets of Harlem.

This chapter suggested a number of criteria for survey designers to consider in deciding what questions to include in their studies and how to go about reducing an array of questions about the same topic into parsimonious and reliable summary indicators for analysis. Readers may want to return to this chapter as they think about how to analyze the data in their own studies. The alternatives are presented here, however, to encourage survey designers to think about these types of analyses early on so that they will know what kinds of items or summary scales to look for or to create in designing their own studies as well as the criteria to use in evaluating them. In fact, it may be desirable to use well-developed scales that have undergone rigorous development and evaluation of the kind described here to measure key study constructs. The next chapter outlines the elements to consider when thinking through the analyses for the study—before asking the first question of a respondent.

Supplementary Sources

For an example of internal consistency reliability analysis, using SPSS, see Norusis (1990, pp. 462–472). An explanation of the steps involved in constructing a summated rating (Likert) scale may be found in Spector (1992). Additional sources of examples of the validity analyses discussed in this chapter include the following: sensitivity and specificity analysis (Hennekens & Buring, 1987, pp. 331–342); factor analysis (Norusis, 1990, pp. 312–346); multitrait multimethod approach (Shortell & Richardson, 1978, pp. 79–83). See Andrich (1988) and Hambleton, Swaminathan, & Rogers (1991) for a discussion of the fundamentals of Rasch models of measurement and Item-Response Theory, and Haley, McHorney, & Ware (1994) for an application of the IRT methodology to scale development.

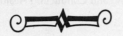

CHAPTER FOUR

THINKING THROUGH THE RELATIONSHIPS BETWEEN VARIABLES

Chapter Highlights

1. An informed approach to survey design includes identifying not only the specific variables that will be used to measure the study concepts but also the relationships between them, which are implied in the study's research objectives and hypotheses.

2. The basis for identifying relevant variables and their interrelationships may be a theory or conceptual framework, previous research, or practical experience.

Before developing the survey questionnaire and approaches to gathering the data, researchers must consider not only the major variables but also their interrelationships that will be examined and why. The study objectives and hypotheses and associated research design are the defining guides for specifying these relationships.

As pointed out in Chapter Two, a theory or conceptual framework, previous research, or practical experience may serve as the basis for delineating the objectives and hypotheses. The analytic thrust (descriptive, analytical, or experimental) as well as the temporal and spatial parameters (cross-sectional, group-comparison, or longitudinal) of the design are meant to mirror and underlie the questions that the study will address (see again Tables 2.2 and 2.3 and Figure 2.1).

Testing Study Hypotheses

As mentioned in Chapter Two, longitudinal or experimental designs allow the investigator to detect more clearly the "cause" of an outcome of interest than do one-time cross-sectional surveys. In one-time surveys the researcher relies on theoretical models of the causal chain of events that lead to certain outcomes and on statistical approaches to testing those models. The process of statistically controlling for other variables in such analyses is comparable to creating equivalence between groups through the random assignment of subjects to an experimental and control condition in a true experimental design. The only condition then that varies between the two groups is the administration of the experimental stimulus, which is analogous to the operation of the "independent variable" in cross-sectional survey analyses. Correspondingly, the sampling design for the study must anticipate the number of cases required to carry out the resulting subgroup analyses.

Discovering the determinants of human behaviors or attitudes requires consideration of a range of complex, interrelated factors. Sociologists in particular have developed and refined approaches for sorting out the most important reasons why people behave the way they do. In the main, these approaches are based on procedures for elaborating study hypotheses (Hirschi & Selvin, 1967; Hyman, 1955; Lazarsfeld, Pasanella, & Rosenberg, 1972; Rosenberg, 1968; Zeisel, 1968). The discussion that follows provides examples of how these approaches can be used to refine the hypotheses that guide the design and conduct of health surveys.

In a chemistry lab students may be given two known compounds and one unknown and asked to identify the unknown compound on the basis of prior assumptions about the reactions that will occur when the chemicals are mixed. Testing study hypotheses is like sorting out the chemistry between two variables when another one is added to the equation. In addition to the main independent and dependent variables, the variables that could be included in a study are termed *test* or *control* variables. They help in examining whether one variable does indeed cause another or whether the relationship observed between the variables is "caused" by some other factor. It is important to identify these other variables in advance of doing a survey to ensure that data are available to examine adequately and accurately the variety of competing explanations for relationships observed between the main independent and dependent variables in a study.

The variables in the hypotheses used here to illustrate the approaches to analyzing health survey data are expressed in terms of dichotomous categorical variables. The same basic logic can be applied, however, to examining the relationships between study variables based on other (higher) levels of measurement. Specific statistical techniques for examining these relationships for different study designs and types of variables are reviewed in Chapter Fifteen.

The first step in developing and testing a hypothesis is to specify the relationship that one expects to find between the main independent and dependent variables of interest. For example, in Table 2.2 the analytical designs were guided by the hypothesis that friends' smoking behavior (independent variable) was predictive of high school seniors' propensity to smoke (dependent variable). The simplest type of statistical procedure for testing the relationship between nominal-level independent and dependent variables is to construct a data table that looks at a cross-classification of the dependent variable Y (whether the senior smokes or not) by the independent variable X (seniors with friends who smoke versus those whose friends do not smoke). (See sample table in Figure 4.1.) If a large proportion (say, 75 percent) of the seniors whose friends are smokers smoke and a smaller proportion (say, 30 percent) of those whose friends are not smokers smoke, then the findings would seem to bear out the study hypothesis.

An approach used by epidemiologists in examining the relative importance of exposure to different health risks (elevated cholesterol levels) in accounting for whether a person has a disease (heart disease) or not, using a case-control design, is the odds ratio (Kleinbaum, Kupper, & Morgenstern, 1982). This ratio can be computed by calculating the ratio of the odds (or likelihood) of exposure among the cases (with the disease) to that among the controls (without the disease) (see Figure 4.1):

$$\text{odds ratio (OR)} = \frac{a/b}{c/d} = \frac{ad}{bc},$$

where,

  a = number of cases exposed (elevated cholesterol level)
  b = number of cases *not* exposed (normal cholesterol level)
  c = number of controls exposed (elevated cholesterol level)
  d = number of controls *not* exposed (normal cholesterol level)

If the variables are not related, their respective odds would be identical (or nearly so) and the ratio of their odds (odds ratio) equal to 1.00 (OR = 1.00). Odds ratios of greater than one indicate a positive covariation between variables (the presence of or the greater the magnitude of an attribute, the *more* likely the other attribute is to be present), while odds ratios less than one reflect a negative or inverse covariation (the presence of or the greater the magnitude of an attribute, the *less* likely the other attribute is to occur).

Odds ratios are most appropriately used with case-control designs to reflect the probability of having a disease or not as a function of having been exposed to selected risk factors. The examples presented in Figure 4.1 and the figures and tables that follow are based on a cross-sectional analytical design. Chi-square tests of differences are reported to document whether there is a statistically significant

FIGURE 4.1. TESTING THE MAIN STUDY HYPOTHESIS.

Theoretical Model and Sample Table

Theoretical Model

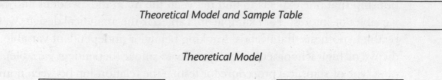

Sample Table

Student Smoking Status (Y)	Friends' Smoking Status (X)		Total
	Some or All	None	
Smoker	*a* 75% (75)	*b* 30% (30)	53% (105) *(a + b)*
Nonsmoker	*c* 25% (25)	*d* 70% (70)	48% (95) *(c + d)*
Total	100% *(a + c)* (100)	100% *(b + d)* (100)	100% (200) *(a + b + c + d)*
odds ratio (OR) = $\dfrac{a/b}{c/d} = \dfrac{ad}{bc} = \dfrac{75*70}{30*25} = \dfrac{5{,}250}{750} = 7.0$			chi-square = 40.6 p = .000

relationship between the independent and dependent variables (as defined in the respective examples). Odds ratios are reported as well to demonstrate the strength of the relationship between a given outcome (smoking or not) as a function of selected risk factors (parents' or friends' smoking), should this be an appropriate analytic strategy given the underlying study objectives and design. (See Chapter Fifteen for further discussion of guidelines for matching the analytic procedures to the study design.)

The strong association of students' smoking behavior with that of their friends is confirmed by the highly significant results for the chi-square test of differences between groups (p = .000) (Figure 4.1). The odds ratio (7.0) for the relationship of friends' smoking status (X) to whether or not a high school student smokes indicates that smokers are seven times more likely than nonsmokers to have friends who smoke.

However, it is possible that other variables (family history of elevated cholesterol or smoking) that might be related to the main (independent and dependent) variables (X and Y) in the study actually account for the relationship observed between these variables. The statistical procedures for examining the impact of these other variables attempt to consider *what if* the influence of these other variables were removed—would the original relationship still exist? This process of removing the influence of these other variables involves not allowing them to vary (or "controlling" them, "adjusting" for them, "stratifying" on them, or holding them "constant") when looking at the original relationship.

The simplest way to control the operation of these other variables is to look at the original relationship between the independent and dependent variables in the study separately for groups of people that have the same value on the variable being controlled. In the cross-classification table of the relationship between friends' smoking behavior (X) and a student's propensity to smoke (Y), the impact of some variable Z could be controlled by looking at that table separately for different categories of Z—for example, students whose parents smoke versus students whose parents do not smoke, students who view smoking as a socially acceptable practice versus those who do not, or minority students versus white students. The variable Z takes on the same value, that is, it is "held constant" within each of the respective categories of Z. Statistical techniques used with higher-order levels of measurement accomplish the same thing through statistically "controlling for" or removing the effects of these other variables.

As in the chemistry example given earlier, three results are possible when the impact of this third factor (Z) is controlled: (1) the original relationship between X and Y disappears, (2) the original relationship between X and Y persists or becomes stronger in one category of Z but not in the other, or (3) there is no change in the original relationship between X and Y. The first result represents an *explanation* or *interpretation* of why the relationship between X and Y seems to be affected so dramatically. The second provides a *specification* of the conditions under which the original relationship is most likely to hold. This is also referred to as "statistical interaction" or "effect modification," meaning that the original relationship between X and Y is different under different conditions defined by the control variable Z. The third outcome is essentially a *replication* of the original study results. These possible outcomes are displayed in Figures 4.2 through 4.5 and are discussed in the following paragraphs.

If the relationship disappears when the effects of Z are removed, it may mean one of two things: (1) X appeared to be linked to Y in the original relationship only because they were both tied to Z, or (2) Z really is an important link in the causal chain between X and Y. In either case, removing the influence of Z affects the relationship between X and Y.

The discussion that follows shows how these relationships can be tested empirically. Which aspect the investigator elects to emphasize depends on the theoretical perspective chosen to guide the collection and analysis of the survey data.

Explanation

One may be interested in further understanding the dynamics of the relationship of having friends who smoke to the likely adoption of smoking among teenagers, as a basis for designing interventions to reduce this occurrence. Based on theory, previous research, or knowledge of the study population, investigators may wish to explore the influence of parents' smoking behavior as well as students' perceptions of the social acceptability of smoking as factors that determine or mediate the impact of peers' smoking practices.

If the investigator views the students' parents smoking behavior as predictive of whether the students have friends who are smokers (Z→X) and of whether they themselves are likely to take up smoking (Z→Y), then the relationship between students' and their peers' smoking behaviors (X→Y) would hypothetically be explained largely by these parental or family influences (Z), as shown in the theoretical model in Figure 4.2.

This model is called *explanatory* because the original relationship can be explained by some other "cause" (Z) for the apparent relationship observed between X and Y. The test variable in this type of model is an *extraneous* or *confounding* variable. It lies outside the direct causal chain between the independent and dependent variables. The original relationship between variables is, as a result, labeled "spurious" because, while it looked as though there was a direct causal relationship between X and Y, the investigator's theory and findings indicate that something else was the real cause of both. Implicitly this extraneous or confounding influence is temporally and instrumentally prior to each of the other factors, that is, the fact that parents smoke is likely to influence the choice of friends who do so as well as set up a predisposition for the student to take up smoking.

The sample tables in Figure 4.2 show how each of these relationships can be tested empirically. First, the relationship between parents' smoking behavior (Z) and friends' smoking status (X), Z→X, is tested (sample table a). The data show that the percentage with friends who smoke is much higher among those with parents who smoke than among those whose parents do not: 67 percent versus 19 percent. These findings establish that parents' and friends' smoking practices are related.

Next, the relationship between the parents' and students' behavior (Z→Y) is examined (sample table b). These data show that 69 percent of the students whose

FIGURE 4.2. ELABORATING THE MAIN STUDY HYPOTHESIS—EXPLANATION.

Theoretical Model and Sample Tables—Explanation

Theoretical Model

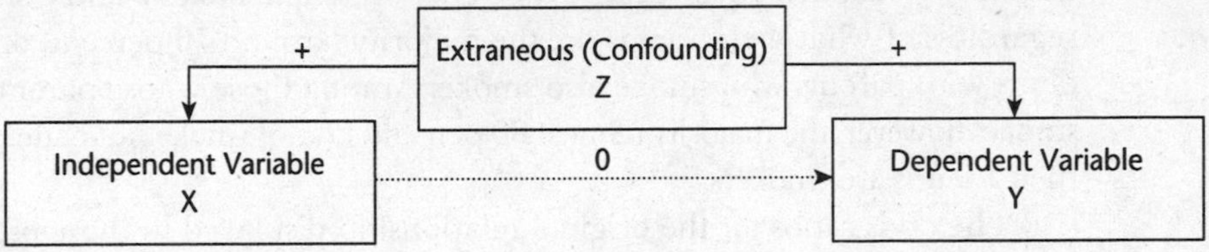

Sample Tables

Table a			Table b		
Friends' Smoking Status (X)	Parents' Smoking Status (Z)		Student Smoking Status (Y)	Parents' Smoking Status (Z)	
	One or Both	Neither		One or Both	Neither
Some or All	67% (87)	19% (13)	Smoker	69% (90)	21% (15)
None	33% (43)	81% (57)	Nonsmoker	31% (40)	79% (55)
Total	100% (130)	100% (70)	**Total**	100% (130)	100% (70)

Table c Z = One or both parents			Table d Z = Neither parent		
Student Smoking Status (Y)	Friends' Smoking Status (X)		Student Smoking Status (Y)	Friends' Smoking Status (X)	
	Some or All	None		Some or All	None
Smoker	69% (60)	70% (30)	Smoker	23% (3)	21% (12)
Nonsmoker	31% (27)	30% (13)	Nonsmoker	77% (10)	79% (45)
Total	100% (87)	100% (43)	**Total**	100% (13)	100% (57)

$OR = \dfrac{60 \times 13}{30 \times 27} = \dfrac{780}{810} = .96$ chi-square = .01   p = .926 $OR = \dfrac{3 \times 45}{12 \times 10} = \dfrac{135}{120} = 1.1$ chi-square = .03   p = .872

parents smoke also smoke compared with only 21 percent of those whose parents are nonsmokers. Parents' smoking practices then influence what their children do.

The final set of tables in Figure 4.2 examines the original relationship hypothesized between their peers' (X) and the students' own behavior (Y), controlling for parental influences (Z), which was found to be related to both, based on the cross-sectional analytic design. The data in sample tables c and d show that, regardless of what their friends do, the majority (around 70 percent) of the students with parents who smoke also smoke. Among those whose parents do not smoke, however, the majority (almost 80 percent) do not smoke no matter whether their friends are smokers.

The odds ratios for the original relationship displayed in those tables controlling for parents' behavior (tables c and d) are close to 1.0, and the chi-square tests of difference not significant, indicating that the relationship between peer and student practices can be largely explained by whether the students' parents smoke or not. These results bear out the important influence that parental role modeling has on student behavior.

Interpretation

However, if the investigator hypothesizes that peers' smoking practices directly influence students' perceptions of the social acceptability of smoking (X→Z) and that this, in turn, predicts whether the student is likely to take up smoking (Z→Y), then a different temporal and causal ordering of variables is suggested. The underlying hypothesis here is that peer influences play an important role in reinforcing whether smoking is an okay thing to do, which leads to a greater chance of teenagers' taking up the practice.

This model reflects an "interpretation" of the direct causal linkages between variables that lead to the outcome of interest: X→Z→Y (Figure 4.3). The control variable that is thought on the basis of the investigator's theory to facilitate an interpretation of why and how X leads to Y is called an *intervening* or *mediating* variable. It theoretically intervenes in or mediates the causal linkage between X and Y.

The investigator may want to go back even further in the causal chain to trace the importance of other determinants of this outcome. For example, there might be an interest in the impact of some variable (Z') antecedent to X (such as race or ethnicity) as a determinant of X (having friends who smoke).

In the example in Figure 4.3, students with friends who smoke are much more likely to believe it is an acceptable practice than those who do not have friends who are smokers: 67 percent versus 19 percent (table a). Those who think it is a socially acceptable practice are also more likely to be smokers: 69 percent versus 21 percent (table b). When controlling for students' perceptions of the social acceptability of smoking (tables c and d), the original relationship between peers'

FIGURE 4.3. ELABORATING THE MAIN STUDY HYPOTHESIS—INTERPRETATION.

Theoretical Model and Sample Tables—Interpretation

Theoretical Model

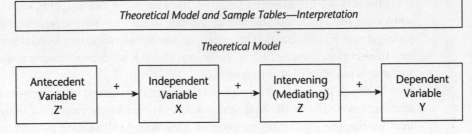

Sample Tables

Table a

Attitude Toward Smoking (Z)	Friends' Smoking Status (X)	
	Some or All	None
Socially Acceptable	67% (87)	19% (13)
Socially Unacceptable	33% (43)	81% (57)
Total	100% (130)	100% (70)

Table b

Student Smoking Status (Y)	Attitude Toward Smoking (Z)	
	Socially Acceptable	Socially Unacceptable
Smoker	69% (90)	21% (15)
Nonsmoker	31% (40)	79% (55)
Total	100% (130)	100% (70)

Table c
Z = Socially Acceptable

Student Smoking Status (Y)	Friends' Smoking Status (X)	
	Some or All	None
Smoker	69% (60)	70% (30)
Nonsmoker	31% (27)	30% (13)
Total	100% (87)	100% (43)

$$OR = \frac{60 \times 13}{30 \times 27} = \frac{780}{810} = .96 \qquad \text{chi-square} = .01 \quad p = .926$$

Table d
Z = Socially Unacceptable

Student Smoking Status (Y)	Friends' Smoking Status (X)	
	Some or All	None
Smoker	23% (3)	21% (12)
Nonsmoker	77% (10)	79% (45)
Total	100% (13)	100% (57)

$$OR = \frac{3 \times 45}{12 \times 10} = \frac{135}{120} = 1.1 \qquad \text{chi-square} = .03 \quad p = .872$$

and students' behavior disappears, as reflected in the odds ratios of around 1.00 and accompanying statistically nonsignificant chi-square results. Regardless of what their friends do, the majority (around 70 percent) of the students who believe smoking is socially acceptable smoke. Among those who do not, however, the majority (almost 80 percent) do not smoke, no matter whether their friends are smokers. In this case, the key link in the causal chain is student attitudes toward the social acceptability of this practice (Z).

Although parental and peer influences are considered separately in the examples provided here, the analyst may want to consider the impact of both in understanding the propensity to become a smoker. Multivariate procedures that permit a number of different factors to be considered as predictive or determinant of a given outcome of interest (such as multiple regression, logistic regression, path analysis, or LISREL, discussed in Chapter Fifteen) could be utilized for this purpose. The same basic logic applies. The investigator, guided by theory, previous research, or practice, must think through the study variables and their hypothesized interrelationships before formulating the survey questionnaire to make sure that the objectives that he or she sets out to accomplish can be achieved.

Interaction or Effect Modification

Another possible outcome when the original relationship between X and Y is looked at for different categories of Z or Z' is that the same relationship remains or grows stronger for some categories of the control variable but not for others. This finding further specifies under what conditions or for whom the hypothesized relationship is likely to exist (Figure 4.4). It may, for example, be important to look at the relationship between peer and student smoking practices for different racial or ethnic groups of students (Z'). Among Hispanic students, the percentage of those who smoke is high among those whose friends are smokers compared with those whose friends do not smoke: 86 percent versus 35 percent. But among African American students the percentage who are nonsmokers is high (almost 80 percent) regardless of whether they have friends who smoke. The odds ratios and chi-square tests of significance for the impact of peer behavior on smoking confirm that it is a major influence among Hispanic students (OR = 12.0, p = .000) but not consequential for African American students (OR = 1.1, p =.872). (This phenomenon of finding that different relationships exist between the independent and dependent variables for different values of a third variable is said to reflect *effect modification* or *statistical interaction* between variables—X and Z' in this case.)

Replication

If the same relationship is found between the original variables when the control variable is considered in the analysis, then the original relationship—in this case,

FIGURE 4.4. ELABORATING THE MAIN STUDY HYPOTHESIS—INTERACTION.

Theoretical Model and Sample Tables—Interaction

Theoretical Model

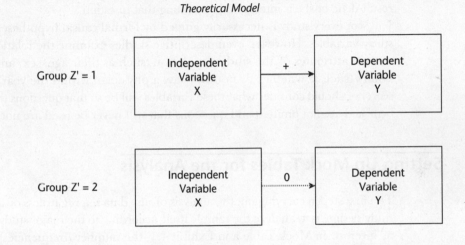

Sample Tables

	Table a Z' = Hispanic			Table b Z' = African American	
Student Smoking Status (Y)	Friends' Smoking Status (X)		Student Smoking Status (Y)	Friends' Smoking Status (X)	
	Some or All	None		Some or All	None
Smoker	86% (75)	35% (15)	Smoker	23% (3)	21% (12)
Nonsmoker	14% (12)	65% (28)	Nonsmoker	77% (10)	79% (45)
Total	100% (87)	100% (43)	**Total**	100% (13)	100% (57)
OR $= \dfrac{75 \times 28}{15 \times 12} = \dfrac{2100}{180} = 12.0$	chi-square = 35.6 p = .000		OR $= \dfrac{3 \times 45}{12 \times 10} = \dfrac{135}{120} = 1.1$	chi-square = .03 p = .872	

between peer and student behavior—is replicated (Figure 4.5). The odds ratios for this relationship, controlling for other factors, are essentially the same (around 7.0, p = .000) as was observed originally (Figure 4.1). The control variable (parental influence, attitudes toward smoking, or race and ethnicity, depending on the model of interest) does not appear to have an effect on the original relationship. The hypothesis that peer behavior directly influences students' smoking practices is not rejected. The investigator will need to explore other possible explanations for this result if he or she is interested in pursuing that question.

Not every study is necessarily guided by formal causal hypotheses between study variables. However, even descriptive studies examine the relationships of certain attributes of the study population (such as their age, sex, and race) to others (such as whether or not they saw a physician within the year). The researcher should consider what these variables will be so that questions that should be asked are not omitted and questions that will never be used are not included.

Setting Up Mock Tables for the Analysis

The first step in carrying out the analysis of any data set, regardless of the type of study design, is to analyze the sample itself according to the major study variables of interest. In Mock Table a in Exhibit 4.1, the number (frequencies) and percentage of people in each category of the major analysis variables can be displayed. One can then see what percentage (and how many) of the sample were smokers; what percentage (and how many) had parents or friends who smoked; and finally, what percentage (and how many) thought smoking was socially acceptable. Univariate summary statistics for describing the distribution of the sample on the variables (such as a mean, median, and standard deviation) are reviewed in Chapter Fifteen. If certain subgroup breakdowns (by race, for example) are important for carrying out the analysis plan for the study, then special efforts may be required in the design of the sampling plan for the study (described in Chapter Seven) to obtain a sufficient number of individuals in the respective subgroups (white, African American, and Hispanic).

Mock Table b in the exhibit allows the researcher to look at a hypothesized relationship between the dependent and independent variables, paralleling the approach to hypothesis testing outlined earlier. In cross-tabular analyses of the kind outlined here and in Figures 4.1 through 4.5 for cross-sectional analytic designs, the percentages should be computed within categories of the independent variable ("friends' smoking status"), that is, each column in table b should sum to 100 percent. The percentages within the table would reflect the percent of students who were smokers among those who had no friends who smoked versus those for whom either some or all of their friends smoked to address the question

FIGURE 4.5. ELABORATING THE MAIN STUDY HYPOTHESIS—REPLICATION.

Theoretical Model and Sample Tables—Replication

Theoretical Model

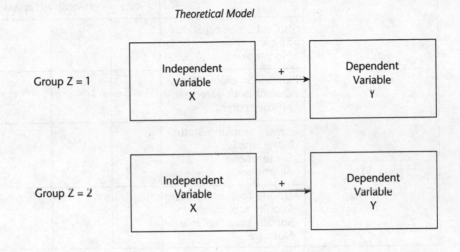

Group Z = 1

| Independent Variable X | + | Dependent Variable Y |

Group Z = 2

| Independent Variable X | + | Dependent Variable Y |

Sample Tables

	Table a Z = 1			Table b Z = 2	
Student Smoking Status (Y)	Friends' Smoking Status (X)		Student Smoking Status (Y)	Friends' Smoking Status (X)	
	Some or All	None		Some or All	None
Smoker	75% (49)	31% (20)	Smoker	74% (26)	29% (10)
Nonsmoker	25% (16)	69% (45)	Nonsmoker	26% (9)	71% (25)
Total	100% (65)	100% (65)	**Total**	100% (35)	100% (35)

$OR = \dfrac{49 \times 45}{20 \times 16} = \dfrac{2205}{320} = 6.9$ chi-square = 26.0 p = .000

$OR = \dfrac{26 \times 25}{10 \times 9} = \dfrac{650}{90} = 7.2$ chi-square = 14.6 p = .000

EXHIBIT 4.1. SETTING UP MOCK TABLES FOR THE ANALYSIS.

Purpose of Analysis	Examples of Mock Tables
To describe the sample	Table a. Characteristics of High School Students.

Table a. Characteristics of High School Students.

Characteristics	Percent (Frequencies)			
	White	African American	Hispanic	Total

Student Smoking Status
  Smoker
  Nonsmoker				

Parents' Smoking Status
  One or both parents
  Neither parent				

Friends' Smoking Status
  None smoke
  Some smoke
  All smoke				

Attitude Toward Smoking
  Socially acceptable
  Socially unacceptable
  Not sure				

To test for relationship between variables (test a hypothesis)	Table b. Student Smoking Status by Friends' Smoking Status.

Table b. Student Smoking Status by Friends' Smoking Status.

Student Smoking Status	Friends' Smoking Status	
	Some or All	None
Smoker Nonsmoker		
Total	100%	100%

To explain relationships between variables (elaborate a hypothesis)	Table c. Student Smoking Status by Friends' and Parents' Smoking Status.

Table c. Student Smoking Status by Friends' and Parents' Smoking Status.

	Parents' Smoking Status			
	One or both parents		Neither parent	
Student Smoking Status	Friends' Smoking Status			
	Some or All	None	Some or All	None
Smoker Nonsmoker				
Total	100%	100%	100%	100%

of whether friends were likely to influence the students to smoke. In contrast, in case-control designs the percentages would be computed within categories of the outcome variable ("student smoking status"), that is, each row in table b would sum to 100 percent. In that case, the data would reflect the percent of students whose friends smoked among students who were smokers ("cases") versus those who were not ("controls") to address the question of whether smokers were more likely to have been exposed to friends who smoke.

It is not imperative that categories be combined or collapsed (as is done here for those for whom *some or all* of their friends smoke). The decision to do so should be based on both substantive and methodological considerations. Are the groups enough alike to warrant combining? Is the number of cases for one of the categories too small to be analyzed separately?

In Exhibit 4.1, Mock Table c shows how a third (control) variable could be introduced into the analysis to see if the relationship observed between friends' smoking status and student smoking status is a function of parents' smoking practices. In this particular example, the relationship examined in Mock Table b is examined separately for whether one or both versus neither parent smokes. This is analogous to the process of examining the relationship between X and Y for different categories of Z displayed in Figures 4.2 through 4.5. More than three variables can be considered in the analysis but some multivariate statistical procedures are better able to handle analyses of a large number of variables than are others. (Specific types of univariate, bivariate, and multivariate analysis procedures are discussed in Chapter Fifteen.)

The number of tables used to report the study findings should be kept to a minimum and each should be clearly related to the study objectives. Chapter Fifteen provides additional guidelines on how to construct mock tables to address different types of study objectives and Chapter Sixteen offers suggestions regarding how to most clearly format and display data tables in the final report of the study.

Special Considerations for Special Populations

Issues that come into play in pursuing the types of analyses outlined in this chapter with special populations revolve around choosing subgroup breakdowns on interest (minorities versus whites *or* whites, African Americans, Hispanics, Asian Americans, Native Americans, or others) and designing the sample to permit a sufficient number of cases of each type to analyze these subgroups separately. Selected demographics (such as age, gender, and race or ethnicity) are frequently used as control variables in sociological and epidemiological analyses due to their assumed social or biologic relevance. These variables are most often cast either in the role of confounder (extraneous) variables, since they affect rather than are affected by other factors *or* in the role of variables for which interaction effects are expected, that is, when the nature or magnitude of the hypothesized relationship between an independent (or predictor) and dependent (outcome) variable is assumed to be different for different groups (for example, males versus females, young adults versus the elderly, or African American versus Hispanic).

Selected Examples

A rich array of hypotheses may be tested and elaborated with the data from the three case studies in Resources A, B, and C. Theoretical models and previous epidemiological and behavioral surveys informed the selection and formulation of questions to include in those studies and, ultimately, the analyses of the resulting data (Grembowski, Milgrom, & Fiset, 1988; Prohaska, Albrecht, Levy, Sugrue, & Kim, 1990; Thornberry, Wilson, & Golden, 1986). Examples of analyses conducted using these data sets are discussed in Chapter Fifteen.

Guidelines for Minimizing Survey Errors

To pick up a clear signal, background noise must be subdued. The same principle applies in ruling out sources of variation other than the main ones that are expected to give rise to a hypothesized outcome. Four main approaches can be undertaken to control for these other factors. Two of them can be implemented in the initial design of the study (randomization or matching of cases and controls, for example); and the other two during analyses of the data (stratified or multivariate analysis). The design-based alternatives were discussed in Chapter Two. This chapter presented the logic of stratifying (or conducting the analyses separately for different subgroups or categories of variables) as a basis for clarifying whether these variables are a source of noise. The use of multivariate analyses will be more fully discussed in Chapter Fifteen.

This chapter introduced the logic and techniques to use in thinking through a plan for collecting and analyzing the survey data. The reader should return to this chapter after giving more thought to the precise questions that will be included in a survey questionnaire. After the data are collected, the reader can use this chapter to review the steps that might be undertaken to analyze them.

Supplementary Sources

For the classic approach to stratified analysis from a sociological perspective, see Hirschi and Selvin (1967), Lazarsfeld, Pasanella, and Rosenberg (1972), Rosenberg (1968), Zeisel (1968), and from an epidemiologic perspective, consult Hennekens and Buring (1987) and Kleinbaum, Kupper, and Morgenstern (1982).

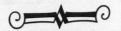

CHAPTER FIVE

CHOOSING THE METHODS
OF DATA COLLECTION

Chapter Highlights

1. Nonresponse and noncoverage are bigger problems in telephone surveys than in personal interview surveys; however, telephone surveys produce data of comparable quality at lower cost.
2. Mail questionnaires cost less than either personal or telephone interview surveys and may offer advantages when asking about sensitive or threatening topics, but nonresponse and constraints on the design of the questionnaire itself are significant problems.
3. Computer-assisted telephone interviews (CATI), computer-assisted personal interviews (CAPI), and computer-assisted self-interviews (CASI) are increasingly being used to collect health survey data.

This chapter provides an overview of the different methods for gathering data in health surveys and the relative advantages and disadvantages of each. The choice of data gathering method will have significant impacts on decisions made at every subsequent stage of a study—designing the sample, formulating the questions, formatting the questionnaire, carrying out the survey, and preparing the data for analysis.

The principal methods for gathering data in surveys are *personal interviews, telephone interviews,* and *self-administered questionnaires* (either by mail or in office, classroom, or other group-administered settings). Sometimes these methods are combined to capitalize on the advantages of each. Since the 1970s, there has been a burgeoning interest in computer-assisted or computerized methods of data gathering (Saris, 1991).

In the discussion that follows, the advantages and disadvantages of the traditional paper-and-pencil approaches to personal interviews, telephone interviews, and self-administered questionnaires will be compared to provide guidance in selecting the approach that might best fit the researcher's objectives and pocketbook. The comparative advantages hypothesized for the computerized alternatives to each of these modes over the paper-and-pencil approach will also be discussed. Finally, the chapter will offer examples of how the respective data gathering methods may be combined in a single study to enhance the unique advantages of each and to reduce the overall costs of the survey.

Criteria for Choosing the Data Collection Method

Three general questions that researchers should ask themselves when deciding upon the approach to use in gathering their data are, Which method is most appropriate, given the study question and population of interest? Which method is most readily available? And, how much money has been budgeted for carrying out the study?

The particular study question or population may suggest that a certain method of data collection must be used or is, at least, highly appropriate. For example, if the investigator is interested in finding out about the health care practices in a low-income Hispanic community, the majority of whose members do not speak or read English or have telephones, then an in-person interview in Spanish may be the only way to do the study. If a company's management is interested in enhancing the candor and confidentiality of responses to a survey that asks employees about health risks resulting from their own behaviors (such as excessive smoking or drinking) or perceived hazards in the workplace, then a mail questionnaire would be more appropriate than personal or telephone interviews. If a drug company wants to get a quick reading on the probable consumer response to alternative nationwide marketing strategies that it is considering for a new sinus headache remedy, then telephone interviews would be the best way to reach the right people in a timely and cost-effective way.

In some instances, certain modes of data gathering may simply not be available to researchers within their institutions or areas or may not be feasible within the proposed scope of their project. For example, projects carried out in large measure by a single student or researcher may necessitate the use of mail or other self-administered questionnaires simply because there is no staff available to carry out personal or telephone interviews with prospective respondents. Again, computerized data collection strategies may seem preferable for a given study, but the firm or organization charged with doing the survey may not have that capability. Very often, the most fundamental determinant of what method is chosen is how much money is available to do the study and what the respective methods of gathering data will cost. As will be seen in this chapter's discussion, there are major disparities between the costs of the different data gathering methods.

The purpose of the study, the availability of a particular method, and its price tag are the overarching questions to have in mind when choosing among the methods.

Computerized Data Collection Methods

Before discussing the relative advantages of personal, telephone, and self-administered forms of data gathering in particular, a description of the computerized versions of each of these methods will be presented.

Computer-assisted telephone interviewing (CATI) was the first widely applied computerized data gathering technology. In the CATI system, the questionnaire is programmed and displayed on a terminal or microcomputer screen. The interviewers call respondents, ask the questions displayed on the screen, and then enter their answers into the computer via the computer keyboard. The earliest CATI systems were developed in the 1970s by Chilton Research Services of Radnor, Pennsylvania, to carry out large-scale market research surveys rapidly and cost-effectively for AT&T and other commercial clients, and by the University of California, Los Angeles, to conduct academic, social science-oriented surveys (Fink, 1983; Shanks, 1983). These prototype systems have been refined and expanded through the years, and many firms and organizations have developed software and associated hardware technologies for carrying out computer-assisted telephone interviews (Bethlehem & Keller, 1991; Freeman, 1983; Freeman & Shanks, 1983; Hofman & Keller, 1991; Palit & Sharp, 1983; Rhoads, et al., 1994; Saris, 1991).

The CATI technology accommodates a broad range of functions in the conduct of telephone surveys. These include selection of the sample by means of a random digit dialing (RDD) approach; the assignment, scheduling, and monitoring of interviews; building in specific probes or help menus that the interviewer can access during the interview; programming the logical sequence for a series of questions; and entering the allowable range of codes for certain items so that the interviewer can correct mistakes during the interview. Interviewers in centralized CATI systems can be linked (or networked) through a host computer that controls and monitors this array of functions. There has been considerable interest in the CATI methodology on the part of the U.S. Bureau of the Census, the U.S. Department of Agriculture, and the National Center for Health Statistics (NCHS) (Gardenier, 1991, 1993; Kindel, 1991; Nicholls, 1983; Pierzchala, 1991; Tortora, 1985), as well as by a number of commercial and academic survey research organizations that carry out national, state, and local health or health-related surveys (Spaeth, 1987, 1990).

Computer-assisted personal interviewing (CAPI) is essentially an adaptation of computer-assisted telephone interview technologies. The CAPI interview is programmed into a portable computer that the interviewer can carry to the respondent's home or other location to conduct the interview. CAPI technology has evolved with the development of smaller and smaller portable computers with sufficient storage to accommodate the complex program for the questionnaire, the data gathered from respondents, and the software needed to run the program.

Notebook and hand-held computers have been used in CAPI studies conducted by the Census Bureau, the National Center for Health Statistics, the U.S. Department of Agriculture, and a variety of other federal, academic, and for-profit survey organizations (Gardenier, 1991, 1993; Kindel, 1991; National Center for Health Statistics and U.S. Bureau of the Census, 1988; Pierzchala, 1991).

The promises and approaches to *computer-assisted self-interviewing* (CASI) have blossomed with the advent of new and innovative information exchange technologies (Appel & Nicholls, 1993; Perron, Berthelot, & Blakeney, 1991; Saris, 1989). Video-CASI and audio-CASI make use of the video and audio capabilities of small portable computers to present the questions on the computer screen (monitor) or via headphones connected to the computer to respondents, who then enter their answers on the computer keyboard or pad. This and related approaches offer particular promise for interviewing special populations (adolescents) about sensitive issues (such as drug or alcohol use or sexual practices) (Camburn & Cynamon, 1993; O'Reilly, Hubbard, Lessler, Biemer, & Turner, 1994).

Other CASI technologies that have been tested or used by the Census Bureau, Bureau of Labor Statistics, the National Center for Health Statistics, and academic and for-profit survey research firms include Touchtone Data Entry (TDE) to answer questions using the numeric keypad of a touchtone phone (Phipps & Tupek, 1991; Rosen, Clayton, & Wolf, 1993); Voice Recognition Entry (VRE), which entails a digitized voice functioning as an interviewer to read the questions, recognize the respondent's vocalizations, and echo them back for confirmation (Blyth & Piper, 1994; Winter & Clayton, 1990); FAX machines or the FAX capabilities of personal computers to transmit survey questions and return responses, and the accompanying processing of the information through computerized optical imaging or optical character recognition (OCR) that translates the text into computer readable form (Rosen & Clayton, 1992; Rowe & Appel,

1993; Walker, 1994); and computer interviewing by mail (CIM), in which a disk with the file containing the questionnaire is sent to respondents, who then insert it into their computer, enter their answers, and mail back the disk when done (Jacobs, Cross, & Smailes, 1994; Saltzman, 1992; Witt & Bernstein, 1992). Computerized networks available through electronic mail (E-mail), the Internet, and related electronic highways offer promising channels, as well as new challenges, for the conduct of computer-assisted self-administered questionnaires and interviews. These methods may greatly facilitate and speed access to potential respondents but they also pose a number of problems to be solved with respect to clearly delineating the target population, calculating noncoverage and nonresponse biases, and protecting the confidentiality of electronically transmitted responses.

The TDE, VRE, FAX, and CIM approaches have principally been used in surveys of businesses or establishments (as in the Bureau of Labor Statistics Current Employment Statistics Survey). The use of computerized self-administered questionnaires generally assumes that respondents have access to a computer in an office, classroom, or other group or institutional setting. This approach has been applied in clinical settings for taking medical histories and administering batteries of psychological tests to patients or study subjects and in behavioral modification programs to provide feedback to get people to stop smoking (Adang, Vismans, Ambergen, Talmon, Hasman, & Flendrig, 1991; Joyce, 1988), in electronic mail surveys of employees or students who have access to computers (Kiesler & Sproull, 1986; Letterie, Morgenstern, & Johnson, 1994), or with panels of individuals enrolled for a particular purpose (as in a Dutch survey of a random sample of households selected for a series of public opinion polls that are provided with a home computer and modem to respond) (Saris, 1991).

CASI will be used more and more as computers become commonplace in homes and work environments. Computer-assisted self-interviewing is a promising youngster that is likely to greatly expand the scope and possibilities of the older generations of data gathering approaches.

Comparison of Personal Interviews, Telephone Interviews, and Self-Administered Questionnaires

Table 5.1 provides a comparison of the advantages and disadvantages of personal interviews, telephone interviews, and self-administered questionnaires at each stage in carrying out a survey. The comparison is based on a synthesis of critiques provided by other survey research methodologists (Dillman, 1978, 1991; Fowler, 1993; Groves, 1990b; Groves & Kahn, 1979; Groves, et al., 1988; Miller, 1991; Salant & Dillman, 1994) as well as on current research on health surveys in particular.

TABLE 5.1. COMPARISON OF PERSONAL INTERVIEWS, TELEPHONE INTERVIEWS, AND SELF-ADMINISTERED QUESTIONNAIRES.

Steps in Conducting Survey	Personal Interviews		Telephone Interviews		Self-Administered Questionnaires	
	Advantage	Disadvantage	Advantage	Disadvantage	Advantage	Disadvantage
Drawing the Sample						
Coverage of population	X			X		X(X)
Response rates						
Calculation	X			X		X
Level (high/low)	X			X		XX
Noncoverage and nonresponse bias	X			X		XX
Accuracy in selecting respondent	X(X)		X		X	
Design effects		X	X			
Formulating the Questions						
General format						
Complex questions	X(X)		(X)	X		XX
Open-ended questions	X			X		XX
Use of visual aids	X			X	X	
Types of questions						
Nonthreatening	X		X		X	
Threatening		X	X		XX(X)	
Formatting the Questionnaire						
Longer length	XX					XX
Control of sequence of response to questions	X(X)		X(X)	X	(X)	XX
Carrying Out the Survey						
Supervision of interviewers	(X)	X	X(X)		−	−
Length of data collection period	(X)	X	X(X)			X
Preparing the Data for Analysis						
Need for editing/cleaning	X(X)		X(X)		(X)	X
Need for imputation of missing values	X		X			X
Speed of turnaround	(X)	XX	X(X)			X
Costs		X	X		XX	

Note: Xs indicate whether it is an advantage or disadvantage to use traditional paper-and-pencil methods and (X)s (with parentheses) whether it is an advantage or disadvantage to use computerized methods. The more Xs, the stronger the advantages or disadvantages. See the text of this chapter regarding the basis for the ratings assigned here. The evaluation of different aspects of drawing the sample is based on the assumption of the following types of designs: personal interviews—area probability sample; telephone interviews—random digit dialing; self-administered questionnaires—list sample mailed survey. These assessments would be different for different designs.

The Xs in the table indicate whether a particular method tends to offer advantages or disadvantages in carrying out selected aspects of the survey. More than one X in these columns indicates that it is a strong advantage (or disadvantage). These Xs reflect comparisons of traditional paper-and-pencil versions of gathering data—in person, by phone, or through self-administered questionnaires (by mail, in particular). In addition, (X)s are used to indicate whether there is an advantage or disadvantage to doing the study hypothesized by means of computer-assisted approaches to gathering data with the respective methods.

Drawing the Sample

Coverage of the Population. A central issue in designing a sample for a survey is making sure that everyone the researcher is interested in studying has a chance of being included in the survey. In sampling terminology, this refers to the extent to which the sample design ensures coverage of the population of interest.

Methods for sampling households in communities and then selecting an individual or individuals within those selected households (area probability sampling) have been used most often in identifying respondents for personal interviews. This sampling methodology generally requires that a field staff go out and list the addresses of all the eligible housing units (businesses or institutions would, for example, be excluded). The units in which the study will be conducted are then systematically selected from all the lists compiled by the field staff using methodologies designed by the study's sampling consultant. With this in-person approach to identifying eligible houses and then contacting them for the interview, the coverage of the study population is generally less of a problem than is the case with the other two methods of data collection. The National Health Interview Survey, as well as many other national health and health care surveys, have used these traditional in-person approaches to sample selection and subsequent data collection. Moreover, in-person field and sampling methods are essential for locating certain hard-to-reach populations that have become of increasing interest in health surveys, such as American Indians and the homeless or drug-using populations that congregate in certain blocks or neighborhoods of a city (Burnam & Koegel, 1988; National Center for Health Services Research, 1987).

With the telephone interview approach, however, certain people will be left out of the study simply because the sample includes only people with telephones. Trewin and Lee (1988) documented the percentage of people with telephones for a number of different countries throughout the world. Estimates varied considerably from almost universal coverage in some countries—97 percent in Canada and 95 percent in Sweden, for example—to 16 percent (less than one in five people) in countries such as Hungary and Mexico. Trewin and Lee also pointed out that coverage varied greatly within countries by region and population sub-group. Younger people, single or divorced people, renters rather than homeowners, the unemployed and blue-collar workers rather than professional workers, low-income households, rural households, and minorities were much less likely to have phones in many countries.

Thornberry and Massey (1988) obtained comparable findings in the United States based on data from the National Health Interview Survey on trends in telephone coverage across time and between subgroups. Using 1985 and 1986 NCHS data, they estimated that approximately 93 percent of U.S. households had phones, a figure that represented a substantial increase in coverage (about 13.0 percent) since 1963. The noncoverage for U.S. households as a whole was estimated to be 7.2 percent. However, the noncoverage rate was higher for people who lived in the South (10.4 percent); in rural areas outside Standard Metropolitan Statistical Areas (SMSAs) (11.0 percent); in one-person households (9.9 percent) or in households with seven or more people (16.3 percent) and for people who were African American (15.6 percent) or some race other than white (10.9 percent); never married (8.1 percent), divorced (9.8 percent), or separated (18.8 percent); unemployed (16.0 percent); or had less than a high school education (around 13 percent). There was also evidence that people in nontelephone households were more likely to have more days when they had to restrict their activities or go to bed because of illness or to have chronic conditions that limited their major activity. Face-to-face interviews with a subsample of people without phones in a Robert Wood Johnson Foundation (1987) national access survey showed that they were also twice as likely not to have any medical insurance coverage as those with phones.

As we will see later (Chapter Seven), there are methods for statistically adjusting for this noncoverage of certain groups to make the telephone survey sample more representative. It is well to remember, however, that such adjustments cannot eliminate all possible biases that may result because of the underrepresentation of these groups in the sample.

Self-administered surveys are generally carried out with individuals who have been identified from lists of relevant candidates for the study, such as members of professional health care organizations, hospital employees, health plan enrollees, and so on. Lists may be the best or, in some instances, the only way to identify these individuals. Coverage problems with such lists may result because they are not kept current, so that new people who would be eligible for the study are not included. In addition, other people's names may be left out or lost because of poor record keeping, some names may be duplicated on the list, and some that seem like duplicates may, in fact, not be. Researchers should be aware of these issues in evaluating a list of individuals to whom questionnaires will be mailed for a study.

In fact, before actually launching the study, researchers may want to include a subset of the list in a pilot or pretest of study procedures to see what problems will be encountered. With respect to computerized self-administered questionnaires—because not everyone has access to computers and many people have a strong case of computer anxiety—the timely and broad application of this method may be limited to surveys of establishments or selected groups of individuals (professionals, patients, or students, for example).

Response Rates. Response rates refer to the proportion of people or organizations selected and deemed eligible for the study that actually completes the questionnaires (see discussion of response rates in Chapter Seven). The three modes of data collection differ in their methods of calculating and interpreting these rates.

There may be problems in calculating the response rates for personal interview surveys if it is difficult to determine whether a household or individual is eligible for the study because of refusal or unavailability to complete a screening questionnaire to determine eligibility. These problems are, however, not unique to in-person interview methods.

The computation of response rates for random digit dialing telephone interviews is particularly troublesome because there may be a large number of phone calls that are never completed because the line is busy, no one ever answers the phone, or a recorded message is always on the line when the number is dialed. The wider use of answering machines, beepers, and car phones further complicates the determination of eligibility for telephone surveys. If budget constraints limit the number of callbacks, it will not be possible to determine whether these numbers are eligible ones—working residential phone numbers, for example, rather than businesses or nonworking numbers. These issues complicate the computation of response rates for telephone interviews compared with personal interviews.

Analogous problems exist in computing the response rates for self-administered mail questionnaires. The questionnaire may not be filled out and returned because the intended respondent refused to answer the questionnaire or because he or she was deceased or had moved and left no forwarding address. The latter could be legitimately excluded as being ineligible for the study if their status were known.

The response rates for personal interviews tend to be the highest, followed by telephone and then self-administered (particularly mail) questionnaires. This means that of those determined or estimated to be eligible for a survey, more tend to respond to the in-person approach. This higher response is attributed to a number of factors—the greater persuasiveness of personal contacts in eliciting cooperation, the smaller probability of breaking off the interview in person compared with over the phone, the interviewer's ability to follow up with the respondent in person, and so on (Groves, 1989; National Center for Health Statistics, 1987a).

The response rates in federally sponsored national health surveys conducted using the personal interview approach have ranged from 85 to over 95 percent. Telephone interviews have response rates that are 70 to 85 percent on average, and mail questionnaires have rates in the 60 percent to 70 percent range or lower (Marcus & Crane, 1986). Response rates tend to be lower in "cold contact" surveys, in which respondents have no prior knowledge that they will be contacted for a study, than in "warm contact" surveys, where respondents are sent a letter, called, or contacted in person before being approached for the actual interview.

Cannell and his colleagues at the University of Michigan conducted an experimental comparison of telephone and traditional in-person methods of administering the National Health Interview Survey. They found that the response rate for the telephone survey conducted by the Survey Research Center at the University of Michigan was 80 percent compared with a rate of 96 percent when the survey was conducted in person by U.S. census interviewers (National Center for Health Statistics, 1987a).

There is also the problem, as with the sample coverage issue discussed earlier, that response rates to surveys using the various approaches may also differ for different population subgroups. For example, evidence suggests that young people, the elderly, the poor and poorly educated, the uninsured, and individuals who have certain disabilities (such as hearing loss) or who tire easily may be less apt to participate in telephone surveys. This may have substantial implications for the representativeness and accuracy of estimates derived from telephone-based health surveys of these groups (Corey & Freeman, 1990; Freeman, Kiecolt, Nicholls, & Shanks, 1982; Herzog & Rodgers, 1988; Kristal, et al., 1993; Marcus & Telesky, 1984; Mishra, Dooley, Catalano, & Serxner, 1993; National Center for Health Statistics, 1987a; Smith, 1990). Further, individuals who have problems with reading in general or with reading and interpreting self-administered questionnaires in languages other than their native tongue may be less likely to respond to mail questionnaires. The people most likely to respond to these types of questionnaires are often educated professionals with a substantial interest in the subject matter of the study.

There is, however, some indication that personal interview response rates have declined in recent years because people have become fearful of admitting strangers into their homes, fewer women are at home during the day to participate in such studies, and more high-security buildings preclude ready admittance. The response rates for major national health surveys such as the National Health Interview Survey have remained high, but the costs per interview have continued to rise because of the numbers of return visits necessary to find people at home or to gain access to high security buildings.

Telephone and mail questionnaires are thought to offer some advantages in contacting hard-to-reach respondents. For example, Goyder (1985) has argued that the "mailed questionnaire . . . and electronic variants such as the telephone survey and direct video interaction are perhaps the optimal methods for surveying postindustrial society; these methods are tailor made for reaching a socially disintegrated citizenry, ensconced in high-rise urban fortresses in which face-to-face contact has been delegitimated, yet still susceptible to the behavioral psychology of a carefully orchestrated series of impersonal contacts and follow-ups by survey researchers" (p. 248).

Nonetheless, answering machines and caller-identification features available to phone customers offer formidable barriers to reaching respondents on the phone. To the extent that households increasingly use these devices to screen calls, lower response rates are likely to result for telephone surveys as well. This consequence may be mitigated to some extent by sending advance letters to potential respondents when addresses are available or can be obtained or by making use of the local news media to publicize and lend legitimacy to the study (Oldendick, 1993; Oldendick & Link, 1994; Tuckel & Feinberg, 1991).

The implications of the differential response rates and coverage of different groups for the accuracy and representativeness of estimates are discussed in the following section.

Noncoverage and Nonresponse Bias.

Noncoverage or nonresponse of certain groups means that estimates for the survey as a whole or for those groups in particular may not be accurate because of these groups' underrepresentation in the study. As noted earlier, comparisons of estimates on selected health status variables between the population with phones and those without indicate that those who do not have telephones are as a group in poorer health and may, in some instances, be less apt to be insured or use health care services at as high a rate as those with phones. If there is a substantial underrepresentation of people without phones or with health and health care characteristics that differ significantly from others in the population, then the characteristics for the population as a whole and for these subgroups in particular may be biased. Many nonphone households are temporarily (or episodically) so because they have not paid the phone bill, for example. The number of households continuously without phone service is generally much smaller in most communities (Keeter, 1995).

For national health surveys of the general population with relatively high coverage and response rates, the estimates for those who have phones do not differ significantly from estimates for the U.S. population as a whole, including those with and without phones. Further, the direction of differences between subgroups does not appear to vary for those with phones and the population as a whole, because most people have phones and most people agreed to participate in these studies. However, if there is an interest in studying certain subgroups, such as the elderly or low-income Spanish-speaking residents along the Texas and Mexico border, the lower telephone coverage or response rates for these groups might combine to introduce substantial biases (inaccuracies) into the data for those that could be reached by phone (Adams-Esquivel & Lang, 1987; Corey & Freeman, 1990; Marcus & Crane, 1986). To the extent that coverage and nonresponse might also be issues for mail questionnaires in general or for selected subgroups, comparable biases could occur (Krysan, Schuman, Scott, & Beatty, 1994). Knowing whom you want to include in your study and whom you cannot afford to leave out, as well as their probable rates of coverage and response to different data collection methods, will provide guidance for choosing the survey method that will provide the most accurate and complete data for those groups.

Accuracy in Selecting Respondent. As will be discussed in Chapter Six, which describes different approaches to drawing samples for a health survey, an interviewer can use several approaches to select one or more respondents from a family for the actual interview. With computer-assisted personal and telephone interviews, the accuracy of the interviewer's selection is enhanced. Computerized algorithms can be designed to reduce the mechanical or clerical errors made by interviewers during this process.

Both the personal and telephone interview approaches offer advantages over mail questionnaires in getting the right person. The researcher has no control over who actually fills out a questionnaire once it is mailed. An individual respondent might ask his or her spouse to fill it out and return it; a doctor or health professional may hand it to a secretary or administrative assistant to complete.

Design Effects. The design effects for a survey, discussed in more detail in Chapter Seven, mean principally that the more the survey departs from a simple random sample design (analogous to drawing numbers from a hat) the larger the sampling (standard) errors are likely to be. The sample designs used for identifying sample households geographically to conduct personal interviews (area probability samples) are often complex and involve a number of stages of selection and several clusters of sampling units—at the county, U.S. census tract, and block and household levels. The design effects for these studies are thus often quite high.

The random digit dialing approach used in many telephone surveys, in which a list of all possible numbers for a given area code and prefix (or exchange) is generated and called, has a very low design effect. Approaches to increasing the proportion of eligible (working, residential) numbers by screening groups of numbers generated in this fashion do increase the design effect of the telephone survey. However, the design effects for most telephone surveys are much lower than those for area probability personal interview-based surveys (Groves, 1989; Marcus &

Crane, 1986). Sampling from lists of potential respondents for self-administered surveys is also relatively straightforward and, for the most part, has low design effects. In general, lower design effects are better, and the sample designs for telephone and self-administered surveys usually offer advantages over personal interview survey designs in this aspect of designing and conducting health surveys.

Formulating the Questions

Questions that involve complex concepts or complicated phrasing or response formats have generally been thought easier to handle in a face-to-face interview with the respondent. The assumptions are that interviewers can make more use of visual cues to determine if the respondent has understood the question and that the respondent feels freer to ask questions to clarify their responses than over the phone. With the advent of computer-assisted interviewing, however, complex questions can be more easily designed and handled over the telephone—and in CAPI interviews as well—because relevant probes, help menus, and complex skip patterns that depend on the respondents' answers to certain questions can be programmed into the questionnaire that the interviewer reads from the computer display screen. However, the development and testing of such questions may require a considerable investment of computer and programming time and resources.

Problems arise when questionnaires filled out by respondents without an interviewer to assist them contain complex questions. Respondents may not understand certain concepts or instructions unaided or they may simply consider the task too difficult and decide not to fill out the questionnaire at all.

One type of question that has been used quite often in surveys is the open-ended question. Here, respondents are asked to provide answers in their own words rather than choose a response from a number of categories provided in the interview or questionnaire. Personal interviews are thought to provide the best opportunity to use these types of questions because both respondents and interviewers feel freer to spend the time to provide and record these answers than they would over the phone. There is evidence that telephone interviews are shorter on average and that the amount of information recorded for open-ended questions is less than in the case of in-person interviews. It is not clear, however, that the accuracy or validity of the answers to open-ended questions is necessarily lessened over the phone simply because people tend to give shorter answers (Bradburn, 1983; Groves, 1989; Groves & Kahn, 1979).

As with complex questions, it is not advantageous to use open-ended questions and response formats on self-administered questionnaires because of respondents' possible unwillingness to take the time to answer them or because of their limited writing skills.

A limitation of telephone interviews compared with personal interviews is that with the latter the interviewer can make use of visual aids (such as cards with response categories listed, containers to show the amount of some food product or beverage the respondent is asked to report the frequency of consuming, and so on). Conceivably such devices could be used in a self-administered questionnaire if their application in the study were made clear to the respondent. Video-CASI and audio-CASI offer the possibility of displaying relevant images and sounds to respondents, which may be of particular utility for people who are illiterate, have low reading levels, or do not speak English. Videotapes are another device that can be used in administering a questionnaire or other stimulus to which study subjects are asked to respond by means of a computerized data entry or a paper-and-pencil format (Albrecht, 1985).

Somewhat different devices may be needed to facilitate complete and accurate responses to threatening or sensitive questions (such as those relating to sexual practices, drinking behavior, or drug use) compared with less threatening items (such as how often the respondent eats breakfast or went to the doctor in the previous year). One of the principal concerns with the advent of the telephone interview was whether equally accurate answers to the range of (threatening and nonthreatening) questions could be obtained with this approach compared with personal interviews.

The early empirical research on the comparability of results obtained from the two methods produced mixed results (Colombotos, 1969; Groves & Kahn, 1979; Hochstim, 1967; Jordan, Marcus, & Reeder, 1980; Klecka & Tuchfarber, 1978; National Center for Health Services Research, 1977b; Rogers, 1976; Siemiatycki, 1979; Singer, 1981). In the major experiment conducted at the University of Michigan that compared the findings from a telephone survey adaptation of the National Health Interview Survey with those from the traditional in-person interview for that study, there were few or no differences in the estimates of health events (disability days, physician visits, and so on) between the two modes. Where differences did exist, they were in the direction of higher rates of reporting of these events by the telephone respondents than by those interviewed in person. This is contrary to other research that suggests people tend to shorten their answers or underreport responses on the phone. The Michigan researchers concluded that reporting of health events may, in fact, be more complete over the phone than in person.

Studies comparing survey data with medical records have demonstrated that patients tend to *underreport* visits, so "more" probably means "better," although no criterion source was used in the Michigan study to evaluate whether telephone or in-person interviewing gave more accurate information. The investigators also point out that higher reporting on the phone may have been the result of the excellent training, experience, and high motivation of the telephone interviewers in the experiment (National Center for Health Statistics, 1987a).

In an experimental application of the National Health Interview Survey to a local area in Florida, researchers at the Research Triangle Institute similarly found that the reporting of health events using the telephone approach was either equivalent to or more accurate and complete than the data obtained in person (Kulka, Weeks, Lessler, & Whitmore, 1984; Weeks, Kulka, Lessler, & Whitmore, 1983).

Health surveys may deal with sensitive or threatening questions. Psychological research literature in general and on health surveys in particular suggests that threatening or sensitive behaviors or characteristics—for example, clinical depression (Aneshensel, Frerichs, Clark, & Yokopenic, 1982); drinking behavior (Mangione, Hingson, & Barrett, 1982); physical disability (Freeman, Kiecolt, Nicholls, & Shanks, 1982); or sexual practices leading to trophoblastic disease (Czaja, 1987–1988)—are reported with *equal or greater* frequency over the phone compared with personal interviews. It is assumed that the respondent enjoys greater anonymity over the phone and is, therefore, more likely to report socially undesirable behaviors and less likely to feel pressure to provide socially desirable responses.

Self-administered questionnaires are thought to offer the greatest anonymity to respondents, followed by telephone interviews (Aquilino, 1994; Fowler, Roman, & Di, 1993; McEwan, Harrington, Bhopal, Madhok, & McCallum, 1992; Schwarz, Strack, Hippler, & Bishop, 1991). A possible advantage of computerized self-administered questionnaires is that respondents may feel that the process is even more depersonalized and less threatening than a paper-and-pencil questionnaire and therefore be more willing to answer candidly (Kiesler & Sproull, 1986; O'Reilly, Hubbard, Lessler, Biemer, & Turner, 1994).

More experimental research needs to be conducted comparing the respective methods for asking both threatening and nonthreatening questions. However, the evidence to date suggests that personal, telephone, and self-administered approaches may produce comparable answers to nonthreatening questions but that the latter method in particular offers advantages over the first two in asking about sensitive or threatening health or health care practices.

Formatting the Questionnaire

Advantages to carrying out a long interview in person are that the interviewer is better able to prevent a respondent from breaking off the interview and to deal with interruptions, respondent fatigue, or lagging motivation as the interview proceeds. In contrast, self-administered questionnaires should, as a rule, be kept short and simple to maximize respondents' willingness to fill out and return them.

Initially it was believed that telephone interviews needed to be brief because of the difficulty of keeping people on the phone for extended periods of time. However, health survey researchers have been successful in achieving good response rates in studies involving complex telephone interviews of an hour or more (Fleming & Andersen, 1986). Presumably health studies have an advantage in this regard; respondents are thought to be more interested, in general, in talking about their health than in talking about the brands of tires they use on their cars or whether they favor the Federal Reserve's current monetary policy, for example.

Evidence of whether computer-assisted interviews tend to shorten or lengthen the interview process is mixed at present. Results probably vary as a function of the particular computerized system adopted (Saris, 1991).

Obviously, both the personal and the telephone interview permit more control over the sequence in which a respondent answers the questions in a survey than does the self-administered questionnaire. When respondents fill out a questionnaire by themselves, they can conceivably answer the questions in any order they choose. The computerized modes of data collection enhance the consistency of the sequence in which questions are asked and answered. If this sequence is programmed into the interview, then the line of questioning can go only in the direction that the program permits.

Carrying Out the Survey

A distinct advantage of centralized telephone interviews is that they allow closer supervision of interviewers' performance in conducting the interview than is possible when individual interviewers are dispersed throughout an area. With computer-assisted telephone interviews in particular, the supervisor can listen in on the interview and actually view the screen through a remote supervisory monitor as the interviewer enters the respondents' answers. This greatly facilitates the supervisor's providing additional interviewer training or instructions as needed, assisting the interviewers if they encounter problems with certain respondents, and reducing the variability across interviews that can be a function of different interviewers' approaches to asking questions (Couper & Groves, 1992a; Edwards, Bittner, Edwards, & Sperry, 1993; Groves & Mathiowetz, 1984; Miller, 1984).

Interviewer supervisors for large-scale field studies carried out by the major survey research firms are provided with computers for routinely reporting the status of their interviewers' progress in the field to their firm's headquarters. With the advent of CAPI systems, possibilities exist for fully recording or monitoring the personal interviews as well, to provide advantages similar to those found in centralized CATI systems.

The length of the data collection period must also be considered. Personal interview-based area probability studies require much longer periods for gathering data than do telephone interviews. Field interviewers may need to make several trips to a residence before they find someone at home. There is also a lag time in getting the completed interview logged and returned to the supervisor and ultimately to field or data-processing headquarters. With centralized telephone interviewing it is possible to follow up with nonresponders at many different times during the day or at night, and there should be minimal lag time in getting the interview processed once it is completed. Because self-administered questionnaires are generally mailed, the field period for such studies is longer, and it is dictated by the initial response to the survey as well as by the number and intervals of planned follow-up efforts.

Computer-assisted modes of data collection promise to shorten the length of the field period for telephone and personal interviews because the data gathered during the interview can be immediately stored in the computer. However, more front-end work is required to develop and test the questionnaire before it goes into the field. Whether time is saved with computerized self-administered questionnaires would depend on the particular data gathering system that is developed and the traditional mode of self-administration (mail or group) with which it is being compared (Nicholls & Kindel, 1993).

Preparing the Data for Analysis

Once the data are collected, the next step is to make sure that they are complete and that any obvious mistakes made during the data gathering phase are identified and corrected. The procedures for this next stage of processing are referred to as data "editing" or "cleaning" and will be discussed in more detail in Chapter Fourteen. Errors that may be identified include following the wrong sequence of questions so that the wrong questions are answered or that questions are left out or have values that are much too high (a thousand physician visits in the year) or low (a six-foot, six-inch adult male reported to weigh seventy-five pounds) either logically or relative to other information in the questionnaire.

Most errors of this kind occur in self-administered questionnaires on which the information may have been recorded in a haphazard or illegible fashion and there is no interviewer available to correct the respondent's mistakes. The quality of personal and telephone interviews is less likely to be affected by errors of this kind.

Computer-assisted modes of data collection are expected to expedite the data editing and cleaning process. Logical or other checks can be programmed in when the questionnaire is designed so that the interviewer or respondent is forced to correct inappropriate answers before proceeding.

Need for Imputation of Missing Values. Another problem arises when respondents refuse to answer certain questions or say they do not know the answer, or when a question is inadvertently left out by the interviewer or the respondent. Once again, this is most likely to be a problem with self-administered questionnaires. Methods for imputing (or estimating) values for the questions for which information is missing can be designed to provide a more complete data set for analysis (see Chapter Fourteen). These procedures, however, rely on certain assumptions about the appropriate basis for assigning values to cases for which the information is missing.

Research comparing the rates of missing values and other errors in computer-assisted methods of data gathering with traditional paper-and-pencil questionnaires generally document rates that are similar or lower for computerized methods of data collection (Couper & Burt, 1993; Dielman & Couper, 1995; Groves, 1983; Groves & Nicholls, 1986; Martin, O'Muircheartaigh, & Curtice, 1993).

Speed of Turnaround. Principally because of the length of the respective field periods and the lack of centralized administration, personal and mail self-administered surveys are also likely to move through the data-processing phase of the study more slowly than telephone surveys. Computerized data collection systems usually make the data coding, processing, and analysis steps simultaneous with the data collection phase of the study. Errors are identified and corrected while the data are being entered, and summary tallies are run on the data as batches of interviews are completed. This, of course, greatly reduces the data processing time required for the survey. However, much more time and effort are required at the beginning of the study to program and double-check all the features to be built into a computerized questionnaire and associated data gathering and data processing steps (House, 1985; Nicholls & Groves, 1986; Saris, 1991).

Costs

The price tag for a particular survey method may be the principal determinant of whether it can be feasibly employed. Personal interview approaches are, for example, more expensive than comparable telephone interview surveys. Depending on the design of the respective types of studies, the overall costs for telephone interviews may be half that of in-person interviews (Groves & Kahn, 1979; Kulka, Weeks, Lessler, & Whitmore, 1984).

The principal components accounting for the differences between the two approaches are the higher sampling and data collection costs for personal interview surveys. There are, after all, staff salaries and travel expenses to be paid when listing and contacting households selected for the study. No such costs are incurred when samples are drawn for either telephone or mail surveys, although funds are of course needed to generate or acquire the list of potentially eligible phone numbers or respondents and then to select those to be included in the final study.

Direct data collection costs are less for telephone surveys than for personal interview studies, but the developmental costs may be higher for some computer-assisted surveys. Mail surveys are the least costly method of gathering survey data.

In summary, as shown in Table 5.1, the telephone and personal interview methods have more advantages than the mail questionnaire approach. The main differences between personal and telephone interview methods are that noncoverage and nonresponse problems are greater in the latter. At the same time, however, costs are much lower and there may be fewer disadvantages in carrying out the survey and coding and processing the data with phone (especially CATI) interviews. Sample coverage and response rates, question and questionnaire design, and data coding and processing issues may be more problematical with mail questionnaires. But they offer a distinct advantage in terms of lower survey costs and they have value as a relatively anonymous method for asking sensitive or threatening questions about health and health care behaviors.

Many health surveys do, in fact, incorporate more than one of these methods—personal interviews, telephone interviews, and self-administered questionnaires—into their study designs to lower survey costs or to optimize the survey design advantages provided by a particular approach. Offering professionals and respondents for surveys of organizations or institutions (such as hospitals or businesses) a choice of response method is likely to increase the overall response rate to the study (Parsons, Warnecke, Czaja, Barnsley, & Kaluzny, 1994; Spaeth & O'Rourke, 1994). In a national telephone survey of access to medical care in the United States sponsored by the Robert Wood Johnson Foundation, personal interviews were conducted with a subsample of respondents who did not have phones to estimate the level of telephone noncoverage and nonresponse bias in the survey (Sudman & Freeman, 1987). In an evaluation of home care programs for ventilator-assisted children in three states, a self-administered questionnaire was sent to families before telephone interviews were attempted; respondents were thus able to fill out on their own more sensitive questions about their families and the stresses felt by the caregivers and had the time to pull relevant information on the child's hospitalizations from bills and other records before being contacted by phone (Aday, Aitken, & Wegener, 1988).

Researchers should consider not only the pros and cons of each method in deciding which approach to use but also how the methods might be meaningfully combined to minimize the costs or maximize the quality of their study.

Special Considerations for Special Populations

The who, what, where, and when questions posed at the outset of this volume take on renewed significance when researchers are choosing methods for gathering survey data. If the major topics to be addressed are sensitive and threatening ones (sexual or drug use practices), then more anonymous methods may be warranted in order to minimize the underreporting of these events. A survey of hard-to-reach or special populations (minority groups, prostitutes, intravenous drug users) would dictate consideration of the noncoverage or nonresponse biases that are likely to attend with different sampling and data collection designs. If timeliness is of particular concern (to inform institutional planning efforts, for example), then approaches (such as CATI) that permit the most rapid collection of high-quality data may be required (Aneshensel, Becerra, Fielder, & Schuler, 1989; Coffey, 1992; Dull, 1990; Marin, Vanoss, & Perez-Stable, 1990).

Selected Examples

Data for the National Center for Health Statistics–National Health Interview Survey was traditionally gathered in person through paper-and-pencil interviews (PAPI). Beginning in the 1990s, selected supplements were administered using computer-assisted personal interviews (CAPI). The 1996 redesign of the NHIS provided for the entire interview (core questionnaire as well as any special supplements) to be administered using CAPI. Substantial methodological research, as well as feasibility testing of these procedures, preceded this decision (Gardenier, 1991, 1993; Kovar, 1990; National Center for Health Statistics and U.S. Bureau of the Census, 1988).

The Chicago AIDS survey was one of the last paper-and-pencil interview telephone surveys conducted by the Survey Research Laboratory at the University of Illinois, which uses the CASES system developed at the University of California at Berkeley (Survey Research Laboratory, 1995). A particular strength of that study was the extensive time and effort spent in developing the approach to asking sensitive questions over the phone, which should undergird the development of these types of items, irrespective of the method (computerized or PAPI) used to gather the data.

The Washington State study of dentists' clinical decision making was based on a widely regarded and utilized approach to mail survey design developed by Don Dillman and his colleagues (discussed in more detail in Chapters Twelve and Thirteen) (Dillman, 1978; Salant & Dillman, 1994). The University of Washington investigators who designed that survey also successfully applied the Dillman methodology in a subsequent national survey of dental professionals, looking at issues of dental malpractice (Milgrom, et al., 1994; Milgrom, Whitney, Conrad, Fiset, & O'Hara, 1995). Mail questionnaires remain a viable and affordable option, especially for targeted populations for whom good lists are available.

Guidelines for Minimizing Survey Errors

The strengths and weaknesses of the alternative approaches to gathering survey data summarized in this chapter highlight the importance and utility of a total survey design framework and associated consideration of the errors that are likely to result from the complex of decisions required in designing a survey

No decision is perfect. Errors are inevitable. Trade-offs accompany the array of decisions required to design and conduct any survey—there may be high response rates but low coverage of drug users in the community from convenience samples of those participating in drug rehabilitation programs or large sampling errors for relatively rare groups in the study population, such as Vietnamese residents living in a clinic's service area. To make conscious and informed decisions that enhance data quality, however, survey designers must take a clear-eyed look at what the trade-offs are likely to be, enlightened by a clear understanding of what the survey is primarily intended to accomplish and sound knowledge of the particular strengths and limitations of the data gathering alternatives available to them.

Supplementary Sources

For a discussion of the pros and cons of personal interviews compared with mail questionnaires, see Dillman (1978, 1991), Salant and Dillman (1994), and Dillman and Sangster (1991); for comparisons with telephone interviewing methods, see Groves (1990b) and Groves, et al. (1988). Saris (1991) provides a useful overview of computer-assisted interviewing approaches.

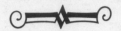

CHAPTER SIX

DECIDING WHO WILL BE IN THE SAMPLE

Chapter Highlights

1. The four basic types of probability sample designs—simple random sample, systematic random sample, stratified sample, and cluster sample—have different features that can be used to minimize costs and reduce sampling errors in surveys.
2. Four criteria for evaluating sample designs include the likely precision (variable sampling error) and accuracy (bias) of the resulting estimates (means or proportions, for example), as well as the complexity and efficiency (cost of minimizing errors) in actually implementing the design.
3. Area probability, random digit dialing, and list samples are the main methods for designing probability samples for personal interviews, telephone interviews, and mail questionnaires, respectively.
4. Probability sampling procedures for locating and sampling rare populations of people include screening, disproportionate sampling, network sampling, and dual-frame sampling.
5. There are four main procedures used in sampling respondents within households—the Kish, Troldahl-Carter-Bryant, Hagan and Collier, and last or next birthday methods.

Sampling is used to decide who will be included in a survey because gathering information on everyone in a population (as is done in the U.S. census) is beyond the scope and resources of most researchers. There will always be random variation in estimates of the characteristics of a population derived from a sample of it because of fluctuations in who gets included in any particular sample. Estimates derived from conducting a census of the entire population of interest would not have these random sampling errors but would be prohibitively expensive to carry out on a frequent basis. Sampling makes gathering data on a population of interest more manageable and more affordable. It enables the characteristics of a large body of people or institutions to be inferred, with minimal errors, from information collected on relatively few of them.

As with all aspects of designing and conducting a survey, attention must be given to ways of minimizing the sources of variable and systematic errors during sampling. The discussion that follows is intended to (1) underline the importance of relating the sample design to the research question being addressed in the study, (2) describe different types of sample designs, and (3) delineate criteria for evaluating alternative designs in the context of economically minimizing survey errors.

Relating the Sample Design to the Research Question

The constant point of reference for any major decisions about the practical steps in carrying out a survey should be the research questions that the study is principally intended to address. The framework introduced in Chapter Two for formulating the research question for the study (see again Table 2.2) can also serve as a guide for the sample design process: the questions it asks are *what* and *who* are the focus of the study, *where* and *when* is it being done, and *why*. In the example provided in Chapter Two, the focus was on the cigarette-smoking behaviors (what) of high school seniors (who) in a large metropolitan high school (where). The timing and frequency of data collection (when) varied, depending on the study design and whether the emphasis was on describing or explaining this behavior or the impact of interventions to alter it (why).

Target Population or Universe

The target population for the survey is the group or groups about which information is desired. This is sometimes referred to as the study *universe*. It is the group to which one wishes to generalize (or make inferences) from the survey sample.

Sample inclusion criteria (such as the civilian noninstitutionalized population of the United States or adults ages eighteen and over) or exclusion criteria (persons living in group quarters or those who speak neither English nor Spanish) are directly reflective of the target population for the study.

Different research designs have fundamental and compelling implications for identifying and sampling from the target population. Cross-sectional designs dictate a look at whether the designated time period for identifying the population (such as clinic users) represents the population over time (patients who had visited the facility over the past year sampled from medical records) or at a specified point in time (patients seen at the clinic on designated days sampled from visit logs). Group-comparison designs argue for careful attention to assuring that the groups that are being compared (racial and ethnic minorities) are systematically and adequately included in the sampling plan. Longitudinal designs must anticipate issues of whether the same or different people will be followed, and what additional steps will need to be taken to assure the comparability of the data gathered over time.

Sampling Frame

The sampling frame is the list of the target population from which the sample will actually be drawn. It is, in effect, the operational definition of the study universe (target population), the designation in concrete terms of who will be included, where they can be located, and when the data will be collected. In the school example, it would be the list of seniors (who) enrolled in city high schools (where) at the beginning or end of the school year (when).

There are often problems with the sampling frames available to researchers, however. A list provided at one point in time may fail to take into account students who drop out of school or new students who have enrolled by the time the study actually begins. There may also be clerical errors in the list; for example, the same student's name may be inadvertently repeated on the list and the names of other students omitted. These and other sampling frame problems are common when trying to match the definition of the desired target population for the study to an actual list of eligible candidates—regardless of the data collection method used (in person, by phone, or through the mail). We will see in later discussions that different types of problems with the sampling frame may be more severe with certain types of sample designs than with others (such as the difficulty of determining whether a sampled phone number is an eligible working residential number when the line is always busy or no one ever answers the phone).

Distinctions are sometimes drawn between the intended (target) population and the actual (study) population because of these sampling frame limitations. Basically, however, the researcher should try to match the basis and process for selecting the sample as closely as possible to the definition of the desired target population or universe for the study. Otherwise, the sample is likely to be plagued with substantial noncoverage biases, that is, individuals who *should* be included but are not.

Sampling Element

The sampling element refers to the ultimate unit or individual from whom information will be collected in the survey and who, therefore, will be the focus of the analysis. The sampling elements for the study should be clearly specified in defining the target population or universe (individuals, households, families, or institutions, for example). In the preceding example, the sampling elements are high school seniors.

In complex sample designs the researcher may need to go through several stages to get at the ultimate sampling element of interest. These successive stages may involve selecting several sampling units, such as cities, blocks within the cities, and households, to obtain the ultimate sampling unit—noninstitutionalized residents of a particular state or of the entire United States, for example. The designation of who to include in the study is also determined by the other aspects of the research question (what, where, when, and why the study is being done). Defining the precise individuals you want to collect information about or from is a central decision that will affect all subsequent approaches to that individual (person or institution), as well as the ways in which the data that are gathered on that sampling unit will ultimately be processed and analyzed.

Sample Design

The decision most critical to shaping the steps in the sample selection process is determining the type of sample design to be used. There are two principal types of sample designs—*probability* and *nonprobability* designs. The basic distinction between the two designs is that the former relies on the laws of chance for selecting the sampling elements, while the latter relies on human judgment.

The probability of entering the sample is directly determined by the sampling fraction used in selecting cases for probability-based designs, where the sampling fraction is equal to the sample size (n) divided by the size of the study universe (N) or n/N. In the example of the high school seniors, a probability sampling method could involve entering the ID numbers for all seniors registered at the school on a computer (N=300) and then creating a program to draw a desired sample of sixty students (n=60) by selecting every fifth name after some randomly assigned starting point. The sampling fraction (or chance) of a student coming into the sample would then be one in five (60/300). A nonprobability sampling approach would be to ask the principal or a group of teachers at the school which students it would be best to include, based on their knowledge of who smokes and their assessment of which students would be willing to cooperate with the project. The probability of coming into the sample on this relatively ad hoc basis cannot be determined.

Nonprobability sampling methods may be of several kinds. *Purposive samples* select people who serve a certain purpose, such as a focus group of employed mothers for a study of employed mothers' needs for child-care services. *Quota samples* focus on obtaining a certain number of designated types of respondents—for example, women between fifteen and forty-four years of age who are shopping in a drugstore. A *chunk sample* is simply a group of people who happen to be available at the time of the study—the people in the waiting room of a big-city emergency room on the night that a researcher decides to collect data on why patients are there and how long they have to wait. Samples can also be drawn from people who volunteer, such as students who respond to an advertisement to participate in a study of the effects of a low-fat diet on weight loss. The chance (probability) of any given individual being chosen, using any of these approaches, cannot be empirically estimated.

The main reason for sampling from a population is to collect information on a subset of individuals or institutions that represents (or is similar to) the entire population of interest. With probability sampling techniques, there are well-developed statistical methods for estimating the range of error and the level of confidence that the results for any particular sample are likely to have in reflecting the real population value. With nonprobability methods, this assessment is simply a judgment call on the part of the researcher. Thus, probability sampling methods allow the researcher to have greater confidence when generalizing to the study's target population.

Nonetheless, nonprobability sample surveys serve a number of useful purposes. Such studies permit in-depth investigations of groups that are difficult or expensive to find (such as prostitutes or homeless runaways). In the early stages of designing standardized surveys, they are helpful in developing and testing questions and procedures with respondents similar to those who will be included in the final study. They also serve to generate hypotheses that could be more fully explored in larger-scale, probability-based sample surveys.

Alternative probability-based sampling methods are described in the following section.

Types of Probability Sample Designs

The principal probability sample designs—*simple random sample, systematic random sample, stratified sample,* and *cluster sample*—are different sampling approaches that are often used in combination in carrying out a survey. The simple and systematic random sample approaches represent relatively simple designs. The stratified and cluster sample approaches are used in complex multistage surveys. In practice, most complex survey designs involve combinations of all four sampling methods. Each of the methods will, however, be discussed in turn, so that their respective advantages and disadvantages can be delineated. See Figures 6.1 (here) and 6.2 (in the following section). In the next section examples of different types of probability samples—for personal, telephone, and mail surveys—will also be presented to demonstrate how these approaches can be used in combination.

Simple Random Sample

A simple random sample is selected by using a procedure that gives every element in the population a known, nonzero, and equal chance of being included in the

FIGURE 6.1. TYPES OF PROBABILITY SAMPLE DESIGNS—RANDOM SAMPLES.

Type of Design	Selected Examples of Drawing Sample				
Simple Random Sample (Select sample through randomly drawing numbers, such that every element in the population has a *known, nonzero, and equal* chance of being included.)	*Random Numbers Table*				
	91567	42595	27958	30134	04024
	17955	56349	90999	49127	20044
	46503	18584	18845	49618	02304
	92157	89634	94824	78171	84610
	14577	62765	35605	81263	39667
	98427	07523	33362	64270	01638
	34914	63976	88720	82765	34476
	70060	28277	39475	46473	23219
	53976	54914	06990	67245	68350
	76072	29515	40960	07391	58745
	90725	52210	83974	29992	65831
	64364	67412	33339	31926	14883
	08062	00358	31662	25388	61642
	95012	68379	93526	70765	10592
	15664	10493	20492	38391	91132

Type of Design	Page 1	Page 2	Page 3
Systematic Random Sample (Select a starting point on a list randomly and then every *n*th unit thereafter, such that every element in the population has a *known* chance of being included.)	1 2 3* 4 5 6*	7 8 9* 10 11 12*	13 14 15* 16 17 18*

sample. The methods used most often for drawing simple random samples are lottery or random numbers selection procedures. In either case, before the sample is drawn, every element in the sampling frame should be assigned a unique identifying number. With the lottery procedure, these numbers can be placed in a container and mixed together, after which someone draws out numbers from the container until the required sample size is reached.

A random numbers sample selection device produces a series of numbers through a random numbers generation process. Each number is unique and independent of the others. Random numbers generation and selection software or published random numbers selection tables can be used in drawing simple random samples. (See an example of a random numbers table in Figure 6.1.)

To identify the ID numbers of the cases to be included in the sample, the researcher must first choose a random place to start on these tables (for example, by closing her eyes and putting her finger on the page, with the number on which her finger lands becoming the starting point). There should also be decision rules, specified in advance, for moving in a certain direction and choosing numbers (for example, she chooses the first two digits of the five-digit random numbers identified by moving from right to left across every row and column of the table after the random starting point, skipping any numbers that fall outside the range of IDs assigned to elements in the sampling frame). The researcher then matches the numbers generated by means of this process with the ID numbers for each element in the sampling frame. The elements with ID numbers that match those chosen from the random numbers table will be included in the sample. This process would continue until the desired sample size is reached.

Systematic Random Sample

Systematic random sample procedures represent an approximation to the simple random sample design. The process is similar to that found in the probability sampling approach that was used for drawing a sample of high school seniors: the researcher selects a random starting point and then systematically selects cases from the sampling frame at a specified (sampling) interval.

The determination of the starting point and sampling interval (k) is based on the required sample size. If, for example, a sample of a hundred students is desired out of a list of a thousand, then the sampling interval would be determined by dividing the total number on the list (sampling frame) by the desired sample size (k = 1,000/100 = 10). This means that the researcher should count down ten cases after starting from the case chosen as the random starting point within the first to tenth interval (between the first and tenth cases on the list) and continue to identify every tenth case until the one hundred cases are selected. In the example in Figure 6.1, the sampling interval is three; that is, one out of every three of the eighteen cases on the list will be selected, resulting in a sample of six cases.

Stratified Sample

The stratified sample approach is used when there is a particular interest in making sure that certain groups will be included in the study or that some groups will be sampled at a higher (or lower) rate than others. With the stratified sampling approach, the entire sampling frame is divided into subgroups of interest, such as city blocks that have high concentrations of Hispanics versus those that have few; health professionals who are members of their national professional association versus those who are not; or lists of phone numbers that have been called previously and are known to be working numbers versus those that have not been called previously. The researcher then uses a simple random or systematic random sampling process to select cases from the respective strata. Some individuals would be selected from *every* stratum into which the sample is divided. (See Figure 6.2.)

FIGURE 6.2. TYPES OF PROBABILITY SAMPLE DESIGNS—COMPLEX SAMPLES.

Type of Design	*Selected Examples of Drawing Sample*		
Stratified Sample (Divide population into *homogeneous strata* and draw random-type sample separately for *all strata*.)	Stratum A	Stratum B	Stratum C
	A1*	B1*	C1
	A2	B2	C2*
Proportionate: same sampling fraction in each stratum	A3*	B3*	C3
	A4	B4	C4*
	A5*	B5*	
Disproportionate: different sampling fraction in each stratum	A6		
Cluster Sample (Divide population into *heterogeneous clusters* and draw random-type sample separately from *sample of clusters*.)	Cluster 1	Cluster 2	Cluster 3
	A1*	A2*	A3*
	B2	C4	A6
	B3*	C3*	B5*
	C1	B4	B1
	A5*	C2*	A4*

The principal reason for dividing the sample into strata is to identify the groups that it is crucial to include based on the purposes of the study. If there are few members of the groups of interest in the target population, a simple random or systematic random sample may result in none or a very small number of these cases being included simply because there is a very small probability that such individuals will be sampled.

Dividing the population into strata and then sampling from each of these strata ensures that cases from all the groups of interest will be included. The proportion of cases selected (sampling fraction) in each stratum should be high enough to capture a sufficient number of cases to carry out meaningful analyses for each group. Another approach to obtaining enough cases for groups that may represent a relatively small proportion of the population as a whole is to draw a higher proportion of cases from that stratum relative to the other strata. Proportionate sampling selects the same proportion of cases from each stratum, while disproportionate sampling varies the proportion (sampling fraction) across strata.

For example, the researcher might decide to sample college professors who are members of a national professional association at a higher rate than professors who are not members by taking one out of five (20 percent) individuals in the member stratum and one out of ten (10 percent) in the nonmember stratum. In this case, members would be sampled at twice the rate of nonmembers. The precise sampling fractions to be used in each stratum should reflect some optimum allocation between strata, based on the amount of variability across cases (standard error) and the cost per case in each stratum. (See Kish, 1965, pp. 92–98, for a description of the procedures for estimating the optimum allocation of cases.)

Cluster Sample

The cluster sample method also involves dividing the sample into groups (or clusters). However, the primary purpose of cluster sampling is to maximize the dispersion of the sample throughout the community in order to represent fully the diversity that exists there while also minimizing costs. This method has traditionally been used in national, state, or community surveys of people who live in certain geographical areas. Clusters of housing units (for example, city blocks containing fifty houses) are identified during the sample design process. Then these clusters are sampled, and either all or a subsample (seven to ten) of the households in the sampled clusters are sampled from each cluster (or city block).

This approach substantially reduces the travel costs between interviews. A simple random sample of households throughout the country or even within a moderate-size community would be prohibitive because of the distances between sampling units, the time and effort involved in following up with people who were not at home at the time of the first visit, and so on. We will see later that there are also advantages in sampling clusters of phone numbers and using these clusters as the basis for identifying sets of phone numbers that are most likely to yield working residential numbers.

However, it is quite likely that a cluster of houses or phone numbers taken from one neighborhood may include people who are more like one another (racially, socioeconomically, and so on) than they are like a cluster of people identified in another neighborhood. As a result, there tends to be more diversity or heterogeneity *between* than *within* clusters. We will see later that this may result in higher sampling errors in cluster sample designs than in random and stratified ones.

Criteria to Evaluate Different Sample Designs

Four primary criteria may be applied in evaluating alternative sample designs: *precision, accuracy, complexity,* and *efficiency.*

Precision refers to how close the estimates derived from a sample are to the true population value as a function of variable sampling error. The standard errors of the estimates (derived from the sample variance) provide an estimate of variable sampling error. Variable error always exists when a sample is drawn because the estimates (means or proportions, for example) for different randomly selected subsets of cases of the same size are likely to differ simply due to chance. Standard errors are higher for smaller samples and more complex (especially cluster) designs (Kalton, 1983).

Accuracy refers to how close the estimates derived from a sample are to the true population value as a function of systematic error or bias. Bias results when certain groups or individuals that are eligible to be included are systematically left out because of problems with designing the sampling frame (excluding new residential construction) or implementing the intended sampling procedures (talking to whoever answers the phone rather than randomly selecting a survey respondent).

Complexity refers to consideration of the amount of information that must be gathered in advance of doing the study, as well as the number of stages and steps that will be required to implement the design. *Efficiency* refers to obtaining the most accurate and precise estimates at the lowest possible cost.

Theoretically, sampling (variable) error cannot be computed for nonprobability sampling designs since the assumptions required for computing it are not met (random selection from a known population with a hypothesized mean and variance). Systematic error (noncoverage bias) is likely to be particularly problematical for nonprobability designs because simple convenience or availability as the primary bases for selection may lead to a very unrepresentative set of cases. The complexity and costs (although not the efficiency) are likely to be less for many nonprobability designs.

Table 6.1 compares the advantages and disadvantages of different probability designs. The simple random sample is the least complex design, but because of the simple randomization process (luck of the draw), some groups (especially those which represent a very small proportion of the population) may not be included at all or in large enough numbers. This design is relatively straightforward to execute but would not be efficient for certain purposes (such as drawing a sample of households throughout a metropolitan area).

The systematic random sample has many of the same advantages and disadvantages as a simple random sample. It would, however, be a particularly useful approach when complete and accurate lists of the eligible study population are available. Biases may nonetheless enter into the systematic sampling process if a periodic ordering of elements in the sample frame exists that corresponds with the sampling intervals for designating selected cases, such as every other case being

TABLE 6.1. ADVANTAGES AND DISADVANTAGES OF DIFFERENT PROBABILITY SAMPLE DESIGNS.

Design	Advantages	Disadvantages
Simple random	• Requires little knowledge of population in advance.	• May not capture certain groups of interest. • May not be very efficient.
Systematic	• Easy to analyze data and compute sampling (standard) errors. • High precision.	• Periodic ordering of elements in sample frame may create biases in the data. • May not capture certain groups of interest. • May not be very efficient.
Stratified	• Enables certain groups of interest to be captured. • Enables disproportionate sampling and optimal allocation within strata. • Highest precision.	• Requires knowledge of population in advance. • May introduce more complexity in analyzing data and computing sampling (standard) errors.
Cluster	• Lowers field costs. • Enables sampling of *groups* of individuals for which detail on individuals themselves may not be available.	• Introduces more complexity in analyzing data and computing sampling (standard) errors. • Lowest precision.

a male veteran followed by his spouse's name, or every seventh house on the blocks in a new residential community being on a corner lot.

Stratified sampling offers a number of advantages. The researcher can ensure that certain groups are systematically included by using disproportionate sampling if needed. Variable sampling error is likely to be less principally because the standard error is computed based on a weighted average of the within-stratum variance, which has less variability (is more homogeneous) by definition than the sample as a whole. However, this design does introduce somewhat more complexity into implementing the sampling plan and analyzing the data than do either simple or systematic random samples.

Cluster sampling greatly increases the efficiency of sampling widely dispersed populations or areas, and it permits sampling of groups of individuals (households, schools, and so on) when information on the number and characteristics of the individuals (ultimate sampling elements) themselves is not directly available. But it is the most complex design and has the lowest precision, principally because the standard errors are based on the variation *between* what are likely to be relatively homogeneous clusters. (This issue will be addressed in more detail in Chapter Seven in discussing sample design effects.)

Putting It Together: Combined Designs

Most probability-based sample designs do, in fact, involve combinations of the array of discrete approaches and procedures just reviewed. Three primary types of designs highlighted here—*area probability, random digit dialing,* and *list samples*—have been used extensively in conducting personal household interviews, telephone interviews, and mail surveys, respectively. The sample design for the three studies for which questionnaires are provided in Resources A to C will be discussed later in this chapter as examples of these approaches.

Area Probability Sample

In area probability samples the emphasis is on selecting certain geographical areas containing the defined target population (the civilian noninstitutionalized population of the United States in the instance of the National Center for Health Statistics–National Health Interview Survey [NCHS–NHIS]) with a known probability of selection. With area probability sample designs, data are usually gathered from the households and individuals included in the resulting sample through personal interviews with everyone living in the household or with selected household members.

Sampling with probability proportionate to size (PPS) is an underlying component of many area probability designs. This approach combines elements of simple random, systematic, cluster, and stratified sampling. A notable public health application of PPS sampling procedures is in the World Health Organization Expanded Programme on Immunization (EPI). That program uses a PPS design for sampling villages and children to estimate the vaccination status of young children in developing countries. It is sometimes referred to as the 30×7 design because it traditionally entails sampling thirty clusters (such as villages) and selecting seven children of the required age within each cluster. This approach can, however, be adopted to whatever number and size of clusters is appropriate to maximize the efficiency of sampling dispersed target populations (Bennett, Woods, Liyanage, & Smith, 1991; Lemeshow & Stroh, 1989). The principal advantage of the PPS approach is that the sample is self-weighting, that is, the resulting distribution of cases on characteristics of interest (such as households in high, medium, or low income areas) directly mirrors the distribution in the study universe.

An example of the steps required to execute a PPS design is provided in Table 6.2. The first step involves estimating the desired sample size (n) needed to meet study design requirements (procedures for estimating sample sizes are discussed in Chapter Seven). In Step 2, a desired cluster size is decided upon (n_c). The criteria that come into play are the trade-offs between saving on data collection costs by sampling groups of households that are close together versus the fact that standard (sampling) errors will increase as the size of these clusters increase. Traditionally, cluster sizes range from seven to ten sampling elements in area probability samples. In Step 3 the number of clusters (c=11) needed to achieve the sample size is computed by dividing the desired sample size (n=77) by the cluster size (n_c=7). In this example, eleven clusters with seven households in each cluster are needed, to yield the desired sample size of seventy-seven households.

Step 4 entails estimating the total number of sampling units in the study universe. This number is derived from census data in those countries for which they are available, updated as appropriate for estimated change since the last census. In areas for which this information is not available, estimates can be provided by knowledgeable people in the community or other relevant sources (tax or school rosters). In Step 5, cumulative totals of housing units in the study universe (N=2,200) are computed, and in Step 6, the sampling interval (k) for identifying clusters is determined by dividing the number in the study universe (N) by the target number of clusters (c): k = 2,200/11=200. The blocks in which every two-hundredth household appear, based on the cumulative listing, will be designated as ones from which a cluster of seven households will be selected. The sampling interval (one out of two hundred) dictates that in Step 7 a random starting point will be identified from the cumulative list of housing units within this interval (the

TABLE 6.2. SAMPLING WITH PROBABILITY PROPORTIONATE TO SIZE (PPS).

Steps	Example
1. Estimate the desired sample size (n).	77
2. Fix the desired cluster size (n_c).	7
3. Calculate the number of clusters (c) needed to achieve the desired sample size: n/n_c.	77/7 = 11
4. Estimate the total number of units in the universe (Col. B, Table) from which the sample will be drawn (N).	2200 Col. B, Table.
5. Calculate the cumulative total of the number of units across *all* clusters in the universe.	Col. C, Table.
6. Calculate the sampling interval (k) for selecting clusters from the universe: N/c.	2200/11 = 200
7. Pick a random starting point (r) to select clusters within the designated sampling interval (Step 6), using a random numbers table.	50
8. Calculate the selection numbers (HU #) for the blocks to be sampled by entering the random starting point, adding the sampling interval, and then repeat the process to identify sampled blocks: $r = HU_1$ $HU_1 + k = HU_2$ $HU_2 + k = HU_3$, etc.	Col. D, Table.
9. Assign cluster numbers to each designated block.	Col. E, Table.
10. Confirm % in strata for sample agree with % in universe.	Col. B, E (%), Table.

A City blocks (or towns)	B Estimated number of housing units	C Cumulative number of housing units	D Selection number	E Cluster number
High				
A	100	100	50	#1.
B	50	150	—	—
C	75	225	—	—
D	150	375	250	#2.
E	200 (575/2200 = 26%)	575	450	#3. (27%)
Medium				
F	250	825	650	#4.
G	125	950	850	#5.
H	50	1000	—	—
I	100	1100	1050	#6.
J	50 (575/2200 = 26%)	1150	—	— (27%)
Low				
K	200	1350	1250	#7.
L	300	1650	1450, 1650	#8., #9.
M	125	1775	—	—
N	150	1925	1850	#10.
O	275 (1050/2200 = 48%)	2200	2050	#11. (46%)

fiftieth household was identified from a random numbers table as the starting point in this example). In Step 8, the sampling interval (200) is added to this initial starting point (50) to identify a housing unit (250) from the cumulative listing. The block in which it appears is selected and this process is repeated to identify the blocks from which the subsequent clusters (up to eleven) will be selected. In Step 9, numbers can then be assigned to each cluster identified in Step 8.

As mentioned earlier, the beauty of the PPS design is that it is self-weighting, that is, the distribution of characteristics (such as income) in the resulting sample parallels the distribution in the study universe. This is confirmed in the example provided, where the distribution of three strata in the study universe is mirrored in the distribution of cases (approximately one-quarter, one-quarter, and one-half, respectively) in the study sample.

Geographic information systems (GIS), which permit computerized mapping of household and population distributions as well as overlaying associated demographic or other characteristics, offer a promising technology for facilitating the design and implementation of area probability samples (Currie, Li, & Wall, 1993; Saalfeld, 1993).

Random Digit Dialing

Three primary approaches are used to develop sampling frames of phone numbers for telephone surveys: *list-assisted frames, random digit dialing,* and *multiple frame* sampling methods (Lepkowski, 1988; Mohadjer, 1988; Voss, Gelman, & King, 1995). Originally, list-assisted frames drew on numbers that were published in phone books. Newer methods employ computerized databases of directory numbers supplemented by other sources that include both listed and unlisted phone numbers (such as motor vehicle registration department lists). The primary supplier of these phone number databases is Donnelley Marketing Information Services (Stamford, Conn.), which publishes most U.S. telephone directories.

The random digit dialing approach is based on a randomly generated set of phone numbers, starting with the area code and exchanges (central office codes) for the area in which one wishes to place the calls. Current and proposed area code and exchange combinations are available on BELLCORE data files produced by Bell Communications Research (BCR) (Morristown, N.J.). Once relevant area code and exchange digits are identified, a random numbers generation procedure is used to create the rest of the digits for the phone numbers to be used in the sample. With this approach every possible phone number in the area has a chance of being included in the study.

The efficiency of this sampling process can be increased by reducing the nonworking, business, or nonresidential numbers that are likely to be generated.

The Waksberg-Mitofsky procedure was developed to facilitate identification of working residential numbers (Waksberg, 1978). In the first stage of sample selection with the Waksberg-Mitofsky procedure, primary sampling units are, in effect, clusters or blocks of a hundred numbers identified by the first eight digits of the phone number: (xxx) xxx–xx00 through (xxx) xxx–xx99. If the first randomly generated number in this block of a hundred numbers is an eligible (working, residential) number when called, then the entire block of numbers will be included in the sample. If not, then that block will be eliminated from the sample. In the second stage of selection (within the selected blocks of one hundred numbers), the remaining series of numbers in the blocks (PSUs) selected are called until the desired sample size is reached.

Criticisms of the Waksberg-Mitofsky procedure have focused on problems and delays at two stages. At the first stage, there are problems and delays in identifying eligible households because of difficulties in getting through to the parties to whom the number is assigned. At the second stage, many numbers within an eligible cluster identified at stage one must be called for what turns out to be a relatively low yield of working residential numbers. Multiple frame sampling methods are used to address these problems through, for example, using information from list-assisted frames to stratify BELLCORE area code-exchange clusters by their likely yield of working numbers or phoning more than one number within a cluster as a basis for disproportionately sampling clusters that are likely to yield a higher proportion of working numbers (Brick & Waksberg, 1991; Brick, Waksberg, Kulp, & Starer, 1995; Casady & Lepkowski, 1991; Potthoff, 1987; Tucker, Casady, & Lepkowski, 1992). Telephone samples can be purchased from commercial firms such as GENESYS (Fort Washington, Penn.) and Survey Sampling, Inc. (Fairfield, Conn.). Address labels can be obtained for the phone numbers to be called through commercial suppliers such as Telematch (Springfield, Va.) for the purpose of sending advance letters to potential respondents.

List Sample

The first step in list sample surveys is to identify a list of potentially eligible respondents, make some judgments about the completeness of the list, consider any problems that may be encountered when sampling from the list (duplicate names, blank or incomplete information on certain individuals, names of people who are deceased or who moved out of the area, and so on), and decide whether the respondents meet the eligibility criteria that have been defined for the study. Once eligibility has been determined, it is necessary to derive the sampling fraction and systematically sample prospective participants on the list.

Procedures for Selecting the Respondent

The preceding discussion has reviewed the major steps involved in designing probability samples of individuals. In this section, alternative procedures for the selection of individuals at what is usually the ultimate stage of sampling will be described—that is, how to choose the individuals to interview once contact with a household has been made and not everyone who lives there is to be interviewed.

There are four principal probability-based approaches to respondent selection. Two involve the use of random selection tables after detailing the composition of the household (Figure 6.3) and two screen for respondents by means of characteristics that are fairly randomly distributed in the population (such as the person who had a birthday most recently) (Table 6.3).

Kish Tables

The first approach was designed by sampling statistician Leslie Kish for use in area probability-based personal interview surveys (Kish, 1965). With this approach, the interviewer requests the names, ages, and (as appropriate) other information for all the members of the household, who are then listed on a household listing table in the order specified. Generally the household head (or whoever is answering the question) is listed first, followed by the other family members from oldest to youngest (see Figure 6.3). Once everyone living in the household has been identified and listed in a specified order (on a chart with numbered lines, for example), the number of the person to interview (identified by the numbered line on which his or her name is listed) can be determined, based on the line number associated with the corresponding number of people in the household on the Kish selection table.

Kish (1965, pp. 396–404) generated a series of eight different selection tables that reflect different designations of the person to choose, given different numbers of people in the household. Each table was to be used with a certain proportion of the cases in a sample. The example of one such selection table (Table D) is displayed in Figure 6.3. These tables can be directly programmed into computer-assisted systems or generated by computer, using procedures Kish developed, and placed on sample assignment sheets in paper and pencil interviews (Waksberg & Mohadjer, 1991). Each ultimate sampling unit then has a preassigned Kish table to use as the basis for deciding whom to interview.

The Kish respondent selection process is a very systematic one for ensuring that all relevant members of the household are identified and have a chance of being included in the sample. There has been increasing concern with the application of the Kish procedure in telephone surveys, however, where there is a greater probability than in personal interviews that certain respondents (such as women or the elderly) will break off the interview immediately if they feel they are being asked an intrusive or tedious series of questions. The other approaches to respondent selection have been designed to address some of these perceived disadvantages of the Kish approach for telephone surveys.

Troldahl-Carter-Bryant (TCB) Tables

With the Troldahl-Carter-Bryant (TCB) procedure, only two questions are asked: (1) how many persons of a certain age (as appropriate to study objectives) live in the household, and (2) how many of these individuals are of a certain gender (Czaja, Blair, & Sebestik, 1982). As with the Kish approach, there are alternative selection tables that can be assigned to a predetermined proportion of the interviews for deciding which age-sex respondent to choose.

Originally, the second question in the TCB procedure asked for the number of males in the household. Research conducted by Czaja, Blair, & Sebestik (1982), however, suggested that the rate of nonresponse was higher when this approach was used and, further, that the proportion of women living alone was also underrepresented. When the respondent was asked about the number of women in the household with the TCB approach, the results for the Kish and TCB methods were very similar. With the TCB approach, however, there may be a tendency to underrepresent individuals between the oldest and youngest in households in which there are more than two individuals of the same sex. Further, there is a general tendency to underrepresent males in telephone surveys because they are less likely to be at home at the time of the call.

Hagan and Collier Method

The Hagan and Collier method of respondent selection is an effort to simplify even further the process for identifying which individuals to interview (Hagan & Collier, 1983). With this approach the interviewer simply asks to speak, for example, with the youngest (or oldest) adult male. If there is no male there, then the interviewer asks for the corresponding female. The researcher must provide precise instructions to the interviewer regarding how to proceed if no one in the household fits that description. There are then some ambiguities in directly implementing the Hagan and Collier approach, and no extensive methodological research is yet available that compares this to other methods of respondent selection.

FIGURE 6.3. PROCEDURES FOR SELECTING THE RESPONDENT—SELECTION TABLES.

Procedure	Methodology
Kish Tables (Ask about all potentially eligible individuals in the household, list them, and then use Kish tables.)	Question: Please state the sex, age, and relationship to you of all persons xx or older living there who are related to you by blood, marriage, or adoption.

List all persons age 18 and over in dwelling unit

Relationship to Head (1)	Sex (2)	Age (3)	Adult (4)	Check (5)
HUSBAND	M	52	2	
WIFE	F	50	4	✓
SON	M	23	3	
DAUGHTER	F	19	5	
HUSB. FATHER	M	78	1	

Number persons 18 or over in the following order:

Oldest male, next oldest male, etc.; followed by oldest female, next oldest female, etc. Then use selection table below to choose respondent.

Selection Table D

If the number of adults in the dwelling is:	Interview the adult numbered:
1	1
2	2
3	2
4	3
5	4
6 or more	4

Troldahl-Carter-Bryant (TCB)
Tables
(Ask how many persons live in the household, how many of them are women, and then use TCB selection charts.)

Questions: (1) How many persons xx years or older live in your household, including yourself?
(2) How many of these are women?

Row B	Col. A			
Number of Women in Household	Number of Adults in Household			
	1	2	3	4 or more
0	man	youngest man	youngest man	oldest man
1	woman	woman	oldest man	woman
2		oldest woman	man	oldest man
3			youngest woman	man or oldest man
4 or more				oldest woman

Note: The intersection of Col. A and Row B determines the sex and relative age of the respondent to be interviewed.

Last/Next Birthday Method

An approach that is gaining increasing acceptance in telephone surveys in particular is the last or next birthday method of respondent selection. With this approach the person answering the phone is asked who in the household had a birthday most recently (last birthday method) or is expected to have one next (next birthday method). This person is then chosen for the interview. (See Questions S1 and S2 in the screening questionnaire in the Chicago AIDS survey in Resource B for an application of the last birthday method of respondent selection, also provided as an example of this approach in Table 6.3.)

Research on this method suggests that overall it is a valid approach to respondent selection, although it does by design tend to capture a disproportionate number of respondents whose birthday is close to the survey date (Forsman, 1993; Lavrakas, Bauman, & Merkle, 1993; O'Rourke & Blair, 1983; O'Rourke & Lakner, 1989; Salmon & Nichols, 1983). Everyone in the household presumably has the same probability of being asked to participate, though as with all respondent selection procedures, reporting error on the part of the respondent who supplies the information on which the selection is based could lead to the exclusion of some persons who should be included. More research is needed to evaluate the application of this approach to different types of household respondents (those of varying races or of different educational and income levels, for example).

Neither the Hagan and Collier nor the next/last birthday approach explicitly asks for the number of people in the household. This information is needed

TABLE 6.3. PROCEDURES FOR SELECTING THE RESPONDENT—RESPONDENT CHARACTERISTICS.

Procedure	Methodology
Hagan and Collier Method (Ask to speak with one of four types of age-sex individuals and if no one of that gender, ask for counterpart of opposite gender.)	Question: I need to speak with (youngest adult male/youngest adult female/oldest adult male/oldest adult female) over the age of *xx*, if there is one.
Last/Next Birthday Method (Ask to speak with the person who had a birthday last *or* will have one next.)	Question: In order to determine whom to interview, could you please tell me, of adults xx years of age or older currently living in your household, who had the most recent birthday? I don't mean who is the youngest, just who had a birthday last.

to determine the probability that any particular individual will be selected and to apply weights to the sampled cases so that they accurately reflect the composition of all the households included in the sample.

Special Considerations for Special Populations

A significant problem in many surveys, and in health surveys in particular, is that the researcher wants to study subgroups that appear with low frequency in the general population (such as selected minority groups, individuals with certain types of health problems or disabilities, patients of a particular clinic or health facility, homeless people, or drug users). There has been a great deal of interest and effort on the part of sampling statisticians to develop cost-effective approaches to increasing the yield of these and other target groups in health surveys (Burnam & Koegel, 1988; Johnson, Mitra, Newman, & Horm, 1993; Kalton & Anderson, 1986; Sasao, 1994; Sudman & Kalton, 1986; Sudman, Sirken, & Cowan, 1988). One of these methods has been touched upon already in this chapter (disproportionate sampling within selected strata). Figure 6.4 describes and provides examples of this and other approaches for sampling rare populations.

Screening

Screening for the subgroups that will be the focus of a study involves asking selected respondents whether they or their households (as appropriate) have the characteristic or attribute (X) of interest. If they answer in the affirmative, they are included in the study. If not, they (or some proportion who say no) are dropped from the study.

This approach can be used quite effectively with either area probability or telephone surveys. Methodologies have been developed that are adaptations of the Waksberg-Mitofsky (Blair & Czaja, 1982; Waksberg, 1978, 1983) approach to screening clusters of telephone numbers. In these approaches, a screening question is asked of the first working residential number in a block of phone numbers (PSU) to see if the sampling unit meets the screening criteria (an African American or Hispanic respondent in the AIDS survey, for example). If it does not, that PSU will be excluded from further calling; if it does, calling will proceed in that PSU. This assumes that there is a higher probability that more eligible households will be clustered in the PSU that met the screening criterion than in those blocks of numbers that did not meet the criterion. This assumption is more likely to be met for certain sets of characteristics than for others.

FIGURE 6.4. PROBABILITY SAMPLE DESIGNS
FOR SAMPLING RARE POPULATIONS.

Type of Design	Methodology	Examples
Screening (Ask respondents whether they/ household have the attribute X and drop those from sample that do not.)	Do you have the attribute X? Yes → Include in Sample No → Drop from Sample	Do you have a chronic illness? Yes → Include No → Drop

Disproportionate Sampling (Assign a higher sampling fraction to stratum that has attribute X.)

Stratum A	Stratum B	Stratum C
A1X	B1	C1X
A2X	B2	C2
A3X	B3	C3
A4	B4X	C4
A5	B5	C5
A6	B6	C6

Sampling Fraction =   3/6   1/6   1/6

Percent black in PSU:
Stratum A: High
Stratum B: Low
Stratum C: Low

Type of Design	Methodology	Examples
Network Sampling (Ask respondents if they know others in *family network,* defined in certain way, who have attribute X.)	Do you have family who have attribute X? Yes → (1) How many? (2) Who and where are they? No → Terminate Interview	Do you have a parent with cancer? Yes → (1) Mother, father, or both? (2) Name(s) and address(es)? No → Terminate Interview

Dual-Frame Sampling (Use a second sampling frame containing elements with attribute X to supplement original frame.)

Frame #1			Frame #2		
1X	7	13	1X	7X	13X
2	8	14X	2X	8X	14X
3	9	15	3X	9X	15X
4X	10	16	4X	10X	16X
5	11	17	5X	11X	17X
6	12X	18	6X	12X	18X

Frame #1:
Area probability sample of clinic's service area

Frame#2:
List sample of clinic patients

In area probability designs interviewers can similarly contact households and ask respondents the screening question as a basis for deciding whether to proceed with interviews in those families. Although area probability screening of this kind is very expensive, the telephone application of this approach has a definite cost advantage over the in-person one. A mail questionnaire would be another cost-effective method for identifying potentially eligible units. Higher nonresponse rates with this method would, however, increase the possibility of bias in identifying who is ultimately eligible for the study.

A particular problem with the screening approach is the possibility of "false negatives." These occur when people who say no to the screening question may in fact have the attribute and might even admit to this later if included in the study and asked the same question again in the course of the interview. The rates of false negatives should be taken into account in thinking through the design of the screening question and in decisions about whether to exclude from the final study all or only a portion of those who say no initially. In general, some proportion of those who say no to the screening question should be included in the sample anyway to permit the rate of false negatives to be estimated.

Disproportionate Sampling

A second approach to "oversampling" certain groups of interest, displayed in Figure 6.4, is the disproportionate sampling within strata discussed earlier. In the example in Figure 6.4, as in the design of the NCHS–NHIS area probability sample, there is an interest in sampling the stratum with a higher concentration of minorities (X), that is, African Americans or Hispanics, at a higher rate. The sampling fraction (number of sample cases divided by number of cases in stratum) in the stratum (A) that has a high proportion of minorities (3/6) is set at three times that of the other two strata (1/6). The optimum allocation of cases between the strata should take into account the expected variability and cost per case within the respective strata. The fact that the sampling fraction is varied across strata will also need to be taken into account in combining cases from the respective strata for analysis. This will be discussed later in describing the procedures for weighting survey data gathered by means of disproportionate sampling techniques.

Commercially available telephone databases contain linked zip code, census tract, and associated demographic data from the U.S. census and other sources that can be used in stratifying phone exchanges for the purpose of disproportionately sampling selected population groups based on place of residence or selected demographic characteristics (race or income, for example) in random digit dialing surveys (Mohadjer, 1988).

Network Sampling

Another method that has been developed and applied in health surveys is network or multiplicity sampling. Health survey sampling statisticians have, in fact, contributed significantly to developing this approach (Czaja & Blair, 1990; Czaja, Snowden, & Casady, 1986; Czaja, Trunzo, & Royston, 1992; Czaja, et al., 1984; Sudman & Freeman, 1988).

Network sampling asks individuals who fall into a sample (drawn by means of conventional probability sampling methods) to use certain counting rules in identifying relatives or friends that have the attribute of interest, most often some medical condition or disability. Respondents are then asked to indicate how many people they know with the condition and where they live. The researcher can then follow up with the individuals named or simply use the information provided to generate prevalence estimates for these conditions in the population.

With network sampling, the probability of any given individual being named is proportional to the number of different households in which the originally sampled persons and the members of their networks, defined by the specified counting rules, reside. This information provides the basis for computing so-called multiplicity estimators for network samples. These estimators reflect the probability that respondents will be named across the multiplicity of networks to which they belong. As with the screening approach, there may be response errors on the part of informants about the occurrence of the condition in their network and in the accuracy of the size of the network they report. The costs of following up with individuals named by the original respondents will also add to the overall expense of the study. Establishment of counting rules for determining the size of the network and construction of the associated multiplicity estimators are relatively complex procedures. This is definitely an approach that requires consultation with a sampling expert.

Dual-Frame Sampling

Dual-frame sampling involves using more than one sampling frame in the design of the sample for the study. In general, one of the frames is expected to have a higher or known concentration of the subgroup of interest, which can then be combined with the other frame to enhance the yield of those individuals in the study as a whole. In the example provided in Figure 6.4, the researcher could conduct an area probability sample of residents in a clinic's service area to gather information on the need for and satisfaction with medical care among community residents. If the study design also calls for comparisons of the access and satisfaction levels of community residents who have used the clinic versus those who have not, it may be necessary to supplement the area probability sample with a list sample of patients who have actually used the clinic. This was the basic sampling design used for an evaluation of the impact of community hospital-based group practices conducted by the author and her colleagues (Aday, Andersen, Loevy, & Kremer, 1985; Loevy, 1984).

As with the multiplicity sampling procedure, it is important in dual-frame designs to consider carefully the probabilities that individuals from the respective frames will come into the sample and to construct appropriately the weights and procedures for computing estimates based on combining the respective samples.

Sampling Mobile Populations

The preceding approaches are the principal methods used for sampling rare and elusive groups. Additional problems arise in identifying universes of highly mobile populations, such as migrant workers, the homeless, or visitors to a health care facility or provider. Nonprobability sampling methods offer one alternative although, as mentioned earlier, significant noncoverage biases may exist in studies employing these approaches.

Probability-based procedures have been developed to attempt to sample mobile and elusive populations. These include methods for sampling in time and space and capture-recapture methods, among others. With the first approach, specific blocks of time at given locations are identified and these are then used to form primary sampling units for a first stage of sampling. At the second stage, systematic random samples of elements (visitors, for example) are drawn within selected time-space blocks (clusters). In the capture-recapture method, which was originally developed for counting wildlife populations, two independent observations are taken at approximately the same time to count the population of interest. The number of individuals observed each time, as well as the number observed at *both* periods, is used to estimate the size of the total population as a basis for deriving a relevant sampling fraction (or fixing a probability of selection) for the sample. Although both theoretical and practical problems exist with these methods, they offer promising alternatives to largely nonprobabilistic designs. (An overview of these and other methods for sampling mobile populations is available in Kalton, 1991; Kish, 1991; and Sudman, Sirken, & Cowan, 1988.)

Selected Examples

Table 6.4 summarizes the sample designs of the three studies with questionnaires included in this book (Resources A, B, and C). They represent three different approaches to sampling—area probability, random digit dialing, and list samples—

for personal, telephone, and mail surveys, respectively. These designs all involve several stages of drawing the respective samples, and different aspects of the methods just described are utilized in each stage.

Area Probability Sample

The first example is a description of the area probability sample for the National Health Interview Survey sponsored by the National Center for Health Statistics, a component of the Centers for Disease Control and Prevention of the U.S. Department of Health and Human Services. The NHIS sample design is revised after each decennial census of the population to take into account changes in the population and its distribution as well as to accommodate changing survey objectives. The NHIS is based on a stratified, multistage area sample. Key objectives in the 1990 NHIS sample redesign implemented in January 1995 were to improve the reliability of estimates for Hispanics and African Americans and for subnational geographic areas, especially for states (Judkins, Marker, & Waksberg, 1994). The NHIS by itself, however, is expected to yield estimates only for a few of the most populous states.

Stage 1. The first stage of selecting the 1995 NCHS–NHIS sample involved dividing the United States into 1,995 primary sampling units (PSUs), each of which was one or more counties or a metropolitan statistical area (MSA), as designated by the U.S. Office of Management and Budget. First, the PSUs for the 52 largest metropolitan statistical areas in the nation were designated as self-representing (SR). SR means these PSUs individually represent themselves in the sample and are included with certainty (had a 100 percent chance of being selected). For the study an additional 43 PSUs, for a total of 95 SR PSUs, were designated as SR. A stratum is considered SR if it is composed of a SR PSU. As part of the process, 142 non-self-representing (NSR) strata were then formed; these strata are represented by one or more sample PSUs that represent both themselves and other PSUs in the stratum. Within the individual NSR strata, for all but 21 of the 142 strata, two PSUs were sampled; for these 21 strata one PSU was selected from each stratum, yielding 263 NSR PSUs; the 95 (52 + 43) SR strata each comprised a PSU, yielding a total of 358 sample PSUs out of a possible 1,995 being chosen. PSUs were selected using a probability proportionate to size (PPS) design, based on their estimated 1993 population size.

Stage 2. In Stage 2 of sampling, the 358 selected PSUs were divided into segments that contained clusters of households and then a stratified subsample of these segments were systematically selected for the sample. In a NHIS sample PSU, two types of segments are typically employed. Area segments are usually used to represent housing units built prior to April 1, 1990 (1990 census), and are based on the survey field staff's enumerating housing units in sampled clusters of house-holds; permit segments are usually used to represent housing units built on or after April 1, 1990, and are based on a sample of records of building permits issued since 1990. The use of a sample of permits is to reduce the unintended variability in number of households in area segment; without a sample of permit samples, occasionally some area segments could contain an unexpectedly large number of housing units where the area included substantial new building since the 1990 census. The segments were stratified based on the concentration of African Americans and Hispanics. Housing units in higher concentration African American and Hispanic census blocks were sampled at higher rates.

Stage 3. In the final stage of sampling, all the households within the selected cluster were contacted. The housing units that were vacant or had been demolished were eliminated from the study. Before data collection, addresses in each area segment had been systematically designated as either an "S" or an "I" unit. For households at an "I" address that were still eligible for the study, information was obtained on all the members of the household through personal interviews with a key informant and as many other household members as were available at the time of the interview for the core NHIS questionnaire for those. In an "S" housing unit, if an African American or Hispanic person were found to reside there after doing the household listing, then the household was retained in the sample. If not, the interviewer ended the interview. In those households for which the full interview was to be completed, a randomly selected adult or child (as appropriate) was chosen as the sample person for the special supplements.

Random Digit Dialing Sample

A modified Waksberg-Mitofsky random digit dialing (RDD) sample approach was used to conduct the University of Illinois Survey Research Laboratory for the Chicago AIDS survey.

Stage 1. In the first stage of sample selection, this procedure created primary sampling units that were, in effect, clusters or blocks of numbers in the Chicago metropolitan area identified by the first eight digits of the phone number. If the first randomly generated number in this block of one hundred numbers was an eligible (working, residential) number when called, then the entire block of numbers was included. If not, then that block was eliminated from the sample. In this survey, there was an interest in oversampling African American and Hispanic respondents. Therefore, an additional eligibility criterion was imposed at this stage of sampling for a subset of the PSUs—that is, to include the PSU only if the first number called yielded an African American or Hispanic respondent (Blair & Czaja, 1982; Waksberg, 1983). This screening was focused on telephone exchanges

TABLE 6.4. SELECTED EXAMPLES OF PROBABILITY SAMPLE DESIGNS.

Area Probability Sample: National Center for Health Statistics Health Interview Survey	Random Digit Dialing (RDD) Sample: Waksberg-Mitofsky Design for Chicago Area Survey on AIDS	List Sample: Dental Clinical Decision-Making Study
Target Population: civilian noninstitutionalized population	*Target Population:* general population in Chicago metropolitan area aged eighteen and over	*Target Population:* general practice dentists providing care to at least 75 Washington Education Association members and their dependents located in one of four counties
Stage 1 (Total PSUs = 358)	*Stage 1*	*Stage 1*
1. Divide the U.S. into 1,995 primary sampling units (PSUs)—a county, a group of counties, or metropolitan statistical area.	1. Implement a random or systematic selection of area code–central office code combinations for area: (312) xxx-.	1. Identify eligible dentists from Washington Dental Service claims.
2. Select the 52 largest MSAs as self-representing (SR) PSUs. Select an additional 43 PSUs as SR in the process of forming strata within individual states for metropolitan and nonmetropolitan areas.	2. Add two random digits to each area code–central office code combination: (312) xxx-xx.	*Stage 2* (Total Dentists = 200)[a] 2. Determine sampling fraction. 3. Draw systematic random sample of eligible dentists.
3a. Stratify other PSUs into 142 non-self-representing (NSR) strata where no stratum straddles two states or straddles metropolitan and nonmetropolitan areas.	3. Prepare list of all possible 8-digit numbers, which become PSUs with clusters of 100 numbers each: (312) xxx-xx00 through (312) xxx-xx99.	
3b. Select 1–2 sample PSUs individually in each NSR stratum (select only 1 PSU in stratum with small population size).	4. Assign last two digits of the number randomly, such as: (312) xxx-xx24.	
Stage 2	5. Dial the resulting number.	
4a. Divide each sample PSU into clusters of segments (a group of housing units usually in the same census block).	6a. Eligible household number—complete the interview. Retain the PSU of 100 numbers.	
	6b. Ineligible household number—terminate the interview. Eliminate the PSU of 100 numbers from further calls.	

4b. Identify two types of segments: (1) area segments expected to have 8 or 12 housing units, determined by listing units in a small geographic area (usually census block); (2) permit area segments, expected to have 4 housing units, determined by records of building permits issued since April 1, 1990 (1990 U.S. census).

4c. Stratify area segments in each PSU into 20 substrata based on joint distribution of blacks and Hispanics.

5. Select a stratified sample of about 6,800 segments containing about 62,000 addresses.

6. Systematically subsample housing units in segments which contain substantially more than the expected number of housing units (usually very rare).

Stage 3

7a. Contact sample addresses. Classify as ineligible addresses corresponding to vacant and demolished housing units. Screen sample households at "S" addresses for a black or Hispanic person and complete interview with households at "S" addresses that have a black or Hispanic member. End interview with households at "S" addresses that have neither a black or Hispanic member. Interview sample households at "I" addresses.

7b. Obtain interviews for 106,000 persons in 42,000 responding households.

Stage 2 (Total Households = 1,540)

7. Randomly assign two new digits to end of cluster of numbers for same or new PSU (as appropriate).

8. Repeat process until desired sample size is reached.

---

[a] All eligible dentists were included, resulting in a census, rather than a sample, of the universe.

in the city of Chicago in particular, which had a larger concentration of minorities than did area suburbs.

Stage 2. In the second stage of selection (within the selected blocks of one hundred numbers), the remaining series of numbers in the blocks (PSUs) selected were called until the desired sample size was reached—a total of 1,540 households in the Chicago AIDS survey.

List Sample

The third example is a list sample of dentists identified in the Washington State Study of Dentists' Preferences.

Stage 1. The first step involved identifying eligible dentists, general practitioners who practiced in a four-county area of Washington State and had provided services to at least seventy-five Washington Education Association members or their dependents between 1984 and 1985.

Stage 2. In the dentists' preferences study, once the list of eligible dentists was determined ($N = 200$), all of them (100 percent) were included in the study. This, in effect, resulted in a census, rather than a sample per se, of the universe of dentists eligible for this study.

Guidelines for Minimizing Survey Errors

P-A-C-E off the steps carefully in designing the survey sample. *P*ay *a*ttention to both *c*ost and *e*rrors. *P*recision (random error), *a*ccuracy (systematic error), *c*omplexity, and *e*fficiency, as well as the match of the sample design to the survey objectives, are the key criteria to keep in mind in evaluating the pros and cons of different designs or combinations of design alternatives.

This chapter has provided an overview of the alternatives for deciding *who* should be selected for the sample. The chapter that follows presents techniques for estimating, adjusting, and evaluating *how many* should be included.

Supplementary Sources

For an overview of sample designs in general, see Fink (1995b), Henry (1990), Kalton (1983), Kish (1965), Levy and Lemeshow (1991), Maisel and Persell (1996), and Scheaffer, Mendenhall, and Ott (1990), and for health surveys in particular, see Cox and Cohen (1985) and Levy and Lemeshow (1980).

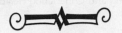

CHAPTER SEVEN

DECIDING HOW MANY WILL BE IN THE SAMPLE

Chapter Highlights

1. The research questions, objectives, and associated research design are the fundamental bases for computing the sample size needed to reliably carry out a study.
2. Design effects reflect the extent to which the sampling error for a complex sample design differs from that of a simple random sample of the same size.
3. Survey response rates are based on the number of completed interviews as a proportion of those cases drawn in the original sample that were verified (or estimated) to be eligible for the study.
4. Sample weighting procedures involve assigning more (or less) weight to certain cases in the sample to adjust for disproportionate sampling or the differential noncoverage or nonresponse to the survey by different groups.

Simultaneous with deciding *who* to include in a sample is the decision about *how many* respondents to include. This chapter discusses how to determine the study sample size, the response rates, the appropriate weighting of sample cases, and the errors associated with sampling them in a particular way.

Relating the Sample Size to the Research Questions and Design

As indicated in Chapter Two, the research questions and associated study design are the primary anchors and guides for the conduct of a survey, including the computation of the desired sample size for the study. The essential focus of descriptive designs is to estimate or profile the characteristics (parameters) of a population of interest. Analytical designs are directed toward testing hypotheses about why certain characteristics or relationships between variables are observed. Experimental studies examine whether a given program or intervention had an intended (or hypothesized) impact. Analytical and experimental designs entail comparisons between groups, often over time, as a basis for exploring the explanations for why an outcome or effect was observed in one situation (for individuals exposed to certain health risks or those randomly assigned to an experimental group) but not in others (among unexposed individuals or members of the control group).

The discussion that follows provides a general overview of the sample size estimation process as well as formulae and examples for common designs and types of estimates. Formulae for other types of designs, tables of sample sizes based on these computations, and computer software for determining sample sizes under certain study designs and assumptions are readily available (for example, see Borenstein & Cohen, 1988; Cohen, 1988; Dean, et al., 1994; Kraemer & Thiemann, 1987; Lemeshow, Hosmer, Klar, & Lwanga, 1990; Lipsey, 1990; Lwanga & Lemeshow, 1991). Lemeshow, Hosmer, Klar, and Lwanga (1990) and Lipsey (1990) were the principal sources for the formulae for computing sample sizes used in Tables 7.1a, 7.1b, and 7.3. The logic and rationale for estimating required sample sizes must be clearly understood, regardless of the specific technologies used in deriving them. Exhibit 7.1 compares the major steps and criteria to use in estimating the sample size for descriptive and analytical or experimental designs.

Computing the Sample Size for Descriptive Studies

A sample is used as a basis for estimating the unknown characteristics of the population from which it is drawn. The standard error is a measure of the variation in the estimate of interest (for example, the proportion of low-income minority women who had seen a doctor during the first trimester of their pregnancy or the mean number of visits for prenatal care overall) *across* all possible random samples of a certain size that could theoretically be drawn from the target population or universe (women living in a particular community). The estimates for all the samples that could (hypothetically) be drawn can be plotted and expressed as a *sampling distribution* of those estimates. As the size of the samples on which the estimates are based increases, sampling theory suggests that this distribution will take on a particular form, called a *normal sampling distribution* (see Figure 7.1).

If the means of all possible simple random samples of a certain size that could be theoretically drawn from a population were averaged, the result would equal the actual mean (μ) for the population as a whole. The standard error (SE) is the standard deviation (or amount of variation on average) of all the possible sample means from this population mean. The greater the variation in the population mean from sample to sample, that is, the larger the standard error associated with this distribution of sample values, the less reliable the estimate can be said to be.

Standard errors may be high because (1) there is a great deal of variation in the elements of the population being studied (wide variations in whether different subgroups go for prenatal care, for example) or (2) the size of the sample used is too small to obtain consistent results when different samples of this size are drawn. Knowing that the distribution of values for all possible samples drawn from a population is theoretically going to take on the shape of a normal sampling

FIGURE 7.1. NORMAL SAMPLING DISTRIBUTION.

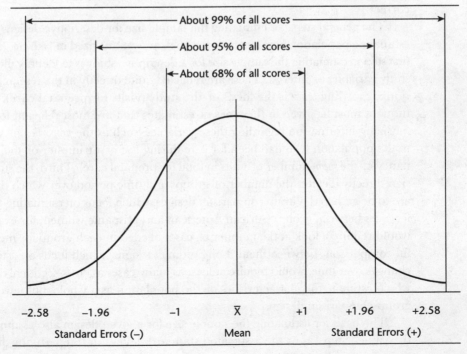

distribution is useful in making inferences about a population from sample data. As Figure 7.1 indicates, for a normal sampling distribution 68 percent of the sample means obtained from all possible random samples of the same size will fall within the range of values designated by plus or minus 1.00 standard error of the population mean, 95 percent will fall within plus or minus 1.96 standard errors, and 99 percent within plus or minus 2.58 standard errors.

In practice, it is not possible to draw all possible samples from a population. Researchers instead draw only one sample, and for large samples they assume a normal sampling distribution of the estimates of interest (percentages and means) and compute the standard error for the estimate from this one sample. Based on the assumption of a normal sampling distribution, they can then estimate the probability of obtaining a particular value for a sample mean by chance, given certain characteristics (mean, variance) of the population.

Some values (those at the ends or tails of the normal distribution) would rarely occur—only 5 percent of the time, for example, for values further than two standard errors from a hypothesized population mean. If the estimate obtained in the study falls at these extreme ends of the distribution, researchers could conclude that the hypothesized population mean was probably not the true value given the small chance of its being found for a sample drawn from that population if the hypothesis were true. Ninety-five percent of the time this assumption would be correct.

The general steps for estimating the sample size for descriptive designs, where estimating population parameters is the goal, are summarized in Exhibit 7.1. The first step in estimating the sample size for a descriptive study is to identify the major study variables of interest. These are reflected quite directly in the research questions regarding *what* is the focus of the study (visits for prenatal care). Then, thought must be given to the types of estimates that are most relevant for summarizing information regarding these variables (such as the *proportion* of women in the population who had been for care during the first trimester of their pregnancy or the *mean* number of visits in total for prenatal care). Third, the study design directly dictates the number of groups and time period over which the data are to be gathered. Group comparison designs, which focus on estimating the differences between groups (African American and Hispanic women, for example), would require a look at the number of cases needed in each group for meaningful comparisons between them. Longitudinal designs, which focus on estimated changes over time, would require at least as many cases as cross-sectional designs, which estimate the characteristics of the population as a whole, but fewer than group-comparison designs.

The basis for estimating the sample size for a given design also assumes that the value (Step 4a) or the associated standard deviation (Step 4b) for the esti-

EXHIBIT 7.1. CRITERIA FOR ESTIMATING
THE SAMPLE SIZE BASED ON THE STUDY DESIGN.

Design:	Descriptive	Design:	Analytical or Experimental

Objective: To estimate a parameter.

Framework: Sampling distribution

Steps:

1. Identify the major study variables.

2. Determine the types of estimates of study variables, such as means or proportions.

3. Select the population or subgroups of interest (based on study objectives and design).

4a. Indicate what you expect the population value to be.

4b. Estimate the standard deviation of the estimate.

5. Decide on a desired level of confidence in the estimate (confidence interval).

6. Decide on a tolerable range of error in the estimate (precision).

7. Compute sample size, based on study assumptions.

Objective: To test a hypothesis.

Framework: Power analysis

Steps:

1. Identify the major study hypotheses.

2. Determine the statistical tests for the study hypotheses, such as a t-test, F-test, or chi-square test.

3. Select the population or subgroups of interest (based on study hypotheses and design).

4a. Indicate what you expect the hypothesized difference (Δ) to be.

4b. Estimate the standard deviation (σ) of the difference.

4c. Compute the effect size (Δ/σ).

5. Decide on a tolerable level of error in rejecting the null hypothesis when it is *true* (alpha).

6. Decide on a desired level of power for rejecting the null hypothesis when it is *false* (power).

7. Compute sample size, based on study assumptions.

---

mate of interest can be specified or obtained. The next steps entail deciding on the level of confidence (Step 5) the investigator would want to associate with the range of values that may contain the true population value (parameter) as well as what would be the desired level of precision (or deviation) around the estimates that are derived from a sample of a specified size (Step 6).

Table 7.1a provides the specific formulae and examples of sample size estimation for a number of common descriptive designs and types of estimates.

Design—Cross-Sectional (One Group), Estimate—Proportion

The investigator might estimate that around half (P = .50 = 50 percent) of the women in the study population are likely to go for prenatal care during the first trimester. It might be deemed reasonable to report an estimate that is precise

TABLE 7.1A. SAMPLE SIZE ESTIMATION—
DESCRIPTIVE STUDIES: SELECTED EXAMPLES.

Design and estimates	Formula	Example
Cross-Sectional (One Group)		
Proportion	$$n = \frac{z^2_{1-\alpha/2}P(1-P)}{d^2}$$ where, P = estimated proportion d = desired precision	$$n = \frac{1.96^2 \times (.50)(.50)}{(.05)^2} = 384$$
Mean	$$n = \frac{z^2_{1-\alpha/2}\sigma^2}{d^2}$$ where, σ = estimated standard deviation d = desired precision	$$n = \frac{1.96^2 \times (2.5^2)}{1^2} = 24$$
Group-Comparison (Two Groups)		
Proportion	$$n = \frac{z^2_{1-\alpha/2}[P_1(1-P_1)+P_2(1-P_2)]}{d^2}$$ where, P_1 = estimated proportion (larger) P_2 = estimated proportion (smaller) d = desired precision	$$n = \frac{1.96^2[(.70)(.30)+(.50)(.50)]}{.05^2} = 707$$
Mean	$$n = \frac{z^2_{1-\alpha/2}[2\sigma^2]}{d^2}$$ where, σ = estimated standard deviation (assumed to be equal for each group) d = desired precision	$$n = \frac{1.96^2[2 \times (2.5^2)]}{1^2} = 48$$

Note:

$Z_{1-\alpha/2}$ = *standard errors* associated with *confidence intervals*:

1.00	68%
1.645	90%
1.96	95%
2.58	99%

Source: Lemeshow, Hosmer, Klar, and Lwanga, 1990.

within plus or minus 5 percent of this value (desired precision, d = .05), that is, 50 percent of the women in the study population plus or minus 5 percent (45 percent to 55 percent) visited a doctor during the first trimester. These estimates should, however, be based on previous research or knowledge of the study population. An example with .50 as the estimate is used here because a .50/.50 split in the proportion who did/did not have a characteristic tends to yield the largest sample size requirements.

As seen in Figure 7.1, the researcher could be confident that 95 percent of the time the sample estimates will fall within 1.96 standard errors $(Z_{1-\alpha/2})$ of the specified population value, if it were the true value. The standard error for a proportion is

$$SE_p = \quad P(1-P)/n \quad \textit{where,} \ P = \text{estimate of proportion}$$
$$\text{in the population}$$

The precision (d = .05), or tolerable deviation of values around the estimate, can be expressed in terms of units of standard errors $[d = (z_{1-\alpha/2}(SE_p)]$. The formula for expressing the desired precision in units of standard errors essentially serves as the basis for deriving (or solving for) the sample size (n) needed to produce this acceptable range of error at a given level of confidence:

$$d = z_{1-\alpha/2}(SE_p) \qquad \textit{where,} \ d = .05 = 1.96 \times SE_p, \text{ when } \alpha = .05$$
$$d = z_{1-\alpha/2}[\quad P(1-P)/n]$$
$$d^2 = z^2_{1-\alpha/2} P(1-P)/n$$
$$n = z^2_{1-\alpha/2} P(1-P)/d^2$$

In the example in Table 7.1a, 384 cases are needed to estimate that the population value is .50 plus or minus .05 with a 95 percent level of confidence if the sample estimate is between .45 and .55.

In Table 7.1b, selected other examples of the sample sizes required to estimate a proportion with a desired level of precision based on the formula for a cross-sectional (one-group) design and assuming a 95 percent level of confidence are provided. The number of cases required increases as the proportion begins to approach .50 (meaning that the sample divides fairly evenly on the estimate or characteristic of interest) and the desired level of precision (the tightness of the allowable range around the estimate) is made more stringent (smaller) (Marks, 1982).

TABLE 7.1B. SAMPLE SIZE ESTIMATION—DESCRIPTIVE STUDIES: SELECTED EXAMPLES.

Estimated Proportion (P)	Desired Precision (d)									
	.01	.02	.03	.04	.05	.06	.07	.08	.09	.10
.01	381	96	43	24	16	11	8	6	5	4
.02	753	189	84	48	31	21	16	12	10	8
.03	1118	280	125	70	45	32	23	18	14	12
.04	1476	369	164	93	60	41	31	24	19	15
.05	1825	457	203	115	73	51	38	29	23	19
.06	2167	542	241	135	87	61	45	34	27	22
.07	2501	626	278	157	101	70	52	40	31	26
.08	2828	707	315	177	114	79	58	45	35	29
.09	3147	787	350	197	126	88	65	50	39	32
.10	3458	865	385	217	139	97	71	55	43	35
.15	4899	1225	545	307	196	137	100	77	61	49
.20	6147	1537	683	385	246	171	126	97	76	62
.25	7203	1801	801	451	289	201	148	113	89	73
.30	8068	2017	897	505	323	225	165	127	100	81
.35	8740	2185	972	547	350	243	179	137	108	88
.40	9220	2305	1025	577	369	257	189	145	114	93
.45	9508	2377	1057	595	381	265	195	149	118	96
.50	9605	2402	1068	601	384	267	197	151	119	97

Note: Design—Cross-sectional (one group); estimate—proportion; confidence interval—95 percent. See formula for this design in Table 7.1a, on which the computations of the sample sizes in this table are based.

Design—Cross-Sectional (One Group), Estimate—Mean

The investigators might also be interested in estimating the average number of visits women had during their pregnancy to within plus or minus one visit ($d = 1$). The projected numbers of visits for prenatal care may range from zero to ten, with some women not expected to go at all and others having as many as ten visits. The standard error for the sample mean is

$$SE_M = \sigma / \sqrt{n} \qquad \textit{where, } \sigma = \text{standard deviation of variable in the population}$$

The basis for deriving the desired n to yield this precision with a given level of confidence parallels that used in estimating the sample size for proportions:

$$d = z_{1-\alpha/2}(SE_m) \qquad \textit{where, } d = 1 = 1.96 \times SE_m, \text{ when } \alpha = .05$$
$$d = z_{1-\alpha/2}\sigma / \sqrt{n}$$
$$d^2 = z^2_{1-\alpha/2}\sigma^2/n$$
$$n = z^2_{1-\alpha/2}\sigma^2/d^2$$

The standard deviation (σ) for the variable of interest will not necessarily be known in advance of doing the study. However, it may be estimated from previously published research and pilot tests or pretests with the target population or related groups. It may also be estimated using the range of likely answers, that is, by dividing the expected range (ten) by four (to reflect the four quartiles of a distribution) to yield an estimated standard deviation of 2.5 for this particular estimate (Marks, 1982).

Applying the formula for estimating the sample size for means in the example in Table 7.1a, twenty-four cases are needed to estimate the number of visits (plus or minus one visit), with a 95 percent level of confidence assuming a standard deviation of 2.5.

Design—Group Comparison (Two Groups), Estimate—Proportion

The researchers may also be interested in having an adequate number of observations to estimate the differences in the proportions (who went for care) for different groups (Hispanic and African American women, for example). Based on knowledge of the subgroups of interest or previous research, they may assume that only 50 percent of Hispanic women will go for prenatal care in the first trimester compared with 70 percent of African American women—a 20 percent difference. The researchers would like to be able to detect this magnitude of difference within a reasonable range of variability (d = .05, or .20 +/− .05 = a range of .15 to .25) with 95 percent confidence.

In estimating the sample size required for estimating differences in the proportions, the standard errors of the proportions for both groups (P_1 and P_2) must be taken into account (see the example in Table 7.1a). The sample size is then obtained using the following formula:

$$n = z^2_{1-\sigma/2}[P_1(1-P_1)] + P_2(1-P_2)]/d^2$$

In the example in Table 7.1a, 707 cases are needed in *each* group to detect a difference of 20 percent between the groups with a 95 percent level of confidence.

Design—Group Comparison (Two Groups), Estimate—Mean

The researcher may also assume that the average numbers of prenatal care visits are likely to differ for Hispanic and African American women in the target community. They would like to be able to estimate this difference with a reasonable level of precision (d = 1 visit) and confidence (95 percent). The formula for estimating the sample size for group-comparison designs is comparable to that for the one-group case, but it uses the combined (or pooled) standard deviation $(2\sigma^2)$ for the two groups:

$$n = z^2_{1-\alpha/2} \, [2\sigma^2]/d^2$$

In this particular example, the standard deviation (σ) for the means for the respective groups is assumed to be the same (2.5). Based on this formula, in the example in Table 7.1a at least forty-eight cases would be needed in *each* group to estimate a difference between the groups to within plus or minus one visit at a 95 percent level of confidence assuming a standard deviation of 2.5 for the sample mean for each group.

Tables for estimating the sample sizes for the types of estimates and designs summarized in Table 7.1a are available in Lemeshow, Hosmer, Klar, and Lwanga (1990) and Lwanga and Lemeshow (1991).

Computing the Sample Size for Analytical and Experimental Studies

Whereas descriptive studies focus on *what* the characteristics (or parameters) of a population are, analytic and experimental studies attempt to understand *why*. They are concerned with testing hypotheses derived from theory or practice regarding the relationship between or impact of certain variables (such as attitudes and knowledge regarding prenatal care or interventions to enhance pregnant women's access to services) on others (the appropriate use of prenatal care).

The theory or assumptions underlying these types of studies generally predict that there will be a statistical association between the variables or significant differences between groups being compared on a characteristic of interest. To set up a statistical basis for testing these assumptions, two types of hypotheses are stated: a *null hypothesis* (Ho) and an *alternative* (or research) *hypothesis* (Ha). The null hypothesis essentially states that there is no association between the variables or differences between groups. The alternative hypothesis states the associations or differences that are expected if the first hypothesis (of no difference) is rejected. The latter more directly mirrors the theoretical or substantive assumptions on which the study is based.

The likelihood of rejecting the null hypothesis is greater the stronger the relationship between variables (knowledge of risks during pregnancy and prenatal care use) or the greater the differences between groups (Hispanic and African American women) that actually exist. However, these relationships can be very difficult to demonstrate empirically if a large amount of sampling or measurement error characterizes the data gathered to test the hypotheses. From a sampling point of view, the key concern is having a large enough number of cases to minimize the variable sampling (standard) error in the estimates. As discussed earlier in this chapter and displayed directly in the standard error formula $[SE = \sigma/\sqrt{n}]$, sampling error can be reduced by increasing the sample size (denominator) or minimizing the random errors in the data collection process (reducing the numerator, either by enhancing the reliability of study measures or by adapting or standardizing the interviewing and data collection process). A larger sample size would be required if the differences to be detected are small (but nonetheless substantively significant) and the random errors around the estimates large.

Table 7.2 displays the likely outcomes of the hypothesis-testing process, which parallels sensitivity and specificity analysis in evaluating the validity of alternative screening procedures (see Chapter Three). In reality, either the null hypothesis (Ho) *or* the alternative hypothesis (Ha) is true, but not both. Inaccuracies and imprecision in the data gathering process could nonetheless result in a failure to empirically confirm the underlying empirical reality.

A Type I error results from falsely *rejecting* the null hypothesis when the hypothesis is actually *true*. Type I error is reflected in the significance level (α) used for delineating values that are very unlikely if the population estimate is a given value (μ) but are nonetheless still possible. The probability of *not rejecting* the null hypothesis when it is *true*, that is, the sample estimate appears within a reasonable range of frequently appearing values given that the hypothesized population parameters are true, is reflected in the confidence interval ($1-\alpha$) set around this estimate.

Type II error (β) refers to the reverse error: *failing to reject* the null hypothesis when it is actually *false*. This type of error becomes particularly critical to consider

TABLE 7.2. TYPE I AND TYPE II ERRORS.

Sample	Population	
	Group 1 & 2 differ (Ho is not true)	Group 1 & 2 do not differ (Ho is true)
Significant difference (reject Ho)	Correct conclusion Probability = $1 - \beta$ (power) (*true +*)	Type I error Probability = α (alpha) (*false +*)
No significant difference (do *not* reject Ho)	Type II error Probability = β (beta) (*false −*)	Correct conclusion Probability = $1 - \alpha$ (confidence) (*true −*)

when differences are assumed to exist but are very small or the errors around the estimates are large. Each alternative hypothesis has a different probability of being accepted or rejected as a function of the differences and errors that are assumed for each. This presents special challenges in thinking through the substantively meaningful relationships that can be affordably detected. The lower the likelihood of a Type II error (β), that is, the less likely one is mistakenly to fail to reject the null hypothesis, the greater the power ($1-\beta$) of the test is said to be. The probability of both Type I and Type II errors decreases as the sample size increases, primarily because the estimates obtained from larger samples are more reliable (have less random sampling variation).

Approaches to estimating sample sizes required to test hypotheses meaningfully require a specification of the null and alternative hypotheses, the expected values for the key estimates as well as the likely sampling variability around them, and suitable levels of significance and power. A widely used convention is to set the significance level at 5 percent ($\alpha=.05$) and power at 80 percent ($1-\beta =.80$), although these may certainly be varied, depending on the desired trade-offs in terms of the respective types of errors (Type I and Type II error), as well as costs.

The alternative hypotheses (Ha) may be stated as either a one-tailed or two-tailed option. One-tailed hypotheses state that associations or differences between groups are likely to be in a certain direction (one group will have more or fewer visits for prenatal care than another, that is, Ha: $\mu_1<\mu_2$). Two-tailed tests simply state that the groups are not the same or equal (Ha: $\mu_1\neq\mu_2$), but they do not dictate the direction of the difference. The sample size requirements for one-tailed hypotheses (based on tests for differences in one direction) are lower than for two-tailed tests (that test for differences in both directions). A one-tailed test is recommended when one has a large measure of confidence in the likely direction of a difference because of a logical or biological impossibility of it being otherwise or because of knowledge of previous research in the area.

In experimental designs, there is a particular interest in detecting the effect (or difference) between experimental and control groups. The effect size (Δ/σ), which essentially reflects the hypothesized difference (Δ) between groups, standardized (adjusted) for the average (or pooled) variation (σ) between groups, provides a basis for calculating the sample size for these types of designs (Cohen, 1988; Lipsey, 1990). This method may also be used in estimating the sample size requirements for analytical designs.

The general steps for estimating the sample size for analytical and experimental designs are summarized in Exhibit 7.1. The first step entails stating the primary null (Ho) and alternative (Ha) hypotheses to be tested. The second and third steps dictate consideration of the statistical procedure to be used in testing the study hypotheses, based on the types of estimates (means, proportions, odds ratios) being considered (Step 2) and the underlying design (such as an analytical group-comparison, case-control, or experimental design) on which the study is based (Step 3). These steps directly dictate the types of analysis it is most appropriate to conduct given the hypotheses and associated design: a t-test or analysis of variance (ANOVA) tests of the differences between means or a chi-square test of differences between proportions between two groups in analytic group-comparison or experimental designs, or the computation of an odds ratio for case-control studies, for example (see Chapter Fifteen).

The fourth step entails providing specific hypothetical values for the estimates of interest (means, proportions, or odds ratios), the likely sampling variation in each, and the computation of the effect size when this approach is to be used in estimating the required sample size. For some estimates (proportions and odds ratios), the sampling variability is implicitly computed in the formulae or approaches used in deriving the sample size estimates and for others (means), this would have to be estimated from previous studies or from the range of the distribution of values on the variable (described earlier).

Steps 5 and 6 entail setting reasonable levels of Type I error and power for economically detecting hypothesized differences.

Table 7.3 provides the specific formulae and examples of sample size estimation for a number of common analytical or experimental designs and types of estimates. Tables for estimating the sample sizes derived from the formulae provided here for analytical designs are available in Lemeshow, Hosmer, Klar, and Lwanga (1990) and Lwanga and Lemeshow (1991). The approach to effect size estimation for experimental designs is principally derived from Cohen (1988); Kraemer and Thiemann (1987); and Lipsey (1990). Selected charts from Lipsey, on which the power analysis for the examples of experimental designs is based, are reproduced in Figure 7.2.

Design—Group Comparison (Two Groups), Ho: P_1-P_2 = 0

The investigators may have specific hypotheses in mind with respect to likely differences between groups (Hispanics and African Americans) in the proportion (of women) who went for (prenatal) care. The first example in Table 7.3 demonstrates two approaches to estimating the sample size required to test alternative hypotheses regarding the magnitude of these differences, assuming a certain power (80 percent) and Type I error or level of significance (.05): (1) a computational formula and (2) effect size estimation.

The example assumes an alternative hypothesis (Ha: P_1-$P_2 \neq 0$) in which P_1 = .70 and P_2 = .50. To solve the equation, these estimates (.70, .50), their average $[(P_1 + P_2)/2 = (.70 + .50)/2 = .60]$, and the standard errors (z) associated with

TABLE 7.3. SAMPLE SIZE ESTIMATION—ANALYTICAL AND EXPERIMENTAL STUDIES: SELECTED EXAMPLES.

Design and Hypothesis	Formula	Example

Group Comparison (Two Groups)

Ho: $P_1 - P_2 = 0$
Ha: $P_1 - P_2 \neq 0$

Formula

$$n = \frac{\{z_{1-\alpha/2}\sqrt{2\bar{P}(1-\bar{P})} + z_{1-\beta}\sqrt{P_1(1-P_1) + P_2(1-P_2)}\}^2}{(P_1 - P_2)^2}$$

where,

$\bar{P} = (P_1 + P_2)/2$
P_1 = estimated proportion (larger)
P_2 = estimated proportion (smaller)

Effect size

$ESp = \phi_1 - \phi_2$

where,

ESp = effect size for proportions
ϕ_1, ϕ_2 = arcsine transformation for proportions (groups 1,2)

Example

$$n = \frac{\{1.96\sqrt{2(.60)(.40)} + .842\sqrt{[(.70)(.30) + (.50)(.50)]}\}^2}{(.70 - .50)^2}$$

$n = 93$

$ESp = 1.982 - 1.571 = .411$

$n = 93$
(see Figure 7.2)

Group Comparison (Two Groups)

Ho: $\mu_1 = \mu_2$
Ha: $\mu_1 \neq \mu_2$

Formula

$$n = \frac{2\sigma^2[z_{1-\alpha/2} + z_{1-\beta}]^2}{(\mu_1 - \mu_2)^2}$$

where,

σ = estimated standard deviation (assumed to be equal for each group)
μ_1 = estimated mean (larger)
μ_2 = estimated mean (smaller)

Effect size

$ES\mu = \dfrac{\mu_1 - \mu_2}{\sigma}$

where,

$ES\mu$ = effect size for means
μ_1, μ_2 = estimated means (groups 1,2)
σ = pooled standard deviation

$\sigma = \sqrt{\dfrac{\sigma_1^2 + \sigma_2^2}{2}}$

Example

$$n = \frac{2(2.5)^2[1.96 + .842]^2}{(6-4)^2}$$

$n = 25$

$ES\mu = \dfrac{6-4}{2.5} = .80$

$n = 25$
(see Figure 7.2)

Case Control
Ho: OR = 1
Ha: OR ≠ 1

Formula

$$n = \frac{\{z_{1-\alpha/2}\sqrt{2\overline{P^*_2}(1-\overline{P^*_2})} + z_{1-\beta}\sqrt{\overline{P^*_1}(1-\overline{P^*_1})+\overline{P^*_2}(1-\overline{P^*_2})}\}^2}{(P^*_1 - P^*_2)^2}$$

where,

(NOTE: "*" here and above refers to proportion (P*) exposed in case-control design.)

P^*_1 = proportion exposed in cases, i.e.,

$$= \frac{(OR)P^*_2}{(OR)P^*_2 + (1-P^*_2)}$$

P^*_2 = proportion exposed in controls

OR = odds ratio

$$n = \frac{\{1.960\sqrt{2 \times 0.3 \times 0.7} + 0.842\sqrt{0.4615 \times 0.5385 + 0.3 \times 0.7}\}^2}{(0.4615-0.3)^2}$$

n = 130

where,

(NOTE: "x" here and above refers to multiplication of terms or "multiplied by").

$P^*_1 = 2 \times 0.3/[2 \times 0.3 + 0.7] = 0.4615$

$P^*_2 = .30$

OR = 2

Note:

$Z_{1-\alpha/2}$ = *standard errors associated with confidence intervals:*

1.00	68%
1.645	90%
1.96	95%
2.58	99%

$Z_{1-\beta}$ = *standard errors associated with power:*

.524	70%
.842	80%
1.282	90%
1.645	95%
2.326	99%

Sources: Lemeshow, Hosmer, Klar, and Lwanga, 1980; Lipsey, 1990.

FIGURE 7.2. SELECTED RESOURCES FOR POWER ANALYSIS.

A. Arcsine Transformations (φ) for Proportions (P)

P	φ	P	φ	P	φ	P	φ
.01	.200	.26	1.070	.51	1.591	.76	2.118
.02	.284	.27	1.093	.52	1.611	.77	2.141
.03	.348	.28	1.115	.53	1.631	.78	2.165
.04	.403	.29	1.137	.54	1.651	.79	2.190
.05	.451	.30	1.159	.55	1.671	.80	2.214
.06	.495	.31	1.181	.56	1.691	.81	2.240
.07	.536	.32	1.203	.57	1.711	.82	2.265
.08	.574	.33	1.224	.58	1.731	.83	2.292
.09	.609	.34	1.245	.59	1.752	.84	2.319
.10	.644	.35	1.266	.60	1.772	.85	2.346
.11	.676	.36	1.287	.61	1.793	.86	2.375
.12	.707	.37	1.308	.62	1.813	.87	2.404
.13	.738	.38	1.328	.63	1.834	.88	2.434
.14	.767	.39	1.349	.64	1.855	.89	2.465
.15	.795	.40	1.369	.65	1.875	.90	2.498
.16	.823	.41	1.390	.66	1.897	.91	2.532
.17	.850	.42	1.410	.67	1.918	.92	2.568
.18	.876	.43	1.430	.68	1.939	.93	2.606
.19	.902	.44	1.451	.69	1.961	.94	2.647
.20	.927	.45	1.471	.70	1.982	.95	2.691
.21	.952	.46	1.491	.71	2.004	.96	2.739
.22	.976	.47	1.511	.72	2.026	.97	2.793
.23	1.000	.48	1.531	.73	2.049	.98	2.858
.24	1.024	.49	1.551	.74	2.071	.99	2.941
.25	1.047	.50	1.571	.75	2.094		

B. Power Chart for σ = .05, Two tailed or σ = .025, One-Tailed

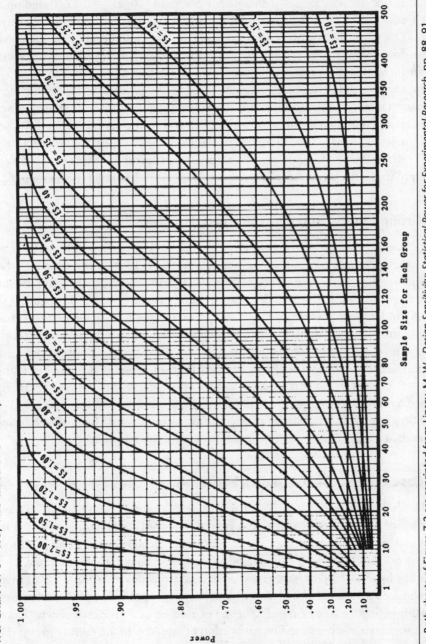

Source: Both charts of Figure 7.2 are reprinted from Lipsey, M. W., *Design Sensitivity: Statistical Power for Experimental Research,* pp. 88, 91, copyright © 1990 by Sage Publications, Inc. Reprinted by permission of Sage Publications, Inc.

a designated confidence interval and power must be specified. For a 95 percent confidence interval, $z_{1-\alpha/2} = 1.96$ and for power of .80, $z_{1-\beta} = .842$. Based on the first example in Table 7.3, around ninety-three cases are needed in each group.

The effect size for proportions is estimated by the differences in the arcsine transformations of the respective proportions. Figure 7.2a provides the arcsine transformations for proportions (arcsine of .70 = 1.982; arcsine of .50 = 1.571). The resulting difference in the estimates used in this example (.411) reflects the estimated effect size (ES_p). Figure 7.2b can then be used to estimate the sample size required in each group to obtain a given level of power (say 80 percent) with a significance level of .05. In this particular example the curve for an effect size of .41 crosses the row for a power of .80 (or 80 percent) at a sample of size around ninety-three, thereby confirming the previous results based on the formula.

Design—Group Comparison (Two Groups), Ho: $\mu_1 = \mu_2$

The second example in Table 7.3 assumes an alternative hypothesis (Ha: $\mu_1 \neq \mu_2$) in which μ_1 equals six visits and μ_2 equals four visits. To solve the equation, these estimates, their estimated standard deviations (2.5 for both groups), and the standard errors associated with a designated confidence interval (95 percent, $Z_{1-\alpha/2} = 1.96$) and power (80 percent, $Z_{1-\beta} = .842$) must be specified. Based on the formula using this example, approximately twenty-five cases are needed in each group.

The effect size for means (ES_μ) is based on the difference between the means estimated for each group (6–4) divided by their pooled standard deviation [$\sigma = \sqrt{(\sigma_1^2 + \sigma_2^2)/2} = 2.5$]. The resulting effect size is .80. Using Figure 7.2b once again, the curve for an effect size of .80 crosses the row for a power of .80 (or 80 percent) at a sample size of twenty-five, assuming a .05 level of significance, thereby confirming the previous results based on the formula.

Design—Case Control (Two Groups), Ho: OR=1

The final example in Table 7.2 is based on a case control design in which the alternative hypothesis is that the odds ratio (OR) is not equal to one, meaning that the risk of disease occurrence (hypertension) is greater for the group that has a given risk factor (smokers) compared with those who do not. In this example, smokers are hypothesized to have twice the risk of nonsmokers (OR = 2.0). The hypothesized odds ratio should be based on previously published or clinical research documenting the role of the risk factors of interest as a predictor of who has the disease and who does not. The proportion of smokers in the control group (P^*_2) is estimated to be .30. The proportion of smokers among cases must be derived based on the estimated odds ratio and proportion exposed (smokers) among the controls. The formula requires that these estimated and derived values, as well as the standard errors used to designate the power and significance level, be entered (Lemeshow, Hosmer, Klar, & Lwanga, 1990, pp. 19–20).

In this example, 130 cases and an equivalent number of controls are needed to detect an odds ratio of 2.0, assuming 30 percent of the controls and 46 percent of the cases are smokers, and power of 80 percent and a significance level of .05.

Computing the Design Effect for the Sample

The size of the sampling errors is also affected by the design of the sample itself. The variances (the standard deviations squared) of estimates obtained from stratified or cluster sample-based designs generally differ from those based on a simple random sample. The ratio of the variance of the complex sample (VAR_{cs}) to that of a simple random sample (VAR_{srs}) is used to quantify the design effect (DEFF) of a specific sample design (Kalton, 1983): $DEFF = (VAR_{cs})/(VAR_{srs})$.

A design effect of 1.3, for example, means that the variance for any estimate based on the sample is 30 percent higher than that derived from a simple random sample. This would reflect a design in which there is some cluster sampling involved. To adjust for the design effect in computing standard errors for more complex sample designs, the standard errors of a given estimate (50 percent) can be computed by means of the formula for a simple random sample (5 percent for a sample of one hundred cases) and then multiplied by the square root of the design effect (1.3). This will result in a standard error of the estimate ($5 \times 1.3 = 5.7$), which more appropriately reflects the complex sample design used in the study.

In a stratified design, cases are drawn from all the strata into which the population has been divided. The standard error for a stratified sample is based on the weighted average of the standard errors *within* each stratum. There will, in fact, be less diversity within each of these relatively homogeneous strata than across the sample as a whole. The net result of taking the weighted average of the standard errors of these relatively homogeneous strata is that the standard errors for a stratified design will be less than those that result from a simple random sample of the same population.

In contrast to a stratified sample, with a cluster design only a sample of clusters is drawn from all the clusters into which the population has been divided. The computation of the standard errors for a cluster design is based on a weighted average of the standard errors *between* the clusters selected for the sample. The more internally homogeneous (or correlated) the cases *within* the respective clusters, the more heterogeneous the means *between* clusters are likely to be. The net result of taking the weighted average of the standard errors *between* relatively homogeneous clusters, then, is that the standard errors for a cluster design will be higher than those based on a simple random sample of the same population. The design effects associated with cluster-type designs may result in their standard errors being two or three times greater than those of a simple random sample.

Most complex survey designs involve combinations of simple random samples and stratified and cluster-type sampling approaches. These designs may also include differential weighting of the sample elements. The design effect for these types of designs—the ratio of the variances on key estimates for the particular sample to that of a simple random sample—will lie somewhere between that of pure stratified and pure cluster-type sample designs.

Statistical procedures have been developed to estimate the standard errors or variances and, from them, the design effects for certain types of sample designs. These procedures include *balanced repeated replication, jackknife repeated replication,* and *Taylor series approximation.* Lee, Forthofer, and Lorimor (1986, 1989) provide an overview of these three alternatives to the analysis of complex sample survey data with particular reference to several large-scale health surveys. These procedures are available in standard software packages to facilitate the computation of relevant design effects. The packages that have been most widely available to general users include SUDAAN (Research Triangle Institute, N.C.); PC–CARP (Department of Statistics, Iowa State University, Ames, Iowa); the CSAMPLE procedure within EPI–INFO, developed for the Centers for Disease Control and Prevention (available from USD, Stone Mountain, Ga.); and WesVarPC (Westat, Inc., Rockville, Md.). In addition, Cohen and his colleagues (Carlson & Cohen, 1991; Carlson, Cohen, & Monheit, 1992; Carlson, Johnson, & Cohen, 1990; Cohen, Burt, & Jones, 1986; Cohen, Xanthopoulos, & Jones, 1988; Cox & Cohen, 1985) have compared the program capabilities, computational efficiencies, and user-friendliness of a number of the standard software packages for computing variances for complex surveys using data from the National Medical Care Expenditure Survey.

Different subgroups and estimates in a study may also have different design effects, principally as a function of the degree of correlation (similarity) within groups that results from sampling clusters of these individuals. Varying design effects for different groups should be taken into account in determining the sample size required for these groups and in adjusting the standard errors of estimates for them during analysis.

Burt and Cohen (1984) have evaluated alternative procedures for estimating the variances, covariances, and associated design effect of variables in a study (the relative variance curve, average relative standard error, and average design effect models) rather than actually running programs to generate design effects for every variable. This reduces the data-processing costs of calculating all these effects directly. Test statistics (such as t-, F-, or chi-square statistics) could be deflated (divided) by an average or estimated design effect as a rough and ready way to accommodate the effects of the complex design on tests of the statistical significance of study findings.

Additional Adjustments in Computing the Sample Size

Once the sample size is computed based on considerations of the study's research questions and design, additional adjustments to this estimated sample size are still needed to assure that the desired target number of cases is obtained (see Table 7.4).

Step 1. Adjust for the Estimated Sample Design Effect

The sample sizes resulting from the computations described in Exhibit 7.1 assume that the sample design is a simple or systematic random sample. If this is not the case, it will be necessary to estimate what the anticipated design effect will be, that is, the impact a more complex design will have on the sampling errors in the survey. Since the actual design effect for a study cannot be computed until after the data are collected, it has to be approximated by examining the design effects for comparable estimates in other studies. The sample size estimate is then multiplied by this factor

TABLE 7.4. ADDITIONAL ADJUSTMENTS IN COMPUTING THE SAMPLE SIZE.

Criteria	Example
1. Adjust for the estimated sample design effect.	DEFF = 1.3 *therefore* $n = 384 \times 1.3 = 499$
2. Adjust for the expected response rate.	Response rate = 80% *therefore* $n = 499 \div .80 = 624$
3. Adjust for the expected proportion of eligibles.	% Eligible = 90% *therefore* $n = 624 \div .90 = 693$
4. Compute survey costs.	Cost/case = $50 *therefore* Total cost = $693 \times \$50 = \$34,650$

Note: This example assumes a beginning sample size of 384, based on the study objectives.

to increase the size of the sample, since the "effective" sample size will be smaller, given the complex nature of the design. Multiplying the 384 cases derived for the first example in Table 7.1a by an estimated design effect of 1.3 (for a design involving some cluster sampling, such as a random digit dialing survey that entails oversampling of selected groups) yields an estimate of 499 cases. This number of cases adjusts for the fact that the design will not be a simple random sample.

Step 2. Adjust for the Expected Response Rate

The next step involves dividing the sample size derived from the preceding steps by the estimated response rate for the study. By thus inflating the number of cases, the investigator adjusts for the fact that a certain proportion of the sample will not respond. An 80 percent response rate is assumed for the example in Table 7.4 (499/.80 = 624 cases).

Step 3. Adjust for the Expected Proportion of Eligibles

This step is similar to the preceding one in that the number of cases derived in Step 2 is divided by the expected portion of cases that will be found actually to be eligible for the survey once they are contacted. The estimated figure here is around 90 percent of the cases (624/.90 = 693 cases). This may be realistic for a list sample survey, in which 10 percent of the individuals are deceased or have moved out of the area since the list was compiled. It would be much lower (25 percent, for example) for a random digit dialing survey, in which a large number of randomly generated phone numbers (say, 2,500) may have to be called to find working residential numbers. The number that must be generated initially (original sample n) in this case would be 624/.25 = 2,496.

Step 4. Compute Survey Costs

This series of steps can be repeated for the major estimates being considered in the analyses, the resulting range of sample sizes reviewed, the costs per case estimated, and the final sample size determined. This last decision is made on the basis of the number of cases it would be ideal to have, whether this number fits with the study budget, and what compromises might have to be made to match the design to the dollars available for the survey.

The results of the computations in Table 7.4 suggest that approximately 700 (693) cases are required to have 95 percent confidence that the hypothesis that about half (50 percent) of the women in the target population went for prenatal care in the first trimester is true, should the value for the sample drawn from the community fall anywhere in the range of 45 percent to 55 percent. The cost per case, assuming the interview is conducted by telephone, is $50. Approximately $35,000 would then be required to carry out the survey.

Calculation of Response Rate

An important approach to evaluating the implementation of a particular sample design is the level of success in actually contacting and collecting information from the individuals or elements to be included in the study. This involves calculating a *response rate* (RR)—the percent or proportion of the cases eligible for the survey with whom interviews or questionnaires were actually completed: $RR=(C/n_{eligible})$ (Kviz, 1977; Hidiroglou, Drew, & Gray, 1993). As will be discussed in the following section, some of the cases that were originally selected for the sample may turn out to be ineligible for a variety of reasons and can therefore legitimately be excluded from the denominator in computing the final response rate.

Table 7.5 portrays the basic elements to be used in computing an overall response rate for area probability, random digit dialing, and list samples. It draws upon the case studies of these different types of sample designs that were described earlier, as well as upon the hypothetical sample of 693 cases derived in Table 7.4.

1. Original Sample Size

The first item of information to consider in computing an overall response rate for a survey is the size of the original sample—the total number of elements originally included in the study—which is 693 cases in this example.

2. Known Ineligible Units

From the original sample are subtracted the elements found ineligible for the survey as the study proceeds ($n = 64$). In area probability samples, this would include housing units that are verified to be unoccupied; households such as businesses or institutional housing that do not fit the criteria of being private residences and are excluded from the definition of the universe; and households that do not fit some screening criterion relevant for the study, such as having family incomes below a certain level or elderly persons living there. For telephone surveys, phone numbers generated through a random digit dialing process that are found to be nonworking numbers or business phones when called would be deemed ineligible. In list samples of individuals, persons who had died by the time of the survey or, if appropriate, moved outside the area encompassed in the study's target population would be declared ineligible and deleted from the denominator in computing the response rate.

TABLE 7.5. CALCULATION OF RESPONSE RATE.

Elements in Response Rate	Type of Sample Design			Example
	Area Probability	Random Digit Dialing	List	
1. Original Sample Size	No. of housing units	No. of assigned phone numbers	No. of elements on list	693
less Ineligible Units				
2. *Known*	Unoccupied unit Institutional housing Doesn't fit screening criteria	Nonworking number Nonresidential number Doesn't fit screening criteria	Deceased Moved outside area Doesn't fit screening criteria Duplicate listings	64
3. *Unknown* (estimate based on proportion of known ineligibles)	Never home	Ring/no answer/ machine Line busy	Moved/no forwarding address	5 ___
equal 4. Eligible Units				624
less 5. Noninterviews	Refusal Break off Too ill (in hospital) Senility/physical problem Language barrier Away for entire field period Never home (estimate)	Refusal Break off Too ill (in hospital) Senility/physical problem Language barrier Ring/no answer/ machine (estimate) Line busy (estimate)	Not returned Moved/ no forwarding address (estimate)	125 ___
equal 6. Completed Interviews				499 ___

7. Response Rate = $\dfrac{\text{No. of Completed Interviews}}{\text{No. of Eligible Units}} = \dfrac{499}{624} = 80\%$

3. Estimated Ineligible Units

As Table 7.5 indicates, however, a problem in each of these types of sampling procedures is that it is often difficult to determine with certainty whether a particular sampling element is ineligible for the study or not. For example, in area probability samples, if no one is ever home when the interviewer makes repeated visits at different times throughout the field period and he or she is unable to determine from neighbors or a landlord whether the housing unit is occupied, then the eligibility of that particular housing unit for the study may be indeterminate (or unknown). The problem of determining eligibility may be even more of an issue for telephone numbers generated through the random digit dialing process if there is never an answer when certain numbers are dialed or the line is always busy. If eligibility for a list sample is linked to the individual's place of residence, questionnaires returned with no indication of the person's forwarding address will be problematical in determining whether that potential respondent continues to be eligible for the study. In these cases, the researcher will have to develop some decision rule for estimating the number of elements for which eligibility cannot be determined directly.

A criterion that can be used in estimating whether those that *could not* be reached are ineligible is to assume that the proportion who *are not* eligible is comparable to the proportion of those who *could* be reached that *were not* eligible (White, 1983). This proportion can be used in approximating the number of cases with unknown status that should be excluded because they are probably ineligible for the study. There may be biases in using this estimate, however, if those who could not be contacted differed in systematic ways (were older, had lower incomes, and so on) from those who were contacted.

There were 55 cases for which eligibility was not known in the original sample of 693 cases. There were then 638 cases in the sample (693 − 55) for which eligibility was known. Of these 638 cases, 64 (10 percent) were found not to be eligible. Applying this same percent to the 55 cases for whom eligibility was not known directly, we would estimate that 10 percent (or 5) of these cases would not be eligible for the survey. The remaining 50 cases were assumed to be eligible but were not interviewed.

4. Eligible Units

The number resulting from subtracting the number of actual and estimated ineligible units ($n = 69$) from the original sample ($n = 693$) is the number of eligible units for the study ($n = 624$), which constitutes the denominator for computing the study's response rate.

5. Noninterviews

Interviews may not be obtained for a number of reasons. The respondents may refuse to participate in the study or break off the interview once it begins. They may be too ill to participate, have mental or physical limitations, or not be fluent in the language in which the interview is being conducted, which would inhibit or limit their participation in the study. Some people may be away during the entire field period. Those who were never home or those in phone and list sample surveys, for whom eligibility could not be determined for other reasons but were estimated to qualify or be "eligible" ($n = 50$, using the approach discussed above) would be included as noninterviews as well. The total number of eligibles with whom interviews were not completed in the example in Table 7.5 was 125.

6. Completed Interviews

The numerator for the response rate is the number of elements eligible for the study with whom interviews or questionnaires are actually completed ($n = 499$).

7. Computing the Response Rate

The final response rate is the proportion that the number of completed interviews represents of the number of units known (and estimated) to be eligible for the study, which is $499/624 = 80$ percent in the example in Table 7.5.

Weighting the Sample Data to Reflect the Population

We saw in the discussion of approaches to sampling rare populations in Chapter Six that the investigator may want to sample some subgroups in the population at different rates to ensure that there will be enough of these individuals without having to increase the overall size of the sample, thus adding to the costs of the study. Also, as just mentioned, there may be problems once fieldwork begins if some groups are less likely to respond than others.

Ideally, however, the researcher wants the sample to mirror as closely as possible the population as a whole. Adjustments for ensuring this correspondence between the distribution of the sample and the population on characteristics of interest involve procedures for *weighting the sample* so that it resembles the population from which it was drawn. Weighting literally involves a process of statistically assigning more or less weight to some groups than others so that their distributions in the sample correspond more closely to their actual distributions in the population as a whole (Kish, 1990).

Two primary types of weighting procedures are discussed here and outlined in Table 7.6. The first set of procedures includes adjustments that can be used if decisions were made when the sample itself was drawn originally that caused it to look different from the population as a whole, such as sampling certain groups at higher (or lower) rates. These include expansion weights (EWEIGHT) to reflect the actual number and distribution of cases in the population and relative weights (RWEIGHT) to readjust the weights to the number of cases to the actual sample size, while maintaining the relative distribution of subgroups within the population.

The second set of procedures is undertaken to adjust for differential non-response or noncoverage for different groups in the population. These include class- or group-specific adjustments based on the respective groups' response rates (RRWEIGHT), and poststratification weighting (POSTWT), that assigns weights to certain subgroups within the sample to bring the distribution of these subgroups in the sample into closer conformity with their known distribution in the population.

Weighting to Adjust for Disproportionate Sampling

The cases may also be weighted to reflect either the actual size of the population from which they are drawn or the number of cases in the original sample.

Weighting to Population Size: Expansion Weights

The sampling fraction (n/N) is the proportion of cases drawn for the sample (n) as a proportion of the total number of elements in the population (N). With multistage designs the overall sampling fraction for a case is a product of the sampling fractions at each stage of the design. If we want the number of people in the sample to mirror the number they represent in the population, we can compute expansion weights for each case based on the inverse of the sampling fraction. This approach is illustrated in Example A in Table 7.6, in weighting the data for a study in which Hispanics were sampled at twice the rate of African Americans.

The sampling fraction for the samples (n) of 900 African Americans and 200 Hispanics, out of 90,000 and 10,000 of these groups in the population (N), respectively, would be 900/90,000 = 1/100 and 200/10,000 = 1/50. Multiplying the number of cases in the *sample* for each group by the inverse of its sampling

TABLE 7.6. WEIGHTING THE SAMPLE DATA TO REFLECT THE POPULATION.

Purpose of Weighting	Method	Example	
To adjust for disproportionate sampling		*Example:* Hispanics are sampled at twice the rate of African Americans to increase their yield in the sample.	
			African American / Hispanic
A. Weighting to population size (expansion weight)	Construct weight that multiplies case by the inverse of the sampling fraction.	N in population n in sample sampling fraction (n/N) expansion weight (N/n)	90,000 / 10,000 900 / 200 1/100 / 1/50 100/1 / 50/1
B. Weighting to sample size (relative weight)	Compute the mean expansion weight and divide case expansion weight by mean expansion weight.	mean expansion weight = N/n = 100,000/1,100 = 90.9 relative weight = case expansion weight/90.9	 100/90.9 / 50/90.9
To adjust for nonresponse and/or noncoverage			
C. Weighting to adjust for response rate (response-rate weight)	Divide case expansion weight by response rate.	response rate (RR) = completed/eligible cases response-rate weight = case expansion weight/RR	.80 / .70 100/.80 / 50/.70
D. Weighting to adjust sample distribution to population distribution (poststratification weight)	(1) Determine population distribution from external data source. (2) Determine sample distribution from survey. (3) Compute poststratification weight (ratio of population to sample distribution): population % ÷ sample %	*Example:* Poor African Americans and poor Hispanics are underrepresented in a telephone survey.	

	(1) Population %	(2) Sample %	(3) Weight
Poor Hispanics	15	5	3.00
Poor African Americans	5	3	1.66
Nonpoor Hispanics	20	20	1.00
Nonpoor African Americans	60	72	.83

fraction would yield the number of each group in the *population:* $900 \times (100/1) =$ 90,000 and $200 \times (50/1) = 10,000$. This is one way of getting back to the actual distribution of each group that exists in the population, even though one group may have been sampled at twice the rate of another. Otherwise, the relative distribution of the cases in the sample (900/11,000 for African Americans; 200/11,000 for Hispanics) would not accurately mirror their distribution in the population.

An example of the use of this approach when only one person is selected to be interviewed in a household (with four people, for example) is to weight the case of the selected sample person by the inverse (4/1) of the proportion this one case represents of everyone in the household (1/4) so that the sample data accurately reflect the composition of all the households in the population from which the sample was drawn.

The assignment of these weights can be carried out through statements in standard statistical packages such as the Statistical Package for the Social Sciences (SPSS) that permit values relevant for specific subgroups {noted in brackets} to be assigned to the individuals in those groups:

expansion weight
IF {African American,Hispanic} EWEIGHT = {expansion weight$_{\text{African American=100,Hispanic=50}}$}

If the population from which a particular sample is drawn is quite large, however, the researcher may not want to use this approach. With standard statistical analysis packages, large sample sizes resulting from weighting the data in this fashion could render the tests of statistical significance virtually meaningless because the computations do not reflect the actual number of observations on which the estimates are based and, with large enough sample sizes, virtually all estimates or the relationships between them are statistically significant.

Weighting to Sample Size: Relative Weights

One way to deal with this problem is to adjust the expansion weights to produce a relative weight that downweights the number of cases to be equal to the actual sample size while maintaining the appropriate distribution of cases produced by the expansion weights. (See Example B in Table 7.6.) The relative weight is constructed by computing the mean of the expansion weights and then dividing the expansion weights for each case by this mean.

The sum of the expansion weights for each group equals the total population N [$\sum (w_i \times n) = N$]. Referring to the example in Table 7.6:

$$\Sigma (w_i \times n) = (100 \times 900) + (50 \times 200)$$
$$= 90,000 + 10,000$$
$$= 100,000$$

To compute the mean expansion weight, divide the sum of the expansion weights (N) by the number of cases in the sample (n): 100,000/1,100 = 90.9. The relative weight is then computed by dividing the expansion weight for each case by this mean expansion weight:

relative weight
COMPUTE   RWEIGHT = EWEIGHT/{mean expansion weight$_{=90.9}$}

Dividing the expansion weight for a given individual by this mean weight yields weighted numbers of cases that are equivalent to the total unweighted sample size, but that is appropriately readjusted for the relative distribution of each group within the target population:

RWEIGHT	*n*	%
90,000/90.9 =	990	90%
10,000/90.9 =	110	10%
Total	1,100	100%

The total number of cases that appears in any particular analysis when this weight is applied reflects the actual number of cases in the study sample (n=1,100), not the population as a whole (N=100,000). The advantage of applying this additional weighting procedure is that it allows the tests of statistical significance to be based on the number of cases from which the sample estimates being examined were actually derived.

The researcher should be sure that all the relevant information required for constructing the final sample weights is fully documented in the course of the study and, when appropriate (such as whether a case represents a Hispanic respondent or not), actually coded on the record for each case.

Weighting to Adjust for Nonresponse or Noncoverage

Problems occurring during the sample design and execution process can cause the characteristics of a sample to differ from the population it was intended to represent. Differential coverage or response to a survey by different subgroups can, for example, account for such differences. Two types of weighting procedures to adjust for these possible sources of bias in the distribution of sample cases include *response-rate* and *poststratification weighting.* Self-weighting samples based on proportionate sampling designs may still require these weighting adjustments to deal with noncoverage or nonresponse bias.

Response-Rate Weighting Adjustments

To adjust for differential response rates (or nonresponse) for each group, the expansion weight computed to adjust for the disproportionate sampling fractions for each group is divided by the group's response rate (Example C in Table 7.6). For example, if the response rates for African American and Hispanics in a study are determined to be 80 percent and 70 percent, respectively, then the expansion weight could be divided by .80 or .70 to adjust for the differential nonresponse before computing the relative weight:

response-rate weight
IF {African American, Hispanic} $RRWEIGHT = EWEIGHT_{\{African American=100, Hispanic=50\}} / \{response\ rate_{African American=.80, Hispanic=.70}\}$

Class- or group-specific response-rate weighting adjustments assume that the original sample can be stratified into different groups for which response rates can be computed.

Poststratification Weighting

Once the sample design is executed and the sample appropriately weighted to adjust for disproportionate sampling or nonresponse of different groups, distributions on selected characteristics of the sample can be compared with characteristics of the population of interest obtained from other sources (census data, clinic records, insurance claims files). If substantial differences are found, then poststratification weights can be applied to the sample to cause it to look more like the population from which it was drawn.

These weights are termed poststratification weights because they are assigned after ("post") designing the sample itself, based on grouping the sample into groups ("strata") for which distributions for the population as a whole are available (see Example D in Table 7.6). Ratios are then constructed by comparing the percentages of the population known to be in each stratum with the percentages reflected in the sample itself. The resulting ratios are the poststratification weights assigned to each case in the sample based on the characteristics used for defining the various strata.

As with the other weighting procedures, each case that appears in the sample then is weighted to increase or decrease its contributions, as appropriate, so that the resulting distribution of cases of this kind in the sample is similar to distributions in the population as a whole. In the example in Table 7.6, poor Hispanics are given a poststratification weight (POSTWT) of 3.00 because they appear to be underrepresented in the sample compared with their known distribution in the population. In contrast, nonpoor African Americans are given a weight (POSTWT) of .83 because they appear to be overrepresented in the sample.

The poststratification weight factor would be multiplied by any other previous weights (*E*WEIGHT, *R*WEIGHT, or *RR*WEIGHT) to produce a final weight (FWEIGHT):

poststratification weighting
IF {group$_x$}   FWEIGHT = _WEIGHT × {poststratification weight$_x$}

Poststratification weighting adjustments assume that a source is available to use as the basis for describing the distribution of the population on the respective characteristics. Census data are often used in making poststratification adjustments for national surveys. A comparable source of information may not be available to investigators, particularly in local surveys. Such adjustments will also not fully correct for biases resulting from substantial nonresponse or noncoverage problems with the sample or for other differences not explicitly incorporated in the poststratification weights.

Special Considerations for Special Populations

Stratification and the disproportionate sampling of concentrated clusters of selected target groups may introduce substantial economies in identifying and sampling rare and special populations, but these practices may also yield significant *dis*economies in the overall efficiency of the sample design due to increased nonresponse bias or sampling (standard) errors relative to costs. The procedures introduced here and in the previous chapter provide useful diagnostics and devices for addressing the sources of variable and systematic errors that are likely to plague surveys of special populations in particular.

Selected Examples

The NCHS–NHIS was designed to include a sufficient number of minority (Hispanic and African Americans) individuals to yield reliable estimates for these populations. The response rates for this study have remained quite high (around 94 percent to 95 percent) over time, although more effort and resources have gone into sustaining these rates in recent years. Expansion weights (termed inflation factors by NCHS), and nonresponse and poststratification weights are all components of the NCHS weighting procedures. Secondary users of the NCHS–NHIS data sets must, however, compute relative weights to readjust the final NCHS sample weights (that expand sample totals to the U.S. population) to the actual sample size (n), as well as run their analyses using software such as SUDAAN or PC-CARP, to adjust the tests of statistical significance for the design effects resulting from the complex nature of the sample design.

Over 7,000 households in the city and suburban areas of the Chicago metropolitan area were screened to yield 1,540 completed interviews in the Chicago AIDS survey (Survey Research Laboratory, 1988). African Americans were oversampled by approximately 15 percent and Hispanics by a factor of two to yield a sufficient number of cases for each group. To increase the efficiency of the design, the disproportionate sampling of minorities was concentrated in the city rather than suburban strata within the Chicago metropolitan area. The overall response rate for the study was 51.4 percent—1,540 completed cases divided by 2,996 "eligible" cases, including 704 households that could not be contacted after repeated attempts. If all of those who could not be contacted were actually *not* eligible (which is unlikely), the response rate would have been 67.2 percent (1,540/2,292). Weights were computed to adjust for the disproportionate sampling of racial and ethnic minorities as well as to assure that the distribution of the sample for certain subgroups (Hispanics, African Americans, and others in the city and suburban areas) conformed to their distribution in the 1980 U.S. census.

The dentists survey essentially entailed a census (rather than a sample) of dentists in the designated target population. The standard deviations (and associated standard errors) derived from the survey sample nonetheless provide useful indicators of the heterogeneity or homogeneity (diversity) within the target population on key attributes of interest (dentists' attitudes toward prevention as a focus of their practice, for example).

Guidelines for Minimizing Survey Errors

Know your fractions: they do, in fact, sum to a large part of the whole in the sample size estimation process. The standard error (SE = $\sigma/\sqrt{n}$), for example, is a key formula that parsimoniously summarizes the average variable sampling error associated with estimates derived from samples of a designated size from a population with known (or at least hypothesized) characteristics. The larger the denominator (sample size) and the smaller the numerator (average variation within a specific sample), the lower the variable error associated with the sample estimates. This formula also provides the foundation for deriving the sample size for many types of designs, that is, solving for "n" solves the "n."

The numerator and denominator and the quantity captured by their arithmetic relationship in computing the design effects, response rate, and weights are similarly little measures that say a lot about both the magnitude and management of variable and systematic errors associated with the number and distribution of sample cases.

Controversies exist in the applied sampling field with respect to whether weighting and other complex design adjustments may, in fact, introduce more rather than fewer errors in the analyses of sample survey data (Korn & Graubard, 1991, 1995; Rao & Bellhouse, 1990). Further, random coefficient (RC) linear regression models, also known as "hierarchical linear models," offer a new and promising alternative to traditional variance-adjustment approaches (based on sample design effects) for analyzing data based on multistage cluster sampling designs (Kreft, 1995). In any case, survey designers should be aware of the sampling issues discussed in this and the preceding chapter and be prepared to ask informed questions of a qualified sampling consultant, if necessary, to resolve how best to proceed.

Supplementary Sources

Lemeshow, Hosmer, Klar, and Lwanga (1990) and Lwanga and Lemeshow (1991) provide formulae, tables, and examples for computing sample sizes for a variety of types of health studies. The use of effect sizes as a basis for sample size estimation is fully described in Cohen (1988), and software for executing this approach is documented in Borenstein and Cohen (1988). Kraemer and Thiemann (1987) and Lipsey (1990) offer some useful and practical adaptations of Cohen's method to an array of analytic and experimental study designs.

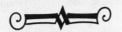

CHAPTER EIGHT

GENERAL PRINCIPLES FOR FORMULATING QUESTIONS

Chapter Highlights

1. The development of survey questions should be guided by practical *experience* with the same or comparable questions in other studies, scientific *experiments* that test alternative ways of asking questions and the magnitude of the errors that result, and theoretical *expectations* about what ways of asking a question will produce what outcomes based on cognitive psychology and other conceptual approaches to total survey design.

2. The criteria for evaluating survey questionnaires include the clarity, balance, and length of the survey questions themselves; the comprehensiveness or constraints of the responses implied or imposed by these questions; the utility of the instructions provided for answering them; the order and context in which they are integrated into the survey questionnaire; and the response errors or effects that result from how the questionnaire is ultimately designed as well as from the characteristics and behavior of the respondents who answer it and the interviewers who administer it to them.

This chapter is the first of four chapters that present guidelines for developing the survey questions and incorporating these questions (or items) into an integrated and interpretable survey questionnaire to be read or presented to respondents. It provides an overview of (1) the preliminary steps to take in identifying or designing the questions to include in a survey, (2) the theoretical approaches to use in anticipating sources of errors in these questions, and (3) general guidelines for question and questionnaire development to minimize errors that can result from the design of the questions or the questionnaire or from the way in which the questions are asked or the questionnaire is administered.

Preliminary Steps in Choosing Survey Questions

First, as has been repeated throughout the preceding chapters, survey researchers should use the principal research question and associated study objectives and hypotheses to guide their selection of questions for their survey. For example, what are the major concepts that the survey designers want to operationalize? Are they the main variables that will be used to describe the study sample and, by inference, the population from which it was drawn, or are they independent, dependent, or control variables to be used in testing an explicit study hypothesis? In other words, how will the concepts actually be used in the analyses, and what is the most appropriate level of measurement to employ in choosing the questions to capture (or operationalize) these concepts?

Second, survey researchers should not try to reinvent the wheel. After thinking through the concepts to be operationalized in their survey, researchers should begin to look for other studies that have dealt with similar topics and assemble copies of the questionnaires and articles that summarize the research methods and results of those studies.

Researchers should next determine whether formal tests of the validity and reliability of specific questions or scales of interest have been conducted. They should also look for any other evidence of methodological problems with these items, such as the rates of missing values or the degree of correspondence of responses to those questions with comparable ones asked in other studies. If possible, researchers should speak with the designers of these studies to gain additional information about how well questions worked in their surveys.

Using seasoned approaches not only provides researchers guidance as to the probable quality and applicability of the items for their own purposes but also enhances the possibility for substantive comparisons with these and other studies and adds to the cumulative body of methodological experience with survey items.

Third, the researcher should consider the type of question each item represents and the best way to ask that particular type of question. Are they questions about factual and objective characteristics or behaviors, about nonfactual and subjective attitudes or perceptions, or about some (subjective or objective) indicators of health status? How respondents think about these different types of questions will vary. For example, respondents may call upon different frames of reference and feel different levels of threat in answering a question about the number of visits they made to a dentist in the year compared with one about their perceived risk of contracting AIDS. The rules for asking questions should take these different cognitive experiences into account in order to discover what the respondent really thinks about the issue.

Fourth, researchers should consider the extent to which the medium (personal interview, telephone interview, or mail questionnaire) affects the message (what does or does not come across to the respondent) in the survey. Respondents in personal interviews are influenced by the implicit or explicit verbal and visual cues provided by the interviewer as well as by the questionnaire that the survey designer provides. With telephone interviews, the medium and hence the message is largely a verbal one, and with mail questionnaires the messages are entirely visual. The intent in designing any survey question is that the message the researcher intended to send comes across clearly to the respondent.

Fifth—and perhaps most important—survey designers should have some idea of the kinds of errors that can arise at each stage in developing survey questions and the approaches to use to minimize or eliminate such errors. In recent years, there has been greater attention to developing and applying theoretical frameworks for identifying and estimating the magnitude of errors of various kinds in surveys. Principles for designing survey questions to minimize such errors are still more often based on experience than on experiments. The following section presents the results of some very recent experiments and also discusses the vast body of experience available to designers of survey questions. The purpose of this section is to suggest how to minimize the errors that inevitably result when people are asked to describe what is in their heads.

Sources of Errors in Survey Questions

Smith (1987) traced many of the changes in how questions have been asked in surveys and public opinion polls. He pointed out that the emphasis in question design has shifted from relatively unstructured inquiries that closely approximated normal conversations to the highly formalized, structured, and standardized protocols of most contemporary studies. According to Smith, these protocols reflect a "specialized survey dialect" far from the "natural language" of normal conversation (p. S105). Other critics of modern survey question design argue that meaning is lost and distortions and inaccuracies result when people are questioned in this way (Beatty, 1995; Mishler, 1986; Suchman & Jordan, 1990).

In fact, the "art" of asking questions, which requires creativity and ingenuity on the part of the survey designer to develop an item that speaks to the respondent in the way that the designer intended, has always been an important aspect of designing survey questions. In contrast, the "science" of formulating and testing hypotheses about whether what the question elicits from respondents is an accurate reflection of what they really *mean* or of the *truth* that the survey designer intended to learn has only begun to emerge.

The first book to inventory the guidelines and principles to use in designing survey questions, aptly titled *The Art of Asking Questions,* appeared almost fifty years ago (Payne, 1951). The principles presented in that book were based primarily on the experience of the author and others in designing and implementing questions in polls and public opinion surveys. However, they were also based on the results of so-called split-ballot experiments, in which different approaches to phrasing or formatting what were thought to be comparable questions were used with similar groups of respondents, and the results were then compared. The simplicity and wisdom of the suggestions in that book continue to make sense to many contemporary designers of surveys and polls and to be confirmed by more formal methodological research on survey question design (Belson, 1981, 1986; Biemer, Groves, Lyberg, Mathiowetz, & Sudman, 1991; Bradburn, Sudman, & Associates, 1979; Converse & Presser, 1986; DeMaio, 1983; Dillman, 1978; Groves, 1989; Kalton & Schuman, 1982; Lessler & Kalsbeek, 1992; Molenaar, 1991; Schuman & Presser, 1981; Schwarz & Sudman, 1992, 1994, 1995; Sheatsley, 1983; Sudman & Bradburn, 1982; Sudman, Bradburn, & Schwarz, 1995; Swain, 1985; Tanur, 1992).

The primary impetus for formalized, empirical research on the accuracy of survey questions began with experimental work by investigators at the University of Michigan Survey Research Center. Their work involved comparisons of survey data and physician record data on health events and health care, as well as studies of the impact of interviewer characteristics and behaviors on responses to survey questions (Kahn & Cannell, 1957; NCHSR, 1978).

With the publication of *Response Effects in Surveys,* Sudman and Bradburn (1974) made a major theoretical contribution to modeling the different aspects of the survey design processes and the various errors that can emerge. In that book, the authors introduced a framework that detailed the role of the interviewer, the respondent, and the task (principally the questionnaire and how it was administered) in the research interview. They also introduced the concept of *response effects* to reflect the differences between the answers obtained in the survey and the actual (or true) value of the variable that the question was intended to capture. These are differences that can result from either the characteristics or the performance of the three principal components of the survey interview.

Subsequent to Sudman and Bradburn's preliminary work, the concept of *total survey design* and an accompanying approach to estimating *total survey errors* from *all* sources in surveys came into prominence in the late 1970s. For example, Andersen, Kasper, Frankel, and Associates (1979) argued that errors in surveys were a function of both the inconsistency and the inaccuracy of data, which in turn resulted from problems with the design and implementation of the sampling, data collection, and data-processing procedures involved in carrying out a survey.

Sudman and Bradburn's concept of "response effects" provided significant conceptual and methodological guidance for identifying and quantifying an important potential source of errors in surveys: people's responses to the survey questions themselves. These errors, it was thought, resulted from interviewers' or respondents' behaviors or the nature of the interview task itself. In 1979 these same researchers and their associates published *Improving Interview Method and Questionnaire Design,* which summarized much of their own research on how to increase the accuracy of reports on sensitive topics (such as drug use, alcohol consumption, sexual behavior, and so on) in surveys, using their response effects framework (Bradburn, Sudman, & Associates, 1979).

There has been an increasing interest on the part of survey methodologists in the design of empirical studies for identifying and quantifying the sources and magnitude of response effects (or errors) in surveys. In 1980 a Panel on Survey Measurement of Subjective Phenomena was convened by the National Academy of Sciences to review the state of the art of survey research, with particular reference to how subjective (nonfactual) questions are asked in surveys (Turner & Martin, 1984). The panel concluded that the lines between subjective and objective questions in survey research cannot always be clearly drawn, since even respondents' answers to factual questions are filtered through their internal cognitive memory and recall processes. With questions on more subjective topics, such as respondents' knowledge about or attitudes on certain issues, understanding *how* they think about the topic may, in fact, be essential to designing meaningful questions to find out *what* they think about it.

Sudman and Bradburn (1974), in their initial formulation of the response effects concept, pointed out that determining the real (or "true") answer to survey questions is more problematical with nonfactual or attitudinal questions than with what are generally thought of as factual or objective questions. The latter assume there is some external, identifiable behavior or event that is being referenced in the question asked. Respondents' reports of these phenomena do not always necessarily agree with these "facts," however.

In estimating the accuracy of respondents' reports on factual questions of this kind, tests of criterion validity are applied (see Figure 3.2 in Chapter Three for a description of this procedure). With this approach, the "facts" that respondents report in the survey questionnaire (such as the number of times they said they went to a particular physician during the year) are compared with a criterion source (the provider's medical records, for example) to estimate just how accurate their answers are. Estimates of respondents' "false positive" or "false negative" responses are then developed to quantify the magnitude of their "overreporting" or "under-reporting" in the study (Marquis, 1978, 1984; Marquis, Moore, & Bogen, 1993).

The accuracy of responses to nonfactual questions can, to some extent, be assessed by means of examining their construct validity—that is, the extent to which the results agree with the theory on which the concepts expressed in the question are based (Kalton & Schuman, 1982). However, it may not always be apparent whether it is the theory or the methods that are at fault if the results are not what was expected theoretically.

Efforts to assess the accuracy of nonfactual questions have, therefore, tended to rely more on split-ballot or other experiments in which different ways of asking subjective questions are used and the results compared. Inconsistencies in the results serve to warn the researcher that the questions may indeed convey different meanings to respondents. The more consistent the results, the more confidence the researcher can have that the questions are substantively comparable (Converse & Presser, 1986; Schuman & Presser, 1981).

Several prominent survey research methodologists have called for the development of a comprehensive theory or set of theories to provide more systematic predictions about which survey design decisions are going to lead to which outcomes and with what magnitude of error (Bradburn, 1982; Groves, 1987, 1989; Schuman & Kalton, 1985). These conceptual frameworks can then guide the development of empirical studies to test theoretically grounded predictions formally, to accumulate and integrate the resulting findings systematically, and ultimately to build a fund of scientific knowledge on which to base survey design decisions.

Contributions of Cognitive Psychology to Questionnaire Design

The theoretical perspectives and concepts of cognitive psychology are viewed as a promising starting point by survey methodologists concerned with developing a science of survey question and questionnaire design and a scientific way to estimate the errors associated with these procedures. In 1983, for example, the Committee on National Statistics with funding from the National Science Foundation, convened an Advanced Research Seminar on the Cognitive Aspects of Survey Methodology (CASM) to foster a dialogue between cognitive psychologists and survey researchers on these issues. The proceedings of that conference, *Cognitive Aspects of Survey Methodology: Building a Bridge Between Disciplines,* pointed out how concepts and methodologies from cognitive psychology could be used to inform the design of surveys in general and health surveys in particular. One example given of this approach was the National Center for Health Statistics–National Health Interview Survey (Jabine, Straf, Tanur, & Tourangeau, 1984).

Tourangeau (1984), in a contributed article in the CASM proceedings, pointed out that there are four main stages identified by the social information-processing frameworks of cognitive psychology that can be used in describing the steps respondents go through in answering survey questions: (1) the *comprehension stage,* in which the respondent interprets the question; (2) the *retrieval stage,* in which the respondent searches his or her memory for the relevant information; (3) the *estimation/judgment stage,* in which the respondent evaluates the information retrieved from memory and its relevance to the question and, when appropriate, combines information to arrive at an answer; and (4) the *response stage,* in which the respondent weighs factors such as the sensitivity or threat level of the question and the social acceptability and/or probable accuracy of the answer, and only then decides what answer to give.

This framework has gained considerable prominence as a basis for designing and evaluating survey questions in order to minimize the errors that are likely to occur at each stage (Biemer, Groves, Lyberg, Mathiowetz, & Sudman, 1991; Tanur, 1992). Bradburn and Danis (1984) pointed out that different types of survey questions may place different demands on the respondent at different stages of the response formulation process. The retrieval stage may be particularly important in asking respondents to recall relatively nonthreatening factual information because of the heavy demands such questions place on their memory of relevant events or behaviors. When asked more threatening or sensitive questions, respondents may decide at the last (response) stage to sacrifice the accuracy of their responses to lower the psychic threat that results from giving answers that are not perceived to be socially acceptable ones. For certain attitudinal questions the *judgments* that the respondents make about the issue (the third stage of the process) may be particularly critical as they think through how they will answer the question.

Cognitive psychologists posit that there are schemata (frameworks or "scripts") that respondents have in their heads and subsequently call upon in responding to stimuli, such as those generated by survey research questions (Markus & Zajonc, 1985). One of the devices used in experimental cognitive psychology laboratories to discover and define these scripts is to ask subjects to think aloud in answering questions that are posed by the researcher—that is, literally to say out loud everything that comes to mind in answering the question, which the researcher can then tape or otherwise record for subsequent analysis. These reflections thus become the data that the investigator uses to arrive at an understanding of the schemata inside people's heads that are called upon in responding to different types of questions.

Further, cognitive psychologists are not concerned only with how a question is asked and the process the respondent goes through in answering it. They are also concerned with the context in which the question is presented and how the associations with other events that respondents make as a result affect their interpretation (or processing) of the question and the information they call forth to answer it. The importance of the context in influencing the schemata called forth by respondents has also been applied in trying to interpret the impact that the context or order (as well as the phrasing) of questions within a survey questionnaire has on how people answer those questions.

As mentioned earlier, the surveys of the National Center for Health Statistics (NCHS) were the particular focus of the 1983 CASM conference. Subsequent to that conference, the NCHS developed a formal program in the Cognitive Aspects of Survey Methodology, building upon concepts and methods suggested at the conference. The NCHS–CASM program provides funding for external researchers who are interested in conducting basic research that uses the principles of cognitive psychology to improve the design of health survey questionnaires (Lessler & Sirken, 1985). The results of these studies are published in the National Center for Health Statistics Vital and Health Statistics Series 6 (NCHS, 1989a, 1989c, 1989d, 1991a, 1992a, 1992d, 1994a). The NCHS also supports a Questionnaire Design Research Laboratory, which employs the concepts and methods of cognitive psychology to test items to be included in NCHS continuing surveys (Fienberg, Loftus, & Tanur, 1985; Lessler & Sirken, 1985). The procedures and results of many of the instrument development activities conducted at the NCHS design laboratory are reported in the NCHS Cognitive Methods Staff Working Paper Series (available through the National Center for Health Statistics, Hyattsville, Md.).

The applications of cognitive psychology have been extended to the design of other major national surveys, such as those conducted by the U.S. Bureau of the Census, the U.S. Department of Agriculture, the Bureau of Labor Statistics, and Statistics Canada (Biemer, Groves, Lyberg, Mathiowetz, & Sudman, 1991; Bureau of Labor Statistics, 1987; Gower, 1994; Jobe & Mingay, 1991; Tanur, 1987). A series of conferences have provided an overview of the concepts and methods from cognitive psychology as they could be applied in making practical decisions about how to ask survey questions (Biemer, Groves, Lyberg, Mathiowetz, & Sudman, 1991; Hippler, Schwarz, & Sudman, 1987; Schwarz & Sudman, 1992, 1994, 1995; Tanur, 1992).

Methods for Developing Survey Questions

The science and art of developing survey questions has matured significantly as a result of advances in the application of the principles of cognitive psychology to question design, an increasing acknowledgment of the value of qualitative and ethnographic research methods, and marketing research techniques for developing questions that best speak the language and convey the meaning intended by respondents. Different question development strategies may point to different types of problems with the instrument and also vary substantially with respect to the costs associated with implementing them (Blixt & Dykema, 1993; Lessler, 1995; Presser & Blair, 1994). An array of procedures are reviewed here. Investigators will not necessarily apply all of these in developing and testing survey items. However, they should be aware of them and consider which or which combination may be most fruitfully applied in assuring that the questions they ask are both sensible and meaningful to respondents.

Group Interviews

Group interviews, and particularly *focus groups,* have been used extensively in marketing research to solicit the opinions of targeted subsets of potential customers for a new product or marketing strategy (Frey & Fontana, 1991). With the increasing recognition that the standardized and scientized language of surveys may not be readily understandable by many respondents, focus groups of (generally six to ten) individuals like those that will be included in a survey (such as caregivers for the elderly, persons with AIDS, intravenous drug users) are invited to provide input at all stages of the instrument development process (Basch, 1987; Desvousges & Frey, 1989; O'Brien, 1993; Schechter, Trunzo, & Parsons, 1993; Trunzo & Schechter, 1993). For example, they may be asked to identify the issues that are of concern to the groups that are the primary focus of the study or what comes to mind when they think of the key study concepts (caregiver stress, safe sex, high-risk behavior) in the early stages of instrument development; review and comment on actual drafts of the questionnaire; and suggest explanations or hypotheses in interpreting study findings once the data are gathered. A number of sources are available to provide guidance for the conduct of focus groups (Krueger, 1994; Morgan, 1993; Stewart & Shamdasani, 1990).

Ethnographic Interviewing

Ethnographic interviewing is another approach, borrowed from traditional qualitative research methods, that may also provide useful guidance at each stage of the instrument development process. In-depth individual interviews may be preferred to focus groups when there is a concern with the reluctance of certain types of respondents (teenagers or those who are less educated) to speak up or to address particularly sensitive or personal topics in a group setting. These interviews may be either relatively unstructured or structured in terms of the questions that are asked of participants. They are often supplemented with participant observation by the investigator, who spends time informally visiting with or observing individuals or groups like those who will be the focus of the study (teenage gang members, pregnant women who go to a public health clinic) (Axinn, Fricke, & Thornton, 1991; Bauman & Adair, 1992; Rubin & Rubin, 1995; Von Thurn & Moore, 1993).

Other Techniques

Other techniques that have been drawn from research in cognitive psychology in particular include *think-aloud strategies, laboratory and field experiments,* and *behavior coding of interviews.*

With *think-aloud* strategies, respondents like those that will be included in the study are administered questions that have been developed to measure study concepts and asked a series of specific probe questions either at the time a question is asked (concurrent think-aloud) or at the end of the interview (retrospective think-aloud) regarding what they were thinking when they answered the questions and how they arrived at their answers. This approach has been used extensively in the NCHS Questionnaire Design Research Laboratory (QDRL) in evaluating questions for the NCHS–National Health Interview Survey (NHIS) supplements, as well as other government-sponsored surveys (Beatty, 1994; Kerwin, 1993a, 1993b; Stussman, 1994). A training manual has been developed by the NCHS QDRL for those who are interested in using this approach (Willis, 1994a). Think-aloud strategies are particularly useful for surfacing the cognitive processes (the framework for approaching the question and basis for calling upon or weighing evidence) that respondents may employ at the various stages of responding to questions identified by cognitive psychologists (Ericsson & Simon, 1993; Fienberg, Loftus, & Tanur, 1985; Forsyth & Lessler, 1991; Jobe & Mingay, 1989; Willis, 1994b; Willis, Royston, & Bercini, 1991).

A disadvantage of the think-aloud strategy, however, is that it does not provide for the systematic manipulation and evaluation of alternative approaches to phrasing questions. *Laboratory and field experiments* attempt to address these weaknesses (Fienberg & Tanur, 1989). In experimental studies a particular theory or set of hypotheses is used to guide the development of distinct options for phrasing or ordering questions, and an experimental design is employed to carry out this study either in a laboratory setting or with respondents like those who will be included in the study through personal, telephone, or self-administered interviews. The National Center for Health Statistics has conducted or sponsored an array of experimental studies of this kind, which provide the foundation for much cognitive research on question and questionnaire design (NCHS, 1989a, 1989c, 1989d, 1991a, 1992a, 1992d, 1994a). Investigators with limited resources or research design expertise may be reluctant to undertake such experiments in developing their own surveys. They should, however, be guided by the insights and guidance provided by the research that has been conducted in this area. The chapters that follow will apply the findings from such studies in detailing the principles for formulating different types of survey questions.

Behavior coding entails a rigorous analysis of the behavior of interviewers and respondents, based on trained coders coding their behaviors by listening to live or taped interviews (Dijkstra & Van der Zouwen, 1982; Fowler, 1989a; Fowler & Mangione, 1990; Oksenberg, Cannell, & Kalton, 1991; Morton-Williams & Sykes, 1984; Sykes & Morton-Williams, 1987). This is a relatively labor-intensive approach, and as a result it is generally based on only a small number of interviews. An alternative approach is to have interviewers focus on recording selected aspects of the respondents' behavior in the course of the interview, such as whether they ask to have the question repeated or clarified, interrupt the interviewer, or ask how much longer it will take (Burgess & Paton, 1993). In either case, the resulting information can be quite useful in identifying and revising questions that seem to create problems for either the interviewer or respondent.

Methods for Testing Survey Procedures

The development of a new product almost always involves a series of tests to see how well it works and what bugs need to be corrected before it goes on the market. The same standards should be applied in designing and carrying out surveys. *No* survey should *ever* go into the field without a trial run of the questionnaire and data collection procedures to be used in the final study. Failure to conduct this trial run is one of the biggest and potentially most costly mistakes that can be made in carrying out a survey. One can be sure that something will go wrong if there is not adequate testing of the procedures in advance of doing the survey. Even when such testing is done, situations can arise that were not anticipated in the original design of the study. The point with testing the procedures in advance is to anticipate and eliminate as many of these problems as possible and, above all, to avert major disasters in the field once the study is launched. The survey design literature variously refers to this phase of survey development as a pilot study or pretest. It may, in fact, encompass a range of activities including evaluating (1) individual questions; (2) the questionnaire as a whole; (3) the feasibility of sampling and data collection procedures; and (4) the procedures for coding and computerizing the data, if time and resources permit. This last step is, of course, imperative for computer-assisted data collection methods, in which the procedures for gathering the data involve direct entry of the respondents' answers into a computerized data system.

Questions

Conventional survey pretests (or pilot studies) have often not incorporated formal procedures for developing and evaluating survey questions, but simply an open-ended debriefing with respondents or interviewers regarding problems they encountered with the draft questionnaire. Research conducted by Hunt, Sparkman, and Wilcox (1982) suggested that formal protocols for asking respondents about problems they had with particular questions were more effective in identifying such problems than was an open-ended, general debriefing. Further, it seemed to be easier for respondents to pinpoint problems with questions in which valid response alternatives were clearly left out than with questions that presented more subtle conceptual difficulties (loaded, double-barreled, or ambiguous questions).

The procedures derived from qualitative research methods and cognitive psychology reviewed earlier provide a much more disciplined look at the effectiveness of survey questions. At a minimum the pretest should determine whether the words and phrases used in a question mean the same thing to respondents as to the survey designers. For example, is it clear to all respondents that "family planning regarding their children" refers to birth control practices and not to planning relative to their child's education or other aspects of their child's development (Converse & Presser, 1986)? Testing should also surface problem items such as loaded, double-barreled, or ambiguous questions or ones in which the entire range of response alternatives is not provided to respondents. A think-aloud strategy with respondents may be particularly useful to clarify what they were actually thinking of when answering the question.

One should also seriously consider excluding questions for which there is a very skewed distribution or minimal variation in the variable or for a particular subgroup of interest (for example, when 99 percent of the respondents give the same answer to a question). Although such a finding may be of substantive importance, it may also signal that the question is not adequately capturing the variation that does exist in the population on the factors it was intended to reflect. If a large number of respondents refuse to answer a question or say they don't know how to answer it, this too suggests that the item probably should be revised and retested.

Questionnaire

Another important task during pretesting is to identify problems that exist with the questionnaire as a whole. How difficult and burdensome do the respondents perceive answering or filling out all the questions to be? Do the skip patterns between questions work properly? Are the transitions between topics logical? Is there evidence that respondents fall into invariant response sets in answering certain series or types of questions? Do large numbers of respondents break off the interview early on or begin to express impatience or fatigue as the interview proceeds? The occurrence of any of these problems should be a signal to the survey designer that he or she needs to redesign all or part of the questionnaire.

Sampling Procedures

The third major aspect of a study that should be evaluated is the feasibility of the proposed sampling procedures. Complex procedures for oversampling certain groups (such as using screening questions or disproportionate, network, or dual-frame sampling methodologies) should be thoroughly tested to make sure that the field staff can accurately execute these procedures. Also, if a large enough pretest can be conducted, this will enable the researchers to estimate whether the probable yield of target cases using the proposed approach will be adequate. Within-household respondent selection procedures, particularly those that require interviewers to ask a number of questions or to go through several different steps, should also be thoroughly tested before being incorporated into the final study.

Ideally the pretest should be carried out with a sample of people similar to those who will be included in the final study. Purposive rather than probability sampling procedures could be useful in netting enough members of subgroups for which special problems in administering the survey questionnaire are anticipated (poorly educated persons, members of non-English-speaking minorities, known drug users, and so on). There would then be an opportunity to see if problems do in fact arise in administering the survey to these groups and to come up with ways of dealing with them before implementing the final study.

Data Collection Procedures

Pretests can also be used to evaluate whether certain procedures can be satisfactorily carried out using the data collection method proposed. An important dimension to assess is the probable response rate to the study. During the final (or dress rehearsal) stage, all the initial contact and follow-up procedures that will be used in the actual study should be implemented and the results evaluated. Findings may indicate that the methods for prior notification of respondents have to be refined, the introduction to the interview redesigned, more intensive follow-up procedures developed, or cash incentives provided.

Data Preparation Procedures

A final technical aspect of the survey design that can be evaluated during the pretest phase is the feasibility of the procedures for coding and computerizing the data. As mentioned earlier, the design and testing of the data entry, file structure, and storage systems for computerized data collection methods are integral parts of the questionnaire design process itself. Planning how the responses to answers obtained will be coded is also useful in evaluating the cost and feasibility of a paper-and-pencil data collection strategy. It is also helpful during the pretest stage of either a computerized or a paper-and-pencil questionnaire to use an open-ended response format in asking questions for which the range of probable responses is not known. The results can then be used to design codes for the questions in the final study.

Survey Cost Estimates

If there is uncertainty about the possible cost of executing certain aspects of a study, the pretest results can be helpful in finalizing its overall budget.

The actual number of cases to include in the pretest should be guided by the resources available to the researcher as well as by the types of questions to be answered with these preliminary studies. A simple test of how well the questionnaire worked, for example, would require fewer resources than evaluations of the entire range of sampling, data collection, follow-up, and coding and data-processing procedures proposed for the final survey. It is generally much more expensive to make changes with computerized data collection procedures subsequent to pretesting, because of the time and expense involved in redesigning *all* the interdependent parts of the survey package. According to one rule of thumb, a dress rehearsal for the study should include between twenty-five and fifty cases. However, the researcher should consider dividing this number of cases (or more cases, if resources are available) among several stages of testing so that there is ample opportunity to test all the changes that are made to the survey instrument or procedures before the fielding of the actual study. With federally sponsored surveys, fewer than ten questionnaires can be piloted or pretested without formal approval of the revised instrument by the Office of Management and Budget.

The section that follows presents the general principles for formulating survey questions that emerge from the practical, empirical, and theoretical mosaic of current health survey research design.

Basic Elements and Criteria in Designing Survey Questionnaires

The basic elements and criteria to consider in designing survey questions and integrating them into a survey questionnaire are summarized in Figure 8.1.

The primary elements of a survey questionnaire are (1) the questions themselves, (2) the response formats or categories that accompany the questions, and (3) any special instructions that appear in the questionnaire or that are associated with a particular question to tell the respondent or interviewer how to address it.

Questions

Words, phrases, and *sentences* are the major elements used in formulating survey questions.

Words. Words are the basic building blocks of human communication. They have been likened to the atomic and subatomic particles that constitute the basis of all chemical elements. Question designers need to be aware that the words and phrases included in a survey questionnaire and the way in which they are combined into the questions ultimately asked can affect the meaning of the question itself, much as different ways of combining elements in a chemistry laboratory can result in very different substantive outcomes (Turner & Martin, 1984).

The fundamental criterion to keep in mind when evaluating the words chosen to construct a survey question is their clarity. There are two major dimensions for assessing the clarity of the words used in phrasing a survey question—the clarity with which they express the concept of interest and the clarity with which they can be understood by respondents (Fowler, 1992, 1995).

First, researchers should consider whether the word adequately captures or conveys the *concept* that the researcher is interested in measuring with the survey question. What is the substantive or topical focus of the question—on the disease of AIDS, for example—and what does the researcher want to learn about it—the respondents' knowledge about, attitudes toward, or behavior in response to the illness? This is the first-order responsibility of researchers in deciding what words to use—clarifying *what* they are trying to learn by asking the question.

The second dimension in deciding upon the words to use in a survey question is whether the words chosen to express the concept are going to make sense to the *respondents*. Health survey designers often wrongly assume that survey respondents know more about certain concepts or topics than they actually do; the same

FIGURE 8.1. BASIC ELEMENTS AND CRITERIA IN DESIGNING SURVEY QUESTIONNAIRES.

Elements	Illustrations	Criteria

Questions

Words   `AIDS`   Clarity

Phrases   `agree` `or` `disagree`   Balance

Sentences   `Do` `you` `agree` `or` `disagree` `that` `AIDS`   Length

`can` `be` `transmitted` `by` `shaking` `hands`

`with` `a` `person` `with` `AIDS` ?

Responses

Open-ended   _____   Comprehensiveness
                 _____
                 _____

Closed-end   xxxxxxxxxx 1   Constraints
                               xxxxx 2
                               xxxxxxxxxxxxxx 3
                               xxx 4

Instructions   (Instructions tell you what to do next or how to   Utility
                        do it.)

Questionnaire

Order and Context

**Questionnaire
Administration**

Response Effects

designers may use words or phrases that have certain technical meanings that are not fully understood by respondents.

Good advice in choosing the words to include in survey questions is, *keep them simple.* Payne (1951), for example, suggested that one should assume an eighth-grade level of education of respondents in general population surveys. For other groups, such as well-educated professionals or low-income respondents, assumptions of higher or lower levels of education, respectively, would be appropriate. The readability of survey questions can be evaluated through specialized software that is available for this purpose as well as through grammar checking options available in major word processing packages (Grammatik, 1991).

Phrases. Just as the process of selecting words and putting them together to constitute phrases and sentences in designing survey questions is a cumulative one, criteria noted in Figure 8.1 can also be seen as relevant to apply at the subsequent stages in designing survey questions. For example, both the individual words that are chosen *and how they are combined into phrases* affect the clarity of their meaning conceptually and to the respondents themselves.

Another criterion that comes into play as the researcher begins to consider the combinations of words—or phrases—that could be used in developing survey questions is the relative balance among these words. The balance dimensions to consider in phrasing survey questions are threefold: (1) whether both sides of a question or issue are adequately represented, (2) whether the answer is weighted (loaded) in one direction or another, and (3) whether more than one question is implied in the phrasing of the question. Asking whether respondents agree with an item rather than implying but failing to provide the equivalent alternative when asking about attitudes toward a topic has been found to lead to different responses from those given when explicit alternatives are provided: "Do you agree or disagree that . . . ?" versus "Do you agree that . . . ?" (Payne, 1951; Schuman & Presser, 1981).

Another dimension of balance in the phrasing of survey questions is whether a question is explicitly "loaded" in one direction or another, such as "Don't you agree that . . . ?" Such a question makes it quite hard for the respondent to register a response that is counter to the one implied. In another form of the loaded question, certain premises or assumptions are implied in how the question is asked: "How long have you been beating your kids?" Recent research on the phrasing of sensitive questions about such behaviors as alcohol or drug use suggests that a survey researcher's deliberately loading questions in this way may elicit more reporting of these kinds of behaviors. In the absence of validating data on such behaviors, overreporting of them is assumed to be more accurate than underreporting. In general, however, survey designers should be cautious in phrasing survey questions to make sure that they do not inadvertently encourage a respondent to answer in a certain way.

A third aspect in balancing the phrasing of survey questions is whether two questions are implied in what is meant to be one: "Do you agree or disagree that AIDS can be transmitted by shaking hands with a person with AIDS or through other comparable forms of physical contact?" Along with the vagueness of the phrase "through other comparable forms of physical contact," there seems to be an additional question that goes beyond asking simply about the results of "shaking hands with a person with AIDS." Questions that have more than one referent of this kind are called *double-barreled questions.* They shoot more than one question at the respondent simultaneously, making it hard for the respondent to know which part of the question to answer and for the survey designer to figure out which aspect of the question the person was actually responding to.

Sentences. As mentioned earlier, clarity and balance are criteria that can be used in evaluating survey questions as well as the words and phrases that compose them. In addition, the length of the resulting sentences becomes an important dimension in evaluating survey questions. Payne (1951) suggested that, in general, the length of questions asked of respondents should be limited to no more than twenty words. Recent research has suggested, however, that shorter questions are not always better questions. People may be more likely to report both threatening and nonthreatening behaviors if the questions asked of them are somewhat longer. The assumption here is that longer questions give respondents more time to assemble their thoughts and also more clues to use in formulating answers. But longer questions may work better in personal interviews than in telephone interviews or mail questionnaires. With telephone interviews, respondents may have trouble remembering all the points raised in a long question and be reluctant to ask the interviewer to repeat it. Respondents filling out a mail questionnaire may feel that the question looks too complicated or will take too long to answer. More guidance for deciding how long questions should be will be provided in subsequent chapters.

Responses

In some ways, discussing the questions asked in surveys apart from the responses they elicit is an arbitrary distinction. The latter are directly affected by, and even in some instances imbedded in, how the former are phrased. However, there are criteria for *how* to answer the question implied in the types of response categories provided or assumed in the question. These criteria are in addition to *what* the question is asking, which is implied by the choice of words and phrases for the sentence used in framing the question. Criteria that are particularly relevant to apply in evaluating how questions should be answered are the comprehensiveness and constraints associated with the response categories that are imposed or implied by the survey question.

The two major types of survey questions are *open-ended* and *closed-end* questions. They differ principally in whether or not the categories that respondents use in answering the questions are provided to them directly. An open-ended question would be, "What do you think are the major ways AIDS is transmitted?" Respondents are free to list whatever they think relevant.

Closed-end variations of this question would involve providing respondents with a series of statements about how the disease might be transmitted and then asking whether they agree or disagree with each statement. Other forms of closed-end responses involve rating or ranking response formats. With a rating format, respondents can be asked to indicate, for each mode of transmission provided in the survey questionnaire, whether they think it is a very important, important, somewhat important, or not at all important means of transmitting the disease. With a ranking response, respondents can be shown the same list of, say, ten items and asked to rank them in order from one to ten, corresponding to their assessment of the most to least likely means of transmitting AIDS.

The open-ended response format can lead survey respondents to provide a comprehensive and diverse array of answers. The closed-end response format applies more constraints on the types of answers respondents are allowed to provide to the question. Each approach has its advantages and disadvantages.

Open-Ended Questions. Using open-ended questions during the pilot or pretest stage of a study offers particular advantages. The researcher can take the array of responses provided in these test interviews and use them to develop closed-end categories for the final study. With this approach the survey designer can have more confidence that the full range of possible responses is included in the closed-end question. However, it is much easier to code and process responses from closed-end questions. Using open-ended questions in this way can then optimize both the *comprehensiveness* of the answers obtained to questions during the development and testing phases of the study and the cost-effective benefits resulting from the *constraints* imposed by the closed-end response format of the final study.

Open-ended questions may still be necessary or useful in the final study if the researcher is interested in the salience or importance of certain issues or topics to respondents (Geer, 1991). Open-ended questions encourage respondents to talk about what is on the top of their heads or what comes to mind *first* when answering the question. To the extent that there is convergence in the answers respondents provide when this open format is used, the researcher can have confidence in the salience of these issues to study respondents. For example, the author and her colleagues, in an evaluation of the impact of home care programs on ventilator-assisted children and their families, asked a series of open-ended questions to elicit information about the major problems *and* benefits the families experienced in having their children at home (Aday, Aitken, & Wegener, 1988). The large numbers of those providing similar responses to these questions underlined the salience of certain issues across the board to such families in caring for their medically complex children.

Closed-End Questions. Survey respondents tend to try to work within the framework imposed by the survey questionnaire or interview task. Providing respondents with only certain types of alternatives for answering a question may mean that some responses that are in respondents' heads are, therefore, not fully reflected in their answers. The number and type of response categories, whether a middle (or neutral) response is provided for registering attitudes, whether an explicit "don't know" category is offered to respondents, and so on will directly affect how they answer the questions (Belson, 1981; Biemer, Groves, Lyberg, Mathiowetz, & Sudman, 1991; Blair & Burton, 1987; Schuman & Presser, 1981; Sudman & Schwarz, 1989). As mentioned earlier, however, coding closed-end questions takes less time than coding open-ended ones and may be more reliable across respondents and interviewers as well. The impact and usefulness of these various closed-end response alternatives for different types of survey questions will be discussed in more detail in subsequent chapters.

Instructions

Instructions form the final building block for the survey questionnaire. Instructions can be part of the question itself or they can serve to introduce or close the questionnaire or make meaningful transitions between different topics or sections within it. The principal criterion to use in evaluating instructions is their utility in ensuring that the question or questionnaire is answered in the way it should be. For example, sometimes the instruction RECORD VERBATIM is used with open-ended questions to encourage the interviewer to capture the respondents' answers in their own words to the maximum extent possible. Instructions are also used alongside response categories to tell the interviewer or respondent the next question to SKIP TO, depending on the answer to that question. Instructions are also useful in guiding the interviewer through the steps for selecting the respondent to interview or in showing the respondent to a mail questionnaire how to fill it out. Instructions are often designated by using parentheses, ALL CAPITAL LETTERS, or some other typeface to set them apart from the questions per se.

Questionnaire

The survey questions and accompanying response formats and instructions are then ordered and integrated into the survey questionnaire itself. The order and context in which the items are placed also has an impact on the meaning of certain questions and how respondents answer them. As mentioned earlier in this chapter, the order and context effects in surveys have been an important focus in the recent applications of cognitive psychology to questionnaire design (Schwarz & Sudman, 1992).

Questionnaire Administration

Sudman and Bradburn (1974) pointed out that various elements can give rise to response effects or errors in the answers actually obtained in a survey. These include (1) the structure of the survey task itself, especially the questionnaire; (2) the characteristics and performance of the survey respondents; and (3) the characteristics and performance of the interviewers charged with gathering the data. With mail questionnaires, errors associated with the interviewer are eliminated. The characteristics of the task and the respondents do, however, take on even greater importance in deciding how to design and administer the questionnaire in order to maximize the quality of the data obtained in the survey. As discussed in Chapter Five, the mode of data collection (in-person, telephone, mail), as well as whether paper-and-pencil or computer-assisted methods are used, can affect how certain types of questions are answered. Instrument development and pretesting procedures should ultimately employ the procedures to be used in the final study (Schechter & Beatty, 1994; Schwarz & Hippler, 1995; Schwarz, Strack, Hippler, & Bishop, 1991).

Special Considerations for Special Populations

Research on conducting surveys of special populations, such as ethnic minorities (Freidenberg, Mulvihill, & Caraballo, 1993; Johnson, et al., 1994; Marin & Marin, 1991; Von Thurn & Moore, 1993), intravenous drug users (Blair, Binson, & Murphy, 1992), teenagers (Stussman, Willis, & Allen, 1993), or the elderly (Herzog & Rodgers, 1989; Jobe & Mingay, 1990; Keller, Kovar, Jobe, & Branch, 1993) document that the approaches to answering questions may well differ for these groups. Problems may also arise in gaining the cooperation of overstudied populations, such as persons dying of AIDS (Albrecht, 1989, 1993; Albrecht & Zimmerman, 1993).

Implementing "warm" procedures (such as ethnographic interviews and focus groups) that involve informal and more intimate contacts with individuals like those to be included in the final study in the early stages of developing the questions before proceeding with more formal ("cold") procedures for evaluating them (think-aloud protocols, structured experiments, behavior coding, or larger scale pretesting), may be particularly useful for designing culturally sensitive and relevant questionnaires (Cassidy, 1994).

Surveys that involve contacts with large numbers of non-English-speaking respondents should have fully translated versions of the questionnaire. It is very important that any translations of the original questionnaire be back-translated by someone other than the first translator. In this way, questions that arise about different interpretations of the survey's words or concepts by different subgroups that purportedly speak the *same* language can be addressed (Aday, Chiu, & Andersen, 1980; Berkanovic, 1980; Marin & Marin, 1991). This alternative language version of the questionnaire should also be fully pretested with respondents similar to those who will be included in the final study before it goes to the field.

Selected Examples

The supplements used in the NCHS–NHIS have undergone extensive testing in the NCHS Questionnaire Design Research Laboratory, using many of the question development and review procedures detailed here: focus groups, think-alouds, laboratory and experimental testing, mini-pretests and pilot studies (published in the National Center for Health Statistics Cognitive Methods Staff Working Paper Series and NCHS Vital and Health Statistics Series 6).

In the Chicago AIDS survey designers were particularly concerned about respondents' willingness to answer extremely sensitive questions over the telephone. An extensive pilot study was therefore carried out before finalizing the study questionnaire (Binson, Murphy, & Keer, 1987). The final questionnaire, which was designed to maximize respondents' cooperation in answering sensitive questions, was based on the results of this pilot study and the general guidelines for asking such questions discussed in Chapter Ten.

The dentists survey questionnaire was sent to three practicing dentists in Seattle, who were then called for feedback on the instrument. In addition, the questionnaire was pretested with twenty dentists who saw members of the Washington Education Association (WEA) as patients but practiced in counties other than those that were the focus of the study. Survey responses were to be linked with dentists' records for WEA patients. The project investigators were concerned with dentists' willingness to participate in the survey, so a $10 incentive was included in the first mailing during the pretest. The pretest survey had a high rate of return, so this incentive was employed in the final study as well. Only minor changes were made in the survey questionnaire itself after pretesting.

Guidelines for Minimizing Survey Errors

The principles and procedures highlighted here are intended to minimize the inaccuracies or inconsistencies in the answers to survey questions—as a function of how the question is posed, the method used to ask it (telephone or personal interview or self-administered), as well as who asks it *and* who responds. The errors subsequently resulting are variously referred to as "response effects" (Sudman & Bradburn, 1974), "measurement errors" (Biemer, Groves, Lyberg, Mathiowetz, & Sudman, 1991), "nonsampling errors" (Lessler & Kalsbeek, 1992), and "observational errors" (Groves, 1989).

A good offense is the best defense in minimizing these types of errors. That is, survey developers should consult previous research regarding the factors that are most likely to give rise to these errors, as well as plan plenty of "preseason practice" by implementing some or a combination of the pretest procedures outlined earlier for designing and evaluating survey questions.

The chapters that follow build upon the principles and criteria introduced here to suggest guidelines for reducing the response errors in health surveys depending on *how* the survey questions are asked as well as on *what* they are asked about.

Supplementary Sources

Sources that provide straightforward guidance on how to compose survey questions to minimize the kinds of errors discussed in this chapter include Foddy (1993), Fowler (1995), Salant and Dillman (1994), and Sudman and Bradburn (1982).

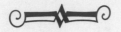

CHAPTER NINE

FORMULATING QUESTIONS ABOUT HEALTH

Chapter Highlights

1. The selection of questions about health for health surveys should be guided by the principles of total survey design.
2. The specific steps for selecting questions about health or other topics for health surveys are as follows: (1) decide how to measure the concepts, (2) relate the concepts to the survey design and objectives, (3) match the scale for the measures chosen to the analysis plan, (4) evaluate the reliability of the measures, (5) evaluate the validity of the measures, (6) choose the most appropriate method of data collection, (7) tailor the measures to the study sample, and (8) decide how best to ask the actual questions.

Deciding how best to measure health may summon much of the same perplexity and diversity of perspective as when the blind people were asked to take the measure of the proverbial elephant. Health surveys have traditionally served a variety of purposes and objectives, and the array of applications in both the public and private sectors continues to multiply. Correspondingly, different disciplines or fields of study or practice dictate different approaches to defining and measuring health as well as variant criteria for critiquing them.

Five major applications of health surveys can be identified, each of which illuminate contrasting perspectives in measuring health. First, health surveys have been widely used in community needs assessment activities or as a basis for planning health programs in a given market or service area. This perspective takes a broad look at the population's health, its determinants, and the various risks for poor health that exist for different members of the community. International and national health agencies, local public health providers, and public and private strategic planners are most likely to design and implement these types of studies (Aday, 1993a; Evans & Stoddart, 1990; Evans, Barer, & Marmor, 1994; McKillip, 1987; Wallace, 1994).

Surveys may also be used to evaluate the impact of experimental or quasi-experimental interventions on the health of affected groups. These studies dictate consideration of indicators of health that are sensitive to change over time or differences between groups to capture meaningfully any effects the programs yield. The RAND Health Insurance Experiment (HIE), an experimental study to evaluate the impact of different types of coverage and associated out-of-pocket costs on utilization and health (Brook, et al., 1979), and the Medical Outcomes Study (MOS), an observational study of the health outcomes of patients with selected illnesses in different practice settings (Stewart & Ware, 1992), have made substantial contributions to research on the measurement of health status and health-related quality of life (HRQOL). These studies have also contributed to informing national health care debates about the appropriateness of different models of financing and delivering services.

A third application of health surveys is for the purpose of gathering data on health plan patients or enrollees regarding their health status, satisfaction, and access to care, as components of "report cards" that are made available to current and prospective enrollees to inform their ultimate choice of plans (GAO, 1994). Patient input is increasingly being touted as an important component in evaluating the quality of care delivered in both inpatient and ambulatory settings (Greenfield & Nelson, 1992). The Health Plan Employer Data and Information System (HEDIS), developed by the National Committee for Quality Assurance (NCQA), an independent nonprofit organization formed to assess the quality of managed care organizations, represents one of the many attempts to standardize how health plans measure and report performance information and indicators (Corrigan, 1995; NCQA, 1993, 1995a, 1995b).

A fourth application of health surveys is epidemiological and clinical research to investigate the determinants or course of disease (based on case-control or cohort designs) and to test the effectiveness of alternative treatments (using randomized clinical trials). The proliferation of managed care in the private sector and the large role the federal government plays in providing coverage (especially for the elderly through Medicare, and the corollary concerns of these payers with the efficiency and effectiveness of services) have generated a burgeoning interest in health and medical care outcomes assessment and accountability. For example, the Agency for Health Care Policy and Research has assumed a role in funding research examining the costs and health outcomes of alternative treatments for an array of health conditions through the Patient Outcomes Research Teams (PORTS) and related projects (Fowler, Cleary, Magaziner, Patrick, & Benjamin, 1994; Goldberg & Cummings, 1994; Hadorn, Sorensen, & Holte, 1995; Hadorn & Uebersax, 1995; Steinwachs, Wu, & Skinner, 1994).

And finally, a fifth application is the use of health status assessment instruments in direct clinical practice to select treatments and monitor patient outcomes. The impetus for this application has been encouraged by the growing interest in evaluating and reporting the performance of health care plans and providers. It also surfaces a unique set of concerns from the perspective of providers regarding the utility, cost, and feasibility of implementing such procedures in the real world of clinical practice (Feinstein, 1992; Wasson, et al., 1992).

Criteria for Developing and Evaluating Measures of Health

A variety of criteria may be applied in developing and choosing measures of health, including *theoretic, psychometric, economic, clinimetric,* and *pragmatic norms.*

Theoretic considerations surface fundamental differences in the definition or conceptualization of health. Those who assume a perspective on the health of a community and the array of factors that influence it, for example, are likely to argue for the importance of gathering data on a broad set of subjective and objective indicators of quality of life (employment, school quality, crime, social support, and so on), based on the implicit assumption that an array of (medical and nonmedical) sectors and interventions are ultimately needed to improve the health of a community (Breslow, 1989). A contrasting perspective on the part of those principally concerned with measuring the effectiveness of *medical care* makes a strong case for distinguishing health-related quality of life measures, arguing that medical care should be held accountable only for those outcomes that it can most directly influence (Greenfield & Nelson, 1992). A related theoretic contrast is reflected in the distinctions drawn by critics of standardized approaches to questionnaire design and administration between the voice of medicine and the voice of the lifeworld (the experiences of everyday life) and their respective influences on how health is ultimately defined and measured (Jylhä, 1994; Mishler, 1986). The voice of medicine, they argue, seeks to elicit the "truth" about an underlying physiological state through decontextualizing and objectifying the language used in the clinical or standardized interview, for example, while the voice of the lifeworld seeks to surface the "reality" of individuals' experiences of health and function as lived in their respective environments through seeking and hearing the stories the patients have to tell in their own words.

Psychometric criteria for evaluating health items, indexes, and scales refer primarily to assessments of the validity and reliability of the measures discussed in Chapter Three. The fields of psychophysics, psychology, and psychometrics provide the theoretical and empirical foundation for this approach. Psychophysics, a field of study that began in the late nineteenth century, explored the application of the measurement procedures relating physical intensities (such as the magnitude of light) to internal sensations (individuals' perceptions of varying intensities of light). It formed the conceptual basis for category scaling techniques, which entail placing a line on a page with clearly defined end points or anchors (perfect health versus death), and asking respondents to rate the desirability of various (health) states in relationship to these anchor points (Froberg & Kane, 1989b).

Economic norms refer to the preferences that individuals have for different health states (levels of functioning) that are likely to influence their choice of treatment alternatives. Economists in particular are concerned with measuring the values (utilities) consumers assign to different options when making purchasing decisions. The conceptual foundation for quantifying these values is rooted in the axioms of utility theory developed by von Neumann and Morgenstern regarding the process of decision making under conditions of uncertainty (Froberg & Kane, 1989b). Approaches to health status measurement based on patients' preferences are receiving increasing attention in the emerging climate of provider accountability for the outcomes of clinical decisions.

Clinometric norms are those raised by practicing physicians as they survey patients in their own practices to assess the effectiveness of the care delivered in general and for individual patients in particular (Feinstein, 1987, 1992). Clinometric criteria may, in fact, conflict with or contradict norms grounded in other schools of thought. Standards of clinical judgment or measures of the pain or distress experienced by patients do not have gold standard points of reference for formally assessing criterion validity but may nonetheless be viewed by clinicians to have a high amount of implicit (face) validity. Some of the most useful clinical indicators of health status, such as the Apgar Score assigned to newborns, include a consciously heterogeneous, rather than homogenous, set of items. Clinicians may therefore be more interested in parsimony than redundancy (and hence reliability) in measuring the health of the patients seen in their busy practice.

A final set of norms are *pragmatic* ones. These include considerations of the cost and complexity of data collection and the ease of interpretation of the profiles or scores used to measure health concepts. These pragmatic concerns take on increasing importance as those who are not necessarily experts in the design and construction of such measures (patients, providers, and policymakers) are called upon either to take the survey, administer it, or interpret the results, as a foundation for deciding a course of action (choosing a health plan, deciding on a type of treatment, or defining the benefits that should be covered in a publicly sponsored health plan).

The relative weight or emphasis assigned to these respective criteria in developing or choosing measures of health is likely to mirror the disciplinary interests and points of view represented by the audiences and purposes motivating the conduct of a given survey. Survey designers must, however, be prepared to shed their disciplinary blinders and consider the applicability of this array of norms in order to maximize the clarity and precision of their own look at health.

Utility-Related Scaling Methods

The fields of psychometrics and economics have most influenced the development of health status measures. The focus of the psychometric approach is to generate *descriptions* of individuals' health states or outcomes, while the economic approach focuses on measuring individuals' *preferences* for these alternative states or outcomes. The Likert and Thurstone scaling methods, and to a lesser extent, Guttman and Rasch scales, have been used in developing psychometric-based summary measures of health status. These approaches to scale development were discussed in Chapter Three with particular reference to their application in developing a major psychometric-based measure of health status, the MOS 36-Item Short-Form Health Survey (SF-36). The principal utility-related approaches to health status measurement are described in this chapter and highlighted in Figure 9.1. Selected examples of major generic health status measures from both traditions, the concepts measured by each, as well as the mode of administration, scaling method, number of questions and scoring procedures are summarized in Table 9.1 (Ware, 1995).

Both types of measures have been employed to measure health-related quality of life (HRQOL) although this construct has been a particular focus of the utility-related measurement approaches (Cella, 1995; Revicki, 1992; Spilker, Molinek, Johnston, Simpson, & Tilson, 1990). Patrick and Erickson (1993, p. 22) define HRQOL as "the value assigned to duration of life as modified by the impairments, functional states, perceptions, and social opportunities that are influenced by disease, injury, treatment, or policy." Both the quantity (length) of life and the quality or health associated with these years of life are central to operationalizing this concept.

FIGURE 9.1. SELECTED UTILITY-RELATED SCALES.

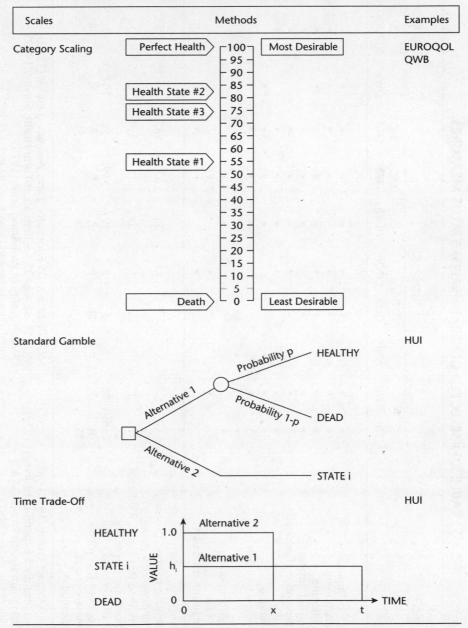

Scales	Methods	Examples

Category Scaling

Perfect Health — 100 — Most Desirable — EUROQOL QWB

Health State #2

Health State #3

Health State #1

Death — 0 — Least Desirable

Standard Gamble — HUI

Alternative 1 — Probability p — HEALTHY

Probability 1-p — DEAD

Alternative 2 — STATE i

Time Trade-Off — HUI

Sources: The "Category Scaling" figure is reprinted from Patrick & Erickson, 1993.

The "Standard Gamble" and "Time Trade-Off" figures are reprinted from *Journal of Health Economics, 5.* George W. Torrance, "Measurement of Health State Utilities for Economic Appraisal: A Review," pp. 1–30, 1986, with kind permission from Elsevier Science—NL, Sara Burgerhartstraat 25, 1055 KV Amsterdam, The Netherlands.

TABLE 9.1. SELECTED GENERAL HEALTH STATUS MEASURES.

Concepts and Characteristics	Psychometric								Utility Related		
	SIP	HIE	NHP	QLI	COOP	DUKE	MOS FWBP	MOS SF–36	QWB	EUROQOL	HUI
Concepts											
Physical functioning	•	•	•	•	•	•	•	•	•	•	•
Social functioning	•	•	•	•	•	•	•	•	•	•	
Role functioning	•	•	•	•	•	•	•	•	•	•	
Psychological distress	•	•	•	•	•	•	•	•		•	•
Health perceptions (general)		•	•	•	•	•	•	•		•	•
Pain (bodily)	•	•	•	•	•	•	•	•		•	•
Energy/fatigue		•	•			•	•	•			
Psychological well-being		•	•				•	•			
Sleep	•		•				•				
Cognitive functioning	•	•			•						•
Quality of life			•		•						
Reported health transition								•			
Characteristics											
Administration method (S = self, I = interviewer, P = proxy)	S,I,P	S,P	S,I	S,P	S,I	S,I	S,I	S,I,P	I,P	S	S,I,P
Scaling method (L = Likert, R = Rasch, T = Thurstone, U = utility)	T	L	T	L	L	L	L	L,R	U	U	U
Number of questions	136	86	38	5	9	17	149	36	107	9	31
Scoring options (P = profile, SS = summary scores, SI = single index)	P, SS, SI	P	P	SI	P	P, SI	P	P, SS	SI	SI	SI

SIP = Sickness Impact Profile (1976)
HIE = Health Insurance Experiment surveys (1979)
NHP = Nottingham Health Profile (1980)
QLI = Quality of Life Index (1981)
COOP = Dartmouth Function Charts (1987)
DUKE = Duke Health Profile (1990)

MOS FWBP = MOS Functioning and Well-Being Profile (1992)
MOS SF–36 = MOS 36–Item Short-Form Health Survey (1992)
QWB = Quality of Well-Being Scale (1973)
EUROQOL = European Quality of Life Index (1990)
HUI = Health Utilities Index-Mark III (1993)

Bibliography:

SIP — Bergner, Bobbitt, Carter, and Gilson, 1981;
Bergner, Bobbitt, Kressel, Pollard, Gilson, and Morris, 1976

HIE — Brook, et al., 1979

NHP — Hunt and McEwen, 1980;
Hunt, McKenna, McEwen, Williams, and Papp, 1981

QLI — Spitzer, et al., 1981;
Wood-Dauphinee and Williams, 1987

COOP — Beaufait, et al., 1991;
Nelson, et al., 1987

DUKE — Parkerson, Broadhead, and Tse, 1990;
Parkerson, Gehlbach, Wagner, James, Clapp, and Muhlbaier, 1981

MOS FWBP — Stewart and Ware, 1992

MOS SF 36 — McHorney, Ware, and Raczek, 1993;
McHorney, Ware, Lu, and Sherbourne, 1994;
Ware, Kosinski, and Keller, 1994;
Ware and Sherbourne, 1992;
Ware, Snow, Kosinski, and Gandek, 1993

QWB — Bush, 1984;
Kaplan, 1989;
Kaplan and Anderson, 1988;
Patrick, Bush, and Chen, 1973

EUROQOL — EuroQOL Group, 1990

HUI — Boyle, Furlong, Feeny, Torrance, and Hatcher, 1995;
Feeny, Torrance, Goldsmith, Furlong, and Boyle, 1993

The basic metric in quantifying quality of life, based on this perspective, is an interval or ratio scale that ranges from 0 to 1, with one being a perfect state of health, 0 being death, with varying states of health represented by the points in between. Raters are then asked to evaluate their preference for alternative states of health compared with others or with death. For example, being able to eat, dress, bathe, and go to the toilet without help, and have no limitations in normal work, school, or play activities might be assigned a value of 1.00. Comparatively, having some limitation in these latter role activities may receive a score of .94. Needing help with all the personal care activities, and not being able to engage in one's normal social roles may lower the rating considerably to .50—reflecting that it is much less preferable than being able to function fully in these activities (1.00) but nonetheless still preferred to death (0) (Patrick & Erickson, 1993, pp. 381–382). It is also possible that some states (such as being in a coma on life support systems) may be deemed worse than death and would then be assigned negative values. The scores derived for each state can then be used as weights applied to the actual or anticipated years of life to compute quality-adjusted life years (QALYS)—an operational indicator of health-related quality of life incorporating both the quality and quantity of years lived (Morrow & Bryant, 1995; Robine, Mathers, & Bucquet, 1993; Torrance & Feeny, 1989).

Although a number of utility-related measures have been developed, three have been most widely used and evaluated in measuring HRQOL: *category scaling, standard gamble,* and *time trade-off* (Feeny & Torrance, 1989; Froberg & Kane, 1989a, 1989b, 1989c, 1989d; Patrick & Erickson, 1993; Torrance, 1986, 1987). The first has its roots in psychophysics and the latter two in economics. The response format and examples of each are portrayed in Figure 9.1.

Category scaling methods are comparable to the Thurstone scaling approach. Raters are asked to assign health states to a point on a scale that ranges between 0 (death) and 100 (perfect health), assuming that the points on the scale can be considered equal intervals. Those assigned closer to the perfect or most desirable state (100) would be preferred to those that are not. Thermometers or comparable metrics are used as devices for registering the relative rating of different health states, levels of function, or pain (EuroQol Group, 1990).

The essence of the *standard gamble approach* is that a choice (having a kidney transplant when there is some probability of the risk of rejection or death, for example) is posed to the respondent. With one of the options (not having the transplant) the health state is certain (probability =100 percent): needing regular kidney dialysis for the rest of one's life. If the transplant is undertaken, however, one of two things might occur: either the patient is returned to normal health and lives for an additional number of years (probability p) or dies immediately because of an autoimmune response to the transplanted organ (probability 1-p).

The choice (alternative 1) to have the transplant is then more of a "gamble" than not having it (alternative 2). The chances of the patient dying (1-p) can be varied—from a very small (10 percent) to a high (70 percent) probability of occurrence, for example, using the standard gamble methodology. If the chances of dying are low, a patient may prefer to have the transplant to avoid the prospect of having to be on dialysis for the rest of her life. If the chances are high, she may be less willing to do so. However, if she views being on dialysis to be a very undesirable alternative, the patient may be willing to risk a high probability (1-p=.70) of death from having the transplant. The probability (p) at which the respondent is "indifferent" (that is, cannot really decide between the two alternatives given the risks) is then assigned as the preference value (.30) for the known consequence (lifetime dialysis). It is much less than the most desired state of perfect health (1.00) but still better than death (0). Variations in the standard gamble can also be used to compare states that are likely to be worse than death or temporary health states (Torrance, 1986).

The concept of probability underlying the standard gamble approach is a complex one and may not be readily understandable by some respondents. The time trade-off method was developed as an alternative that would be simpler to implement and interpret. In contrast to the standard gamble method, the respondent is asked to choose between two alternatives that are certain rather than between one certain and one chance outcome. Essentially, raters are asked to indicate how many years of life they would be willing to give up to be in a healthier state compared with a less healthy one.

Referring to the example of the choice of having a kidney transplant (alternative 2) or not (alternative 1) in this model, the patient is offered an alternative of having the transplant and living a certain number of years (x=10) of the estimated remaining years of life (t=20) in a relatively healthy state, compared with living out his or her life (twenty years) on dialysis. With the time trade-off methodology, the number of years of healthy life (x) is varied until the respondent is indifferent (unable to choose between them): for example, the person may reach a point of not being able to choose when the trade-off becomes gaining five years of life (x) in relatively good health with the transplant versus living the full twenty years (t) on dialysis. The preference for living in this state (h) can be computed (x/t) based on these trade-offs (5/20=.25). A score of .25 reflects a low evaluation of the transplant compared with not having it given the few years of healthy life gained (Torrance, 1986).

Preferences and valuations, based on these approaches, provide the foundation for utility-related scales of health-related quality of life. Respondents can be asked their current state of health or level of functioning and the ratings (or weights) derived from these respective approaches can then be used in assigning overall HRQOL scores.

The reliability and validity of these and other approaches to constructing the preferences for treatment alternatives and associated health outcomes has been examined to a limited extent in the literature (Froberg & Kane, 1989b; Patrick & Erickson, 1993; Torrance, 1986, 1987).

Intra- and inter-rater reliability (the consistency within and between raters), as well as test-retest reliability, are the most relevant forms of reliability analyses for these measures. There is no expectation that the varying stimuli (states) presented to respondents will have high intercorrelations (internal consistency reliability). In general, the intra- and inter-rater and test-retest reliability of these approaches have been found to be variable but acceptable (.70 or higher), although as might be expected the test-retest reliability diminishes the longer the time between measurements (Froberg & Kane, 1989b).

Content and construct validity are most applicable to these types of measures. Strictly speaking, there is no "gold standard" against which these judgments can be compared to evaluate their criterion validity. Studies of health-state preferences differ widely in the format and content of health states that are presented to raters, and the content validity of these scenarios is rarely discussed. The convergent validity among the different methods and the hypothetical associations of these preferences with other variables have been neither extensively examined nor supported in the literature. The category rating scales appear to be the easiest for raters to understand and yield the most valid scale values (Froberg & Kane, 1989b).

Methodological concerns with these approaches relate to who is asked to do these ratings (general population, patients, health professionals) and the extent to which the ratings might differ for different groups; the impact of how the question is framed, the content of the descriptions of the health states, and the risk-aversiveness of respondents on responses provided; and the paucity of comprehensive validity analyses (using the multitrait multimethod approach, for example) comparing the various methods (Aaronson, 1989; Cella, 1995; Gill & Feinstein, 1994; Katz, 1987; Froberg & Kane, 1989a, 1989b, 1989c, 1989d; Mulley, 1989; Rutten-van Mölken, Bakker, van Doorslaer, & van der Linden, 1995; Torrance, 1986, 1987). As these types of measures are increasingly used in making critical policy and clinical choices, the need for collaborative and effective partnerships between and among researchers from the disciplines of psychometrics, economics, and cognitive psychology in resolving these controversies takes on a heightened importance.

Steps in Developing and Evaluating Measures of Health

The discussion that follows applies the principles of survey design discussed in other chapters to illustrate the total survey design approach for deciding which questions on health and other topics to include in a health survey.

Deciding How to Measure the Concepts

A primary consideration in deciding which questions to ask in a health survey is the conceptualization of health that best operationalizes the research questions to be addressed in the study (see Table 3.1 in Chapter Three). If there is an interest in profiling a population's overall health status, then general health status measures such as the MOS-SF-36 may be most appropriate. If the focus is on eliciting patient preferences for the health states that might result from alternative treatment choices, then utility-based scales such as the Health Utilities Index (HUI) may be the health status measure of choice.

A number of overviews of health status measures are available (Bergner, 1985; Bergner & Rothman, 1987; Bowling, 1991; Brook, ct al., 1979; Cella, 1995; Elinson & Siegmann, 1979; Hansluwka, 1985; Keith, 1994; Larson, 1991; Lohr, 1989, 1992; Lohr & Ware, 1987; McDowell & Newell, 1987; Patrick & Bergner, 1990; Patrick & Deyo, 1989; Patrick & Erickson, 1993; Rabkin, 1986; Stewart & Ware, 1992; Ware, 1987, 1995; Wilkin, Hallam, & Doggett, 1992).

Multidimensional Concept of Health. As mentioned earlier, health is a complex and multidimensional concept. The World Health Organization (WHO) has defined health as a "state of complete *physical, mental,* and *social* well-being and not merely the absence of disease or infirmity" (World Health Organization, 1948, p. 1). Comprehensive efforts to conceptualize health and develop empirical definitions of the concept have tended to distinguish the physical, mental, and social dimensions of health reflected in the WHO definition (Ware, 1987, 1995).

Ware has characterized physical health as "the physiologic and physical status of the body" and mental health as "the state of mind, including basic intellectual functions such as memory and feelings" (1986, pp. 205–206). He also points out that questions about feelings toward one's body (whether it hurts or how happy one is about it) relate to the interface between mental and physical health.

Although physical and mental health indicators clearly "end at the skin," to use Ware's phrase, indicators of social well-being extend beyond the individual to include the quantity and quality of his or her social contacts with other individuals. There is evidence that the number and nature of such contacts influence individuals' physical and mental health. Also, whether individuals can perform appropriate social roles and thereby be productive members of society is the bottom line in evaluating the impact of their physical and mental health on their overall social well-being. In Ware's conceptualization, social functioning is considered a correlate or outcome of health as measured by physical or mental health indicators, but *not* a core indicator of health per se. Orth-Gomer and Unden (1987) provide a review of many of the measures of social support used in population surveys.

In arriving at the kinds of health questions to ask in health surveys, researchers need to decide which dimensions of health—physical, mental, or social—they want to study. If they want to focus on more than one dimension, they must determine what the various dimensions convey, separately or together, about the target population's health.

Positive Versus Negative Concepts of Health. Another conceptual consideration that influences how health might be measured is that health status can be defined in either positive or negative terms (Twaddle & Hessler, 1977). Examples of positive indicators of health include criteria such as norms for age- and sex-specific measures of height or weight or a scale of positive mental health. As for negative indicators, death may be said to reflect the total absence of health, measured by total or disease-specific mortality (death) rates. Concepts of morbidity serve to define the middle range of a continuum defined by theoretical positive and negative end points that mark the total presence or absence of health. Health providers and patients may, of course, apply different criteria in defining morbidity and associated health status.

Provider Versus Patient Concepts of Health. The assessment of the presence or absence of *disease* relies on clinical or diagnostic judgments of the underlying medical condition (Twaddle & Hessler, 1977). Efforts to identify diseases in the target population of a survey would be obtained by administering physical exams or tests, such as taking participants' blood pressure or administering a glucose-tolerance test, as is done in the NCHS–Health and Nutrition Examination Survey. Another approach would be to ask respondents or their physicians to report diagnosed conditions, as in the NCHS–National Health Interview Survey and the NCHS–National Ambulatory Medical Care Survey, respectively. Comparable mental health diagnoses can be obtained by sampling clinic records or asking mental health professionals to provide this information for the clients they see in their practices.

An approach to defining morbidity based on conceptualizing it as *illness* tends to rely more on the individuals' own perceptions of their physical or mental health than on provider or medical record sources or respondents' reports of clinically diagnosed conditions. The emphasis here, then, is on the person's perceptions rather than on provider judgments. Questions about symptoms that people experienced during the year or their perceptions of their health—whether they consider it to be excellent, good, fair, or poor and how much they worry about their health—are questions that respondents, not providers, can best answer. These questions tap the person's subjective experience of the illness.

Different individuals' perceptions of the same underlying medical condition may vary as a result of cultural or subgroup differences in how illness is defined or because of individual variations in the thresholds of pain or discomfort felt to be experienced. There is evidence that these perceptions are indeed correlated with provider diagnoses of certain types of diseases, such as chronic and severe morbidities (Krause & Jay, 1994; Pope, 1988).

Asking questions to get at people's perceptions of their mental or physical health may tap something different from what providers would say about their health (Hall, Epstein, & McNeil, 1989). The choice of approach should be guided by conceptual considerations of which ways of measuring health make the most sense given the aspects of health the investigator wants to learn about from the study and from whose point of view.

A third approach to estimating morbidity is in terms of the individual's ability to perform certain functions or activities. These indicators are based on behavioral, rather than perceptual or clinical, criteria. Morbidity characterized in this way is sometimes referred to as *sickness* rather than "illness" or "disease" to suggest its connections with the "sick roles" people assume when they perceive themselves to be ill. The sick role makes it socially acceptable for them to change or limit their usual activities in certain ways because of illness (see Resource A, Section D).

Many physical health indexes and some psychological ones build on patient or provider reports of individuals' level of functioning as behavioral indicators of health. The sequential stages of alteration in functioning can be expressed as impairment, disability, and handicap (McDowell & Newell, 1987; WONCA Classification Committee, 1990).

Impairment refers to reduced physical or mental capacities that result from some organic disturbance or malfunction, such as impaired vision. Many impairments can be corrected (by wearing glasses, for example). If impairments are not corrected, disability (a restriction on a person's ability to perform his or her normal physical or social roles or functions) may result. Handicaps reflect situations that result in social disadvantages (such as social stigma or loss of one's job) arising from the person's disability. It is important to point out that the same condition may impact differently on different people's level of functioning. A broken arm may be a disability for a lawyer but a handicap for a professional baseball player. The health-related quality of life concept attempts to identify the non-medical, social, and behavioral consequences of underlying disease states (Wilson & Kaplan, 1995).

Researchers need to decide whether *behavioral* indicators of health are important for their purposes and, if so, what level of functioning it is most appropriate to capture with these measures and for whom.

Generic Versus Disease-Specific Concepts of Health. Another important distinction to consider in selecting relevant measures of health status is generic versus disease-specific indicators (Bergner & Rothman, 1987; Patrick & Deyo, 1989). Generic measures encompass an array of relevant dimensions of health and quality of life (such as general perceptions of health, psychological function, physical/role function, social function, and so on) that are relevant across disease or illness categories. Disease-specific measures are those that are most relevant to measuring the health impact of specific conditions (such as cancer, arthritis, or chronic back pain). Disease-specific measures may be particularly useful in measuring the responsiveness of patients to interventions in a clinical practice setting and generic measures for profiling the needs of a population in a program's service area.

Relating the Concepts to the Survey Design and Objectives

Next, researchers should consider the particular study design being used in their survey (Table 2.1 in Chapter Two) and the types of research questions that can be addressed with the design (Table 2.2 and Figure 2.1 in Chapter Two). Different methodological criteria should be emphasized in choosing health indexes for different types of study designs (Kirshner & Guyatt, 1985).

Cross-Sectional Designs. Cross-sectional survey designs are often used to estimate the prevalence of disease or the need for certain health services or programs in the target population. Researchers must decide, for example, whether disease-specific or generic health status measures are appropriate in gathering data on the target population. Disease-specific measures are appropriate for assessing the health of a patient population that has a particular disease or condition and generic measures for assessing health across a variety of populations or patients. Designers of needs assessment surveys must clearly define the needs they are trying to assess in deciding which health questions to ask in their study.

Group-Comparison Designs. Kirshner and Guyatt (1985) point out the importance of *discriminative criteria* in selecting health indexes for group-comparison designs. This type of design allows researchers to detect real differences between groups. Researchers then need to ask which groups are the focus of the survey and if the instrument is sufficiently discriminating to detect meaningful degrees of difference on the relevant health dimensions *between* these groups.

For example, one type of functional status indicator would be required if the study focuses on comparisons between different age and sex groups in a general population survey, while another type would be required for a study comparing the same groups in a survey of the institutionalized elderly. The indicators chosen would need to have very different scales for measuring physical functioning for these different groups. Health indexes that measure the ability to feed or dress oneself or walk, such as Katz's Index of Independence in Activities of Daily Living (Katz,

Ford, Moskowitz, Jackson, & Jaffe, 1963), would be appropriate for the institutionalized elderly sample but not for the general population sample, because the majority of the persons in the latter sample would be able to perform these tasks.

In comparing the major subgroups of interest within these respective types of samples, and particularly within the general population sample, researchers may need to consider the appropriate roles (working, going to school, for example) for different age groups in collecting information that can be meaningfully compared between them. This is the approach used in the National Center for Health Statistics–National Health Interview Survey (NCHS–NHIS) in collecting information on the major activity limitations of people of different ages (see Resource A, Section B).

Longitudinal Designs. With longitudinal designs Kirshner and Guyatt (1985) point out the importance of considering *predictive criteria.* That is to say, the individual items and the summary scales developed from them should predict changes in certain criterion measures over time. One would, for example, expect health questions in surveys inquiring about the numbers and types of medical conditions to be associated with subsequent mortality rates for a cohort of individuals being followed over time in epidemiological surveys.

In conducting longitudinal studies of this kind, survey researchers need to be particularly sensitive to the extent to which variations in the health indicators could be affected by other external factors in the environment, as well as to the fact that changes in the questions in successive waves of the study could introduce errors in detecting true changes in these indicators over time. For example, using National Center for Health Statistics survey data, Wilson and his colleagues (Wilson, 1981; Wilson & Drury, 1984) pointed out the impact of some of these factors on interpreting trends in illness and disability. Improved diagnostic and treatment techniques for a selected illness can lead to a higher survival rate of people with the disease and, hence, a higher, rather than lower, prevalence of the disease over time. Increased access to medical care can result in more "prescribed" days of disability (limiting one's usual routine because of illness) or to the diagnosis of previously undiagnosed conditions. Changing the survey methodology to increase the reporting of health events will also reduce the comparability of survey results with data from previous years.

Measuring changes in health indicators requires that investigators be aware of the factors to which those indicators are sensitive and whether they are the "true" changes that the investigators are interested in measuring or simply "noise" that confounds the interpretation of any differences that are observed over time.

Experimental Designs. "Evaluative" criteria should be applied in the development or choice of health indexes for surveys used in experimental studies. These criteria determine whether the indicator is sensitive to detecting the changes hypothesized to result from some clinical or programmatic intervention (Guyatt, Deyo, Charlson, Levine, & Mitchell, 1989; Kirshner & Guyatt, 1985).

The researcher should consider what changes in an individual's health, such as specific levels or types of physical functioning for people with rheumatoid arthritis, are predicted to result from the intervention—the use of a new drug or physical therapy regimen, for example. Further, health promotion interventions that focus on producing "good health" may require indicators that define the positive end of a continuum conceptualized as the presence or magnitude of health or well-being, while more treatment-oriented interventions may require that the negative end of the continuum—the presence or magnitude of "illness"—be defined.

Health measures in experimental or quasi-experimental designs should be scaled to be responsive to different levels or types of interventions and at the same time should not be subject to large random variation between questionnaire administrations.

Matching the Scale for the Measures Chosen to the Analysis Plan

The third major set of considerations in deciding the types of health questions to ask in surveys is the level of measurement and type of summary scale that would be most appropriate to use in asking or analyzing the questions. As discussed in Chapter Three, variables can be nominal, ordinal, interval, or ratio levels of measurement (Table 3.1). There are also a variety of devices for condensing the information from several different questions into a single summary or scale score (Figure 3.3 and Table 3.4). Ultimately, and perhaps most importantly, the kinds of analysis that can be conducted with the data are a function of how the variables are measured (see Chapter Fifteen). In deciding how to ask the questions, then, the researcher should give considerable thought to what he or she wants to do with the data once they are collected.

Level of Measurement. Researchers might decide that a simple classification of individuals into categories—those who can climb stairs or dress themselves versus those who cannot—is adequate for their purposes. If so, asking questions that rely on nominal dichotomous responses (*yes* or *no*) would be sufficient. Typologies can also be constructed on the basis of cross-classifications of these variables— can climb stairs *and* dress oneself; can climb stairs but *not* dress oneself; can dress oneself but *not* climb stairs; or can do *neither*.

If finer discrimination is required to detect varying levels of functioning for different individuals, then a question or scale with an ordinal level of measurement would be more appropriate. For example, the study subjects could be rank-ordered according to whether they can perform more or fewer functions or seem to be more or less happy with their lives. A variety of ordinal summary devices could be used if this type of discrimination is desired: simple indexes that add up the number of tasks the subjects can accomplish; Likert-type scales that summarize scale scores reflecting the extent to which they can perform these tasks; or Guttman scales for which the total score reflects the actual profile of various tasks the person may be able to perform.

Ratio or interval measures or summary scales, such as the Thurstone Equal-Appearing Interval scale, provide more information for the researcher to use in order to estimate not just whether the "health" of certain individuals is better than that of others but also how much better. Building in this level of discrimination in choosing questions to include in the study could be particularly important in experimental or quasi-experimental designs in which the investigator is interested in determining the magnitude of improvement that results from different levels (or dosages) of an experimental treatment applied to study subjects. Utility-related measures generally assume a cardinal (interval or ratio) level of measurement (Torrance, 1986, 1987).

Number of Items. A related measurement issue in choosing the questions to include in a health survey is whether the survey designer wants to use a single-item or a multi-item scale to measure the health concept of interest. There are advantages and disadvantages to each approach. Single items are easier and cheaper to administer and are less of a burden for the respondents to answer. Health variables based on one or only a few questions may, however, be less reliable than multi-item scales that more consistently capture a larger part of the concept.

However, there are some disadvantages in asking a number of different questions. For example, a single score summarizing across a variety of dimensions can be hard to interpret substantively and may also not adequately capture differing patterns of responses to different dimensions or indicators of the concept.

Both single-item and multi-item approaches to asking questions about people's health are used in health surveys. One question used with considerable frequency as an indicator of overall health status asks whether a respondent thinks his or her health is excellent, good, fair, or poor. The precise wording of this question has varied in different surveys. The current NCHS–NHIS survey asks, "Would you say (PERSON's) health in general is excellent, very good, good, fair, or poor?" (Resource A, Section G, Question 4). In previous NCHS–NHIS studies, the question was, "Compared to other persons (PERSON's) age, would you say that (his) (her) health is excellent, good, fair, or poor?" (National Center for Health Statistics, 1985c, pp. 42–44). This measure tends to be a particularly sensitive indicator of the presence of chronic and serious but manageable conditions, such as hypertension, diabetes, thyroid problems, anemia, hemophilia, and ulcers (Pope, 1988) and to be correlated with individuals' overall utilization of physicians' services (Andersen, Aday, Lyttle, Cornelius, & Chen, 1987). This question also captures the point of view of the person's own experiences and perceptions.

Many of the individual questions from the NCHS–NHIS that ask whether people were unable to perform age-appropriate roles because of an "impairment or health problem" (Resource A, Section B) or had to restrict their usual activities more than half a day because of "illness or injury" (Resource A, Section D) are used quite often as single-item indicators of health status.

Many health status indicators, however, are based on a number of different questions and may capture various dimensions of health (physical, mental, and social) as well as provide a summative evaluation of health as a whole.

Evaluating the Reliability of the Measures

An important methodological criterion to consider in evaluating any empirical indicator of a concept is its reliability. Methods for evaluating the test-retest, interrater, and internal consistency reliability of survey measures were described in Chapter Three (see Figure 3.1).

Survey designers should review information of this kind when deciding whether the measures they are considering are reliable enough for their purposes. More precise (reliable) measures are required when the focus is on estimates for particular *individuals*—such as changes in physical functioning of individual patients as a result of a clinical intervention—than when looking at differences between *groups*, especially groups for which substantial differences are expected to exist. An example of the latter would be the degree of social functioning for handicapped versus nonhandicapped children.

As mentioned earlier, reliability will probably be lower for single-item than for multi-item indicators of health. The reliability of certain measures may be less for socioeconomically disadvantaged groups (those with less income or lower levels of education) or individuals whose impairments (such as poor sight or hearing) limit their ability to respond adequately to certain types of survey forms or questions.

If information is not available on measures that others have formulated or for new items or scales developed for a survey, then survey designers can assess the reliability of those questions through pilot studies or split-ballot experiments before fielding their study questionnaire, if time and resources permit.

Evaluating the Validity of the Measures

Validity—the accuracy of empirical measures in reflecting a concept—is another important methodological criterion to consider in evaluating survey questions. Approaches for assessing the content, criterion, and construct validity of survey measures were summarized in Chapter Three (see Figure 3.2). Often, however, data on the validity of survey questions are limited.

The place to start in examining the validity of health status measures is their content: Do the items seem to capture the domain or subdimension of health (physical, mental, or social health or health in general) that is the focus of the study? Researchers should systematically scrutinize the items being considered and try to determine whether the items seem to capture adequately and accurately the major concept or subdimension of health that they are interested in measuring. Factor analysis and multitrait multimethod analyses are also useful in making more sophisticated quantitative judgments about whether the items adequately discriminate one concept from another (see the discussion in Chapter Three). In general, valid measures are those that accurately translate the concept they are supposed to measure into the empirically oriented language of surveys.

Choosing the Most Appropriate Method of Data Collection

Once researchers have clearly delineated the major questions they want to address with a study, the ways in which the questions will be conceptualized and measured, and the probable validity and reliability of the measures they will use to summarize the data, they should give thought to practical implementation decisions, such as how they will go about collecting their data.

Certain indicators require certain forms of administration (by expert raters, interviewers, or self-administered formats) (McDowell & Newell, 1987). If researchers are thinking about using one of these measures, they need to consider whether it is appropriate to use the method used originally in designing and administering the scale or to adapt it to their study. They also need to consider the implications that a change will have for the overall reliability and validity of the resulting data.

The burden (time, effort, and stress) on respondents in participating should always be taken into account when deciding on the numbers and kinds of questions to ask in health surveys. Researchers also need to consider both the personal and pecuniary costs and benefits of different data collection approaches (such as those outlined in Table 5.1 in Chapter Five) and whether certain methods of gathering the information are more appropriate than others, given *who* is the focus of the study.

Tailoring the Measures to the Study Sample

A related practical issue in deciding the kinds of questions to ask and how to ask them is the type of sample that will be drawn for the study. Generic health status questions may be more suitable for general surveys of the noninstitutionalized population, while disease-specific questions may be more appropriate for samples of hospitalized patients.

Further, it may be necessary to design and test screening questions to ask of family or household informants so that people with certain types of medical conditions can be oversampled, if they are a particular focus of the study. To be most efficient for this purpose, such questions should have good criterion validity, that is, high levels of specificity and sensitivity and, correspondingly, few false positive or false negative answers (see Figure 3.2 in Chapter Three).

Deciding How Best to Ask the Actual Questions

In deciding exactly how to phrase the questions that will be included in a survey, researchers should follow the principles outlined in the preceding chapter and in Chapters Ten and Eleven. They should consider the precise words, phrases, and resulting sentences to be used; the instructions to be provided with them; and the possible effect of the order and format in which they appear in the questionnaire on people's propensity to respond reliably and accurately.

Certain questions about physical, mental, or social health—such as whether respondents are incontinent or have had feelings that life was not worth living—may be highly sensitive and threatening. In asking these types of questions, survey designers should consider the principles outlined in Chapter Ten for asking threatening questions.

Special Considerations for Special Populations

Considerations that come into play in measuring the health of special populations are numerous. Different cultural, racial, or ethnic groups may experience and express illness in different ways (Alonso, Anto, & Moreno, 1990; Badia & Alonso, 1995). It is therefore particularly important to employ culturally sensitive and relevant approaches to item and instrument development to capture these variant meanings. Translations of standardized health status questionnaires that an investigator would like to use or adapt may (or may not) be available. Even if they are, the reliability and validity of the scale should be assessed and compared with the estimates provided for the English and translated versions on other studies. The results may well differ.

Furthermore, one size does not fit all for certain health status questions across age groups, such as the functional impact of disability for children, adults, and the elderly. In addition, some types of questions or modes of administration will be particularly burdensome or problematical for those whose health one might be most interested in measuring—the elderly or people with low levels of literacy or cognitive, physical, hearing, or visual impairments, for example. Thought must then be given to strategies that are appropriate for facilitating obtaining information from these populations (amplified audio data collection techniques, the use of proxies, or observational rather than respondent report methods).

Selected Examples

The Chicago AIDS survey and the Washington State dentists survey did not have the measurement of health status or health-related quality of life as a primary focus. This is, however, a central component of the NCHS–NHIS. Many of the questions in the NHIS core, and particularly the supplements, have undergone extensive testing through the center's cognitive research laboratory or extramural research program (NCHS, 1987c, 1988c, 1989d, 1992b, 1992d, 1994c; Salovey, Smith, Turk, Jobe, & Willis, 1993; Schechter, 1993, 1994). The development of the disability supplements was, in fact, grounded in an intensive series of question development and assessment activities program (Hendershot, 1990; Simpson, 1993; Simpson, Keer, & Cynamon, 1993; Verbrugge, 1994). Though the NCHS–NHIS does capture a diverse battery of health status measures, critics have argued that it should also incorporate more widely used standardized scales or approaches to measuring health (Patrick & Erickson, 1993).

Guidelines for Minimizing Survey Errors

This chapter identified a variety of norms that might be applied in selecting and evaluating measures of health status. The best advice to minimize both the systematic and variable errors in measuring health is, in fact, to be aware of what a given perspective might either illuminate *or* fail to surface. Disciplinary or methodological parochialism may shed light on parts of the proverbial pachyderm, but the essence and magnitude of the beast as a whole may well be hidden or distorted in the viewing.

Supplementary Sources

See the following sources for a more comprehensive treatment of health status measurement: Bowling (1991), Larson (1991), McDowell and Newell (1987), Patrick and Erickson (1993), and Streiner and Norman (1991).

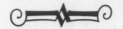

CHAPTER TEN

FORMULATING QUESTIONS ABOUT DEMOGRAPHICS AND BEHAVIOR

Chapter Highlights

1. In selecting the sociodemographic and socioeconomic questions to ask people in health surveys, researchers can start with items comparable to those in the National Center for Health Statistics–National Health Interview Survey or related federally sponsored health surveys and either adapt them or develop new ones as needed to enhance their relevance for a given study purpose or population.

2. In developing factual, nonthreatening questions about behaviors, researchers should try to reduce "telescoping" errors (overreporting) by using devices such as bounded recall and errors of omission (underreporting) by means of aided recall, diaries, or respondent record checks, as well as cognitive survey research techniques, to design and implement the survey questionnaire.

3. Rules for developing sensitive questions about health behaviors should focus on how to reduce the kind of underreporting that results from respondents' feeling threatened when acknowledging they engaged in those behaviors.

This chapter presents rules for writing questions to gather facts about the target populations of surveys. Three types of questions will be considered: (1) questions about demographic characteristics and both (2) nonthreatening questions and (3) threatening questions about health and health care behaviors of survey respondents and their families. Different tasks and respondent burdens are associated with different types of questions. Questionnaire designers should take these differences into account in formulating their questions, as well as in evaluating items that others have developed.

Questions About Demographics

It is not always necessary to start from scratch in developing questions about the basic sociodemographic and socioeconomic characteristics of study respondents and their families. Important advantages of using standardized items of this kind are that they (1) reduce the time and effort needed to develop and test such questions, (2) permit direct comparisons of the sample of a given survey with the results from a variety of other studies, and (3) in some instances, have documented evidence of their reliability or validity in previous studies.

In selecting the sociodemographic and socioeconomic questions to use in health surveys, those asked in the National Center for Health Statistics–National Health Interview Survey (NCHS–NHIS) or related federally sponsored health surveys provide a useful place to start. Using items from these studies offers several advantages: (1) the National Health Interview Survey follows the guidelines or requirements of the Office of Management and Budget (OMB) and other federal statistical agencies (such as the Bureau of the Census) and (2) any modifications to those items are a result of careful methodological and substantive reviews of alternative ways of asking the question. Nevertheless, the researcher should think about whether using questions identical to those in other surveys makes sense given the emphases of a particular survey. Modifying questions to operationalize fully a major concept of interest to the investigator or adapting questions to a particular mode of data collection or study population would certainly be appropriate.

Examples of the majority of items to be discussed appear in the 1995 NCHS–National Health Interview Survey in Resource A of this book. When appropriate, relevant modifications, such as those used when data are collected over the telephone, are mentioned. The question numbers of relevant items in the questionnaires in the resources at the end of this book are cited in the heading that introduces each item in the following discussion.

Household Composition (Resource A, Section A, Questions 1, 2, 4)

An important change has occurred in the procedures for identifying individuals who live in a sampled household and their relationships: national surveys now start with the "reference person" rather than with the "head of the household." The reference person is defined as "the person or one of the persons who owns or rents this home." Questions about the relationship of others in the household are then asked of this designated reference person. This convention was adopted by the U.S. Bureau of the Census for the Current Population Survey and other surveys to reflect better the nontraditional composition of many U.S. households and the emerging sensitivity on the part of many American families to identifying any one member as the head of the family.

The core National Health Interview Survey questionnaire gathers data on everyone in the household. All persons seventeen years or over are asked to take part in the interview if they are at home. Any person nineteen years or over or of any age if ever married may respond for other related family members who are not present at the time of the interview. Selected individuals may, however, be sampled for the special supplements in any given year. For example, only one adult family member (eighteen years or over) was interviewed for the 1995 supplements to the NHIS on health practices related to the Year 2000 Health Objectives for the Nation and AIDS Knowledge and Attitudes and a supplement on Immunization was asked for a sample child under six years of age. Procedures for selecting particular respondents to be interviewed, once the composition of the household is determined, were described in Chapter Six.

Age and Sex (Resource A, Section A, Question 3)

The question used in the National Health Interview Survey to find out people's ages is, "What is (PERSON's) date of birth?" In addition, interviewers are asked to confirm, "What then is (PERSON's) age?" and, if necessary, reconcile the responses. Sudman and Bradburn (1982) suggest that if age is one of many independent variables in the analyses, then a simplified question, "In what year were you/was (PERSON) born?" would be sufficient (p. 178).

In a study comparing methods that conform closely to the NCHS–NHIS and Sudman and Bradburn approaches with other ways of asking people's age, Peterson (1984) found that all the questions tended to yield fairly accurate responses. However, he found that asking "How old are you?" resulted in the greatest number of refusals to answer (9.7 percent) and that asking people to put themselves into age categories—eighteen to twenty-four, twenty-five to thirty-four, and so on—resulted in the highest percentage of inaccurate responses (4.9 percent) among the methods that were compared. Based on these findings, either the NCHS–NHIS or Sudman and Bradburn approaches would seem to be the best means of minimizing reporting errors when people are asked their age.

A person's sex is generally recorded on the basis of observation. However, the question may have to be asked for family members who are not present at the time of an in-person interview or directly of the household respondent in a telephone interview—"Please tell me (PERSON's) sex"—if not apparent from the person's name or other information provided during the interview.

Marital Status (Resource A, Section L, Question 7; Resource B, Question 49)

For every person fourteen years of age or older, the National Health Interview Survey asks, "Is (PERSON) now married, widowed, divorced, or has (PERSON) never been married?" The designers of the Chicago AIDS survey recognized the importance of an alternative to these traditional categories for the purposes of that study, and thus added "not married but living with a sexual partner" as a response category. Survey designers need to consider the importance of adding such a category to reflect this growing group of "mingles" (couples living as if married, though single) in their study.

Race and Ethnicity (Resource A, Section A, Questions 5, 6; Resource B, Screening Questionnaire, Question S5)

Classifying individuals according to their racial and ethnic identities is one of the most difficult and controversial issues to address in surveys as well as in other vital statistics and health and demographic reporting systems. The approaches used in the NCHS–NHIS conform with the directives for asking these questions issued for federally supported surveys by the Office of Federal Statistical Policy and Standards (Office of Management and Budget, 1994).

In the National Health Interview Survey, respondents are given a card with a numbered list of racial groupings and asked, "What is the number of the group or groups which represents (PERSON's) race?" The categories provided are 1–White, 2–Black/African American, 3–Indian (American), 4–Eskimo, and 5–Aleut, or an array of Asian and Pacific Islander (API) groupings (Chinese, Filipino, Hawaiian, Korean, Vietnamese, Japanese, Asian Indian, Samoan, Guamanian) and other races (categories 6 to 16). If respondents say yes to more than one of these categories, they are asked to indicate, "Which of these groups . . . would you say BEST represents (PERSON's) race?" In the past, NCHS asked interviewers simply to observe and record whether they thought the respondent was white, African American, or another race. The interviewer is still asked to do this, but the information is used only if the question about self-reported race is not answered. A troublesome issue that remains under discussion is how to classify mixed-race individuals.

The NCHS–NHIS classification of ethnicity focuses on classifications of Hispanic subgroups. Respondents are handed a card and asked, "Are any of those groups (PERSON's) national origin or ancestry? (Where did [PERSON's] ancestors come from?)" The list provided is as follows: 1–Puerto Rican; 2–Cuban; 3–Mexican/Mexicano; 4–Mexican American; 5–Chicano; 6–Other Latin American; 7–Other Spanish. If the respondent says, yes, that one of the groups applies, he or she is asked, "Please give me the number of the group."

In previous NCHS surveys, the question regarding Hispanic ancestry was asked after the question on race. There was, however, a tendency for Hispanic individuals not to answer the race question or to indicate their race as "other." Methodological research has documented that missing values on the race question are reduced and that Hispanics born in the United States especially are more likely to identify themselves as white when the Hispanic identity item is placed first. Martin, DeMaio, and Campanelli (1990) argue that this is because U.S.-born Hispanics may have implicit rules for reporting race, such as, "Apply the U.S. racial category 'white' to describe Hispanic persons with more 'roots' in the United States, but only after acknowledging Hispanic identity" (p. 565).

Hispanic surname lists have also been used as a basis for identifying persons with Hispanic ancestry in the census and other federal surveys (Judkins, Massey, & Smith, 1992; Passel & Word, 1980; Perkins, 1993). There has been considerable controversy about whether to classify individuals of Hispanic heritage as "La Raza," "Hispanics," or "Latinos" (Hayes-Bautista, 1983; Hayes-Bautista & Chapa, 1987; Trevino, 1987; Yankauer, 1987) and about the numbers and kinds of subcategories to use in identifying subgroups within this population (Trevino, 1982, 1988; Westermeyer, 1988). There is substantial evidence that "Hispanics" do differ from "non-Hispanics" and that there is variability in the health status and health care practices of subgroups of Hispanics according to whether they identify themselves as Puerto Rican, Cuban, Mexican/Mexicano (Mexican American, Chicano), or some other category (other Latin American, other Spanish) (Delgado & Estrada, 1993; National Center for Health Statistics, 1984; Schur, Bernstein, & Berk, 1987). Comparable controversies exist regarding the sociocultural meanings of terms used to designate African Americans (colored, Negro, black, African American) (Smith, 1992) as well as those identifying the growing and heterogeneous array of Asian and Pacific Island subpopulations within the United States (Yu & Liu, 1992).

The self-reports of racial and ethnic identification used by NCHS represent the widely accepted "official" approaches to gathering such information as well as efforts to respond to both the methodological and sociocultural issues surrounding these designations. In a telephone interview in which no materials are sent to respondents in advance, the racial and ethnic categories used in the respective questions have to be read to respondents. The telephone version used in the AIDS survey combined the racial and ethnic questions into one to facilitate oversampling certain groups in that study. Survey respondents were asked, "What is your racial background?" and then classified by the interviewer on the basis of the responses they provided. (See Resource B, Screening Questionnaire, Screener Forms 2 and 3, question S5.)

Education (Resource A, Section L, Question 2)

For everyone five years of age or older in the NCHS–NHIS, the following question is asked to elicit information about years of schooling: "What is the highest grade or year of regular school (PERSON) has ever attended?" Respondents are then asked, "Did (PERSON) finish the (NUMBER) [grade/year]?" The term *regular school* is used to exclude time spent at technical or trade schools from the years of school reported. This two-part question is recommended by the Bureau of the Census to reduce the upward bias that results from asking simply, "What is the highest grade or year of regular school (PERSON) *completed?*" Individuals can be classified according to the number of years of education they received or the type of school they graduated from (elementary school, high school, or college).

Employment Status (Resource A, Section D, Question 1; Section L, Question 5; Resource B, Question 51)

The questions used in the NCHS–NHIS to find out about employment status parallel to those used in the U.S. Bureau of the Census Current Population Survey. In the National Health Interview Survey the basic screening question about whether the person is working or not appears at the beginning of a series of questions that ask if people had to limit their usual activity in the last two weeks because of an impairment or health problem. People eighteen years or older are asked, "Did (PERSON) work at any time at a job or business, not counting work around the house? (Include unpaid work in the family [farm/business])." If not, the respondent was asked, "Even though (PERSON) did not work during those two weeks, did (PERSON) have a job or business?" A series of follow-up questions are used to determine for those who were not working whether they were "looking for work" or "on layoff from a job."

The survey designer may need to decide if the amount of detail provided by the NCHS questions is necessary, given the purposes to which the data will be put. The approach used in the Chicago AIDS survey represents a simplified alternative that is used in many surveys. This question asks, "Are you currently employed?" and, if so, "Are you *self*-employed?" If not employed, the person is asked, "Are you . . . retired, disabled, a student, keeping house, temporarily unemployed, or not looking for paid employment?" In addition, sometimes those who say they are working are asked, "Is that full-time or part-time?" Individuals can then be classified according to whether they are employed (full-time or part-time), unemployed, or not in the labor force.

Occupation (Resource A, Section L, Question 6; Resource B, Question 51)

The questions asked in the NCHS-NHIS about the type of job and industry in which people are employed are used to code occupations according to guidelines developed by the U.S. Bureau of the Census. A series of questions are asked, including "For whom did (PERSON) work?"; "What kind of business or industry is this?"; "What kind of work was (PERSON) doing?"; "What were (PERSON's) most important activities or duties at that job?"; "Was (PERSON) an employee of a PRIVATE company, a FEDERAL government employee," and so on. The questions asked in the Chicago AIDS survey represent a streamlined version of this series for surveys conducted by phone. Both the NCHS–NHIS and telephone interview version of the question assume that a formalized coding scheme and trained occupation coders are available to encode systematically the information provided by respondents. On the one hand, asking individuals an open-ended question about what their occupation is may yield insufficient detail to code accurately many responses. On the other hand, asking them to fit themselves into precoded categories of occupations designed by the researcher may result in considerable variability based on how different individuals *think* their job should be coded.

Occupation as well as education and income are traditionally used to construct measures of socioeconomic status (SES). The researcher choosing an approach for asking about occupation—or wondering whether to include such a question at all—must weigh the costs and benefits of asking it.

Income (Resource A, Section L, Question 8; Resource B, Question 56)

Questions about income are some of the hardest to get good data on in surveys and generally result in the highest rates of refusals by survey respondents. The NCHS–NHIS makes use of several devices to maximize the quality and completeness of the information obtained on this question.

A "split-point" form of asking the question, in which the respondent is asked whether family income is above or below a certain amount, has been found to reduce the threat to the respondent and, hence, to make him or her more willing to answer (Locander & Burton, 1976). The NCHS question asks, "Was the total combined FAMILY income during the past twelve months—that is, yours, (READ NAMES . . .) more or less than $20,000?"

To increase the accuracy of reporting, a detailed list of items that should be included in this family income figure is also provided: "Include money from jobs, social security, retirement income, unemployment payments, public assistance and so forth. Also include income from interest, dividends, net income from business, farm, or rent, and any other money income received." In addition, the importance of the information and how it will be used is underlined by this probe: "Income is important in analyzing the health information we collect. For example, this information helps us to learn whether persons in one income group use certain types of medical care services or have certain conditions more or less often than those in another group."

Depending on whether the respondent reported a family income of more or less than $20,000, different cards with a number of income categories identified by different letters are handed to the respondent who is then asked, "Of those income groups, which letter best represents the total combined FAMILY income during the past twelve months (that is, yours, [READ NAMES . . .])? Include wages, salaries, and the other items we just talked about." NCHS uses rather detailed categories, based on $1,000 intervals for those who report income under $20,000, to make it easier to code the poverty-level status of respondents. If necessary, the probe mentioned earlier is used to encourage respondents to answer the question.

The income question used in the AIDS survey differs from that used in the NCHS–NHIS. It is based on a split-point version of a question that was found to yield the best data overall of several approaches used in asking about income over the phone (Locander & Burton, 1976). However, this version of the question does not include any of the definitions or probes used by NCHS. In addition, the skip patterns for the detailed split points used in asking about income require that the interviewers be well trained in administering this technique. Using this approach would be less problematical with computer-assisted telephone interviews, however, because relevant skip patterns could be preprogrammed for the interviewer.

The approach used in the NCHS–NHIS applies a number of devices to enhance the quality and completeness of the family income data. The Chicago AIDS survey suggests some compromises that may be made in asking such questions over the phone. How much and what to ask to get this or other information in any given survey must be dictated by the perceived importance of a certain item for analysis of the data as well as by the cost and quality trade-offs that the researcher may find it necessary to make.

Nonthreatening Questions About Behaviors

Methodological research on survey question design has demonstrated that different cognitive processes come into play when people answer factual questions about their previous behaviors or experiences depending on how threatening they perceive the questions to be. Sudman and Bradburn (1982) suggest that one test for determining whether a question is potentially threatening is to consider whether the respondent might think there is a "right" or "wrong" answer in terms of what a "socially acceptable" response would be. Questions about alcohol consumption or sexual practices—as in the NCHS–NHIS and Chicago AIDS surveys—could be considered threatening. Some respondents may feel that other people would frown upon these activities. Questions about whether people went to a doctor or were hospitalized in the year may be seen as less threatening because they put the respondent at less risk of being criticized for behaving one way or the other.

Formulating answers to *nonthreatening* questions about past behaviors relates to the second stage of the question-answering process identified by Tourangeau (1984)—the memory and recall of relevant events. The two major types of memory errors that occur in surveys are that the respondent reports too much (overreporting) or too little (underreporting) relative to their actual experiences based on comparisons with some external criterion source, such as provider medical records or third-party payer forms.

Overreporting and Underreporting Errors

The problems that may lead to overreporting or underreporting occur in situations where respondents (1) *telescope*, that is, include events from outside the time period being asked about in the question or (2) *omit* events that should have been included within the reference period. A respondent's ability to recall events is a function of the time period over which the events are to be remembered (past two weeks, six months, or year, for example) and of the salience or significance of the event to the person (being hospitalized, for example, is a more salient event for respondents than the number of times they ate carrots in the last year). Manipulating the recall period for the target behaviors can result in opposite effects in terms of telescoping and omission errors. The shorter the recall period, the less likely respondents are to omit events but the more likely they are to telescope behaviors from the surrounding periods of time into this shorter reporting period. In contrast, the more salient an event the less likely it is to be omitted, but the more likely it is to be incorporated into the time period about which the question is asked even when it occurred outside that period.

The NCHS–NHIS uses several different recall periods to facilitate the construction of estimates of individuals' health behaviors. For example, respondents are asked whether they saw a doctor in the previous two weeks and, if so, how often (Resource A, Section E) as well as whether they contacted a physician during the previous year and, if not, what the last time they saw a doctor was (Resource A, Section G, Question 3). In that survey, interviewing is conducted with subsamples of respondents throughout the year. With appropriate weighting procedures, the two-week estimates can be annualized to reflect the rates for the year as a whole. These estimates are usually what are reported as the NCHS estimate of the numbers of visits Americans make to physicians annually. The question with the longer recall period is used to make estimates of the time interval (in years) since a physician was *last* seen, because many people may not have seen a physician in the last two weeks but may have done so over the course of the year or the last several years. Methodological research has documented that the accurate recall of physician visits, as well as of hospitalizations, decays (diminishes) substantially for annual as opposed to shorter periods of recall. For example, the net underreporting of hospitalizations for a twelve-month recall has been estimated to be around 10 percent compared with 5 percent when using a six-month time period (Jobe, Tourangeau, & Smith, 1993; Jobe, et al., 1990; Makuc & Feldman, 1993).

These findings point up the importance of considering the frame of reference that respondents use when asked to recall events and the devices that can be applied in developing questions to minimize both underreporting and overreporting errors in survey reports of health events.

Cognitive Survey Research Procedures

Cognitive research on surveys in general and health surveys in particular has documented the importance of more fully understanding the thought processes in which respondents engage in answering factual questions, as well as the factors that constrain or enhance recall, as a basis for deciding how best to design such questions (Herrmann, 1994; Jobe, Tourangeau, & Smith, 1993; Schwarz & Sudman, 1994).

Respondents' memory and reporting of events are influenced by both the structure of the task (questions or questionnaire) and the techniques (or schemata) they may call upon in answering them. A basic assumption underlying cognitive survey research is that respondents are "cognitive misers," that is, they will try to minimize the thought and effort needed to complete a task (respond to a question) by looking for clues (or a frame of reference) from the stimulus (item) that is presented to them or from convenient and familiar rules of thumb based on their previous (specific and general) experiences.

One of the most important frames of reference derived from the question itself, for example, is the response categories that are provided to answer it. Substantial methodological research has documented that the distributions of answers people give to questions about the number of times they engage in a particular behavior is influenced by the format and range of values provided in the response categories (Blair & Ganesh, 1991; Bless, Bohner, Hild, & Schwarz, 1992; Gaskell, O'Muircheartaigh, & Wright, 1994; O'Muircheartaigh, Gaskell, & Wright, 1993b; Schwarz, 1990; Schwarz & Bienias, 1990; Schwarz, Strack, Müller, & Chassein, 1988). For example, respondents who were given a high frequency scale regarding the number of times they watch TV on average each week (ranging from up to ten hours to more than twenty-five hours) were more likely to report a higher rate of TV watching than those provided a low frequency scale (up to two and a half to more than ten hours). This tendency is greater for relatively frequently occurring (or mundane) behaviors (eating certain foods regularly) than for rare (or salient) events. A questionnaire design alternative to deal with this problem is to use an open-ended rather than a closed-end response format, especially when it is unclear what frequency range for a question may be most fitting for a given study population.

Cognitive survey researchers have also helped to surface the internal schemata or approaches respondents use in answering questions. Respondents may actually try to recall and count the specific events (episodes) that occurred relatively infrequently during the reference period (three or fewer times), but they are much more likely to use various estimation strategies for events that occurred more often. An array of hypotheses have been explored in both laboratory and field settings to attempt to identify these strategies.

For example, respondents may set limits (or bound) their answers based on previous experiences or an implicit or implied comparison with others; they may round their estimates to prototypical values (such as seven, fourteen, or thirty days); they may think of a kind of autobiographical timeline or landmark public or private event (a presidential election or the birth of their first child) as a point of reference; disaggregate (break down) the task into a series of simpler tasks (the different reasons for their child going to see a doctor) and then sum or impute a summary (total visits to the doctor) based on these discrete computations; or they may consider what they typically do or what they know they "should" do (get a pap smear or mammogram) (Blair & Burton, 1987; Burton & Blair, 1991; Huttenlocher, Hedges, & Bradburn, 1990; Jobe, Tourangeau, & Smith, 1993).

Trying to recall accurately specific episodes, especially frequently appearing events, may lead to the underreporting of these events, whereas employing estimation strategies can result in overreporting. Research has, however, suggested that when the approach to asking questions attempts to take into account the heuristic or devices that respondents use in trying to answer a question, then more accurate reporting can result (Czaja, Blair, Bickart, & Eastman, 1994; Mooney & Gramling, 1991; NCHS, 1989a, 1989d, 1991a, 1992a, 1992d, 1994a).

Employing cognitive interviewing and think-aloud strategies during the instrument development stage is a good way of surfacing the ways respondents go about answering a question (see Chapter Eight). There is also evidence from research on the recall of visits to a physician (Jobe, et al., 1990; Means & Loftus, 1991; NCHS, 1989a), the use of preventive procedures (Bowman, Redman, Dickinson, Gibberd, & Sanson-Fisher, 1991; NCHS, 1994a), and diet (Buzzard & Sievert, 1994; Davis & DeMaio, 1993; Kohlmeier, 1994; Lee-Han, McGuire, & Boyd, 1989; Smith, Jobe, & Mingay, 1991a, 1991b), that when respondents are provided greater opportunity for free recall of relevant events, use explicit cognitive techniques (think-aloud, timeline, or the decomposition of their answer into parts) in choosing how they come up with an estimate, or are given more time for responding, they provide more accurate answers.

Bounded Recall Procedures

The primary device used to reduce overreporting of health events as a result of telescoping events from other time periods—especially those that took place before the date specified in the interview—is the bounded recall procedure. This procedure was developed for continuous panel surveys, where respondents could actually be interviewed at the beginning and end of the time periods referenced in the survey questionnaire. The first interview would serve to identify events that occurred *before* the interview period so that they could clearly be eliminated if the respondent later reported that they occurred during the period *between* the first and second interviews. This bounded recall device was used in panel surveys conducted in connection with the 1977 National Medical Care Expenditure Survey (NMCES) and the 1987 National Medical Expenditure Survey (NMES) in which summary reports of what respondents said during the previous interview were provided to interviewers. Interviewers could then use these reports to make sure that events were not reported a second time as well as to complete certain questions through information that had become available since the previous interview (such as hospital or doctor bills).

Sudman, Finn, and Lannom (1984) developed and tested an adaptation of the bounded recall procedure for a cross-sectional survey using several of the questions asked in the National Health Interview Survey. This study involved an adaptation of the National Health Interview Survey questions about disability days, days spent in bed, physician visits, and nights spent in a hospital for a personal interview survey of a probability sample of Illinois residents. Respondents were administered questions about their health behaviors in the *previous* month (the inclusion dates being referenced were specified) and were then asked about corresponding events in the *current* calendar month. After adjustments for the numbers of days on which reporting was based, the results showed that the events reported in the current (bounded) month were less than the previous (unbounded) month and that comparable NCHS–NHIS estimates fell in between these two estimates. The authors concluded that "the use of bounded recall procedures in a single interview reduces telescoping" and that if the comparable NCHS–NHIS questions were explicitly bounded they might produce lower estimates as well (Sudman, Finn, & Lannom, 1984, p. 524). Subsequent research has documented that asking people about the same procedure twice, first in connection with a given reference period (physical exam within the last six months) and then in connection with the reference period of interest (within the last two months), can also reduce overreporting (Loftus, Klinger, Smith, & Fiedler, 1990).

Memory Aid Procedures

The main question design devices used to reduce errors of omission help jog the respondent's memory or recall of relevant events. They include using aided recall techniques, records, and diaries.

Aided Recall Techniques. These methods are the simplest of the three memory aid devices and place the least burden on respondents. They basically provide explicit cues to aid respondents in recalling all the events they should recall in thinking about the question. Clues are included in the questions about physician visits to make sure respondents explicitly consider visits that they may have made to a number of different physician specialists as well as those with a nurse or someone else working for the doctor: "[D]id (PERSON) see or talk to a medical doctor? {Include all types of doctors, such as dermatologists, psychiatrists, and ophthalmologists, as well as general practitioners and osteopaths.}(Do not count times while an overnight patient in a hospital.)"; "[D]id anyone in the family receive health care at home or go to a doctor's office, clinic or hospital, or some other place? Include care from a nurse or anyone working with or for a medical doctor. Do not count times while an overnight patient in a hospital" (Resource A, Section E, Questions 1, 2).

Methodological studies comparing these versions of the questions with those in which memory aids were not provided showed that larger numbers of visits were reported in general, and for the types of providers listed, in the version in which aids were used (NCHS, 1985c).

Question 7 in the Chicago AIDS questionnaire (Resource B) is another example of an aided recall procedure. In that question respondents were asked, "Where have you seen information or heard about AIDS?" The interviewer then recorded all the sources they mentioned, such as television, radio, a newspaper, and so on. There were some ten sources that the survey designers were interested in learning about. For the sources that the respondent did not mention in response to the first question, they were asked, "Have you seen any information or heard about AIDS from (READ ANY CATEGORIES NOT CIRCLED IN Q. 7A)?" In this way, the investigator could learn the salient sources to respondents and also give them some assistance in identifying others from which they might have received information about AIDS but had forgotten to mention.

Records. A second memory aid recommended to reduce the underreporting of health events is to ask respondents to consult personal records, such as checkbooks, doctor or hospital bills, appointment books, or other sources during or in advance of the interview to aid them in answering certain questions. The large-scale national surveys carried out by NCHS, the Agency for Health Care Policy and Research, and the Center for Health Administration Studies employed this technique, generally by sending a letter in advance of a personal interview to inform respondents about the study and to encourage them to have relevant records handy when the interviewer came.

This device is less useful for telephone surveys, especially those such as the AIDS survey that are based on random digit dialing techniques. These techniques provide no advance warning to either the interviewer or the respondent about *who* will fall into the study and, therefore, no opportunity to encourage them to get relevant information together beforehand. There is also a much greater opportunity for the respondents to terminate the interview or refuse to cooperate when called back a second time after being asked to check their records. As mentioned in Chapter Six, computerized databases linking phone numbers to addresses are commercially available, however. Though it would add to the time and cost of doing the survey, such databases can be used to identify mailing addresses for sending an advance letter, if it is particularly useful to do so.

Encouraging respondents to check record sources is a very useful approach with mail surveys. Many dentists or their receptionists, for example, probably needed to consult their records to accurately report the number of different types of services provided during a "typical week," as was requested in the Washington State Study of Dentists' Preferences (Resource C, Question 20).

Diaries. A third technique to aid respondents' reporting of events is the use of a diary in which they can record these events on a regular basis, as they occur. In the NMCES and NMES surveys described earlier, respondents were asked to use calendars provided by the researchers to record certain relevant health events when they occurred (they took a day off work due to illness, had an appointment with the doctor, had a prescription filled, and so on). The respondent then consulted the diary when interviewed about these events (Wright, 1991).

Log-diaries have been used in the National Ambulatory Medical Care Survey and other physician surveys in which doctors and their staffs are asked to record selected information about a sample of patients who come into their office during a particular period of time. In these instances, diaries were the major data collection devices. Diaries are useful for recording information on events that occur frequently but may not have a high salience to respondents (such as recalling what one ate). Two of the biggest problems in identifying the nutritional content of the foods people eat relate to the accuracy of recall in what was eaten even twenty-four hours prior to an interview and to the representativeness of this one day for eating habits in general. Asking respondents to record what they eat over a several-day period can help reduce errors of this kind.

Study participants often perceive keeping diaries to be burdensome and time-consuming, and this may result in inaccurate or incomplete information being provided. In addition, monitoring and processing diaries can be expensive (Verbrugge, 1980). For some types of studies—as in the food-intake example—it may be the best or even the only way to gather the required information. In this case the researcher will need to consider the trade-offs in terms of the cost and quality of gathering data in this way and if incentives to study participants to maximize cooperation might be helpful.

Threatening Questions About Behaviors

Different rules need to be considered when formulating threatening questions about health and health care behaviors. Tourangeau (1984) suggests that, at the final or response stage of answering a question, considerations other than the facts come into play as respondents contemplate the answers they will provide. In the face of threatening questions respondents may decide to provide a less than honest response if they think their answer will cause them to be viewed either as "deviant" or, at a minimum, as behaving in a socially "undesirable" way. Various researchers have suggested a number of devices in designing threatening questions for reducing these tendencies on the part of respondents (Bradburn, 1983; Bradburn, Sudman, & Associates, 1979; Bradburn & Danis, 1984; Lee, 1993; Sudman & Bradburn, 1982; Tourangeau, 1984). Their suggestions are presented in terms of each of the building blocks that were outlined in Chapter Eight for constructing survey questions: words, phrases, sentences, responses, instructions, questions, and questionnaires.

Words

The words used in phrasing threatening questions should be familiar to the respondent. The approach employed in the AIDS survey represents a compromise to using individual respondents' own words for sexually explicit behaviors in a survey conducted over the phone. For example, Question 41 (Resource B) asks, "In the past five years, have you engaged in anal intercourse—that is, rectal intercourse?" The instructions provided to interviewers about how to handle that question during the interview advise them: "Synonyms for 'anal intercourse' include 'rectal intercourse,' 'sodomy,' 'butt fucking,' 'ass fucking,' and 'cornholing.' If *R* [respondent] uses those phrases, you can respond, 'That's another way to say it'; you are *not* to offer or use or repeat the synonyms."

The language used in the final questionnaire was arrived at after careful piloting and pretesting with a sample of people similar to those who would be included in the final study (Binson, Murphy, & Keer, 1987). If respondents used terms other than those used in the questionnaire, they were advised that their own words were also "okay," but the interviewer himself or herself used the standardized phrasing in asking respondents about the behaviors.

Phrases

Concerning the balance of the phrasing to use with threatening questions, Sudman and Bradburn (1982) suggest that it may, in fact, be better to "load" the questions to reduce a tendency for respondents to underreport socially undesirable behavior when answering such questions. One approach to loading a question deliberately is to suggest that others also engage in the behavior. For example, a statement of this kind is provided in the Chicago AIDS survey in an introduction preceding a series of questions about different sexual practices: "People practice many different sexual activities, and some people practice things that other people do not" (Resource B, Question 40).

A second approach to loading a question to reduce the underreporting of what may be perceived to be undesirable behaviors is to suggest that people in authority support these behaviors. An example of this technique is used in Question 21 of the AIDS survey: "Some government health officials say that giving clean needles to users of illegal drugs would greatly reduce the spread of AIDS. Do you *favor* or *oppose* making clean needles available to people who use illegal drugs as a way to reduce the spread of AIDS?"

A third approach is to ask the question so as to imply that the person does engage in the behavior by asking *how often* he or she engages in it, not *if* he or she does. For example, a question in previous NCHS–NHIS surveys asked, "In the past two WEEKS . . . , on how many days did you drink any alcoholic beverages such as beer, wine, or liquor?" People who said they had not had at least one drink in the past year were skipped out of the question. However, those who were asked to report about their behaviors in the past two weeks were asked in terms of "How often?" rather than "Did you?" It was thus somewhat harder for them to deny having drunk an alcoholic beverage during this period, if they had. However, a response category was provided for those who had said "none." A risk in asking questions in this way is that people who do not engage in these behaviors might be offended by what seems to be a built-in assumption that they did engage in what they believed would be perceived to be socially unacceptable practices.

Sentences

Another way to reduce the underreporting of what are thought to be socially undesirable practices is to make the sentences used in asking them longer rather than shorter. There are several examples of this approach in the AIDS questionnaire (Questions 36, 40, 43). In these instances, several sentences of explanation about the question are read to respondents before they are asked to respond directly themselves. There is evidence that longer questions increase the reported frequencies of socially undesirable behavior by some 25 to 30 percent compared with shorter questions (Bradburn, Sudman, & Associates, 1979). A longer question gives the respondent more time to think about the question, provides a fuller explanation of what is being asked and why, and is generally thought to underline the importance of answering it.

Responses

Another technique recommended to increase the reporting of behaviors that are traditionally underreported is to use open-ended rather than closed-end response formats. With closed-end formats respondents may assume there is a ceiling on what they should report or perceive based on the ranges provided and that they must be odd people if the frequency with which they engage in the behaviors meets or exceeds that limit. For example, the questions in the NCHS–NHIS about number of cigarettes, on average, smoked each day (Resource A, Section IV, Part A, Question 4) is open-ended in format. It asks the respondent "how many" without providing categories for them to use in responding.

Instructions

Another useful device in designing questionnaires is to build in transition sentences or introductions at points when the topic being addressed changes. This may be particularly important when introducing threatening topics so that the respondent is forewarned about what is coming next and given an opportunity to decide how he or she wants to respond. Both the AIDS and NCHS–NHIS surveys make frequent use of this device. For example, in introducing a series of questions about sexual practices in the AIDS survey, the interviewer is told to say: "So that we can help prevent the spread of AIDS, we need to know more about the sexual practices and drug use patterns of the general public in the Chicago area. Some of these questions need to be rather detailed and personal. If you prefer not to answer a question, please tell me, and I will simply go on to the next question. We appreciate your cooperation in answering these questions" (Resource B, Question 36).

Questionnaire

Other suggestions about asking threatening questions relate to the order and context in which they appear in the questionnaire. For example, Sudman and Bradburn (1982) suggest that when asking about undesirable behaviors, it is better to ask whether the person had *ever* engaged in the behavior before asking about his or her current practices. For behaviors that are perceived to be socially desirable ones, they advise asking about current practices *first*. They argue that respondents will also be more willing to report something in the distant past first because past events are less threatening. Interviewers should then progress toward asking them about current behavior.

This device was used in the NCHS–NHIS in asking a series of questions on the topic of smoking. Respondents were asked, "Have you smoked at least 100 cigarettes in your entire life?"; then, "Around this time LAST YEAR, were you smoking cigarettes everyday, some days, or not at all?; followed by, "Do you NOW smoke cigarettes everyday, some days, or not at all?" (Resource A, Section IV, Part A, Questions 1 to 3).

Survey designers may thus need to consider a combination of strategies to reduce the threat perceived by respondents in answering questions about socially undesirable events and to increase the reporting of these events—asking them how often they engage in some behavior now after moving them through a somewhat less threatening sequence of questions about whether they ever engaged in it.

It is also desirable for threatening questions to appear at the end of the questionnaire, after respondents have a clearer idea of what the study is about and the interviewer has had an opportunity to build a rapport with them. Such questions could also be imbedded among questions that are somewhat threatening or sensitive so that they do not stick out like sore thumbs. For example, one of the most sensitive questions in the AIDS questionnaire—"Do you think of yourself as heterosexual, homosexual, or bisexual?"—appears toward the end of the questionnaire, following a series that asks about the respondent's religious preference and before standardized questions about race and income (Resource B, Question 54). All these questions may, to some extent, be considered sensitive ones. But placing the question about sexual orientation after questions relating to religious preference may suggest to the respondent that it is all right for people to have different sexual preferences, just as it is all right to have different religious preferences— and thereby reduce the threat some may feel in answering. This is an example of the "art" of thinking through the placement of such questions; the "science" of how to do it is far from well developed at the present time.

Questionnaire Administration

Field procedures that can help reduce the threat of sensitive questions include relatively anonymous methods, such as using self-administered questionnaires rather than personal or telephone interviews or asking a knowledgeable informant rather than the individuals themselves to provide the information (Hay, 1990; Johnson, Hougland, & Clayton, 1989; Johnson, Hougland, & Moore, 1991; Makkai & McAllister, 1992; Martin, Anderson, Romans, Mullen, & O'Shea, 1993). There is evidence that respondents may be more inclined to report threatening behaviors *for* others than *about* themselves. There is also evidence that individuals are more willing to report such behaviors about themselves when they perceive that their anonymity is well ensured (Sudman & Bradburn, 1982).

A device to maximize the anonymity of respondents' reporting of threatening events is the randomized response technique (Fox & Tracy, 1986; Warner, 1965). This technique involves giving the respondent a choice of answering either a threatening or a nonthreatening question: "In the past five years, have you used a needle to inject illegal drugs?" or "Is your birthday in August?" The respondent is then told to use a randomization device, such as flipping a coin, to decide which question to answer—if "heads," to answer the first question and if "tails," the second. The interviewer or test administrator will neither see nor be told the results of the coin toss and, hence, which question the respondent was supposed to answer. Researchers, however, would be able to compute the probability of a particular (yes) response to the nonthreatening question. Any departure from this probability in the actual responses can be used to estimate the proportion of responses to the threatening item.

The randomized response technique does not enable responses to be linked to individual respondents, which limits the explanatory analyses that can be conducted with other respondent characteristics. There are few studies validating the technique and evidence exists that some respondents are still likely to "lie," but it is difficult to determine how many and who they are. Further, the procedure may seem like a complex one to respondents, many of whom may be suspicious and therefore reluctant or unwilling to cooperate in answering the question (Beldt, Daniel, & Garcha, 1982; Edgell, Himmelfarb, & Duchan, 1982; Fox & Tracy, 1986; Orwin & Boruch, 1982; Umesh & Peterson, 1991).

Health surveys have always dealt with sensitive topics. This focus has become even more pronounced in recent years, with morbidities such as AIDS, mental illness, and drug and alcohol abuse coming increasingly to the public's attention. More research needs to be conducted to examine the reliability and validity of the variety of mechanisms for asking questions about threatening topics.

In the absence of substantial methodological research in this area at the present time, however, the best advice is to (1) try devices that seem to have worked in other studies; (2) attempt to validate aggregate estimates on the behaviors for which data are gathered against other data—if available; (3) conduct pilot studies using split-ballot alternatives of the questions to see if they agree—when time and money permit; and (4) ask respondents directly at the end of the interview which questions they thought were particularly threatening. This last step makes it possible to determine if respondents' perceptions of threat are associated with different rates of reporting behaviors and, if so, to take this into account when analyzing and interpreting the findings.

Special Considerations for Special Populations

Asking people of color or ethnic minorities to indicate their race, ethnicity, or ancestry or to respond to questions about whether they engage in what are thought to be "socially undesirable" practices (substance abuse, high-risk sexual behaviors) does, in fact, place them in a kind of double jeopardy. Such questions are often difficult or troublesome to answer in general because of the categories that are presented for responding or the fear of either informal (social rejection) or formal (legal recourse) sanctions if answered honestly. The historical and contemporary realities of racism and xenophobia further confound both the message and the meaning of asking such questions of minority groups (Mays & Jackson, 1991). Methodological research suggests that racial and ethnic minorities tend to underreport sensitive behaviors and respond differently to vague quantifiers (such as "very often") when answering questions about the frequency with which they have engaged in these or other behaviors (Aquilino & Lo Sciuto, 1990; Fendrich & Vaughn, 1994; Ford & Norris, 1991; Schaeffer, 1991). These findings argue for greater cultural sensitivity and the implementation of cognitive survey development strategies in designing and evaluating such questions in general and for minority subpopulations in particular.

Selected Examples

The cognitive research laboratory at the National Center for Health Statistics, which has directly influenced the design and redesign of the National Health Interview Survey, has also served as a crucible for testing an array of theoretical propositions about the cognitive processes in which respondents engage in answering challenging or sensitive survey questions. The protocols developed for those studies, summarized in detail in the reports emanating from them, do in fact yield guidelines that others may want to use or test in their own studies on related health topics. The principles, as well as the principals (University of Illinois, Survey Research Laboratory investigators), involved in the development of the sensitive and challenging questions asked in the Chicago AIDS survey also contributed to the design and conduct of a number of NCHS cognitive research laboratory studies (NCHS, 1994a).

Guidelines for Minimizing Survey Errors

The simple and useful proverb "Square pegs do not fit well into round holes" has merit and meaning in designing survey questions that ask people to fit themselves into categories describing who they are or how often they do things that they may not readily reveal even to their closest confidants. As amply documented in this chapter, respondents will try to place themselves into the categories survey designers construct. These categories may, however, be ill-fitting ones and the survey respondents' presentation of themselves and their experiences may be distorted as a result. It is well then to encourage respondents like those to be included in the survey to define the contours of their thinking about the topics to be covered in the study before developing the questions that are presumably intended to reveal them.

Supplementary Sources

For additional information on developing demographic and threatening and non-threatening behavioral questions, see Fowler (1995), Lee (1993), and Sudman and Bradburn (1982).

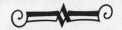

CHAPTER ELEVEN

FORMULATING QUESTIONS ABOUT KNOWLEDGE AND ATTITUDES

Chapter Highlights

1. Rules for formulating questions about people's knowledge of different health or health care topics should focus on how to minimize the threat that these questions may pose and the tendency of respondents to guess when they are not sure of the "right" answer.
2. In formulating attitude questions, it is particularly important to be aware of any previous research on the specific items being considered and of general methodological research on the response effects associated with alternative ways of asking *or* answering this type of question.

This chapter presents guidelines for formulating questions about knowledge of and attitudes toward health topics. These types of questions are more subjective than the ones discussed in Chapter Ten because they ask for judgments or opinions about—rather than simple recall of—facts.

Important assumptions underlying cognitive survey research on knowledge and attitude questions are that they are systematically stored in long-term memory and that answering them is a product of the four-stage process identified for answering survey questions in general: interpreting the question, retrieving relevant beliefs and feelings, applying them in making appropriate judgments, and finally selecting a response (Tourangeau & Rasinski, 1988; Tourangeau, Rasinski, & D'Andrade, 1991). For opinion or attitude questions, the third stage of replying to the question (the judgment stage) may be particularly relevant. At that stage respondents evaluate the information retrieved from memory and its relevance to answering the question and then make subjective judgments about what items of information should be combined, and how, to answer it (Bradburn & Danis, 1984; Tourangeau, 1984). Guidelines for formulating such questions focus on the means for accurately capturing and describing these judgments.

Knowledge questions have a somewhat more objective grounding than attitude or opinion questions because some standard or criterion for what constitutes a "right" answer is presumed to exist. Researchers should, however, think through the "correct" or "most nearly correct" answer to such questions and how they will be scored *before* asking them. If it turns out that more than one answer is correct or that the correctness of a given answer is open to question, then the respondents' answers may be more appropriately considered their opinions or attitudes on the matter than an indication of their knowledge relative to some standard of accuracy. In contrast, "the terms *attitude, opinion,* and *belief* all refer to psychological states that are in principle unverifiable except by the report of the individual" (Sudman & Bradburn, 1982, p. 120).

Questions About Knowledge

Questions concerning knowledge about the risk factors for certain diseases or methods to prevent or treat them have long been important components of health surveys. With the increased emphasis in the public health and medical care community on the impact of individual beliefs, knowledge, and behavioral change on reducing the risks of certain diseases, such as cancer, hypertension, and AIDS, questions of this kind have been asked with growing frequency in health surveys. For example, many of the Year 2000 Health Objectives for the Nation are concerned with health promotion and disease prevention activities related to smoking, alcohol consumption, obesity, lack of exercise, poor diet, and so on. Programs for effecting changes in these and other behaviors that put people's health at risk require information about the general knowledge of the risks associated with the practices, attitudes toward them, and current or anticipated behaviors in those areas.

Surveys used to gather information for developing or assessing the performance of these programs are sometimes referred to as knowledge, attitude, and behavior (KAB) surveys. The 1995 National Center for Health Statistics–National Health Interview Survey (NCHS–NHIS) is an example of a KAB study of the American public to find out about health practices related to achieving the Year 2000 Health Objectives for the Nation (see Resource A).

In the absence of effective medical interventions to treat AIDS, major public health education programs have been directed at informing the public in general and high-risk target groups in particular about the practices that put people at risk of getting the disease and the alternatives that can reduce that likelihood. KAB surveys have been an important component of the needs assessment and program-planning activities associated with these efforts.

Since 1987 NCHS has had a supplement to the National Health Interview Survey in which a subsample of respondents are asked a series of questions about their knowledge of and attitudes toward AIDS. Since that survey began, the NCHS Advance Data Series has issued monthly reports that trace changes in the American public's attitudes and knowledge about the disease. This survey, like a number of polls conducted in recent years on this topic (Singer, Rogers, & Corcoran, 1987), provides longitudinal data on the nationwide effectiveness of major federal, state, and local AIDS education activities. The Chicago AIDS survey (Resource B) was, as mentioned earlier, the baseline study for a major AIDS education demonstration project in that city. Other studies have used surveys to assess adolescents' knowledge, attitudes, and beliefs about AIDS to inform the development and implementation of school health education programs for a high-risk group of sexually active adolescents near a "high-density AIDS epicenter" in San Francisco (DiClemente, Zorn, & Temoshok, 1986) and to obtain information from physicians in or near such areas regarding their knowledge of the disease, their attitudes toward homosexuals in general and treating AIDS patients in particular, and their technical and clinical management of AIDS patients (Lewis, Freeman, & Corey, 1987; Richardson, Lochner, McGuigan, & Levine, 1987).

Questions

In considering the specific questions to ask to find out about people's knowledge of a health topic, survey designers should start with questions that others have asked. Consideration should then be given to whether (1) methodological studies are available that document the internal consistency or test-retest reliability of such questions; (2) items asked of one population group are relevant and appropriate to ask in a survey of a different group; (3) using the items in a different order or context in a different questionnaire might affect how people respond to them; and (4) new items will have to be developed to capture more sophisticated knowledge of the disease and the risk factors associated with it as the scientific and clinical understanding of the illness itself advances.

At a minimum, knowledge questions are useful for finding out who has heard of the disease or diseases that are the focus of a health survey. In the Chicago AIDS survey, for example, a key screening question asked early in the questionnaire is, "How much have you heard or read about the health condition AIDS

(Acquired Immune Deficiency Syndrome)? Have you heard or read a lot about AIDS, some, or nothing at all?" (Resource B, Question 6). Those who reported that they had heard "nothing at all" about AIDS were skipped out of the subsequent detailed questions that asked about respondents' knowledge, attitudes, and behaviors with respect to the disease.

It is also advisable to ask more than one question to capture people's knowledge or understanding of the issue. Simply asking, "Do you know what causes (DISEASE)?" tells you very little about the state of awareness of those who say yes. Also, as in any testlike situation, when people are asked to answer questions on what they "know" about an issue, those who are not sure of the right answer are likely to guess. If only one question is asked, there is a 50 percent chance that the person will get the right answer by guessing. People's summary performance on a number of items is thus a better indication of their overall knowledge of the topic. For example, in the NCHS–NHIS survey respondents are asked a number of questions regarding their knowledge about the risk factors and modes of transmission for AIDS (Resource A, Section V, Questions 4 and 5).

The main reason people claim to know more than they actually do when asked such questions is to prevent themselves from being viewed as ignorant on the topic. To reduce this threat, Sudman and Bradburn (1982) suggest phrasing knowledge questions as though they were intended to elicit the respondents' opinions about, rather than their knowledge of, the issue or using phrases such as, "Do you think . . . ?," "Do you happen to know . . . ?," or "Can you recall, offhand . . . ?" The device of phrasing knowledge questions so that they sound more like opinion questions is used in the NCHS–NHIS survey (Resource A, Section V, Questions 4 and 5).

Responses

When numerical responses are required to answer knowledge questions, Sudman and Bradburn (1982) also recommend that the question be asked in an open-ended fashion so as not to provide clues about the right answer and to make it harder for respondents to guess if they are not sure of the answer.

Questionnaire Administration

Another way to reduce the threat of knowledge questions is to use nonverbal procedures, such as self-administered questionnaires. In this case, explicit "don't know" responses can also be provided for the respondents to check if they are not sure of the right answer. However, using self-administered forms of asking such questions is more appropriate in supervised group-administered data gathering sessions than in unsupervised situations or in mailed questionnaires where respondents might cheat by looking up or asking someone else the answer.

A method for estimating whether respondents are overreporting their knowledge of certain topics is to use "sleepers"—fictional options—when asking respondents whether they are knowledgeable about various aspects of a topic (Bishop, Tuchfarber, & Oldendick, 1986; Sudman & Bradburn, 1982). For example, when conducting a marketing study about the brand names of different headache remedies or the penetration of a new advertising campaign, this device can be used when asking respondents if they have heard of various health care plans or medical delivery organizations. When the respondents who say they "know" about the fictitious or nonexistent alternatives are identified, their records can be excluded from the analyses or their responses to the sleeper questions coded as "wrong answers" when scores of their knowledge of the topic are constructed.

Questions About Attitudes

The same advice in phrasing knowledge questions applies to attitude questions: (1) use questions others have developed and tested and (2) think through how you will scale or analyze the items before including them in your study. As indicated earlier (Chapter Three), considerable developmental effort is often required to design reliable scales for summarizing individuals' attitudes on an issue. Therefore, researchers should begin with items that others have developed and used, particularly those for which reliability and validity have already been tested. Different types of scaling methods, such as the Likert, Guttman, Thurstone, and Rasch techniques, also make different assumptions about how attitude items should be phrased and about the criteria to use in selecting the final items to incorporate in the scale. Researchers should determine which of these approaches they want to use in summarizing the data for the attitude items relating to a particular topic *before* making a final decision about the questions to ask in their survey. As with factual questions, if respondents perceive a large burden in assembling or evaluating the evidence to use in answering attitudinal items, they are likely to engage in *satisficing* behavior; that is, they fail to draw upon all the relevant input or engage in the cognitive work to process and integrate the information required to provide a complete or unbiased response (Krosnick, 1991).

Rules of thumb presented here to mitigate the satisficing tendency when asking attitude questions once again follow the outline for formulating survey questions described in Chapter Eight: words, phrases, sentences, responses, questionnaire, and questionnaire administration (see Figure 8.1).

Words

Sudman and Bradburn (1982) point out that "attitudes do not exist in the abstract. They are about or toward something, and that something is often called the *attitude object*" (p. 121). It is important, then, in choosing the words for attitude questions to be clear about the object or focus of the evaluations sought from respondents. For example, if researchers have an interest in learning about respondents' attitudes or opinions toward smoking, they should clarify whether the focus is on cigarette, cigar, or pipe smoking; smoking anywhere or in the workplace, restaurants, or airplanes; the direct or passive effects of smoking; and so on. Perhaps all these dimensions are of interest to the investigator, in which case a series of attitude items could be asked about the topic. The point is that researchers should clarify *what* they want to learn before presenting a question to respondents.

The impact of the choice of words on the way in which people respond to attitude questions has been documented by split-half experiments, in which minor changes in wording have resulted in varying distributions on what are thought to be comparable questions. One example is the use of the words *forbid* and *allow* in public opinion polls that ask whether respondents think the government should "forbid" or "allow" certain practices: "Do you think the government should *forbid* cigarette advertisements on television?" versus "Do you think the government should *allow* cigarette advertisements on television?" There is some indication that because "forbid" sounds harsher than "allow," respondents are more likely to say no to allowing the practice than yes to forbidding it. The impact of this change in wording may be greater for more abstract issues or attitude objects (such as free speech or Communism) than for concrete ones (such as X-rated movies or cigarette advertising on television) (Hippler & Schwarz, 1986; Schuman & Presser, 1981).

Phrases

Another important issue in designing attitude items is the phrasing used in those items. Some evidence suggests that formal balancing of the alternatives for responding to attitude or opinion items, such as asking respondents whether they agree *or* disagree with or support *or* oppose an issue is warranted so that both alternatives for answering the questions are provided and it is clear to the respondent that either answer is appropriate. For example, "Do you *favor* or *oppose* making clean needles available to people who use illegal drugs as a way to reduce the spread of AIDS?" (Resource B, Question 21).

However, it is more difficult to choose a clearly distinct and balanced *substantive* counterargument or alternative in asking respondents' attitudes toward an issue: "Do you feel a woman should be allowed to have an abortion in the early months of pregnancy if she wants one, *or* do you feel a woman should not be allowed to end the life of an unborn child?" (Schuman & Presser, 1981, p. 186). Some people, for example, may feel that having an abortion "later" in the pregnancy would be acceptable. For those individuals, the alternative in the second half of the questions is not the balanced or equivalent alternative to the option described in the first half.

Similarly, problems can emerge with double-barreled or "one-and-a-half-barreled" questions, in which more than one question is introduced or implied in what questionnaire designers present as a single question. In this situation, it is not clear to respondents which question they should be answering or how they should register what they see as different answers to different questions. Sudman and Bradburn (1982), therefore, suggest using unipolar items (with one substantive alternative) if there is a possibility that bipolar items (with two alternatives) do not really capture independent (and clearly balanced) dimensions.

For example, in the dentists survey, some practitioners may have had trouble deciding the extent to which they agreed or disagreed with the statement, "The primary focus of dentistry should be directed at controlling active disease rather than developing better preventive service" (Resource C, Question 17d). For some dentists both approaches may be important, while for others other aspects of dental therapy may be more important. However, if respondents said they disagreed or strongly disagreed with the statement it would not be clear whether they thought neither approach was important—that *both* should be the "primary focus of dentistry"—or that, as the survey designers intended, they thought "better preventive service" was a *more appropriate* focus than "controlling active disease." Interestingly, this item (Resource C, Question 17d) was eliminated in a factor analysis of this and other items in the dentists survey (Questions 17a to 17f) to identify the major dimensions of practice beliefs (Grembowski, Milgrom, & Fiset, 1990a).

Sentences

The length of the question or series of items used in attitude questions can also affect the quality of individuals' responses. There is evidence that a medium-length introduction to a question (sixteen to sixty-four words), followed by a medium-length question (sixteen to twenty-four words) or a long question (twenty-five or more words), yields higher-quality data than either short introductions followed by short questions or long introductions followed by long questions. Also, the quality of responses to batteries of items—those that contain a list of questions to be answered using the same response categories (such as yes or no; agree, disagree, uncertain; and so on)—also tends to decline as the number of items increases. The "production line" nature of such questions may lead to carelessness on the part of the interviewer or respondent in asking or answering them (Andrews, 1984).

Responses

Considerable research has been conducted on the appropriate response formats to use in asking attitude questions. In general, the use of open-ended response formats is discouraged except during the preliminary or developmental stages of designing new questions. It is difficult to code and classify open-ended verbatim answers to nonfactual, attitudinal questions. The results will, therefore, be less consistent and reliable across respondents—and interviewers—than when standardized, closed-end categories are used.

Sometimes, open-ended questions are designed for the interviewer to "field-code." With field-coded questions, the respondents are asked the question by means of an open-ended format. However, precoded categories are provided for the interviewer to classify the response into closed-end codes. This technique reduces the time and expense associated with the coding and processing of open-ended answers and it also makes it possible to check the reliability of interviewers' coding. This approach is not recommended for use with subjective, attitudinal questions because of the errors and inconsistencies that can result when interviewers try to fit what respondents say into such categories (Schuman & Presser, 1981; Sudman & Bradburn, 1982).

Avoiding "Yea-Saying." A methodological issue that has been raised with some frequency when considering appropriate closed-end response formats for attitude items is the problem of yea-saying. This refers to the tendency of respondents to agree rather than disagree with statements as a whole *or* with what are perceived to be socially desirable responses to the question (Bachman & O'Malley, 1984; Bishop, Oldendick, & Tuchfarber, 1982; Schuman & Presser, 1981).

A number of different solutions have been suggested for identifying and dealing with this tendency. One method for identifying the tendency is to include both positive and negative statements about the same issue in a battery of items; for example, "People with AIDS deserve to have the disease" as well as, "People with AIDS *do not* deserve to have the disease." If respondents say they agree with both items, or comparable alternatives for other items, this obviously suggests a tendency toward yea-saying.

One solution to mitigating this response tendency is to use a "forced choice" rather than an agree-disagree format in asking such questions (Bishop, Oldendick, & Tuchfarber, 1982; Schuman & Presser, 1981). The latter format involves asking respondents whether they agree or disagree with statements such as, "How much a baby weighs at birth is more likely to be influenced by the mother's *eating habits* during pregnancy than by her *genetic background*." With a forced choice format respondents would be asked instead, "Which, in your opinion, is more likely to account for how much a baby weighs at birth—the mother's eating habits during pregnancy *or* her genetic background?"

Other devices for reducing the yea-saying tendency relate to the order and form of response categories provided to respondents. Sudman and Bradburn (1982), for example, suggest that rather than asking respondents to "circle all that apply" in a series of statements about various attitudes toward a topic, they should be asked to say yes or no (does it apply to them or not) for *each* item. They are then forced to think about every item separately and not just go down the list and check those that "look good." This is good advice for other types of questions as well, because if the respondent or interviewer is asked to circle or check *only* those that apply, it is not always clear whether those that were not checked did not apply, were skipped over by the respondent or interviewer when reviewing the list, or were missed simply because the respondent did not give much thought to the items.

Sudman and Bradburn (1982) also recommend that when survey designers provide a list of alternatives for individuals to use in answering a question, the "*least* socially desirable" alternative should appear *first* in the list; for example, "In terms of your own risk of getting AIDS, do you think you are *at great risk,* at some risk, or at no risk for getting AIDS?" (Resource B, Question 29). Otherwise, the respondent may choose the more desirable response right away without waiting to hear the other possible responses. The precise effect that the order of the response categories has on how respondents answer questions is far from clear, however. Some studies suggest that people tend to choose the first category mentioned (primacy effect), others the last category mentioned (recency effect), and still others the categories toward the middle of the list (Krosnick & Alwin, 1987; Payne, 1951; Schuman & Presser, 1981; Sudman & Bradburn, 1982). In self-administered surveys respondents tend to choose the first option, while in personal or telephone interviews they are more likely to pick the last one (Salant & Dillman, 1994).

Incorporating positively and negatively worded items or using a forced choice format does not necessarily assure that acquiescence will be reduced. In fact, it may produce other response effects (such as tending to choose the first or last option in a forced choice question) (McClendon, 1991). If there is concern about the effect that phrasing or ordering the responses in a certain way may have on respondents' answers to certain questions and if no methodological research has been done on these items, researchers may consider conducting their own split-half experiments during the piloting or pretesting stages of their study if time and resources permit. The Marlowe-Crowne Social Desirability Scale is also used to identify respondents who may be distorting their answers to survey questions in a socially desirable direction; it asks a series of questions thought to reflect this tendency. Attitudinal items that are found to have a high correlation with this measure can then be eliminated (Bradburn, Sudman, & Associates, 1979; Crowne & Marlowe, 1960).

Measuring Attitude Strength. An important issue in measuring people's attitudes is determining the strength with which the attitudes are held. This is measured through scales for *rating* or *ranking* the order of people's preferences for different attitudinal statements about a topic.

With *rating scales,* respondents are asked to indicate the level of intensity they feel about the statements along the dimensions provided by the researcher. One example would be asking respondents whether they strongly agree, agree, disagree, or strongly disagree with statements about how dentistry should be practiced (Resource C, Question 17). Again, on a scale of 1 to 5, with 5 being extremely ashamed of having a disease and 1 not at all ashamed, respondents can be asked to indicate how ashamed they would be of contracting different illnesses (Resource B, Question 34).

With *ranking formats,* respondents are asked to rank-order their preferences for different alternatives. For example, a major component of the Washington State Study of Dentists' Preferences in Prescribing Dental Therapy asks dentists to rank-order the top three patient, technical, and cost factors they consider in choosing among alternative dental therapies (Resource C, Questions 1 to 16).

An important issue to address in designing rating scales is *how many* categories or points should be provided in such scales. A large number of points (7 to 10) may, for example, permit the greatest discrimination in terms of attitude strength or intensity. But increasing the numbers of categories will make it harder for the respondent to keep all the responses in mind, particularly if verbal labels (such as strongly agree, agree, and so on) rather than numerical labels ("On a scale from 1 to 5 . . .") are used to identify the respective points along the scale. Research suggests that scales with 5 to 7 points are more valid and reliable than those with only 2 to 3 categories, although the gradations of opinion reflected in the verbal labels used with these formats may be difficult for certain groups (those for whom English is a secondary language or the elderly, for example). For detailed discrimination (along a 10-point scale, for example) numerical scale categories are recommended.

Research has suggested that verbally labeling only the end points of the scale and allowing the intermediate points to take their meaning from their relative position between the end points results in higher-quality data than labeling every point of such scales for those with seven or fewer categories (Alwin & Krosnick,

1991; Andrews, 1984; Sudman & Bradburn, 1982; Tillinghast, 1980). However, more respondents are likely to endorse the lower (less positive) range of an 11-point scale that ranges from 0 to 10 compared with a scale that ranges from −5 to +5, even though the endpoints have the same verbal labels—"not at all satisfied" and "very satisfied." The explanation for this finding is that the 0 to 10 scale is implicitly viewed by respondents as unipolar—the extent to which the feeling is present—and the −5 to +5 scale as bipolar—the extent to which it is present (+1 to +5) *or* absent (−1 to −5). Respondents are therefore more reluctant to register the absence of any positive feelings invited by the negative (less positive) end of the bipolar rating scale (Schwarz, Knäuper, Hippler, Noelle-Neumann, & Clark, 1991; O'Muircheartaigh, Gaskell, & Wright, 1993a; Schwarz & Hippler, 1991; Smith, 1993).

Verbal scales used in personal interview surveys (such as *completely, mostly, somewhat satisfied*) are often converted to numerical scales in telephone interviews ("On a scale of 1 to 5, where 5 is completely satisfied, and 1 is not at all satisfied, how satisfied are you with. . . ."). It may be easier for respondents to keep the numerical scale, rather than the complex-sounding verbal labels (strongly agree, agree, uncertain, disagree, strongly disagree), in their heads in answering questions over the phone. Another device that is frequently used in telephone interviews is to ask whether the person agrees with, disagrees with, or is uncertain about a statement, and then, if they say they agree or disagree, to ask whether they agree or *strongly* agree (or disagree or *strongly* disagree). In personal interviews, cards with the response categories printed on them can be handed to the respondents to facilitate the use of even a large number of verbal response categories. Other numerical devices that have been used to get respondents to register their opinion on an issue include providing pictures of thermometers or ladders for them to use in indicating how "warmly" they feel about the issue or where they "stand" on it (Sudman & Bradburn, 1982).

A related issue in designing rating formats is whether a neutral or middle alternative or "don't know" or "no opinion" option should be explicitly provided for those respondents who do not have a strong attitude, one way or the other, on the topic. Research suggests that when such alternatives are explicitly provided, the proportions of those who say they don't know or don't have an opinion is naturally higher (Bishop, 1987; Kalton, Collins, & Brook, 1978; Presser & Schuman, 1980; Schuman & Presser, 1981).

People who express an opinion when the neutral or no opinion options are not provided but who opt for these categories when they are available are called "floaters." They are more likely to have lower levels of involvement in the issue (assign it less importance or have less interest in it) (Bishop, 1990; Gilljam & Granberg,

1993; Hippler & Schwarz, 1989). Research indicates that the relative percentages (or proportions) of respondents who choose the other categories are not affected by explicitly adding these options. Even though the addition of such alternatives may not affect the overall distribution of positive and negative responses, it is recommended that they be provided so that respondents do not feel forced to choose a category. Instead they are allowed to indicate that they have no opinion or no strongly felt opinion—one way or the other—on the topic, if that *is* the way they feel about it (Andrews, 1984; Sudman & Bradburn, 1982).

The other major type of response format used in obtaining information on the strength of people's opinions on a topic is the ranking scale. As mentioned earlier, a primary focus of the dentists study (Resource C, Questions 1 to 16) is to ask dentists to rank the factors that enter into their choices of alternative clinical procedures. Such rankings can occur, however, only when respondents can see or remember all the alternatives. Sudman and Bradburn (1982) suggest that respondents can handle no more than two to three alternatives at a time over the phone. Even with self-administered or in-person interviews, in which visual devices or cards can be used to rank-order the options, they recommend that no more than four or five alternatives be provided.

In the dentists survey, respondents were asked to rank the factors that influenced their choices with respect to three broad sets of factors (patient, technical, and cost factors) and then indicate which among all the factors were the most important in their decision making. This two-stage approach is useful for reducing the burden on the respondent of rank-ordering a large array of choices.

Paired comparisons of different alternatives have also been widely used in studies that ask respondents to choose among competing options. This approach is, for example, implicit in the utility-related approaches to estimating the preferences for different treatment alternatives, such as having a kidney transplant to be restored to normal health but confronting a three in ten chance of dying from the transplant versus not having it and continuing in a less desirable health state on dialysis (see the discussion in Chapter Nine).

However, if respondents are asked to make a large number of comparisons this method can lead to considerable fatigue on their part and a resultant failure to concentrate on the choices they are making. Even when fully participating in the process, people may not always make entirely consistent choices across items.

In a comparison of rating and ranking methods for eliciting people's value preferences for the characteristics children should have, Alwin and Krosnick (1985) concluded that neither method was necessarily superior to the other for that purpose. However, they did point out that the ranking method clearly forced the respondent to compare and contrast alternatives and choose between them, whereas the rating technique did not. Researchers thus need to decide whether explicitly asking respondents to make such choices is necessary given what they want to learn about their attitudes on a topic.

Questionnaire

A final issue to consider in asking attitudinal questions in surveys is the order in which such questions should appear. There is evidence that people respond differently to questions about their general attitudes on a topic (such as abortion), depending on whether they are placed *before* or *after* a series of questions that tap more specific attitudes on the issue (whether abortion is warranted in the instances of rape, incest, a deformed fetus, risk to the mother's health if she carries the baby to term, and so on). In general, it is recommended that the more general attitude items be asked before the specific ones. Otherwise, respondents tend to feel that they have already answered the question or to assume that the general question refers to other (or residual) aspects of the issue that they were not asked about in detail earlier (Mason, Carlson, & Tourangeau, 1994; Schwarz & Bless, 1992; Schwarz, Strack, & Mai, 1991; Schuman & Presser, 1981; Sudman & Bradburn, 1982; Tourangeau, Rasinski, & Bradburn, 1991).

Previous questions can influence respondents' answers, especially if they are on a related topic and the respondents view the issue as important but do not have a well-formed opinion about it. This may be a particular concern in surveys that ask questions about attitudes (toward breast cancer) and related behaviors (breast self-exam and mammography screening) (Tourangeau, Rasinski, Bradburn, & D'Andrade, 1989a, 1989b). Survey developers should consciously consider the context in which such questions are asked when designing the survey questionnaire. There might be an interest in prompting respondents' recall of specific events (problems in getting medical care) before answering certain attitudinal questions (satisfaction with their regular provider) but not others (their opinion of pending national health care reform legislation). If there is not a clear rationale for ordering the questions, then it might be useful to conduct a split-ballot experiment to examine the impact of changing the order in which they appear in the questionnaire on survey responses.

Questionnaire Administration

Although proxy interviews may be sought for demographic or factual questions, it is not generally advisable to do so for knowledge or attitude items because they are uniquely intended to reflect the respondent's subjective, internal states or feelings, and not necessarily an objective, external reality readily observable by others (Lavizzo-Mourey, Zinn, & Taylor, 1992).

Special Considerations for Special Populations

Yea-saying response tendencies have been observed among minority and poorly educated respondents in particular (Aday, Chiu, & Andersen, 1980). This may be caused by a general tendency to give more socially desirable responses but it may also reflect difficulty in discriminating among the fine gradations of opinion implied by the response categories provided or cultural or linguistic ambiguities in what is meant or intended by the question. The cognitive survey development techniques reviewed in Chapter Eight would be useful in detecting these problems early on and formal tests of the reliability and validity of the resulting summary scales (reviewed in Chapter Three), stratified (broken out) by major subgroups of interest, would document the extent to which these problems exist, once the data are gathered.

Selected Examples: Patient/Consumer Satisfaction

As has been cited throughout the chapter, an array of knowledge and attitude questions illustrating the principles detailed in this chapter are reflected in the three surveys for which questionnaires are provided in Resources A through C. Selected knowledge and attitude summary scales based on these studies were highlighted in Chapter Three.

Although not a focus of these three surveys, questionnaires to tap patient and consumer satisfaction are increasingly being utilized to assess the performance and quality of health care services delivery. Patient satisfaction is viewed as a unique and patient-centered indicator of success in attending to the nontechnical as well as technical aspects of care (Agency for Health Care Policy and Research, 1995; Cleary & McNeil, 1988; Fitzpatrick, 1991a, 1991b; Lewis, 1994; Williams, 1994). Further, many of the principles for designing attitudinal questions in general come into play in developing these measures. A balanced response scale in which both positively and negatively worded items are used is recommended to minimize an acquiescent response set. Item response formats may take one of several forms of a Likert-type scale to tap satisfaction with different dimensions of care: direct (very satisfied, satisfied, neither satisfied nor dissatisfied, dissatisfied, very dissatisfied), indirect (strongly agree, agree, uncertain, disagree, strongly disagree), or evaluative response formats (excellent, very good, good, fair, or poor). Research has suggested that the evaluative rating scale may, in fact, be superior to the direct scaling method in measuring patient satisfaction because the resulting scores tend to be less skewed (toward higher levels of satisfaction), to have greater variability, and to be more likely to reflect the patient's intentions regarding seeking care (Sherbourne, Hays, & Burton, 1995; Ware & Hays, 1988).

The content, number of items, and response format used for selected scales of general satisfaction with medical care, physicians, and hospitals that have been employed extensively in developing report cards or other reports on provider performance are highlighted in Table 11.1 (Davies, Ware, & Kosinski, 1995; Gold & Wooldridge, 1995). In addition, a number of sources provide a review and synthesis of the major conceptual and empirical approaches to measuring patient satisfaction (Hall & Dornan, 1988; Hall, Milburn, & Epstein, 1993; Linder-Pelz, 1982; Pascoe, 1983; Pascoe, Atkinson, & Roberts, 1983; Ross, Steward, & Sinacore, 1995; Strasser, Aharony, & Greenberger, 1993).

The impetus for the first generation of satisfaction measures came primarily from a desire within the health services research and policy communities for valid and reliable methodologies for assessing the performance of the U.S. health care delivery system. The Medical Care Satisfaction Questionnaire, developed by Barbara Hulka and her colleagues, and John Ware and Associates' Patient Satisfaction Questionnaire have been used extensively in soliciting both patients' and the general population's satisfaction with medical care in national, state, and local surveys. The Visit Satisfaction Questionnaire, used in the Medical Outcomes Study (described in Chapter Three), measured patient satisfaction with specific visits to providers across the array of delivery settings that were the focus of that quasi-experimental health services evaluation.

The impetus for the second generation of satisfaction measures (such as the Group Health Association of America Consumer Satisfaction and related National Committee for Quality Assurance Surveys) emanated from a growing interest on the part of the corporate provider community (particularly large-scale managed care organizations) in obtaining consumer assessments of the quality of care received from member providers (Davies & Ware, 1988a, 1991; NCQA, 1993, 1995a, 1995b). The results of patient satisfaction surveys on plan performance were to be incorporated into report cards summarizing both clinical indicators and patient assessments of quality that could be used in marketing health plans to prospective consumers.

The Picker/Commonwealth Program for Patient-Centered Care, supported by the Commonwealth Fund, provided support for the development of scales of hospital patients' satisfaction with care (Patient Judgment System and Patient Comment Card) that could be used in assessing the quality of inpatient care from the perspective of those receiving the services.

The literature is replete with scales to assess satisfaction with a variety of other health-related programs or services: breast cancer screening (Cockburn, et al., 1991); genetic counseling (Shiloh, Avdor, & Goodman, 1990); health maintenance

TABLE 11.1. SELECTED PATIENT SATISFACTION MEASURES.

Concepts and Characteristics	Physician					Hospital	
	MCSQ	PSQ I,II	PSQ III	VSQ	GHAA	PJS	PCC
Concepts	Professional competence Personal qualities Cost/Convenience	Accessibility, convenience Availability of services Continuity of care Finances Interpersonal aspects Technical quality Facilities General satisfaction	Interpersonal manner Communication Technical quality Financial security Time spent with MD Access to care General satisfaction	Physician access Telephone access Office wait Appointment wait Time spent with MD Communication Interpersonal aspects Technical quality Overall care	*Services* Access Finances Technical quality Communication Choice, continuity Interpersonal care Outcomes Care overall General satisfaction *Plan* Services covered Information from plan Paperwork Costs of care Plan overall	Admissions Daily care Information Nursing care Doctor care Auxiliary staff Living arrangements Discharge Billing Total process	Admissions Nurses Doctors Quality of food Privacy Information Family and friends Discharge Hospital quality Total process
Characteristics Number of questions	41	PSQ I = 80 PSQ II = 68	50	9	1st ed. = 35 2nd ed. = 35 (services) 14 (plan)	PJS-46 = 46 PJS-41 = 41 PJS-20 = 20 PJS-10 = 10	General - 9 Specific - 9
Response scale	Strongly agree Agree Uncertain Disagree Strongly disagree	Strongly agree Agree Not sure Disagree Strongly disagree	Strongly agree Agree Not sure Disagree Strongly disagree	Excellent Very good Good Fair Poor	Excellent Very good Good Fair Poor	Excellent Very good Good Fair Poor Don't know	Excellent Very good Good Fair Poor No contact

MCSQ = Medical Care Satisfaction Questionnaire (1970)   GHAA = Group Health Association of America Consumer Satisfaction Survey (1st, 2nd ed.) (1987)
PSQ I,II = Patient Satisfaction Questionnaire, I,II (1975)   PJS = Patient Judgment System (1987)
PSQ III = Patient Satisfaction Questionnaire, III (1984)   PCC = Patient Comment Card (1991)
VSQ = Visit Satisfaction Questionnaire (1985)

Bibliography:	
MCSQ	Hulka, Zyzanski, Cassel, and Thompson, 1970; Hulka, Kupper, Daly, Cassel, and Schoen, 1975; Zyzanski, Hulka, and Cassel, 1974
PSQ I,II	Davies, Ware, Brook, Peterson, and Newhouse, 1986; Doyle and Ware, 1977; Marquis, Davis, and Ware, 1983; Ware, 1978; Ware and Snyder, 1975; Ware, Snyder, Wright, and Davies, 1983; Ware, Wright, Snyder, and Chu, 1983
PSQ III	Marshall, Hays, Sherbourne, and Wells, 1993; Safran, Tarlov, and Rogers, 1994
VSQ	Rubin, Gandek, Rogers, Kosinski, McHorney, and Ware, 1993; Ware and Hays, 1988
GHAA	Allen, Darling, McNeill, and Bastien, 1994; Davies and Ware, 1988a, 1988b, 1991; National Committee for Quality Assurance, 1993, 1995a, 1995b
PJS	Hays, Larson, Nelson, and Bataldan, 1991; Meterko, Nelson, and Rubin, 1990; Nelson, Hays, Larson, and Batalden, 1989; Nelson and Larson, 1993; Rubin, 1990
PCC	Nelson, Larson, Davies, Gustafson, Ferreira, and Ware, 1991

Source: Information on PSQ I,II, and III, VSQ, and GHAA adapted from Table 1 (pp. 85–86) in Gold and Wooldridge (1995).

organizations (Weiss & Senf, 1990); mental health services (Elbeck, 1992; Elbeck & Fecteau, 1990; Hansson, Björkman, & Berglund, 1993; Myers, Leahy, Shoeb, & Ryder, 1990; Ricketts, 1992); nursing (McDaniel & Nash, 1990; Megivern, Halm, & Jones, 1992; Scardina, 1994; Turner & Matthews, 1991); and pharmacy services (MacKeigan & Larson, 1989).

Guidelines for Minimizing Survey Errors

Asking questions to find out deep-seated opinions and feelings is somewhat like digging for buried treasure. One must know where and how to look as well as what previous explorations might have surfaced. The objective of the undertaking (the concept to be measured) must be clearly defined, the tools (questions and response categories) for extracting it honed, and the environment (order and context) in which it is embedded taken into account. Existing maps (previous research) as well as tailored scouting expeditions (pilot studies or split-ballot experiments) may both be needed to surface the gems that are the object of the inquiry.

Supplementary Sources

Other sources to consult on attitude scale construction include DeVellis (1991), Nunnally and Bernstein (1994), and Oppenheim (1992).

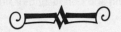

CHAPTER TWELVE

GUIDELINES FOR FORMATTING THE QUESTIONNAIRE

Chapter Highlights

1. The format, order, and context in which questions are asked should all be considered in making final decisions about the form and content of the survey questionnaire.
2. Researchers should test and evaluate different approaches to formatting or ordering questions during the pilot and pretest stages of the study if they are not sure which approach will work best in their study.

This chapter presents guidelines for formatting and ordering questions in a survey questionnaire. Three issues in particular will be addressed: (1) the techniques for displaying the questions in mail, telephone, personal interview, and computerized questionnaires (format); (2) the order in which the questions appear; and (3) their relationship to other questions in the survey questionnaire (context). Each of these three factors affects the clarity and meaning of the questions and thus the respondent's ability or willingness to answer the questions reliably and accurately.

Format

Different modes of data gathering (mail, telephone, personal interview, or computerized) present somewhat different clues to the respondent about how to proceed with the survey questionnaire. Mail or self-administered questionnaires are often reliant solely on the clarity and appeal of the visual presentation of the questions, response categories, and accompanying instructions. With telephone interviews, auditory signals and the quality of the communication between the interviewer and respondent are central. In personal interview situations, visual and auditory stimuli as well as the norms of conversational and interpersonal interaction implicit in the exchange between the interviewer and respondent all come into play in encouraging or facilitating a response. As discussed in Chapter Five, computerized data collection methods (CAPI, CATI, and CASI) present unique challenges and opportunities in the questionnaire design and administration process.

With self-administered questionnaires, the principal criterion to consider in evaluating the instrument is whether the respondent can understand and answer the questions without having someone present to clarify or explain them. In telephone surveys, a key consideration is whether a question is likely to be understood if it were read exactly as it is written. In personal interview surveys, greater use can be made of visual aids (such as showing respondents a card with the response categories for a question listed on it or encouraging them to check relevant records before answering). Computer assisted data collection methods enhance the availability of an array of audio and visual cues to respondents and interviewers for understanding and answering questions. Advance letters are useful to provide prospective respondents information about a survey before they are actually contacted for the interview. (The content and format of these letters are discussed in Chapter Thirteen.) The introduction to a telephone survey is especially critical for enlisting respondents' cooperation. Salant and Dillman (1994, p. 127) recommend a brief businesslike introduction that includes the interviewer's name, the organization and city from which he or she is calling, a one-sentence description of the survey, and a conservative estimate of how long the interview will take.

Exhibit 12.1 highlights the major do's and don'ts in formatting survey questionnaires in general. This chapter's discussion pinpoints their particular relevance and the adaptations required for different data gathering methods. The examples in the exhibit are based primarily on Sudman and Bradburn's (1982) conventions for developing paper-and-pencil telephone and personal interviews. Adaptations for mail or self-administered surveys recommended by Don Dillman's Total Design

Method for mail questionnaires are highlighted in the discussion that follows (Dillman, 1978; Dillman, Sinclair, & Clark, 1993; Salant & Dillman, 1994). The dentists questionnaire in Resource C is based on Dillman's guidelines for mail surveys; the AIDS survey in Resource B is based primarily on Sudman and Bradburn's approach for interviewer-administered questionnaires. Proprietary computer-assisted data gathering software packages have their own languages and protocols for designing and formatting a survey questionnaire, although many of the same basic principles apply when using these approaches (Saris, 1991).

Assign Numbers to Each Question

All questions should be numbered to provide clear referents to every item in the questionnaire for interviewers, respondents, data-processing staff, and analysts. Subparts of a question should be indented and assigned letters, which are then attached to the main question number, such as Q. 20a., b., c., d. (see Resource B). Some skip patterns or other instructions within the questionnaire may also require that particular questions be identified by number. Incorporating the question number into the names of analysis variables when constructing and documenting the data file for the study provides a clear road map to the source questions for those variables. Computerized data collection systems, in particular, require that each item on the questionnaire be identified through unique questions or code numbers.

Use a Vertical Response Format for Closed-End Responses

Another important rule of thumb that has been recommended for formatting closed-end response categories is to use a vertical format for the categories. In a vertical format, the categories and corresponding response codes are presented in list form, one right after the other (Resource B, Question 3a):

Too much 1

Not enough 2

Right amount 3

Don't know 8

This is in contrast to a horizontal format: Too much . . . 1 Not enough . . . 2 Right amount . . . 3 Don't know . . . 8. Dillman (1978) and Sudman and Bradburn (1982) point out that it is much easier for the respondent or interviewer to get confused and circle the wrong code for a response category when the horizontal format is

EXHIBIT 12.1. DO'S AND DON'TS OF QUESTIONNAIRE DESIGN.

Do	Don't
1a. Assign numbers to each question.	*Don't leave off the question number.*
b. Use letters to indicate subparts of a question when it has more than one part.	*Don't leave off the letter for subparts of a question.*

1a. If a center to treat people with AIDS was going to be set up in your neighborhood, would you *favor or oppose it?*

Favor (Skip to Q. 2) 1
Oppose 2

(If "oppose"):
1b. Why is that?

1a. If a center to treat people with AIDS was going to be set up in your neighborhood, would you *favor or oppose it?*

Favor (Skip to Q. 2) 1
Oppose 2

(If "oppose"):
Why is that?

---

2. Use a vertical response format for closed-end responses.

White 1   African American....2   Hispanic....3

White 1
African American...........2
Hispanic.......................3

Don't list closed-end responses horizontally.

---

3. Use numerical codes for closed-end responses.

Don't use alphabetic codes or blank lines to place X or check on, for closed-end responses.

In general, would you say that your health is...
(Read categories and circle number for answer.)

Excellent 1
Good...........................2
Fair 3
Poor?...........................4

In general, would you say that your health is...

Excellent ____
Good ____
Fair ____
Poor ____

---

4. Use consistent numerical codes and formats.

Don't use different numerical codes and formats for comparable responses to different questions.

Yes..............................1
No................................2
Don't know 8

1 Yes   2 No   3 Don't know

1. Yes
2. No
8. Don't know

5. **Align response codes.**

   Yes 1
   No 2
   Don't know 8

   White 1
   African American 2
   Hispanic 3

   Note: Dillman puts response code immediately to the left of the answer.

6. **Provide clear instructions for open-ended items.**

   What was your blood pressure the last time you had it checked?

   RECORD HIGH VALUE: _____
   (systolic reading)

   RECORD LOW VALUE: _____
   (diastolic reading)

7. **Provide clear special instructions.**

   (Ask males only):
   Did you use a condom?

8. **Provide clear skip instructions.**

   8a. Do you smoke cigarettes?

       Yes **(Ask Q. 8b)** 1
       No **(Skip to Q. 9)** 2

   8b. How many cigarettes do you smoke per day on average?

   RECORD NUMBER OF CIGARETTES: _____

9. **Phrase full and complete questions.**

   What is your age? *or*
   What is your date of birth?

Don't **vary alignment of response codes on a page.**

   Yes 1
   No 2
   Don't know 8

   White 1
   African American 2
   Hispanic 3

Don't **just leave a space with no instructions for the answer.**

   What was your blood pressure the last time you had it checked?

   _____

Don't **have instructions about how to answer questions in same typeface and format as question.**

   Ask males only:
   Did you use a condom?

Don't **leave out explicit skip instructions.**

   8a. Do you smoke cigarettes?

       Yes 1
       No 2

   8b. How many cigarettes do you smoke per day on average?

Don't **simply use words or headings to elicit information from respondents.**

   Age? _____

EXHIBIT 12.1. DO'S AND DON'TS OF QUESTIONNAIRE DESIGN, cont'd.

Do	Don't

10. Use a forced choice format for a list.

Should an employer be allowed to require job applicants to be medically tested for... (Circle answer for yes or no to each.)

	Yes	No
a. V.D.?	1	2
b. Using illegal drugs?	1	2
c. High blood pressure?	1	2
d. Having AIDS virus?	1	2

11. Use column format for a series with the same response categories.

	Strongly agree	Agree	Disagree	Strongly disagree
a	1	2	3	4
b	1	2	3	4
c	1	2	3	4
d	1	2	3	4
e	1	2	3	4
f	1	2	3	4
g	1	2	3	4

Note: Dillman suggests that words/phrases for the categories be repeated within columns for a mail questionnaire.

Don't ask respondent to indicate "all that apply" if they could indicate more than one response.

Should an employer be allowed to require applicants to be medically tested for... (Circle all that apply.)

a. V.D.?	1
b. Using illegal drugs?	2
c. High blood pressure?	3
d. Having AIDS virus?	4

Don't repeat a string of questions with same response categories.

a. Male homosexuals are disgusting.

Strongly agree	1
Agree	2
Disagree	3
Strongly disagree	4

b. Male homosexuality is a natural expression of sexuality.

Strongly agree	1
Agree	2
Disagree	3
Strongly disagree	4

12. **Use column format for a series with comparable skip patterns.**

    1. Did you go to see any of the following providers in the past twelve months, from (date) to (date)? (Read list and circle number for yes or no.)

	Yes	No
a. Dentist?	1	2
b. Chiropractor?	1	2
c. Psychotherapist?	1	2

    Don't fail to clearly link a series of questions to subsequent dependent items.

    For each provider *marked yes in Q. 1:*

    2. How many times did you go see a (provider) during this period? (Record number.)

    ____ times
    ____ times
    ____ times

    1. Did you go to see any of the following providers in the past twelve months, from (date) to (date)? (Read list and circle number for yes or no.)

	Yes	No
a. Dentist?	1	2
b. Chiropractor?	1	2
c. Psychotherapist?	1	2

    2. How many times did you go see this type of provider during this period? (Record number.)

    ____ times

13. **Put all parts of a question on the same page.**

    Don't split a question between pages, particularly when skip instructions are part of the question.

14. **Allow plenty of space on the questionnaire.**

    Don't crowd the questions and space for recording the answers.

15. **Carefully consider the appearance of the questionnaire.**

    Don't just start the questions on page 1 without introducing the study, identifying the sponsoring organization, and so on.

EXHIBIT 12.1. DO'S AND DON'TS OF QUESTIONNAIRE DESIGN, cont'd.

Do

Don't

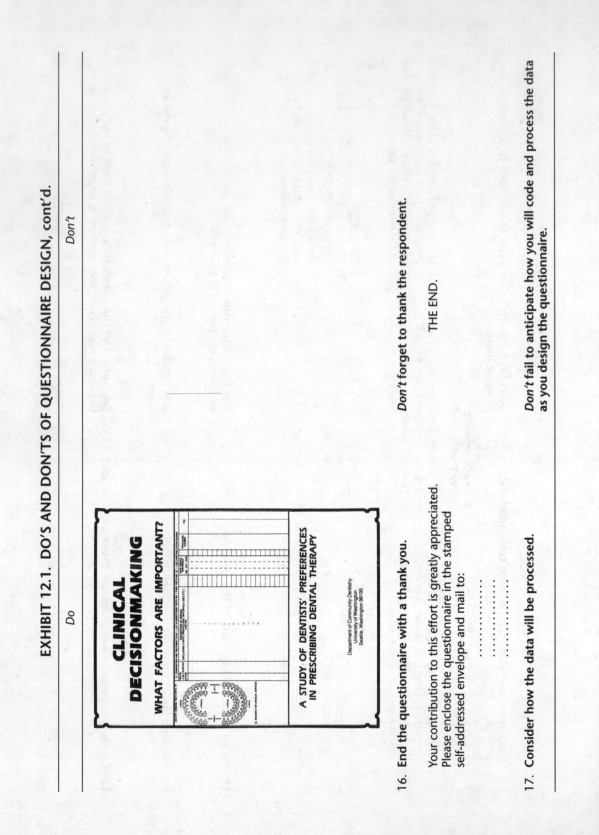

CLINICAL DECISIONMAKING

WHAT FACTORS ARE IMPORTANT?

A STUDY OF DENTISTS' PREFERENCES IN PRESCRIBING DENTAL THERAPY

Department of Community Dentistry
University of Washington
Seattle, Washington 98195

16. End the questionnaire with a thank you.

Your contribution to this effort is greatly appreciated. Please enclose the questionnaire in the stamped self-addressed envelope and mail to:

. . . .
. . . .
. . . .

17. Consider how the data will be processed.

Don't forget to thank the respondent.

THE END.

Don't fail to anticipate how you will code and process the data as you design the questionnaire.

used (for example, circling "1" for "Not enough" in the previous example). On a mail questionnaire, one may want to use a code of "4" rather than "8" for the "Don't know" response because some respondents may be confused by the jump from "3" to "8."

Use Numerical Codes for Closed-End Responses

Using numerical codes rather than alphabetic letters (alphanumeric characters) or putting an "X" next to the category that best represents the respondent's answer are the recommended methods for closed-end response categories. The likelihood of error with the "X-marks-the-spot" method is greater because of the misplacement of the "X" in relationship to the lines provided beside the answer categories and because it is not as easy to input the data when response codes are not directly available on the questionnaire. Numerical response codes are also likely to yield fewer problems in coding and processing the data than letters (a, b, c, d, and so on) because some statistical software packages present problems in handling these types of codes. They are also more limiting in terms of the number of unique codes (the twenty-six letters in the alphabet) that can be employed.

Use Consistent Numerical Codes and Formats

Another recommendation is to follow a consistent pattern in assigning code numbers to comparable response categories for different questions. Assigning the same code numbers to comparable response categories for different questions throughout the questionnaire (for example, yes = 1; no = 2; respondent refused = 7; respondent doesn't know answer = 8) and using a consistent pattern for the placement of response codes for comparable types of questions (such as along the right margin in Questions 3 and 4 in Resource B) reduce the uncertainties for interviewers and respondents about which code to use in answering questions with similar response formats.

Research has suggested that in mail surveys respondents may answer in terms of the first categories on the list (primacy effect), while in telephone or personal interview surveys they are more likely to respond in terms of the later categories (recency effect) (Ayidiya & McClendon, 1990; Salant & Dillman, 1994). Procedures for minimizing these effects include reducing the number of categories presented to respondents, varying the order of presentation of the categories in interviewer-administered surveys, and (in personal interviews) showing cards to respondents with the response categories listed. Computer-assisted data collection methods offer particular advantages in addressing this issue, particularly in their ability to randomize the order in which options are presented to respondents.

Align Response Codes

Align the response codes to be circled or checked along the right margin for telephone or personal interviews (see Questions 1 to 10 of the AIDS telephone survey, Resource B), to the left of the response categories for mail questionnaires (see Questions 21 to 25 of the dentists survey, Resource C), and in line with counterpart codes for questions that precede or follow. Dillman recommends placing the response codes to the left of the categories in self-administered questionnaires because it is easier for the respondent to circle them there. Placing the codes along the right margin in interviewer-administered surveys is likely to result in fewer errors on the part of trained interviewers than might be the case with respondents who fill out the questionnaire themselves. In addition, it facilitates subsequent inputting of the data directly from the questionnaire. With self-administered questionnaires, the ease and accuracy of respondents' recording their answers is primary, while with an interviewer-administered instrument, more weight can be given to formatting the questionnaire to facilitate data processing.

The labels for response codes can also be column headings for answers to a series of subparts to a question. These labels should be placed directly over the codes to which they apply (as in Question 31 in Resource B):

Q. 31 . . . please tell me how afraid you are of . . .

	Not at all afraid				*Extremely afraid*
a. getting diabetes?	1	2	3	4	5
b. getting cancer?	1	2	3	4	5

. . . *and so on.*

Provide Clear Instructions for Open-Ended Items

For open-ended items, clear instructions should be provided about how the information should be recorded. It may be particularly important to specify the units to be used in responding, such as visits, patients, or procedures (see Question 20 of the dentists questionnaire, Resource C).

Provide Clear Special Instructions

Any instructions relating to how the question should be answered or the skip patterns to be followed should appear next to the response category or question to which it refers (see Resource B, Questions 40a to 40c). It is helpful to set off these instructions from the questions by putting them in all capital letters (Dillman) or italics (Sudman and Bradburn):

40a. In the past five years, have you engaged in vaginal intercourse?

Yes 1

No (*Skip to Q. 41a*) 2

(ASK FEMALES ONLY):

b. Did your partner/partners use a condom . . . .

always, ... 1

sometimes, or 2

never? 3

(ASK MALES ONLY):

c. Did you use a condom . . .

always, ... 1

sometimes, or 2

never? 3

Dillman's Total Design Method for mail questionnaires recommends that the questions be set apart from the response categories by spelling out the latter in all capital letters (Dillman, 1978). (See Resource C.) Instructions should be fully written out when first used in the questionnaire ("Circle the number of your answer"), reduced in length later ("Circle number"), and eventually omitted.

Provide Clear Skip Instructions

Both the respondent and the interviewer need to be instructed clearly with respect to where to go next when the answer to a particular question (as Question 40a earlier) dictates the other questions they should answer. Dillman recommends that arrows (as in Questions 23 and 31 of the dentists questionnaire, Resource C) be used in self-administered questionnaires, although clear instructions in parentheses beside the response code to which it applies is also a useful strategy (see Questions 19a, 20a, 21a in the Chicago AIDS survey, Resource B). In computer-assisted data collection, the relevant skip patterns or probes are programmed into the interview. As in paper-and-pencil questionnaires, these steps should be checked and double-checked before the questionnaire goes into the field to ensure that the instructions are directing the interviewer or respondent as they should.

Phrase Full and Complete Questions

Often single words or incomplete sentences are used in posing survey questions, such as "Age?" or "Occupation?" Such terse terminology is likely to be insufficient for the respondent to gain a clear understanding of how the question should be answered. Complete sentences should be used to clarify fully and precisely the information that is needed: "What is your age?" or "What is your date of birth?"

Use a Forced Choice Format for a List

Questionnaires often ask respondents or interviewers to circle a code for all relevant answers among a series of categories provided. The danger of this approach is that it is not always entirely clear what *not* circling an answer may mean. For example, it might mean (as intended) that it did not apply to the respondent. But it might also indicate that the respondent was not sure and left it blank or that it was inadvertently overlooked either by the respondent or the interviewer (Rasinski, Mingay, & Bradburn, 1994).

Use Column Format for a Series with the Same Response Categories

Often a series of survey questions (especially those relating to respondents' attitudes toward a particular topic) have the same response categories (such as strongly agree, agree, disagree, not sure, disagree, or strongly disagree). To economize on the amount of space required for responding to these questions and to facilitate the ease of recording the responses, a column format for arraying the questions and response categories is recommended. With interviewer-administered questionnaires, numbers (such as 1 through 5) can be assigned to the response codes or continuum (see Questions 31 to 33 in the AIDS survey, Resource B) and the interviewer can be instructed to circle the number that corresponds to the respondent's answer. Dillman, however, recommends that in mail surveys the actual phrases representing the response categories be provided for the respondent to circle (see Question 17 in the dentists survey, Resource C). This is thought to provide a somewhat more concrete approach for respondents to use in answering the questions, because having to relate the numbers to the response category headings may be confusing to individuals who are not used to filling out survey questionnaires. Dillman also recommends that the basic question be repeated and set off with lines to provide a kind of cap for it directly above the response categories (see Question 17, Resource C), with leaders (or dots) running from each of the statements to which the respondent is asked to reply to its corresponding answer categories.

When a series of questions are asked about multiple household members or events, parallel vertical response columns should be used for recording the answers to the same question for each respondent. (In the NCHS–NHIS questionnaire shown in Resource A, for example, there are identical response columns provided for each member of the household.) The name of each person, as well as other relevant demographic information about him or her, should be recorded at the top of the columns on the inside of the cover pages of the bookletlike questionnaire. The interior pages of the questionnaire should be shorter so that the demographic information remains visible at the top as these interior pages are turned. The questions and relevant answer columns for the respective respondents should appear on these shortened pages. With computer-assisted questionnaires, comparable response categories for each respondent can be called up on the computer terminal screen by the interviewer when it is time to collect information on that person.

Use Column Format for a Series with Comparable Skip Patterns

On some occasions, a series of questions may have a comparable skip pattern, such as asking how many times a particular type of health professional was seen after first asking questions about whether that type of provider was consulted or not (see item 12 in Exhibit 12.1). Once again, a column format, with the relevant questions and instructions serving as headings for the respective questions would be appropriate. This has many of the same advantages as mentioned earlier for a series with the same response categories. It also assures that the answers to any follow-up questions are clearly linked to the preceding (screener) questions. This is a relatively complex format, and it is not generally recommended for use in self-administered survey questionnaires.

Put All Parts of a Question on the Same Page

Questions and accompanying response categories should never be split between pages; the respondent or interviewer would have to flip back and forth to answer the question or might assume that the question ends on the first page and, therefore, fail to consider certain responses. Nor is it desirable to split subparts of a question, particularly if the same skip patterns or instructions apply to all parts of the question. With computer-assisted questionnaires, *segmentation* may be a problem, meaning that the interviewer loses sight of the context in which the discrete questions that appear on the computer terminal are being asked (House, 1985; House & Nicholls, 1988; Saris, 1991). Adequate information should therefore be provided on each computer screen to guide the interviewer in dealing with the question or the sequence of questions in which it appears.

Allow Plenty of Space on the Questionnaire

There should be sufficient space provided in the questionnaire for responding to open-ended questions. Large and clear type should be used in printing the questionnaire or displaying the questionnaire on a terminal screen. Also, the questions should not be crowded together, either on the printed page or on the computer terminal. Dillman recommends that white space, rather than dividing lines, be used to separate questions in a self-administered survey and that space be provided at the end of a mail questionnaire for any additional comments respondents may wish to offer (see end of dentists questionnaire, Resource C) (Dillman, 1978; Salant & Dillman, 1994).

Carefully Consider the Appearance of the Questionnaire

Dillman's Total Design Method places considerable emphasis on the appearance of questionnaires, particularly that of mailed self-administered forms. It is generally desirable to put paper-and-pencil questionnaires into booklets to permit ease in reading and turning pages and also to prevent pages from being lost. In Dillman's initial formulation of the booklet format, he recommended the following conventions: condense in size ($6\frac{1}{2}$ x $8\frac{1}{4}$ inches), principally to save on mailing costs; use 12-point elite type and photoreduce (79 percent), to provide more white space; and print the booklet on white or off-white 16-pound bond paper to assure that it can be copied on both sides (Dillman, 1978). Based on experience with this approach in an array of studies and the increased availability of efficient word processing technologies, he and his colleagues now suggest that regular legal size ($8\frac{1}{2}$ x 14 inches) paper be printed on both sides and then folded and stapled into a booklet and that it is not necessary to photoreduce the type. In fact, it may be desirable to have larger typefaces for self-administered questionnaires sent to certain populations (the elderly or others who may have trouble reading small type). No questions should be printed on the front or back cover pages of the questionnaire (Salant & Dillman, 1994). The cover page should have an "interest-getting title" and "a neutral but eye-catching illustration" (Dillman, 1983, p. 362) in addition to the name and address of the study sponsor. No detailed questions should appear on the back cover of the questionnaire. Space may, however, be provided for any additional comments the respondents may wish to provide on the subject as well as the address to which the questionnaire should be returned.

Colored covers or sections of the questionnaire can be helpful in drawing a respondent's attention to the questionnaire or in identifying different parts of the instrument that should be used for different respondents (Phipps, Robertson, & Keel, 1991). Thus, the cover and back page of the dentists study questionnaire were orange, and the three screening forms used in the Chicago AIDS survey were all different colors (yellow, blue, and green). The title of the study, the date, and the name of the organization or individual conducting the study should also appear on the first page of the questionnaire to identify clearly the topic and sponsorship of the survey.

It is helpful in interviewer-administered surveys to provide spaces for the interviewer to record the time that the interview began and ended, particularly during the pilot or pretest stages of the survey, so that the time it will take on average to do the interview can be estimated. With computer-assisted interviewing, the length of the interview can be logged automatically. The number of pages or amount of time for an interview will be influenced by the topic, the respondent's interest in it, the burden and complexity of the questionnaire itself, and the mode of data collection being used. As discussed in Chapter Five, interviewer-administered questionnaires can usually be longer than self-administered ones. Lengthy questionnaires may in particular affect the response rates to mail questionnaires (Burchell & Marsh, 1992). Dillman (1978) recommends that self-administered questionnaires be no longer than twelve pages. For topics not especially salient to the respondents, the questionnaire should be much shorter. Sudman and Bradburn (1982) recommend no more than two to four pages.

End the Questionnaire with a Thank You

Questionnaires should always end with a thank you to respondents for their time and effort. Mail surveys should include instructions about where to mail the questionnaire.

Consider How the Data Will Be Processed

Thought should be given to how the data will be coded and computerized at the time the questionnaire is being designed. With computerized questionnaires, relevant coding and editing specifications can be built into the questionnaire. Deciding how data from paper-and-pencil questionnaires will be entered into a computer during the period the questionnaire itself is being designed is important for making sure that the data will be available in the form in which they will be needed. The trade-off in making all these decisions at the start, of course, is that it takes longer to get the questionnaire actually designed and tested. Procedures for coding and computerizing the data will be discussed in more detail in Chapter Fourteen.

Order

The order in which questions are asked in the questionnaire affects respondents' willingness to participate in the study as well as the interpretation of the questions by those who do agree to be interviewed.

The form and content of the study's introduction, which is read to respondents in interviewer-administered surveys or which respondents themselves read in self-administered questionnaires, should be carefully designed and pretested. Andrews (1984) suggests that medium-length introductions (sixteen to sixty-four words), rather than very short or very long ones (less than sixteen words or more than sixty-four, respectively), are likely to elicit the best response. The introduction should state who is conducting the study and for what purpose, the topics that will be addressed in the interview, and the length of time it is expected to take.

It is important that the first question be a relatively easy one for the respondent to answer, that it be on an interesting, nonthreatening topic, and, ideally, that it relate to the focus of the study as set forth in the introduction. The first questions asked in the Chicago AIDS survey are, for example, "In general, would you say that your health is excellent, good, fair, or poor?" and "How much do you worry about your health? Do you worry about it a great deal, somewhat, or not at all?" (Resource B, Questions 1, 2). These are relatively easy questions about something that is interesting to most people (their health) and they establish a relatively nonthreatening start for the series of questions about more sensitive health issues that follow. Similarly, in the redesign of the National Center for Health Statistics–National Health Interview Survey (NCHS–NHIS) in 1982, the question about whether or not people had been hospitalized within the year was moved to the beginning of the questionnaire to establish clearly the health and health care focus of the study early in the interview (Resource A, Question 1, Introduction and Hospital Probe page).

It is generally advisable to make the first question a closed-end one so that more structure is provided to the respondent for answering it. This question could, however, be followed by a related open-ended question if the topic is such that respondents are likely to be interested in elaborating on or explaining their answer to the previous question. Mail questionnaires, however, should never begin with open-ended questions because this would give respondents the impression that filling out the questionnaire will be a lot of work. As indicated in Chapter Five, the number of open-ended questions asked in self-administered questionnaires should be kept to a minimum.

Ideally, it is best to ask personal demographic questions—such as the respondent's or household member's age, sex, race, and income—at the end of the interview, after there has been an opportunity to convey clearly the purpose and content of the study and after the interviewer has established rapport with the respondents. Dillman (1978) particularly recommends this be done in mail questionnaires. But, as in the Chicago AIDS survey, it is often necessary to ask these as screening questions early in the interview in order to decide who to interview or to oversample certain population subgroups (see Resource B, screening questionnaires). In that case, the rate of breakoffs and refusals subsequent to asking these questions should be carefully evaluated during the pretest of the questionnaire, and the questions or other aspects of introducing the study to respondents should be redesigned to try to maximize cooperation.

For topics that have higher salience or when asking both general and specific questions about attitudes, it is advisable to ask general questions *before* specific ones. In contrast, for general questions about people's behaviors, particularly questions that might be less salient to respondents or that rely on the recall of specific events, asking detailed questions about these experiences *first* might help them recall the details needed to answer the more general question. For example, in the NCHS–NHIS, questions about people's health in general and their total number of visits to a physician in the year (Resource A, Section G) follow a series of questions about what limits they may have had to place on their normal activities because of illness and injury and how often they visited a physician during a two-week period preceding the interview. This approach provides respondents with an opportunity to recall specific details about their experiences before they are asked to answer a more general question that summarizes them. It should be pointed out, however, that whenever individual items from other studies are used in a survey, the context for these items (the questions that precede and follow) may well differ and this could affect the comparability in how respondents answer the questions.

Research applying the principles of cognitive psychology to questionnaire design has suggested that people tend to use autobiographical schemata in responding to survey questions, particularly those that require the recall of a series of events over time (Bradburn, Rips, & Shevell, 1987; Schwarz & Sudman, 1994). In designing such questions, researchers should phrase the question or series of questions in such a way that respondents are asked to respond in chronological order—either from the present backward in time or from some point in time in the past to the present. It may also be helpful to identify a salient autobiographical event of either a personal nature ("Since you were married . . . ") or a public nature ("Since the last presidential election . . . ") that can serve as an anchor point for respondents to use in recalling these events.

In general, it is advisable to group together questions related to the same topic. Also, as mentioned in Chapter Eight, transitional phrases or instructions should be provided when new topics are introduced so that the shift does not seem an abrupt one to respondents and they have an opportunity to think about the topic before being called upon to answer a question about it.

Consideration should also be given to arranging the order and format of questions so that respondents do not fall into an invariant pattern in responding to the items—sometimes referred to as a *response set*—because of boredom or the burden of providing discriminating answers to the questions. For example, a series of questions might ask respondents to report whether or not they saw certain providers in the year and, if so, how many times. If a great many questions in the questionnaire are of this kind, the respondent may get wise and decide to start saying no when asked if they had certain types of experiences because they realize they can avoid answering many other questions if they do so. Varying the format and placement of such questions is thus important for enhancing the interest and variety of the questionnaire, as well as for reducing the chance of respondents' falling into these types of patterns in responding to the questionnaire.

It is advisable to design some sort of device for reviewing the flow of questions in the questionnaire and how they relate to one another before mocking up the questionnaire itself so that the logic and utility of the order in which the questions are asked can be evaluated and the skip patterns that depend on how certain questions are asked are clear. Designing a flowchart that explicitly reflects the order in which questions are asked and the questions to which respondents are directed on the basis of answers to prior questions, is, for example, a very useful device for designing and verifying the appropriate order and format of the survey questionnaire. Such flowcharts are imperative in designing computer-assisted data collection instruments and strongly advised in thinking through the arrangement of questions in paper-and-pencil questionnaires, especially those that have large numbers of items or complex skip patterns.

Context

The study of context effects in survey questionnaires is a new area of methodological research that draws heavily on the concepts and theories of cognitive psychology (Hippler, Schwarz, & Sudman, 1987; Schwarz & Sudman, 1992; Tourangeau & Rasinski, 1988).

Tourangeau and Rasinski have pointed out that each of the stages in responding to a question (comprehension, retrieval, estimation/judgment, and response) can be affected by the questions that precede it. They suggest that earlier questions can provide information for the respondent to use in understanding the questions that follow. Earlier items can also prime respondents to consider particular types of beliefs that they might then call upon later as they try to retrieve their opinion on a related issue. The earlier questions can also provide some norm or standard of comparison for respondents to use in making a judgment about the right answer to the current question. Finally, in the response stage, respondents may feel that their answers should be consistent with attitudes or information they provided earlier in the questionnaire.

The context of survey questions becomes problematical when people answer what seems to be the same question differently, depending on the content and order of other questions in the questionnaire. This would, of course, be a particular issue in using and comparing the same items between different surveys. It is advisable for survey designers to build in a split-ballot experiment or a think-aloud feedback strategy in evaluating different versions of the questionnaire during the pilot or pretest stages of the study if they think that context effects might be a problem in their study.

Special Considerations for Special Populations

The form and format of survey questionnaires must acknowledge and take into account the capacities of potential respondents—aurally, visually, and cognitively. Different modes of gathering data rely and call upon different aptitudes on the part of survey respondents. The choice of method for formatting and presenting survey questions should therefore seek to optimize or match the unique strengths of a given method with the special capabilities of those of whom the questions are asked.

Selected Examples

As indicated throughout this chapter, the surveys in Resources A, B, and C drew heavily on many of the principles detailed here for designing and formatting survey questionnaires. The NCHS–NHIS presents special challenges because of gathering data on all household members as well as including lengthy supplements for selected respondents. The 1996 redesign of the NHIS was intended to streamline and focus the content of the survey as well as optimize the applicability and utility of computer-assisted means of gathering the data.

The Chicago AIDS survey reflects adaptations required for telephone interviews, as in Questions 31 to 35, that employ a convention of using numbers, "On a scale from 1 and 5," with the end points defined (extremely or not at all *afraid* of getting an illness, extremely likely or not all *likely* to get it) rather than using verbal labels for each point of the scale. Another adaptation in telephone interviews with questions that ask the extent to which a respondent agrees with a statement or was satisfied with aspects of their experience, for example, is to break the question into two parts, "Do you agree or disagree?" or "Were you satisfied or dissatisfied?" and then ask, "Do you (dis)agree or *strongly* (dis)agree?" and so on.

Guidelines for Minimizing Survey Errors

Clarity, coherence, and consistency are sound principles to keep in mind in configuring the format, order, and context of survey questions, respectively. The content and format of the questions, response categories, and instructions must provide clear guidance to survey respondents and interviewers regarding how to answer them. Ideally, the order in which questions are posed should reflect an underlying coherence in the concepts and the topics addressed in the questionnaire and their interrelationship. The context in which items are imbedded should be governed by a self-conscious logic with respect to how preceding questions may influence those that follow.

Supplementary Sources

The reader is referred to Dillman (1978), Salant and Dillman (1994), Fowler (1995), and Sudman and Bradburn (1982) for guidance on the design and formatting of paper-and-pencil questionnaires and to Saris (1991) for an overview of the issues in developing computer-assisted instruments.

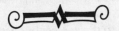

CHAPTER THIRTEEN

MONITORING AND CARRYING OUT THE SURVEY

Chapter Highlights

1. Field procedures for carrying out a survey include deciding how to introduce the study to respondents, how to follow up with nonrespondents, when to schedule the initial and follow-up contacts, how to keep track of the results of those contacts, whether to provide cash incentives to respondents, whether to allow respondents to serve as proxies for other people, and what documentation to provide for these procedures.

2. The process of hiring interviewers for a personal or telephone interview should include a consideration of the applicants' physical, social, personal, and behavioral characteristics.

3. Interviewers should participate in a training session that provides a general introduction both to survey interviewing and to specific aspects of the study that interviewers will be carrying out.

4. Interviewer supervisors should monitor the following quality control tasks: (1) field editing; (2) interview validation; (3) interviewer observation; and (4) retrieval of missing data.

5. Survey management involves assuming responsibility for the overall conceptual development of the study, scheduling and overseeing the tasks required to carry out the survey, monitoring quality at each stage of the study's design and

execution, and monitoring expenditures relative to the project budget over the course of the study.

6. Computer-assisted modes of data gathering require a great deal of front-end planning but can greatly expedite data collection, monitoring, and quality control.

This chapter presents the steps for testing and implementing the procedures needed to carry out surveys designed according to the principles discussed in the preceding chapters. In particular, it describes the steps involved in (1) specifying the field procedures, (2) hiring interviewers, (3) training them, (4) supervising the fieldwork for the survey, and (5) managing the survey as a whole. When applicable, specific procedures used in the conduct of personal, telephone, mail, and computer-assisted surveys will be discussed.

Survey designers should consider the criteria discussed in this chapter whether they are hiring or training their own interviewers or evaluating the quality of the field operations of outside firms. If researchers decide to contract with an outside firm, they should request documentation on that firm's procedures for carrying out studies.

Specifying the Field Procedures

Before they begin to implement their survey, designers need to consider the nature of the first contact with respondents about the study.

Advance Notice

It is desirable to provide advance notice of a survey either through the news media, key informant and community contacts, or relevant professional or organizational sponsors in the targeted communities. Interviews preceded by a letter or other contact are called "warm contacts." Those in which no prior notice is given to respondents are "cold contacts." Respondents tend to be more cooperative when they are given advance notice that they will be contacted for an interview.

Personal. In personal interview surveys, such as the National Center for Health Statistics–National Health Interview Survey (NCHS–NHIS), respondents are usually sent an advance letter that describes the study, intended to decrease the element of surprise when the household is contacted as well as lend legitimacy to the survey effort. It is also desirable for the interviewer to wear a printed project name tag and carry a signed original letter from the survey director that explains the purpose of the study and can be left with the respondents.

Telephone. Most telephone surveys, especially those based on a random digit dialing sampling approach, are cold contact surveys. However, databases in which the phone numbers are linked to names and addresses can be utilized to identify potential respondents for the purposes of sending an advance letter to the addresses associated with targeted phone numbers to increase the response rate to the survey.

Mail. Mail surveys to special populations, such as groups of health professionals, can be preceded by a general announcement in professional newsletters or journals. In the revised and updated Dillman Total Design Method, it is recommended that an advance letter be sent one week before mailing the actual survey (Salant & Dillman, 1994). The letter should notify respondents that the survey will be coming, briefly state why the study is being done, and convey that their participation would be greatly appreciated.

The Dillman method also points out the importance of the cover letter for eliciting respondent cooperation in mail surveys (Dillman, 1978; Salant & Dillman, 1994). Such letters should be addressed and sent to the specific individuals selected for the study (rather than to "Dear Dentist," for example), have the current date, and be signed with a blue ballpoint pen. It is particularly important to try to identify a specific individual to whom the questionnaire should be sent in conducting surveys of businesses or other organizations (Paxson, Dillman, & Tarnai, 1995). The letters should, at a minimum, explain the social usefulness of the study, why the recipients and their participation are important, the procedures that will be used to ensure the confidentiality of their responses, the incentives or rewards for participating, and what to do or whom to contact if there are questions about the study. The cover letter should conclude with a thank you for participating.

Examples of advance letters and cover letters for personal, telephone, and mail surveys are provided in Chapter Eight of *How to Conduct Your Own Survey* (Salant & Dillman, 1994). The cover letters and reminder postcard used in the dentists survey appear in Resource C.

Schedule for Contacts

Another important issue in designing the fieldwork for personal and telephone interview surveys is when to schedule contacts with the selected sample units. The spring and fall are better for finding people at home than are the summer and winter months (Vigderhous, 1981). Launching a general population survey during major holiday periods, such as between Thanksgiving and New Year's Day, should be avoided because of the strong possibility that people will be away from home during those periods.

Personal. Research to determine the times that yield the highest rates of interviews with respondents suggests that weekday evenings and weekends, especially Sundays, are the best times to contact households (Weeks, Jones, Folsom, & Benrud, 1980; Weeks, Kulka, & Pierson, 1987).

Telephone. It is not efficient to let the phone ring more than four times, because most calls (97 percent) are answered within four rings (Smead & Wilcox, 1980). Answering machines are increasingly in use in U.S. households either primarily to assure that messages are received while the family is away ("connectors") or primarily to screen unwanted calls ("cocooners") (Oldendick, 1993; Tuckel & Feinberg, 1991). Urban households, those with higher family incomes, and younger adults are more likely to have answering machines, although once contacted, most are willing to grant the interview (Oldendick, 1993; Oldendick & Link, 1994; Tuckel & Feinberg, 1991; Xu, Bates, & Schweitzer, 1993). Piazza (1993) found that the best times to complete interviews in households with answering machines were Saturday morning from 9:00 A.M. to 10:00 A.M. and Monday through Thursday evenings after 6:00 P.M. Generally messages were not left on the answering machine but information was gathered from the outgoing message itself that might provide useful hints about the characteristics of household members (age, gender) in subsequent callbacks.

Mail. Dillman and his colleagues recommend a systematic series of timed contacts to elicit the fullest participation in a mail survey, which are described in detail in the discussion that follows (Dillman, 1978; Salant & Dillman, 1994).

Procedures for Follow-Up Contacts

An important aspect in carrying out a survey is following up with respondents who are not available or do not respond to the first contact. Different protocols for following up may be appropriate with different methods of data collection.

Personal. Returning to households to get a personal interview when respondents were not at home on the first visit can be expensive because of the time and travel involved. In the NCHS–NHIS, there is no specified upper limit of interviewer contacts at a household in order to obtain an interview, although the majority are completed within six contacts (Kalsbeek, Botman, Massey, & Liu, 1994). Many researchers or survey research firms may have to limit the number of callbacks because of budgetary restraints. They must then consider the probable trade-offs in nonresponse rates relative to survey costs in deciding how many calls to allow interviewers to make. The location of interviewers' initial assignments and the protocols for recontacting households should be carefully designed so that the probable yield for each interviewer contact is maximized.

Telephone. Recontacts can be made more cost effectively in telephone surveys than in personal interviews. The Chicago AIDS survey, for example, provided for a maximum of ten attempts. Only one attempt was to be made during an interview shift, unless a busy signal or some other indication that the respondent was at home was obtained. When the line was busy, interviewers were advised to call the number a maximum of three times three minutes apart (Survey Research Laboratory, 1987b). A minimum of at least three callbacks at different times of the day and days of the week should be budgeted, although more are quite likely to be required to achieve a high response rate.

With both personal and telephone interview surveys, all contacts and their outcomes should be recorded. A system of codes to record the disposition of each call, as well as forms on which interviewers can record this information, should be developed, so that a systematic accounting of the status of each case throughout the field period can be made. Different follow-up strategies may also be warranted for different outcomes. When respondents break off an interview or refuse to participate, it is often advisable to reassign the case to a different interviewer, to a core group of interviewers whose principal job is to work with reluctant respondents, or to an interviewing supervisor. For respondents who are not home at the time of the call or whose line is busy, specific call-scheduling protocols can be used to decide which interviewer should make the follow-up call and when. Most computer-assisted telephone interviewing (CATI) systems do, in fact, have computerized call scheduling and assignment procedures built into their basic data collection system.

Mail. Dillman's total survey design approach to mail surveys provides a systematic set of procedures to maximize the survey response rate (Salant & Dillman, 1994):

First: Send a personalized, advance letter to everyone selected for the study.

Second: One week later, mail a personalized cover letter with somewhat more detail about the study, a questionnaire, and stamped return envelope.

Third: Four to eight days later, send a follow-up postcard to thank everyone who responded and to ask those who have not to do so.

Fourth: Three weeks after the first questionnaire is mailed, send a new personalized cover letter to those who have not responded indicating that "We have not yet heard from you" and including a replacement questionnaire and stamped return envelope.

Methodological research has borne out the effectiveness of a systematic follow-up strategy for achieving good response rates, particularly in combination with sending even a modest (one to two dollar) monetary incentive with the initial mailing (Armstrong & Lusk, 1987; Church, 1993; DeLeeuw & Hox, 1988; James & Bolstein, 1990; Heberlein & Baumgartner, 1981; Mullen, Easling, Nixon, Koester, & Biddle, 1987; Perneger, Etter, & Rougemont, 1993; Tedin & Hofstetter, 1982; Yammarino, Skinner, & Childers, 1991).

Dillman and his colleagues recommend the following additional procedures if there is a concern about whether the standard four-step process will yield the desired response rate: enclose a monetary incentive with the initial mailing; call respondents a few days after mailing the replacement questionnaire; do a fifth mailing using two-day priority mail to signal the importance and urgency of a response (Salant & Dillman, 1994). Dillman no longer advises using certified mail because of complaints registered by respondents about having to go to the post office to pick up the survey materials.

The dentists' survey employed Dillman's mail survey design and implementation procedures. It also benefited from suggestions by Sudman on the design of mail surveys of reluctant professionals: (1) point out the professional benefits given their time and effort involved in participating, (2) be sensitive to confidentiality issues, and (3) allow respondents room for written comments rather than offer a forced choice format exclusively (Sudman, 1985). A check for $10 was also included in the initial mailing to dentists as an incentive for them to participate. Those who failed to respond to follow-up mailings were contacted by phone and asked to return the questionnaire if they wished to participate in the study. An overall response rate of 78 percent was achieved in the study, which is a quite good rate of return for mail surveys.

Incentives to Respondents

Survey designers may want to consider the cost-effectiveness of offering incentives to respondents to participate in a study. Research suggests that monetary incentives, particularly when transmitted with an initial mailing or offered before conducting an interview, increase response rates without biasing study results (Berry & Kanouse, 1987; Church, 1993; Furse & Stewart, 1982; Gunn & Rhodes, 1981; Hubbard & Little, 1988; James & Bolstein, 1990; Mizes, Fleece, & Roos, 1984; Nederhof, 1983; Peck & Dresch, 1981; Perneger, Etter, & Rougemont, 1993; Willimack, Schuman, Pennel, & Lepkowski, 1995; Yu & Cooper, 1983). Nevertheless, criticisms have been made of such incentives, principally because of concerns about setting unfortunate or unaffordable precedents for the field (National Center for Health Services Research, 1977a; Sheatsley and Loft, 1981).

The Office of Management and Budget (OMB) forbids the offering of blanket financial incentives to respondents in federally sponsored surveys. The 1995 Paperwork Reduction Act required an explanation for a decision to provide any payment or gift. Requests must be submitted to OMB and cases are decided on an individual basis. Compensation or remuneration is usually provided when particularly burdensome or time-consuming requests are made of study participants, who might not otherwise agree to participate in the study.

One type of nonmonetary incentive that some groups (such as members of a professional group being surveyed) may find appealing is the survey results. A return postage-paid postcard can be provided or respondents can be asked to indicate on the outside of the return envelope for the questionnaire if they would like to have a copy of the finished survey; in this way they do not have to record their names and addresses on the questionnaire itself.

Another approach that has received attention in recent years in mail, telephone, and personal interview surveys is the foot-in-the-door technique. This approach involves a two-stage strategy in which respondents are asked to respond to a relatively small initial request (such as being asked to answer a brief series of questions about health or exercise practices over the phone) and then to participate in a larger data collection effort, which is the real focus of the study (for example, a more extensive series of questions on their use of health care facilities). Research on the effectiveness of this method has produced mixed results. Some studies have shown that it increases respondents' participation in the larger effort, while others have shown the opposite (Fern, Monroe, & Avila, 1986; Furse, Stewart, & Rados, 1981; Groves & Magilavy, 1981; Hippler & Hippler, 1986; Hornik, Zaig, Shadmon, & Barbash, 1990). More research is needed then to clarify when or with whom this foot-in-the-door technique might be most useful.

Proxy Respondents

Another issue to consider when gathering survey data is whether respondents should be allowed to provide the interview or fill out the requested information (that is, act as proxies) for other individuals who were selected for inclusion in the study. Proxies are used, for example, when parents are interviewed about their children's health or health care practices.

Personal. Concerns have been raised that proxies may tend to underreport information for the individuals for whom they are asked to respond. However, research conducted on the National Health Interview Survey has suggested that proxy reporting does not necessarily lead to underreporting. Mathiowetz and Groves (1985) and Mosely and Wolinsky (1986) point out that whether proxy respondents tend to report more *or* fewer health events for themselves than for others depends on their particular health characteristics and whether the study design itself is set up to select proxies who tend to have better or poorer health than those for whom they provide information. Proxies for patients with functional disabilities tend to report that the patients have greater limitations in instrumental activities of daily living (taking medication, using the telephone, shopping, preparing meals, doing housework, and so on) than do the patients themselves (Magaziner, Simonsick, Kashner, & Hebel, 1988).

Telephone. Telephone surveys that gather information on everyone in the family from the person who happens to be at home at the time of the interview sometimes yield results that suggest that proxies tend to report more health problems for themselves than for others. Those who happen to be at home at the time may well be sicker than those who are not. In those surveys in which healthy respondents are asked to respond for those who are too sick to respond for themselves, the opposite is likely to be true. Further, as indicated in Chapter Ten, proxy respondents are less likely to underreport sensitive health behaviors for others than are those individuals themselves.

Mail. In the dentists' preferences survey, potential respondents were told that they could have their receptionist or office manager fill out factual questions that might involve having to consult their practice records (Resource C, Questions 19 to 43). These proxies were not, however, permitted to answer the questions that related to the criteria that the dentists used in making clinical judgments or to their attitudes toward and beliefs about the practice of dentistry.

Cognitive research on the level of agreement between self-reports and proxy reports suggests that the information processing strategy underlying how the questions are phrased (recalling specific episodes versus estimating the number of events), the order and context in which they are asked, and the extent to which the proxy and self-report respondent talk to each other about the activity or attitude being referenced all influence the convergence of proxy and self-reports (Bickart, Blair, Menon, & Sudman, 1990; Bickart, Menon, Sudman, & Blair, 1992; Menon, Bickart, Sudman, & Blair, 1995). More research is needed to document the quality of proxy reports and the factors that contribute to differences between proxy and sample person responses (Moore, 1988).

In general, however, it is not advisable to ask someone to answer attitudinal, knowledge, or other perception-oriented questions for others. Proxy respondents who say they are knowledgeable about a selected individual's behaviors will probably do a good job of reporting this information for him or her, although it is advisable to ask additional questions in order to understand the extent to which the proxies have actually spent time with the sample persons or discussed the matters being referenced with them.

Documentation of Field Procedures

Survey designers should provide written documentation of the specific field procedures to be used in carrying out the survey. In personal and telephone interview surveys, these procedures can serve as resources for training interviewers as well as a reference for interviewers to consult in addressing problems or questions that arise in the course of the study.

Manuals of field procedures generally contain information similar to that found in the interviewer manual of the Chicago Area General Population Survey on AIDS (Survey Research Laboratory, 1987b) (see Resource B). This manual describes the purpose and sponsorship of the study and tells the respondents whom to contact and how if they want more information about the project. It describes the sample design and, when appropriate, gives detailed instructions about how to carry it out. It includes the project time schedule, who the primary supervisor for the project will be and how to reach him or her, procedures for gaining the cooperation of and establishing rapport with respondents, and a sample of questions respondents might ask about the study and instructions on how to answer them. There is also a description of the data collection forms and procedures to use in registering the status of cases that are in process as well as those that did not result in completed interviews. The manual gives a brief overview of the screening and questionnaire materials, and, finally, includes detailed question-by-question specifications that provide definitions for words or phrases used in the questionnaire.

Hiring Interviewers

The process of hiring interviewers for a personal or telephone interview survey should include consideration of applicants' physical, social, personal, and behavioral characteristics. Physical characteristics include age, sex, race, physical condition, physical appearance, and voice quality. Social, personal, and behavioral characteristics encompass experience and work history, education, intelligence, personality, attitude and motivation, adaptability, and accuracy (Couper and Groves, 1992b; Weinberg, 1983).

Physical Characteristics

With respect to the desirable *age* for interviewers, some preference exists for mature individuals (twenty-five to fifty-five years of age). Research conducted on the performance of interviewers in collecting complex utilization and expenditure data in the National Medical Care Expenditure Survey (NMCES) showed that older interviewers (40 years of age or older) were likely to have lower rates of missing information for selected questions (Berk & Bernstein, 1988). This finding may, however, be confounded with other characteristics of the interviewer, such as his or her experience or commitment to the job.

Most interviewers are women. Results of a national telephone survey of consumer attitudes conducted at the University of Michigan showed that turnover rates and nonresponse rates were higher for male than female interviewers and that there was a systematic tendency for male interviewers to obtain more optimistic reports from respondents about their perceptions regarding the economic outlook for the nation. There were, however, no significant differences in the rates of missing data, per-minute interview costs, or responses to factual questions between male and female interviewers (Groves & Fultz, 1985). There are some assumptions in the survey research field that respondents are more likely to open their doors or continue with an interview over the phone, as well as to respond to questions about sensitive or embarrassing issues, when contacted by a female interviewer. However, the choice of male or female interviewers should be guided primarily by the survey's subject matter and data collection design, and thought should thus be given to whether the sex of the interviewer is likely to be of any particular significance in the context of that particular study.

Another issue here is how respondents will respond to an interview conducted by someone who is not of their own race. Research suggests that this may be an issue in surveys dealing with explicitly racial topics (such as studies of attitudes about the effect of the sexual practices of different racial or ethnic groups on their risk of contracting AIDS or other sexually transmitted diseases) (Campbell, 1981; Cotter, Cohen, & Coulter, 1982; Reese, Danielson, Shoemaker, Chang, & Hsu, 1986; Schaeffer, 1980; Weeks & Moore, 1981). These studies show that minority respondents tend to provide more deferential or socially desirable responses to such questions when interviewed by a majority-race interviewer. If the subject matter of the survey deals directly with racially related topics, some thought should thus be given to matching interviewers and respondents along racial and ethnic lines. If a study is targeted to a particular racial or ethnic population subgroup (such as residents of an inner-city barrio), respondents may be more responsive to interviewers with similar sociocultural backgrounds. It would be important to talk with community leaders about these issues before hiring and assigning interviewers to such areas.

In personal interviews, it is important that an interviewer present a neat, pleasant, and professional appearance to respondents so that they feel comfortable admitting him or her to their home.

Oksenberg and her colleagues (Oksenberg, Coleman, & Cannell, 1986) have conducted research on the impact of telephone interviewers' voice quality on refusal rates. Interviewers with the lowest refusal rates tended to have higher-pitched voices and greater ranges of variations of pitch, spoke more loudly and quickly, and had clearer and more distinct pronunciation. They were also rated as more competent overall and as taking a more positive approach to the respondent and the interview than those with higher refusal rates. Attention should thus be given to evaluating the overall quality of telephone interviewers' voices during hiring and training. The information and impression conveyed by the interviewers over the phone are the only clues respondents have about whether the study is legitimate and, if they agree to cooperate, how they should approach answering the questions that are asked of them.

Social, Personal, and Behavioral Characteristics

Evidence of a responsible work history is generally a useful criterion to consider in hiring interviewers. Since many women use interviewing as a way of entering or reentering the work force after a number of years as full-time homemakers, it is appropriate to find out about relevant volunteer or nonsalaried work experience.

Previous experience as an interviewer or in seemingly related areas (sales or fundraising) does not necessarily indicate that a person will be a good interviewer in a given study. Different researchers or survey research firms may have different interviewer training protocols or data collection norms and procedures. Training for a new study or with a different organization may involve unlearning old habits, which might be hard for some people to do. Also, a sales or missionary zeal is not appropriate to surveys, which attempt to capture as accurately and objectively as possible what the respondent thinks or feels about a topic. Further, respondents might refuse to cooperate if they feel that the interviewer is trying to sell them something (Weinberg, 1983). Training, commitment, and the accrual of relevant experience within a given study appear to be consequential correlates of interviewers' performance (Berk & Bernstein, 1988; Couper & Groves, 1992b; Groves, Cialdini, & Couper, 1992; Edwards, et al., 1994; Parsons, Johnson, Warnecke, & Kaluzny, 1993).

Most interviewers have at least a high school education. It is sometimes desirable for interviewers to have some college education as well, particularly if the concepts or procedures used in a study are complex or require some degree of analytical or problem-solving ability. Too much education can be a liability, however, because highly educated individuals may feel overqualified for the job and become bored or careless as a result.

A related quality to look for in interviewers is native intelligence, although survey interviewing ordinarily does not call for exceptionally high levels of intellectual ability. The capacity to read and understand written materials, to make sound and intelligent decisions, and to express themselves clearly verbally and in writing sums up the qualities to look for when hiring interviewers.

An interest in talking and listening to people is also a useful personality trait for an interviewer to have (Weinberg, 1983). In addition, interviewers should not be easily turned off by others' lifestyles and attitudes. Moser and Kalton (1972) suggest that "the interviewer's personality should be neither overaggressive nor overly sociable. Pleasantness and a businesslike manner [are] the ideal combination" (p. 286).

Interviewing is demanding work; having people slam the door in your face or hang up the phone when you call can be part of the daily experience. Further, there is often the frustration of making repeated calls to a home and never finding the person there. Interviewers should, therefore, be highly motivated for the job and be adept at figuring out how to make the best use of their time to finish the required interviewing task and to deal with difficult or frustrating situations in the field.

Another important prerequisite for a successful interviewer is adaptability and flexibility with respect to working hours. A survey of hospital executives might require interviewers to contact and interview them during a regular nine-to-five business day. In contrast, interviewing middle-class couples in a high-rise security complex might involve getting through a security guard or phone-answering machine or making calls during weekend or evening hours.

A willingness to try to enter or record accurately the answers provided by respondents is another important quality for an interviewer. Illegible handwriting or sloppy recording of responses, as well as failure to ask certain questions of respondents, can result in problems throughout all the subsequent stages of coding and processing the questionnaire. Computer-assisted modes of data collection help to mitigate these problems.

Many of the qualities just discussed are hard to quantify on job applications or intake interviews. They are, however, the things to look for in deciding who will *probably* make a good interviewer. The task of ensuring that interviewers are qualified does not end with the hiring process. Interviewers must undergo a training period during which they are taught the general norms and guidelines of the particular firm or researcher in charge of the project, as well as the specific requirements of the survey in which they will be involved. In addition, their performance should be carefully evaluated *before* they conduct their first interview with an actual respondent, and the quality of their work should be monitored on a continuing or sample basis throughout the entire field period for the study.

Training Interviewers

Interviewer training usually involves both a general introduction to survey interviewing and fieldwork techniques and procedures and a review of the specific aspects of the study that the interviewer will be carrying out. General and study-specific interviewer manuals are important resources for the respective types of training (Fowler, 1993; Fowler & Mangione, 1990). The following excerpt from Weinberg's chapter in the *Handbook of Survey Research* (1983, pp. 344–345) indicates that a typical study-specific interviewer training agenda address the following topics:

"1. Presentation of the nature, purpose, and sponsorship of the survey
 2. Discussion of the total survey process
 3. Role of the professional survey interviewer (including a discussion of the ethics of interviewing—confidentiality, anonymity, and bias issues)
 4. Role of the respondent (helping respondent learn how to be a respondent)
 5. Profile of the questionnaire used (identification of types of questions and instructions, answer codes, precolumning numbers for data processing, and so on)
 6. Importance and advantages of following instructions (examples of disadvantages to interviewer when instructions are not followed)
 7. How to read questions (including correct pacing, reading exactly as printed and in order, conversational tone)
 8. How to record answers (for each type of question)
 9. How and when to probe (definition and uses of probes for each type of question)
 10. Working in the field or on the phone (preparing materials, scheduling work, introduction at the door or on the phone, answering respondent's questions, setting the stage for the interview)
 11. Sampling (overview of types of samples, detailed discussion of interviewer's responsibilities for implementation of last stage of sampling on specific survey)
 12. Editing (reviewing completed questionnaires for legibility, missed questions, and so on)
 13. Reporting to the supervisor (frequency and types of reports required)"

The training sessions in both the Chicago AIDS survey and the NCHS–NHIS Health Promotion and Disease Prevention surveys incorporated many of these elements. The NCHS–NHIS is conducted by U.S. census interviewers, most of whom are part of a regular corps of interviewers who participate in the annual NCHS–NHIS.

Resources and techniques for interviewer training include (1) written resource materials, (2) lectures and demonstrations, (3) home study, (4) written exercises,

(5) role playing, (6) practice interviews, and (7) coding of interviewer behavior. As mentioned previously, a study's interviewer manual contains the main written resource materials for a study. Interviewers are encouraged to read and study these materials at home before the training session and to refer to them during training and in the field, as needed. Lectures and demonstrations are commonly used in interviewer training sessions. The NCHS provides a verbatim interviewer instruction guide for trainers to read to interviewers. It is also helpful to demonstrate an actual interview so that interviewers can get a sense of how it should be carried out. Group discussions also afford interviewers the opportunity to take an active role in raising questions or clarifying their understanding of aspects of the study. Written exercises on the more complex features of the questionnaire (such as the process of sampling within-household respondents) also help reinforce an interviewer's ability to handle those issues.

Round-robin interviewing and role playing are very useful devices in training interviewers. An interviewer might administer the questionnaire to a supervisor or another interviewer who reads his or her answers from a script in which different aspects of an interviewing situation are presented. It may be desirable to have more than one script so that the interviewers can role play a variety of different situations. This activity enables the supervisor to observe each interviewer's style of interviewing and provide feedback as appropriate.

The culminating—and perhaps most important—component of the interviewer training process is the opportunity to conduct a practice interview with an actual respondent. Interviewers may be asked to interview a friend or family member, for example, to get a feel for how an interview should go. The interviewer should then administer the interview to one or two other respondents who are recruited on either a paid or voluntary basis. The supervisor can review the interviewers' performance during these trial runs. If satisfactory, the interviewers can then be assigned to the field. If their performance is not acceptable, however, the interviewers can be retrained on those aspects of the study with which they seem to be having problems and asked to do one or two more practice interviews. If their performance is still not satisfactory, this could be grounds for dismissal from the project. Potential interviewers should, of course, be advised at the time they are recruited for the study that dismissal could be an outcome of training.

As mentioned in Chapter Eight, it may also be useful to observe and code systematically the behavior of interviewers to identify those who are having particular problems for the purposes of screening for hiring, devoting special attention to what are identified to be weak spots during training, or retraining or strengthening interviewer performance as the study proceeds (Edwards, et al., 1994).

The length of the formal training period varies from study to study. The number of days of training should be based principally on (1) the complexity of the questionnaire and associated field procedures and (2) the level of interviewer experience with comparable studies. In most academic, professional survey organizations, training is generally two days at a minimum. In complex national surveys, a week or more of initial and supplementary training may be necessary. Billiet and Loosveldt (1988) documented that the effects of five half-days of interviewer training were particularly significant for factual questions that required a great deal of activity on the part of the interviewer, such as giving instructions, probing, or providing feedback to the respondent. Other research has indicated that interviewers who received less than one day of basic interviewer training were much more likely to display inadequate interviewing skills than those who received two or more days of training (Fowler, 1993; Fowler & Mangione, 1990).

Standardized survey interviewing practices have been emphasized as the norm of the survey research trade for over forty years (Cannell, Miller, & Oksenberg, 1982; Fowler & Mangione, 1990; Hyman, 1955; Kahn & Cannell, 1957; National Center for Health Services Research, 1978). In standardized interviewing, interviewers use identical methods to the maximum extent possible in carrying out field procedures, asking questions, probing, and recording responses.

For example, researchers at the University of Michigan have conducted extensive research that suggests that incorporating certain procedures into the interviewing process leads to higher rates of reporting of health events. In using this approach, interviewers first read verbatim instructions to the respondents at the beginning of the interview to clarify the purpose of the study and how respondents should go about providing complete and accurate information. Respondents were also asked to sign an agreement that committed them to do their best to give accurate answers to the questions. Finally, interviewers were given a set of objective criteria for evaluating the quality of respondents' answers and explicit statements to read to provide positive reinforcement and feedback for responses that were judged to be "good" ones. The researchers concluded that these techniques increased the *quantity* of events respondents reported compared with interviews in which these techniques were not used. Explicit criterion sources were not, however, used to directly evaluate the *accuracy* of these results. The findings of the study are therefore not conclusive in documenting that more reporting as a result of using these techniques necessarily means better reporting (Cannell, Miller, & Oksenberg, 1982; Fowler & Mangione, 1990; National Center for Health Services Research, 1978).

However, there has been criticism of the artificiality of the standardized interviewing process and the impact that it might have on the accuracy and completeness of answers that respondents provide (Mishler, 1986; Smith, 1987; Suchman & Jordan, 1990). Mishler (1986), for example, is particularly critical of the practice of conducting standardized interviews, which he sees as a "stimulus-response" approach to data gathering. He argues that interviews should be conducted and analyzed as narrative accounts (or stories) that respondents are asked to tell in their own natural language. Otherwise, the real meaning of the questions and answers to respondents is lost to the investigator. Narrative analysis procedures originally developed in the field of sociolinguistics can then be used to analyze the resulting data. These procedures involve looking at the narrative accounts provided by respondents in response to a question as stories for which semantics, syntax, and pragmatics can be examined as a way of understanding what respondents meant, how they said it, and how the social context of the interview itself affected the stories.

The application of the principles of cognitive psychology in the early stages of developing a more standardized instrument is a constructive and useful approach to addressing these concerns. "Focused" or "conversational" interviewing, in which interviewers are given the opportunity to rephrase the questions to make sense to respondents, if needed, is also an alternative for gathering relatively straightforward factual data (Merton, Fiske, & Kendall, 1990). Interviewers must, however, be trained to distinguish "deviation" (a query that is equivalent in meaning to the original question) from "error":

Original: What is the *highest* grade or year of school you have completed?
Deviation: How many years of school have you *finished?*
Error: How many years were you in school?

In either case, investigators should be clear about the approach they want to use in carrying out the interviews in their study and make sure that the interviewing staff is trained accordingly.

Supervising Field Work

Another important aspect of carrying out a survey is to have well-trained interviewer supervisors. Supervisors are generally involved in training the interviewing staff. They are also in charge of notifying local newspapers and relevant community leaders or agencies about the study, overseeing the scheduling and assignment of interviews to interviewers, implementing the quality control procedures, and writing the time, effort, and expense reports for the interviewing staff. There is generally a ratio of one supervisor to every ten interviewers in field interviews although fewer supervisors are needed in centralized telephone interviewing facilities (Weinberg, 1983). In most firms, interviewer supervisors are former interviewers who came up through the ranks and have a great deal of experience in carrying out and overseeing different types of surveys.

There are four important quality control tasks that supervisors are generally in charge of monitoring: (1) field editing, (2) interview validation, (3) interviewer observation, and (4) retrieving missing data (Weinberg, 1983).

Field Editing Questionnaires

In performing this task, supervisors examine the questionnaire before it is sent to data processing to make sure that the interviewer has not made any major mistakes in carrying out the interview. Interviewers are also encouraged to examine the questionnaire before turning it in so that they can get back to the respondent right away if needed. Supervisors sometimes edit a sample of interviewers' work as it is returned or coordinate the transmission of the questionnaires to a staff of editors and then provide feedback, as necessary, to the interviewers on their performance. Supervisors' field editing role is largely eliminated with computer-assisted personal and telephone interview systems.

Validating Completed Interviews

A quality control procedure that may be particularly important in personal interview surveys is the validation of completed interviews. Validation requires the supervisor or a senior interviewer to call back a sample of the cases assigned to an interviewer and then to directly ask the individuals if they participated in the original interview or to readminister sections of the questionnaire to them. If significant inconsistencies are discovered during this process, other interviews completed by that interviewer could then be checked. Verification that interviewers have falsified cases should result in their immediate dismissal. All their cases should then be validated and, if necessary, assigned to another interviewer. Telling interviewers that their interviews will be validated in this way will probably eliminate any tendency toward curbstoning—that is, an interviewer's figuratively sitting on a curb to fill out the questionnaire. A particular advantage of telephone interviews is, of course, that there can be constant monitoring throughout the field period of the placement and outcomes of calls made by interviewers, virtually eliminating curbstoning in telephone-based studies.

Observing Interviewers

Interviewers can also be observed during the field period. For example, a supervisor can accompany an interviewer to the field to conduct a personal interview or can ask the interviewer to tape-record the interview. In telephone interviews, the supervisor can actually listen in as the interview is being conducted. Observing interviewers in at least one of these ways may be a useful retraining device for interviewers who are encountering problems in the field. It also communicates to the interviewing staff the importance of maintaining consistently high standards throughout the field period.

Following Up to Obtain Missing Data

A fourth major quality control procedure is a protocol for deciding when respondents should be contacted and for what kind or magnitude of information missing when the questionnaire is returned from the field. In general, a list of critical questions should be compiled and incorporated into the field and interviewer training materials. Interviewers should be encouraged to make sure that those questions have been answered before leaving the respondent's home. If they have not been answered, however, a procedure should be developed for deciding who should follow up to get this information, how, and within what period of time. Computer-assisted personal and telephone surveys offer a greater opportunity to build these types of checks into the design and conduct of the interview itself and to deal with any problems that arise while the interviewer is still on the phone or with the respondent.

Managing the Survey

Overall management of a project includes responsibility for formulating the tasks, schedule, and budget, as well as monitoring expenditures over the course of the study.

Schedule

If researchers are carrying out the survey themselves, the principal investigator will have overall responsibility for both the conceptual design of the study and administrative oversight of the project itself. If it is a large-scale study, specific operational tasks may have to be delegated to a study director, assistant study director, field manager, or other project staff. If the project's principal investigator (PI) contracts with a survey firm, he or she will not have direct responsibility for the actual execution of the study. The PI or the PI's delegate, however, should have the opportunity to provide input and monitor quality at each stage of the survey's development and receive regular progress and financial reports on the project.

The major activities and timeframe for the Chicago AIDS survey—a paper-and-pencil telephone survey—are summarized in Table 13.1 (Survey Research Laboratory, 1986). The schedule provided for a substantial commitment of time and effort at the beginning of the study to develop, review, and revise the survey questionnaire. Given the sensitive nature of the subject matter addressed, there was a particular concern with adequately pretesting the questionnaire and providing ample opportunity for the study's advisory group and the Survey Research

TABLE 13.1. SCHEDULE FOR CHICAGO AIDS SURVEY.

Activity	Number of Weeks	Dates
Draft questionnaire	4	7/1–7/29
Get approval from Advisory Panel and SRL QRC	2	7/30–8/13
Revise questionnaire	1	8/14–8/21
Pretest	2	8/22–9/5
Revise questionnaire	1	9/8–9/15
Get approval from Advisory Panel and SRL QRC	1	9/16–9/23
Revise questionnaire	1½	9/24–10/6
Duplicate questionnaire	1	10/7–10/14
Conduct interviews	6	10/15–11/30
Code/enter data—total of 8½ weeks	2½ after interviews	10/15–12/12
Produce data tape/diskettes	1	12/15–12/22

Source: Survey Research Laboratory, University of Illinois, 1986.

Laboratory's Questionnaire Review Committee (SRL QRC) of survey design experts to review and comment on any subsequent revisions. Around 7,000 households were contacted and screened over the six-week data collection period to yield 1,540 completed interviews. Data coding and entry commenced when the field period began and continued for two and one-half weeks beyond this period.

The schedule was adequate for completing the respective types of activity but did not provide flexibility for accommodating unexpected delays. The contractor was interested in completing the data collection before the public health department launched a series of AIDS education initiatives. However, SRL submitted a supplementary proposal for a pilot study involving 150 interviews, to be conducted in parallel with the pretest, to evaluate the feasibility of asking particularly sensitive questions. This was approved and resulted in the actual start date for the conduct of the interviews being extended by three weeks. If the survey had been executed using CAPI, more time would have been required at the beginning of the study to program the questionnaire and associated sampling and data collection procedures but less time would have been needed at the end to produce a clean data tape.

Budget

Perhaps the most important aspect shaping the scale and scope of a survey is the amount of money available to do it. Researchers should clearly specify each of the major tasks associated with carrying out the study (sampling, data collection, data entry, and analysis); the personnel, services, equipment, supplies, and other items required for each of these tasks; the unit costs of the required resources or services;

and any general institutional overhead costs associated with the survey. If the researcher contracts with a survey research firm, the potential contractor should provide a detailed budget for each of the tasks that the firm will be responsible for carrying out. Accounting systems using spreadsheet software should be set up to monitor carefully the expenditure of project funds, relative to the original budget, throughout the course of the study.

The Survey Research Laboratory budget for the Chicago AIDS survey is summarized in Table 13.2 (Survey Research Laboratory, 1986). A two-stage sampling scheme (described in Chapter Six) was employed to screen over 7,000 telephone numbers in the Chicago metropolitan areas to yield approximately 1,500 completed interviews with 800 whites, 500 African Americans, and 200 Hispanics. The interview was estimated to be thirty minutes long. Bilingual interviewers were hired to assist with the Spanish-language interviews. All interviewers attended a study-specific training session, and new interviewers were required to attend one

TABLE 13.2. BUDGET FOR CHICAGO AIDS SURVEY.

Category			Amounts
Salaries			
Principal investigator	$ 9,360		
SRL staff	8,453		
Research assistants (RAs)	14,244		
Salaries subtotal		$32,057	
Wages (interviewers, students)		20,207	
Fringe Benefits			
13.235% of salaries, excluding RAs	2,358		
0.26% of wages, including RAs	90		
Benefits subtotal		2,448	
Expenses (supplies, telephone, etc.)		11,079	
Modified Total Direct Costs		$65,791	
Indirect Costs			
10% of MTDC	6,579		
22% of RA salaries less benefits	3,134		
Indirect costs subtotal			9,713
Computer center charges			283
(for sampling, data processing)			
Total			$75,787

Source: Survey Research Laboratory, University of Illinois, 1986.

day of general interviewer training in addition. Up to ten contacts at different times of the day and week were budgeted. Data processing estimates assumed the questionnaire was thirty pages long, contained 250 closed-end items, two open-ended items (including occupation), and five "other-specify" variables. Trained coders and SRL proprietary software were employed in coding and processing the data. A coding supervisor checked a minimum of 10 percent of the coded interviews, and the valid ranges of codes for each question, skip patterns, and logical edits were checked using the SRL software.

The original study budget provided for a pretest yielding thirty completed interviews, some with members of each subgroup (whites, African Americans, and Hispanics), including Spanish-speaking respondents. The proposed pilot study added approximately $10,000 to the costs of the study, including indirect costs.

The average cost per completed interview for the Chicago AIDS paper-and-pencil telephone survey, including the pilot study, was then approximately $55 (in 1986 dollars).

As has been emphasized throughout this book, survey designers need to think through clearly what they want to do *before* they knock on doors or call to conduct an interview. They also need to realistically consider what they can afford to do—*before* they start. Running out of money before the study is finished means that something does not get done—either well *or* at all.

Sample budgets for personal, telephone, and mail surveys are shown in Chapter Four of Salant and Dillman (1994).

Computer-Assisted Data Collection Systems

A variety of computer-assisted data collection systems are available that are also designed to handle the array of data collection and monitoring tasks reviewed here. Programs used by large-scale governmental and private survey research organizations include commercially available packages, such as Autoquest (Microtab Systems Pty Ltd., Australia), Blaise (Central Bureau of Statistics, The Netherlands), CASES (Computer Assisted Survey Methods, Berkeley, Calif.), and Ci3 (Sawtooth Software, Sequim, Wash.), among others, as well as proprietary software tailored to meet the needs of a specific organization, such as Cheshire (Westat, Inc., Rockville, Md.). Many of these systems, which were initially developed for computer-assisted telephone interviewing, are increasingly being adapted and applied to computer-assisted personal and self-interview modes of data gathering. Computer-assisted data collection (CADAC) methods are essentially becoming the fundamental tools of the trade for governmental, academic, and commercial data collection organizations.

Substantial investments are required to purchase, maintain, and update these systems. Survey researchers must carefully evaluate whether and what type of such a system would best meet their needs in the most cost-effective manner (Saris, 1991; Survey Research Center, 1990). For many, paper-and-pencil methods, especially mail surveys, may still be the preferred and affordable approach. Regardless of whether CADAC systems or paper-and-pencil questionnaires are used to gather the data, successful survey implementation compels the systematic planning and monitoring of the data collection and monitoring procedures reviewed here.

Special Considerations for Special Populations

Considerations of the demographics of data collection personnel often come into play when hiring interviewers or deciding which types of interviewers should be dispatched to interview in certain areas or with certain types of respondents. A broader look at the diversity and fit of personnel and procedures at all levels of designing and implementing the data collection process is, however, required, particularly in developing surveys of groups that do not mirror the modal demographic categories (racial and ethnic minorities or gay men with HIV/AIDS, for example). Input from individuals like those who are to be the focus of the study (as senior study personnel, members of community or technical advisory panels, participants in the pretest and accompanying questionnaire and procedures development process, as well as field staff and interviewers) is likely to yield the most fitting and informed approach to gathering data on those populations (McGraw, McKinlay, Crawford, Costa, & Cohen, 1992; Rhodes, 1994).

Selected Examples

Detailed general and study-specific training and field procedures manuals have been developed by the University of Illinois Survey Research Laboratory (1987b, 1994a, 1994b) and the National Center for Health Statistics (U.S. Bureau of the Census, 1994a, 1994b, 1994c), for the Chicago AIDS survey and the National Health Interview Survey, respectively. The interviewer manual for the AIDS survey is provided in Resource B.

The cover letters and postcard reminder used in the dentists survey are included in Resource C. In this particular survey, the University of Washington Institutional Review Board required a more detailed statement than Dillman traditionally recommends of the benefits and costs to respondents of participating. The survey designers dealt with this requirement by including a general information sheet on the study, instead of overloading the cover letter with this information. This is an option for investigators confronting comparable institutional demands.

Guidelines for Minimizing Survey Errors

To wind one's way through the data collection process successfully compels envisioning the forest as well as spotting the trees. The array of components in implementing a survey can be viewed as steps along a well-marked path. Fortunately, prominent and productive general and health survey research methodologists have provided useful guideposts for signaling the proper course. These include Don Dillman (Washington State University); Seymour Sudman (University of Illinois) and Norman Bradburn (University of Chicago); Charles Cannell (University of Michigan) and Robert Groves (University of Michigan and University of Maryland); and their respective and numerous colleagues. The schools of thought represented in the corpus of the work of these major investigators and their associates provide particularly useful guidance in thinking systemically and theoretically about the interrelatedness of the steps in carrying out a survey, and how best to maximize the quality of the data resulting.

Don Dillman's Total Design Method is rooted in exchange theory and a consideration of the rewards and costs presented to respondents in answering a survey questionnaire (Dillman, 1978). His more recent recommendations incorporate a consideration of the influence of survey design and administration on a variety of types of errors (coverage, sampling, and measurement error), in addition to nonresponse error, which was the central focus of his pioneering contributions in mail survey design (Salant & Dillman, 1994).

Sudman and Bradburn, as mentioned in Chapter Eight, introduced the notion of response effects in surveys—departures from accuracy that may be influenced by characteristics of the instrument, the interviewer, the respondent, or their interaction (Sudman & Bradburn, 1974). This concept has been elaborated and extended and its empirical origins more fully examined in the substantial body of methodological research conducted by these researchers and their colleagues (Bradburn, Sudman, & Associates, 1979; Sudman & Bradburn, 1982). Most recently, they have undertaken a fruitful extension of their previous inquiries in exploring the contributions of cognitive psychology to understanding the effects of question and questionnaire design on survey responses (Schwarz & Sudman, 1995; Sudman, Bradburn, & Schwarz, 1995).

University of Michigan investigators Charles Cannell and Robert Groves and their associates have argued convincingly for the formulation of a fuller theoretical understanding of the interplay of the array of factors that influence respondents' participation in the survey process and the role that interviewers play in encouraging participation (Cannell, Miller, & Oksenberg, 1982; Couper & Groves, 1992b; Groves, Cialdini, & Couper, 1992; Groves, et al., 1988). Groves' formulation of the components and costs of survey errors in the context of a total survey error perspective provides a particularly helpful anchor and benchmark against which the complex decisions involved in designing and implementing surveys can be evaluated (Biemer, Groves, Lyberg, Mathiowetz, & Sudman, 1991; Groves, 1989).

Supplementary Sources

For additional detail on designing personal or telephone surveys, see Frey and Oishi (1995), Lavrakas (1993), and Stouthamer-Loeber and van Kammen (1995). For mail and self-administered surveys, see Bourque and Fielder (1995) and Mangione (1995). Dillman (1978) and Salant and Dillman (1994) are useful references for designing the data collection procedures for both interviewer- and self-administered surveys.

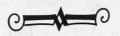

CHAPTER FOURTEEN

PREPARING THE DATA FOR ANALYSIS

Chapter Highlights

1. Coding survey data involves translating answers into numerical codes that can then be used in computer-based data analyses.
2. Data may be entered into a computerized medium (such as magnetic tapes or disks) through either transcriptive or direct data entry procedures.
3. Both range and consistency checks should be conducted to detect and clean (or correct) errors in the data once the data have been computerized.
4. Before analyzing the data, researchers must decide how to deal with questions for which responses are missing because the respondent neglects to provide the information or the interviewer fails to ask the question properly.
5. External data sources can also be used to estimate information for analytical variables of interest in the survey.
6. Analysts should anticipate other data transformations that may be required before implementing the analysis plan.

The rapid development and growth of computer technologies have had a significant impact on the design, implementation, and analysis of surveys. In particular, the evolution of microcomputers has made possible the development of computer-based systems for collecting, processing, and analyzing survey data

(Bourque & Clark, 1992; Madron, Tate, & Brookshire, 1985; Saris, 1991; Schrodt, 1987). Computer-assisted personal, telephone, and self-administered data gathering methods were described in Chapter Five. Many surveys still use paper-and-pencil data collection methodologies but almost all survey designers now rely on computers in preparing and executing their analyses. Computers, however, have their own technical languages for translating and interpreting information. Survey designers therefore need to know how to process (or transform) the information collected from survey respondents into the symbols, language, and logic of computers if they are to make effective use of this powerful and important technology.

This chapter presents approaches for (1) coding or translating survey responses into numerical data, (2) entering these data into a computer, (3) cleaning or editing the data to correct errors, (4) imputing the answers that either respondents or interviewers fail to provide, (5) using information from other sources to estimate values for certain analytical variables of interest, and (6) anticipating transformations of the data that may be required before executing the analysis plan.

Coding the Data

Coding the data involves translating the information that survey respondents provide into numerical or other symbols that can be processed by a computer. Different approaches are generally involved in coding closed-end and open-ended survey questions. With closed-end questions, for example, response categories are provided to respondents or interviewers to use in filling out the questionnaire. It is advisable that numerical codes be assigned to each of these categories, with instructions to circle or check the number that corresponds to the respondent's answer to that question (CIRCLE THE NUMBER THAT CORRESPONDS TO YOUR ANSWER):

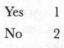

Yes   1
No   2

Failure to associate a code with an answer on the questionnaire (for example, simply placing a line or box to check by each response on a paper-and-pencil questionnaire) will make errors more likely when this response is translated into numbers that can be entered into a computerized data file. With computerized data collection systems, the codes assigned to particular response categories are programmed so that a response is automatically coded when it is entered (punched in on a keyboard by the interviewer or respondent). While nonnumeric characters (such as letters of the alphabet) can also be used as codes or symbols for respondents' answers, it is generally advisable not to do so because they may cause problems when used in certain analysis software packages.

As discussed in Chapter Eight, open-ended questions ask respondents to use their own words in answering. These questions thus yield verbatim or narrative information that has to be translated into numerical codes. Open-ended questions are sometimes asked in pilot studies to elicit responses that can be used to develop categories for coding the data from these questions or to derive closed-end answer formats for the questions in the final study.

To develop codes for open-ended questions, researchers draw a sample of cases in which the question was asked. The actual number of cases to review will vary (say, from twenty-five to one hundred), depending on the sample size for the study as a whole and the variability anticipated in responses to the questions across respondents. The answers to the questions should be reviewed in light of the concepts or framework to be operationalized in the survey. It may be important to code the answers using a number of dimensions to capture complex study concepts. In an evaluation of home care programs for ventilator-assisted children, a conceptual framework based on program goals was used to classify responses to a question asked of key program and advisory board personnel about the criteria they thought should be used in evaluating the success of the programs (Aday, Aitken, & Wegener, 1988).

Survey designers should consider whether answers reflect broad groupings as well as whether specific responses seem to cluster within general dimensions or even form separate subdimensions within them. For example, in the study of ventilator-assisted children, the answers to an open-ended question asked of families about what they perceived their greatest problems or concerns to be in caring for their children at home tended to cluster in three broad areas: issues related to the child's long-term development and survival; problems associated with the stress on the family and other caregivers; and technical issues such as setting up or maintaining needed equipment, making necessary home repairs, or obtaining required financing. These broad groupings were then used as the basis for organizing and classifying respondents' specific answers. Responses that fit within each of these categories were identified and numerical codes were assigned to each. The distribution of responses in the three broad groupings, as well as the specific responses within each, were tabulated in reporting the answers to this question.

Survey designers should thus be involved in developing codes for open-ended questions because they presumably can specify the most useful form and content of the data for subsequent analyses. Once an initial coding scheme has been developed and a sample of answers has been coded by means of this scheme, another coder should be asked to classify the same responses using the same codes independently. Discrepancies between the two coders should be discussed and the coding scheme then revised as necessary or appropriate training or validation procedures developed to ensure a standardized approach to the treatment of respondents' answers across coders.

Special coding staffs are often trained to deal with open-ended questions or questions about people's occupations or about their symptoms or medical conditions. For example, in the National Center for Health Statistics–National Health Interview Survey (NCHS-NHIS), a detailed series of questions are asked about the jobs people hold and their occupations are then coded according to a scheme developed by the Census Bureau. Medical conditions reported in the NCHS–NHIS are coded by means of a modified version of the World Health Organization's International Classification of Diseases coding scheme.

Closed-end questions that ask respondents or interviewers to write in or specify "other" responses not explicitly reflected in the response categories represent a special case of open-ended coding. Coders may be asked to record these responses in a separate file (in which the questionnaire ID number and response are recorded) or, in computerized data collection systems, space may be provided to input such responses, which are then stored in separate files for subsequent coding or processing. These responses can be periodically reviewed to see if some answers appear with sufficient frequency to warrant developing unique codes to distinguish them from the "other" responses.

Interviewers may also be asked to do field coding of survey responses. With field-coded questions respondents are not provided a list of categories from which to choose but are asked the question and the interviewer codes their answers, according to precoded categories available only to the interviewer. This is an alternative to entirely open-ended coding (which is often costly and time-consuming to do). It can, however, introduce response errors if the interviewers are not accurate or consistent in using the codes provided. With computer-assisted (especially telephone) interview methods, respondents' verbatim answers can be recorded and interviewers' coding independently validated by the interviewing or coding supervisor.

Like survey interviewers, survey coders should be well trained and their work checked periodically. They should also be provided with clear instructions (documentation) for coding each question in the survey and dealing with problems that arise during coding.

The key source document for coding survey data is the survey codebook. The codebook provides detailed instructions for translating the answers to each question into codes that will be read by the computer, and it notes any special instructions for handling the coding of particular questions. These codebooks should be developed for paper-and-pencil surveys. They are generated by commercial and proprietary software used to set up computer-assisted data collection (CADAC) or data entry (CADE) procedures.

The column or columns required to reflect the answers to a question are referred to as the *data field* or the *field size* for that question in the data file. The codebook for the survey usually contains general instructions for approaching the coding process as well as the following specific information for each data field: the questions from which the data were gathered, the codes or numbers to be used in coding answers to these questions, and any special instructions required for coding the item.

The names and descriptive labels for variables constructed from a question can also be incorporated into the codebook to facilitate the preparation of documentation for these variables in designing programs to analyze the data (VARIABLE NAMES and VARIABLE LABELS statements in SPSS, for example). Directly incorporating the original question number into the names or labels developed for variables based on these items of course makes it easier to relate the variables used in the analyses to the source questions on which they are based.

The codes are the numbers that have been assigned to or developed for each of the response categories for closed-end or open-ended questions, respectively. Once again, attention can be given to developing mnemonics for the labels that can be used in documenting what each of the codes means later when the analysis program is designed (VALUE LABELS statements in SPSS).

Finally, special instructions or information may be needed in coding a particular item, such as which questions should be skipped if certain answers are given to that question, whether answers to this question should agree with other answers in the questionnaire, or whether this is a critical question about which respondents should be recontacted if they provide incomplete or unclear information.

In general, the first few columns of a record should contain study and respondent ID information. It is desirable to zero-fill multiple-column fields—for example, coding three days of the disability during the year as "003" in a three-column field for that question—because it is easier to keep track of columns in which data are being entered and some software packages handle blanks differently from zeros in processing the data. Verbatim responses to open-ended questions or "other" responses besides those listed for closed-end items can be coded by means of categories developed for this purpose or listed verbatim for the researcher to refer to later. Uniform conventions for coding different types of missing data should also be developed and documented in the codebook:

Type of Missing Data	Length of Field (Column)		
	1	2	3
Respondent refused to answer	7	97	997
Respondent did not know answer	8	98	998
Question skipped (error)	9	99	999

The codebook should be used as the source document for training coders. Coding supervisors should routinely check samples of the coders' work throughout the study and assist them in resolving any problems that arise in coding particular cases.

Entering the Data

Survey data must be entered onto a medium that can be read by a computer. These media include magnetic tape and disk storage space in the body (hard drive) of the computer (or portable diskettes or compact disks in the case of microcomputers). Cards were one of the earliest media used for entering information in a form that could be read by computers. Such cards traditionally had eighty columns. Within each column various digits (0 through 9) could be physically punched with a keypunch machine to represent the code for the field (or part of the field) of information for a given question on the survey questionnaire. However, computer cards have been replaced by such media as magnetic tapes and disk storage space on mainframes, minicomputers, and microcomputers.

There are two main types of data entry—*transcriptive* and *source data*. *Transcriptive data entry* involves coding the data onto a source document, which is then used as the basis for entering the information into a machine- or computer-readable medium. The main types of transcriptive data entry utilize transfer sheets, edge-coding, and punching directly from a precolumned questionnaire. In *source data entry* the data are coded and entered directly into a machine-readable medium. Source data entry methods include optical mark readers, computer-assisted interviewing, and computer-assisted data entry (CADE) (Karweit & Meyers, 1983). Source data entry techniques are newer methods that evolved in response to the increasing computerization of surveys.

Transcriptive Data Entry

Transfer sheets are sheets that are generally ruled off into a series of columns that reflect the format for the data file. Working from the survey questionnaire and codebook, coders assign codes for each question and these codes are then entered in the appropriate columns of the transfer sheets. The transfer sheets are in turn used as the basis for entering data onto a computerized medium, such as a database software.

Edge-coding involves reserving space along the margin of each page of a questionnaire—space in which the codes for the answers to each question can be recorded. This space is generally headed with the statement, "Do not write in this space—for office use only." The column numbers for each question are indicated beside or underneath boxes or lines. The codes corresponding to the answers to each question are then recorded in the boxes or on the lines.

Entering data from a precolumned questionnaire is similar to edge-coding in that the questionnaire itself serves as the basic source document for coding and entering the data. With precolumned questionnaires, however, the location for the answer to a particular question is clearly indicated, generally along the right margin and as close as possible to the response categories for the question on the questionnaire itself. The numbers in boxes along the right margin of the NCHS–NHIS questionnaire (Resource A) correspond to the fields of a data file in which the answers to the questions are entered directly from the questionnaire. For closed-end items, then, the code for the response category that has been circled or checked on the questionnaire is the code that should be entered in the computer for that question. For open-ended questions, coders can write in the codes that have been developed and documented in the codebook, codes that represent the answers to that question, beside the corresponding column number for the question on the questionnaire. Although it is not required, some survey research firms continue to precolumn the questionnaire when entering the data by means of computer-assisted data entry systems (described in the following section).

All three of these transcriptive data entry approaches assume that a codebook has been designed to identify the fields into which the data for a particular question should be recorded. The questionnaires should always be carefully edited before being sent to coding, and the codebook should be used as the basis for identifying the appropriate codes to assign to the answers that respondents have provided. The three transcriptive data entry methods differ principally in the extent to which coders have to transfer information reported in the questionnaire to another location or source for entering. Transfer sheets require transfer of the greatest amount of information and precolumned questionnaires the smallest amount. The more complex the information to be transferred, the more possibilities for errors to occur. Precolumned questionnaires should be carefully designed so that it is clear what information is to be entered in what fields and what conventions are to be used to provide additional instructions to the data entry personnel for entering this information (such as using red pencils to strike through the columns to be left blank because a question was legitimately skipped or editing responses to a question when the respondent mistakenly circles more than one response code).

Electronic spreadsheet packages such as LOTUS or EXCEL or database management systems such as DBASE or ACCESS can be used to enter the data onto a computerized file. These software packages are readily available to most microcomputer users and are relatively easy to use. They do not, however, have procedures for data checking and cleaning built in as standardized features, as do the proprietary data entry packages.

Transcriptive data entry methods, especially transfer sheets, have been supplanted by computer-assisted source data entry approaches.

Source Data Entry

Source data entry methods largely eliminate the intermediate step of coding or transferring information to another source or location before entering it onto a computerized medium (Bourque & Clark, 1992).

One type of source data entry makes use of optical mark readers that read a pattern of responses to boxes or circles that have been penciled in to reflect the respondent's answer to the question. This approach has been used widely in administering standardized tests to students in classroom settings. The type and complexity of questions that can be asked using this approach are limited. This approach also depends heavily on the willingness of respondents or interviewers to record carefully the answers in the spaces provided and on the availability of the equipment required for reading the "mark sense" answer format used in this approach.

Two other direct data entry methods offer much more promise for computerizing survey data and have gained greater prominence with the increasing computerization of the entire survey data collection and analysis process. These are computer-assisted data collection (CATI, CAPI, and CASI) and computer-assisted data entry (CADE) approaches. The computerized telephone, personal, and self-administered data collection methods, along with the relative advantages and disadvantages of each in coding and computerizing survey data, were described in Chapter Five.

Computerized data entry is simply a variation on these data gathering approaches (Pierzchala, 1990). In it, paper-and-pencil questionnaires are used to gather the data and programmed approaches are used to enter the data into a computerized medium for analysis. With this approach a question (or prompt) displayed on a computer terminal video screen asks for the code that should be entered for the response to that question in a given case. Using the survey's codebook and the completed questionnaire, the coder determines the appropriate code and types it in at the terminal keyboard. The screen then prompts the coder to supply the next item of information and so on until relevant codes for every item in the questionnaire have been entered. The format of the prompts may either be in terms of a *form* that mirrors the survey questionnaire or a *spreadsheet* that takes on the appearance of the record for a given respondent, with each row being a respondent and the columns fields of data for each respondent. As with computer-assisted data collection methods, checks can be built into the program to signal discrepancies or errors that seem to exist when the data are entered for a given question, and decision rules can be programmed in or applied to deal with these problems. Further, computer-assisted data entry packages require that the appropriate questions and instructions be programmed and tested *before* the data are entered.

Most large-scale survey firms have designed their own proprietary data entry packages or purchased computer-assisted data entry (CADE) software for this purpose. SPSS (Chicago), SAS (Cary, N.C.), BMDP (Los Angeles), and EPI-INFO (Stone Mountain, Ga.) have data entry and management components that are fully integrated with their statistical analysis packages. An advantage of many of these packages is that they have statistical analysis procedures within their family of programs that can then be executed on the data by means of the associated data entry software package.

Cleaning the Data

Data cleaning refers to the process for detecting and correcting errors during the computerization of survey data. There are two major types of computerized error checking: *range checking* and *contingency checking.*

Range Checking

Range checking refers to procedures for verifying that only valid ranges of numbers are used in coding the answers to the questions asked in a survey. For example, if the codebook shows that answers to a question are either yes or no (coded as 1 and 2, respectively), then a code of 3 for this question would be in error. Decision rules have to be developed for dealing with these errors—by consulting the original questionnaire to determine the correct answer, assigning a code based on the responses to other questions, or assigning a missing value code (such as 9) to indicate an indeterminate response to the item, for example. Because of the time and expense involved, individual questionnaires in the NCHS–NHIS are not pulled to resolve any discrepancies that are discovered once the data are computerized. Instead, decision logic tables are prepared to guide data editing and cleaning, and all problems of the same type are resolved in a consistent manner. These decision logic tables then become a part of the permanent data-processing record for the data set.

Contingency Checking

A second major type of data cleaning is termed *contingency checking.* In this type of cleaning, responses are compared *between* related questions. For example, if a question or series of questions should be skipped because of the answer provided to a prior (filter) question (about the person's age, for example), a series of steps can be programmed to check whether or not these questions have been answered. More substantive contingency checks between questions can also be built into cleaning the data. Individuals who said they saw a doctor five times during the year for treatment associated with a particular chronic condition would be expected to report at least this many doctor visits *in total* when asked about all the times they had been to a doctor in the past year. As with the range-check cleaning procedures, decision rules should be developed for resolving any errors that are detected when these contingency checking procedures are used.

The advantage of the computer-assisted data collection and data entry procedures described earlier is that both range and contingency checks can be built in and major problems can be identified and corrected at the time the data are actually being entered. In the past, when transcriptive data entry procedures were used, most data cleaning was carried out after the data were collected and entered, which often meant that a large number of problems had to be resolved long after the study was out of the field. Nevertheless, if the data are particularly complex or more extensive checking is desired, the researcher may still want to develop and execute supplementary data-cleaning procedures after they are entered. To do this, he or she would use the basic computer-assisted data entry checking procedures. However, extensive checking of this kind will greatly increase the cost of the study and delay the final analyses of the data.

Another approach to checking the accuracy of data entry that is particularly appropriate for transcriptive data entry procedures is to verify all or a sample of the data entry for the questionnaires. This means asking another data entry clerk to punch in the information for the questionnaires on the computerized medium a second time. If any discrepancies occur in repunching the data, they should be flagged and any problems resolved. If certain data entry clerks have high error rates when their work is verified in this way, they may have to be retrained or even removed from the study if their performance does not improve.

Imputing Missing Survey Data

Survey respondents often may not know or may refuse to provide answers to certain questions (such as their total income from all sources during the past year) or interviewers may inadvertently skip questions during an interview. When there are a large number of cases with missing information on a particular question, the result can be biased (or inaccurate) estimates for the variables based on that question or the elimination of cases with missing data from analyses that examine the relationships of this variable to other variables in the study.

Techniques have therefore been developed to impute values on those variables for which data are missing, using information from other cases in the survey. These include deductive, cold-deck, hot-deck, statistical imputation, and multiple imputation procedures (Anderson, Basilevsky, & Hum, 1983; Kalton & Kasprzyk,

1986; Little & Rubin, 1989; Madow, Nisselson, & Olkin, 1983; Rubin, 1987). Although these techniques vary in complexity, they all attempt to take typical values for the sample as a whole or subgroups within it or for comparable cases for which data *are not* missing. They then use the values derived from these sources to arrive at estimates for the cases for which the data *are* missing.

Decisions about whether or not to impute missing data should be dictated by the importance of the variable in the analyses, the magnitude of the missing information, the time and costs involved in the imputation process, and the study resources available for this process. In general, priority should be assigned to imputing data for the major variables in the analysis. Major variables for which information is missing on 10 percent or more of the cases could be the principal candidates for imputation. Researchers would then have to determine which types of imputation procedures would be most appropriate, how long the process would take, and how much it would cost. Final decisions about imputation would depend on the availability of trained project staff and funds. Also, if the proportion of missing values for a given item is substantial (25 percent to 50 percent or higher), the investigator should consider excluding the variable from the analysis altogether.

The basic premise of imputation is that fewer biases are introduced by estimating reasonable values for cases for which data are missing than by excluding them from the analyses altogether. To test whether this assumption is correct, researchers can compare two estimates to a criterion source: (1) the estimate for analyses in which cases with missing values are included and (2) the estimate for analyses in which values are imputed (or assigned). This comparison should indicate which estimate is closer to the "real" value. In the absence of such a validating source, researchers can also compare the results for the variables *excluding* cases that had missing values with the results obtained by *including* those cases for which values have been imputed. This comparison could at least provide some indication of whether the substantive results of the study would vary if different approaches to handling these cases were used.

Deductive Imputation

Deductive imputation is similar to editing a questionnaire and filling in those questions for which information is missing (such as the sex of the respondent) by using other information in the questionnaire (his or her name).

Cold-Deck Imputation

Cold-deck imputation procedures use group estimates, such as means, for the sample as a whole or for subgroups within it as the source of information for the values to assign to those cases for which data are missing.

In *overall mean imputation,* for example, the overall mean for the study sample as a whole on the variable of interest is estimated for everyone for whom information is available, and this mean is then assigned to each case for which information is missing.

Class mean imputation is a refinement of the overall mean imputation procedure. With this procedure, the entire sample is divided into a series of classes or groups based on a cross-classification of relevant variables (family size and occupation, for example). The mean on the variable of interest (family income) is then computed for each subgroup resulting from this cross-classification using the data for those for whom the information is available. This value is then assigned to all the people in that group for whom it is *not* available.

Hot-Deck Imputation

Hot-deck procedures use the actual responses provided by particular individuals in a study as a basis for assigning answers to those persons for whom information is missing.

One of the simplest hot-deck procedures is that of *random overall imputation.* With this procedure, a respondent is selected at random from the total sample for the study, and the value for that person (his or her income, for example) is assigned to all those cases for whom this information is missing.

Random imputation within classes is similar to random overall imputation except that the former procedure takes the selected respondent's value from a randomly chosen respondent within certain classes or groups of respondents (by age, sex, and race, for example). This means that the value chosen is taken from someone in the study for whom the variable of interest (such as income) *is not* missing and who matches the characteristics of the person for whom a value is being estimated (an African American female twenty-five to forty years of age, for example).

A *sequential hot-deck imputation* procedure is basically a variation of the random imputation within classes procedure. It begins with a set of groups and then assigns a value to each group by means of one of the cold-deck procedures described earlier. The cases in the file are ordered sequentially so that, as far as possible, cases that are related in some way (clustered in the same U.S. census tract or phone exchange, for example) appear together. The first record within the group for which values are to be imputed (for example, African American females twenty-five to forty years of age) is examined. If it is missing, then the preassigned (cold-deck) value replaces the missing value. If a real value exists for this first case, it replaces the cold-deck value for this imputation class. The next record is examined. If it is missing, the new hot-deck value is used to assign a value to the case; if it is real, the hot-deck value is replaced. The process continues sequentially until all missing values are replaced by real values donated by the case preceding it within the same class or group.

Hierarchical hot-deck imputation procedures attempt to deal with problems that can arise with the sequential hot-deck procedure when, within an imputation class, a record with a missing value is followed by one or more records with missing values. In such instances, there will not be enough donor cases to match with real values within a class or a number of cases might be assigned the *same* value from the *same* donor case. In the hierarchical procedure, respondents and nonrespondents are grouped into a number of subclasses (age by sex by race) based on cross-classifications of broader groupings (age, sex, race). If a match cannot be found in one of the more detailed subclasses (age by sex by race), the subclasses are then collapsed into one of the broad groupings (age only) and a match is attempted at that level.

Statistical Imputation

Two other data imputation procedures that rely on statistically generated values are *regression imputation* and *distance function matching*. With the regression procedure, a regression equation is used to predict values on the variable for which information is missing; in the distance function matching procedure, a nonrespondent is assigned the value of its nearest neighbor, where "nearest" is defined in terms of a statistically derived distance function (Kalton & Kasprzyk, 1986). An advantage of hot-deck methods is that they deal more effectively with estimating categoric (or nominal) data since they borrow real (rather than estimated) values from donor cases.

Multiple Imputation

An important limitation of many of these approaches to imputation is that they may introduce other errors through, for example, reducing the variance as well as increasing the bias of the resulting estimates by providing only one imputed value to replace the missing value, derived from information from the subset of cases for which information *is* available (which may differ from those for whom it is missing). Multiple imputation generates more than one acceptable value for the items that are missing, creates different complete data sets using these different imputed values, and then combines the estimates resulting from these multiple iterations. (See Little and Rubin, 1989 and Rubin, 1987 for a discussion of this approach.)

The hot-deck, regression, and multiple imputation approaches have been used most often in large-scale national health surveys. The hot-deck and regression methods tend to generate similar distributions and results. Research has demonstrated that multiple imputation does address the variance and bias problems associated with these single-imputation methods, but additional development of the software to implement this method is required to permit its widespread adoption (Ezzati-Rice, Fahimi, Judkins, & Khare, 1993; Ezzati-Rice, Khare, Rubin, Little, & Schafer, 1993; Khare, Little, Rubin, & Schafer, 1993; Lepkowski, Landis, & Stehouwer, 1987; Mathiowetz, 1993; Schafer, Khare, & Ezzati-Rice, 1993; Thran & Gillis, 1992; Winglee, Ryaboy, & Judkins, 1993).

It is not necessary to impute values for all the variables that may have missing values but only for those which are of key analytic importance and have a large number of (10 percent or more) missing values.

Experienced programmers can design or adapt programs to implement these various procedures. If the programming expertise or resources needed to implement these procedures successfully are not available, however, researchers may need to rely on the simpler deductive or cold-deck imputation procedures to estimate missing data on key study variables. It is advisable that flags (or special codes) be developed and entered into the data file to identify the imputed variables for each case in the file. Analyses could be replicated, including and excluding the "made up" data, to see what effect imputing versus leaving out cases with missing information has on the substantive interpretation of the findings.

Estimating Survey Data

"Imputation" makes use of data internal to (from) the survey to construct a complete set of information on the analysis variables in the survey. "Estimation" implies the use of data external to the survey to construct analysis variables *not* directly available in the survey.

For example, an investigator may want to estimate the total charges for physician and hospital services that respondents reported receiving. The respondents themselves, however, may have little or no information on the charges for these services, especially if the providers were reimbursed directly by a third-party public or private insurer through which the respondent had coverage. The researcher could ask the respondent for permission to contact the providers directly to obtain this billing information or use data available from the American Medical Association, the American Hospital Association, or other sources on the *average* charges for these services in the community, state, or region in which the study is being conducted. The data obtained from these external sources could then be used to estimate the "total charges" for the services that study respondents reported receiving.

Anticipating the Analysis of the Data

A first step, before analyzing survey data, is to generate basic descriptive statistics to profile the characteristics of the sample as a whole or selected subgroups within it. In addition to providing a profile of the members of the sample, the frequencies alert the researcher to (1) whether there is a large proportion of missing values for a particular variable, which could preclude the analysis of that variable or suggest the need for procedures to impute values for the cases for which values are missing; (2) whether there are too few cases of a certain kind to conduct meaningful analyses for that group or whether it would make sense, in some cases, to combine certain groups for the analyses; and (3) whether there are outliers, that is, cases with extremely large or extremely small values on a variable compared with the rest of the cases. The researcher may want to consider excluding these outliers or assigning them a maximum value for certain analyses.

If there is a concern with possible nonresponse bias in the survey sample, this is the stage at which analyses could be run comparing the composition of the survey sample with the original target population on selected characteristics for which corresponding data on the study universe are available. Response-rate or post-stratification weighting adjustments, as well as any other weights required to adjust for disproportionate sampling, could be computed and added to the data file (see Chapter Seven).

If the intent is to develop summary indexes or scales to operationalize the major study concepts, then reliability and validity testing of these scales may also be undertaken before using them in analyses to address the principal study objectives or hypotheses. It may be particularly useful to conduct internal consistency reliability analysis or factor analysis of multi-item scales to confirm their coherence or to drop items from the final summary scale, if warranted (see Chapter Three).

It may be necessary to transform the data in other ways as well to make sure the data better fit the assumptions required for a particular analytic procedure. A highly skewed distribution of a key study variable may, for example, require a logarithmic or other arithmetic transformation to assure it better matches the (normal) sampling distribution required for certain procedures (such as multiple regression).

There are also conventions for converting nominal or ordinal variables into "dummy" (interval) variables for the purposes of using them in regression procedures that assume an interval or interval-like level of measurement (Polissar & Diehr, 1982). For example, if one wanted to use a four-category race and ethnicity variable as a predictor in a regression equation, four different dichotomous (interval-like) variables would need to be created to reflect whether the respondent was a member of one of the racial categories or not:

original race variable (nominal)

RACE: 1 = White; 2 = African American; 3 = Hispanic; 4 = Other

dummy variables (interval-like)

RACE1:   1 = White; 0 = African American, Hispanic, or Other
RACE2:   1 = African American; 0 = White, Hispanic, or Other
RACE3:   1 = Hispanic; 0 = White, African American, or Other
RACE4:   1 = Other; 0 = White, African American, or Hispanic

One of the dummy variables can then be chosen as the reference category (the group to which the other groups are compared). To effect this using regression analysis, that variable (RACE1, which designates whites, for example) would not be included as a predictor variable but all of the other dummy variables representing different categories of race and ethnicity (RACE2, RACE3, RACE4) would be. The regression coefficients for these variables would then effectively examine the effect of being a member of the respective minority groups (African American, Hispanic, or other), compared with being a member of the white majority, on predicting the outcome of interest (seeing a physician in the year).

The study design and objectives may also require systematically linking data from other sources (medical records or insurance claims, for example). This step should be anticipated early on, required permissions obtained, and adequate information gathered to match data from survey respondents accurately with information from these other sources.

Once the data are coded, computerized, and cleaned and missing data are imputed or estimated, the resulting data set should then be ready for analysis (Chapter Fifteen).

Special Considerations for Special Populations

Special populations may present special challenges during the coding, cleaning, editing, and imputation processes. In surveys of diverse populations, open-ended questions are apt to yield a comparably diverse array of responses that must be accommodated in the coding schemes for these questions. Questions that respondents had trouble interpreting or answering will surface as having high rates of missing values. Differential item (question) nonresponse rates compound the concerns with the effects of imputing (or not imputing) data on the bias (systematic error) in the survey estimates.

If there is a concern with the quality and completeness of the data that are likely to be obtained for certain subgroups, then the pretest and pilot study phases of the study should be expanded to allow adequate testing of the questionnaire, as a basis for revising or deleting those questions that are particularly problematic prior to the final study.

Selected Examples

In the NCHS–NHIS, data were entered from the precolumned survey questionnaire (Resource A). In the Chicago AIDS survey (Resource B), data were entered by means of a proprietary direct data entry software program developed by the Survey Research Laboratory at the University of Illinois (Survey Research Laboratory, 1987a). The dentists' preferences study (Resource C) used RBASE 5000 database management software on an IBM PC-AT microcomputer. (Notice that neither of these latter two questionnaires was precolumned.) Each survey was subjected to standardized cleaning checks and editing.

Guidelines for Minimizing Survey Errors

Systematic errors (or bias), especially item nonresponse, are of principal concern at this stage of survey implementation. Random errors can occur during the coding and data entry process. These errors, however, can be minimized through adequate training and supervision of the data collection and processing staff; development and implementation of quality control monitoring systems; and reverification of data that have been input by reentering them, in the instance of paper-and-pencil questionnaires.

More troublesome are those variables for which information is missing (either the interviewer or respondent did not record an answer or the respondent did not know how or refused to answer). One can choose to exclude cases with missing data from analyses using the affected variables *or* impute values for those cases using the cases for which data are available. Nonetheless, the cases that have complete information may differ from those that do not. To attempt to minimize the possible biases in the estimates generated from the data, the investigator can use several different approaches to imputation and document whether the substantive results emanating from the various methods are confirmed.

Supplementary Sources

For an overview of data processing in general, see Bourque and Clark (1992); for computer-assisted interviews in particular, see Saris (1991).

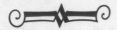

CHAPTER FIFTEEN

PLANNING AND IMPLEMENTING
THE ANALYSIS OF THE DATA

Chapter Highlights

1. A measurement matrix shows how the items asked in a survey questionnaire will be used to create variables to address the study's objectives and hypotheses.

2. Univariate statistics, such as measures of central tendency (mode, median, and mean) and dispersion (percentiles, range, and standard deviation), are used to describe the distribution of a single variable in a study.

3. Bivariate statistics enable the researcher to test hypotheses about the existence or strength of the relationship between *two* variables.

4. Multivariate statistics permit tests of hypotheses about the relationships between *two or more* variables while controlling for other variables.

5. The criteria for selecting the appropriate statistical procedures is based on the variables and the relationships between them implied in the study's research objectives and hypotheses.

6. Constructing mock tables designed to show how the data will be reported forces researchers to specify the types of information they need to collect and what they will do with it *before* they begin the study.

This chapter provides an overview of the process for developing an analysis plan for a study. A well-articulated analysis plan that describes what the researcher plans to do with his or her data is a way of making sure that all the data needed to answer the principal research questions will be gathered and that those items for which there is no clear analytical purpose will not be asked.

Failure to develop an analysis plan is the weakest point in the design of most surveys. Often both experienced and inexperienced survey designers do not have a clear idea of how they will use all the information they gather or they find that they wish they had included other items once they start to analyze it. A clear picture of the variables that will be constructed from the questions asked in the survey and the procedures that will be used in analyzing them provides an invaluable anchor and point of reference for the researcher in deciding what to include in the survey questionnaire. This chapter places particular emphasis on determining which procedures are most appropriate for which types of study designs and variables.

Constructing a Measurement Matrix

In the process of developing and finalizing the survey questionnaire, the analyst should construct a matrix that displays how each item in the survey will be used to address the major study concepts. An example of this measurement matrix for the dentists' preferences survey (which is shown in Resource C) is provided in Table 15.1.

This kind of matrix, at a minimum, lists each question and identifies the major study concept the item is intended to operationalize, the level of measurement it represents, and the objective or hypothesis it most directly addresses. Other information can be added to the matrix as well, such as an indication of the transformation of survey items or the construction of indexes or scales to measure key study constructs; other studies or scales from which the questions were drawn; and what is known (if anything) about their reliability and validity.

This matrix is intended to discipline the investigator to consider how each survey item is useful as well as whether other items may need to be added to address the study objectives adequately. Analysts should give thought to alternative ways of measuring the concepts they incorporate in their studies as well as the types of simple or complex variables they would like to construct for an empirical examination of the relationships between these concepts. The level of measurement that study variables represent has important implications for the choice of analytic procedures and for transformations in the form of the variables that may be required to use certain procedures.

The primary research objectives for the dental preferences study are summarized in Table 2.3 (see Chapter Two). The measurement matrix for this study (Table 15.1) displays how each item in the survey questionnaire would be used

TABLE 15.1. MEASUREMENT MATRIX BASED ON
DENTAL CLINICAL DECISION-MAKING STUDY.

Question	Concept	Level of Measurement	Objective
1–4	Factors influencing preferences for therapies: crown versus amalgam/composite buildup	ordinal	1,2,3
5–8	Factors influencing preferences for therapies: root canal versus extraction	ordinal	1,2,3
9–12	Factors influencing preferences for therapies: fixed bridge versus removable partial denture	ordinal	1,2,3
13–16	Factors influencing preferences for therapies: prophylaxis versus subgingival curettage/ periodontal scaling	ordinal	1,2,3
17	Practice beliefs (Likert scale)	ordinal (interval)	3
18	Practice characteristics: busyness of practice	ordinal	3
19	Practice characteristics: number of visits in typical week	interval	3
20	Practice characteristics: number of procedures in typical week	ratio	3
21	Practice characteristics: average appointment delay (days)	ordinal	3
22	Practice characteristics: average waiting time (minutes)	ordinal	3
23	Practice characteristics: patient recall system (yes/no) (type)	nominal nominal	3 3
24	Practice characteristics: dentist advertises	nominal	3
25	Practice characteristics: dentist provides advance information on treatment costs	ordinal	3
26	Patient characteristics: % living in areas with fluoridated water	ratio	3
27	Patient characteristics: % age distribution	ratio	3
28	Patient characteristics: % employment distribution	ratio	3
29	Patient characteristics: % insurance distribution	ratio	3
30	Practice organization: dentist employment arrangement	nominal	3
31	Practice organization: general or specialty practice (general/specialty) (type of specialty)	nominal nominal	3 3
32	Practice organization: years in practice arrangement	interval	3

TABLE 15.1. MEASUREMENT MATRIX BASED ON DENTAL CLINICAL DECISION-MAKING STUDY, cont'd.

Question	Concept	Level of Measurement	Objective
33	Practice organization: number of dental operatories	ratio	3
34	Practice organization: number of full-time and part-time employees	ratio	3
35	Practice organization: % of time in four-handed dentistry	ratio	3
36	Practice organization: takes time to explain complicated dental procedures	ordinal	3
37	Practice organization: use computer in practice		
	(yes/no)	nominal	3
	(tasks)	nominal	3
38	Practice organization: do own lab work or not	nominal	3
39	Practice organization: fees for common procedures	ratio	3
40	Practice characteristics: dental school attended	nominal	3
41	Practice characteristics: year received degree	interval	3
42	Practice characteristics: average hours worked per week	interval	3
43	Practice characteristics: weeks worked in the year	interval	3
ID	County of practice	nominal	2

Note: See Table 2.3 for study objectives and Resource C for study questionnaire.

to operationalize the major study concepts reflected in these objectives (factors influencing preferences for particular therapies, practice beliefs, practice characteristics and organization, and patient characteristics).

Objective 1 for the survey was concerned with describing the importance of technical, patient, and cost factors in influencing preferences for particular therapies. Objective 2 compared the influence of these factors for dentists practicing in different counties (identified in the case ID number), and Objective 3 analyzed the relative importance of an array of predictors in understanding the factors influencing dentists' preferences.

The questions asked in the dentists survey are a mix of nominal, ordinal, interval, and ratio measures. Ratio measures are principally distinguished from interval measures based on whether a zero value is a theoretically possible response to the question (number of times a specific procedure was performed each week).

As indicated in the matrix, a Likert summary scale will be created to summarize a series of measures intended to capture the dentists' practice beliefs (Questions 17a to 17f). The individual items are clearly ordinal level measures (based on a scale indicating whether respondents strongly agree, agree, disagree, or strongly disagree with the item). However, methodological research in the social and behavioral sciences suggests that it is acceptable to treat these types of ordinal items, and the summary scales produced from them in particular, as interval-level data to permit their use with more powerful statistical procedures (DeVellis, 1991; Nunnally & Bernstein, 1994).

Reviewing Potential Analytic Procedures

Alternative analysis techniques are presented here to acquaint the researcher with (1) the basic types of procedures available to answer a given research question, (2) how they can be used to answer that question, and (3) which procedures are most appropriate to use with what types of data. This chapter also outlines the criteria to apply in deciding what type of statistical procedure best addresses the questions that the study was designed to answer.

The major dimensions to take into account in weighing the relevance of different types of procedures for one's study purposes, reflected in the tables and figures summarizing these procedures (Tables 15.2 and 15.3 and Figures 15.1 to 15.3), include the applicability of descriptive versus inferential statistics; univariate, bivariate, and multivariate analyses; parametric versus nonparametric procedures; tests of the existence of an association as well as measures of the strength of an association; and whether the design is based on independent or related samples.

Descriptive Versus Inferential Statistics

Descriptive statistics simply summarize the characteristics of a particular sample. Inferential statistics enable the researcher to decide, on the basis of the probability theory (sampling distribution) underlying a given test statistic, the level of confidence that he or she can have in inferring the characteristics of the population as a whole on the basis of the information obtained from a particular sample.

Test statistics are inferential rather than descriptive. Test statistics are used to test statistically how often the differences or associations observed between two (or more) groups are likely to occur by chance if a hypothesis about this relationship is true for the populations from which the groups were drawn. Different test statistics are used with different statistical procedures. Test statistics (such as the chi-square, t-test, and F-test statistics) are assumed to have specific types of "sampling distributions," which are based on the size and randomness of the sample for the study, the level of measurement of the study variables being tested, and the characteristics of the population from which the sample was drawn.

Application of the normal sampling distribution for testing hypotheses about the characteristics of the population is discussed in Chapter Seven. An analogous process is involved in testing hypotheses by means of test statistics that have other types of sampling distributions. Appropriate adjustments should be made to the test statistics when complex sample designs are used (Lee, Forthofer, & Lorimor, 1986, 1989).

Since the "truth" of a theoretical hypothesis can never be known with certainty when researchers use methods based on the probability of occurrence of the hypothesized result, statistical hypotheses are generally stated in terms of a "null" hypothesis; that is, there is said to be "no" difference or association between the variables. This is in contrast to the substantive research (or alternative) hypothesis, which states the relationship that one would expect to find given the theories or previous research in the area. If an association *is* found in a particular sample, the researcher would conclude that the null hypothesis of *no* difference or association hypothesized between groups is probably *not* true for the populations from which these groups were drawn.

Univariate, Bivariate, and Multivariate Analyses

Univariate statistics (such as frequencies, percentages, the mode, median, and mean) are useful descriptive statistics for profiling the characteristics of survey respondents. Bivariate statistics focus on examining the relationship between two variables and multivariate statistics on the relationship among an array of variables. These procedures are used directly in testing and elaborating study hypotheses, respectively (for which mock tables were displayed in Exhibit 4.1, Chapter Four).

Parametric Versus Nonparametric Procedures

Parametric statistics make certain assumptions about the distribution of the variables in the population from which the sample was drawn. Many of the parametric test procedures assume a normal distribution in the parent population and a simple random sample of a minimum size (generally at least thirty cases). Nonparametric procedures do not. Further, more nonparametric procedures deal principally with analyses of nominal- or ordinal-level variables, whereas parametric procedures generally assume at least interval or ratio data (Conover, 1980).

Existence Versus Strength of Association

Researchers should also decide whether they are principally interested in testing for the simple *existence of a relationship* (or association) between two variables or groups of interest, as displayed in mock tables (see again Exhibit 4.1 in Chapter Four), or the *strength of the relationship* (or association) between the two variables, or both. An array of statistical procedures and associated tests of significance (such as chi-square, *t*-tests, and analysis of variance) are used to test for the existence of a relationship between variables. Correlation coefficients appropriate to the level of measurement of the respective variables—most of which range between 0 and 1.0 or - 1.0 to + 1.0—can be used to measure the strength and direction of the relationship between variables (or groups).

Independent Versus Related Samples

Another factor to consider in reviewing potential analysis procedures is the basic *study design* for the survey—in particular, whether the groups (or samples) being compared are independent of one another or not. With longitudinal panel designs, the groups being compared at different points in time are not independent. In fact, they include the same people. Similarly, retrospective designs may contain some case-control features, such as looking at people before and after they became ill or matching those with and without the illness on other relevant characteristics. In those instances as well, the samples are correlated (or dependent) and tests appropriate to the related samples should be used. In cross-sectional surveys or other studies in which there is no effort to reinterview the same people or match and compare individuals, tests for independent samples are appropriate. Researchers must take into account whether the samples (or groups) being compared are correlated or not when choosing a particular procedure; some correlations between groups may already be built in because of the way in which the sample was drawn. The procedures used with related samples take any preexisting overlap between them into account in computing the statistics to test the relationships between such groups.

The reader should consult standard statistics and biometry texts for more information on a particular statistical technique of interest. (See sources listed at the end of this chapter.) There are a number of excellent statistical software packages available for use with mainframes, minicomputers, and microcomputers. These include SPSS, SAS, BMDP, STATA, EPI-INFO, and MINITAB. MINITAB is often used as an instructional package for teaching basic statistics. SPSS, SAS, BMDP, and STATA are powerful and versatile packages that contain a variety of analysis procedures. However, SPSS not only has a range of applications similar to the other packages but also documentation and commands that are somewhat more accessible to users with little computer experience. EPI-INFO is readily available in the public domain and offers a wide range of applications for epidemiological research. The decision about which package to use should be based on the user's familiarity with a particular package, what is available at the institution in which the research is being conducted, and whether unique features of a particular package better satisfy the requirements for a given type of analysis. If a complex sample design was used in the study, then the analyses will need to be run using the software and procedures for handling associated design effects described in Chapter Seven.

Using Univariate Statistics to Describe the Sample

The first step in carrying out the analysis of any data set—regardless of the type of study design—is to analyze the sample by each of the major study variables of interest. Investigators may or may not report the basic distributions of and summary statistics on the study variables in their final report of the study. This documentation does, however, provide the starting point for determining what the data look like preparatory to constructing any other analytical variables or pursuing subsequent subgroup analyses. There have to be enough cases, for example, to carry out certain analytical procedures in a meaningful way.

Univariate statistics are summary measures used to describe the composition of one variable at a time, such as how many people with certain ranges of income, levels of perceived health, or numbers of physician visits constitute the sample. The particular types of univariate statistics to use depend on the level of measurement of the respective variables. The basic types of univariate statistics are summarized in Table 15.2.

Frequencies

Frequencies refer to the number and percent of people with certain characteristics. We saw in Chapter Three that regardless of the level of measurement of any particular variable, numerical codes can be assigned to each category or value that is relevant for describing someone in the sample. For nominal variables, such as marital status, the codes simply identify categories of individuals—people who are currently married, widowed, divorced or separated, or never married, for example. For ordinal variables, the codes represent rankings on the level of the variable, such as the extent to which people think they are likely to get a certain illness on a scale of 1 to 5 (as in Question 32 in the AIDS survey shown in Resource B), in

TABLE 15.2. USING UNIVARIATE STATISTICS TO DESCRIBE THE SAMPLE.

	Levels of Measurement		
Type of Univariate Statistic	Nominal Marital Status	Ordinal Perceived risk of AIDS	Interval or Ratio Number of M.D. visits (those with 1+)
Examples			
Frequencies (number and percent of people in sample with the characteristics)	Values % (n) 1–Married 30% (30) 2–Divorced 20 (20) 3–Separated 10 (10) 4–Widowed 0 (0) 5–Never married 40 (40) Total 100% (100)	Values % (n) 1–Not at all 30% (30) 2 20 (20) 3 10 (10) 4 0 (0) 5–Extremely 40 (40) Total 100% (100)	Values % (n) 1 30% (30) 2 20 (20) 3 10 (10) 4 0 (0) 5 40 (40) Total 100% (100)
Measures of Central Tendency			
Mode (most frequent value)	5	5	5
Median (value with half of cases above and half below it)	Not applicable	2.5	2.5
Mean (Average) (sum of values/total n)	Not applicable	Not applicable	$[(1 \times 30) + (2 \times 20) + (3 \times 10) + (4 \times 0) + (5 \times 40)] \div 100 = 3$
Measures of Dispersion			
Range (maximum – minimum value)	Not applicable	Not applicable	$5 - 1 = 4$
Variance (average difference between each value and mean, as follows...) $\dfrac{\text{Sum (value - mean)}^2}{n - 1}$	Not applicable	Not applicable	$\dfrac{[30 \times (1-3)^2 + 20 \times (2-3)^2 + 10 \times (3-3)^2 + 40 \times (5-3)^2]}{99}$ $= 3.03$
Standard Deviation (square root of variance)	Not applicable	Not applicable	$\sqrt{3.03} = 1.74$

which 1 represents their assessment that they are not at all likely to get the disease and 5 their belief that they are extremely likely to do so.

With interval scales, the codes refer to equal points along some underlying continuum, such as units of temperature. With ratio scales, however, some absolute zero reference point (the total absence of the characteristic, such as having no or "zero" visits to a physician in the year) can be a valid value for the variable. (In the example in Table 15.2, the analysis is limited to those who had at least one physician visit in the year.)

Frequencies refer to how often individuals with the given attribute appear in the sample and what percentage (or proportion) they represent of all the individuals in the study. As discussed in Chapter Fourteen, codes can also be assigned to represent data that for some reason are missing for an individual respondent.

In addition to providing a basic profile of the members of the sample, the frequencies alert the researcher to (1) whether there is a large proportion of missing values for a particular variable, which could preclude the analysis of that variable or suggest the need for procedures to impute values for the cases for which values are missing; (2) whether there are too few cases of a certain kind to conduct meaningful analyses for that group or whether it would make sense, in some cases, to combine certain groups for the analyses; or (3) whether there are outliers, that is, cases with extremely large or extremely small values on a variable compared with the rest of the cases. The researcher may want to consider excluding these outliers or assigning them a maximum value for certain analyses.

Running frequencies on variables for which different values are possible (number of disability days in the year) can produce a long list of values. However, univariate statistics are available to summarize these frequency distributions in a more parsimonious fashion.

Measures of Central Tendency

Measures of central tendency help the researcher identify one number to represent the most typical response found on the frequencies for a variable. There are three principal measures of central tendency—*mode, median,* and *mean.* Which measure to use to summarize the frequencies on a survey variable depends on the variable's level of measurement.

Mode. The mode or modal response is the response that occurs most often in the data, that is, the one that has the highest frequency or percentage of people responding. The modal response for each of the variables for which frequencies are displayed in Table 15.2 is five (40 percent of the one hundred respondents).

Median. A second type of univariate summary measure is the value that would split the sample in half if one were to order people in the sample from the highest to the lowest values on some variable of interest (such as lining up students in a class on the basis of their height). This measure—the median—assumes at least an ordinal level of measurement so that study participants can be ranked (or put in order) on the attribute. It would, for example, not make sense to put individuals identified through categories of a *nominal* variable into some order representing more or less of a characteristic such as race, sex, marital status, region of the country, and the like. Sometimes the median value will have to be interpolated (or interpreted) as the midpoint between two values—in Table 15.2, for example, 2.5, which lies between the values of 2 and 3, is the median value—to specify most precisely the point both below and above which exactly half (50 percent) of the cases fall.

Mean. The most commonly used expression of the mean is the arithmetic mean. As indicated in the example in Table 15.2, the arithmetic mean is computed by adding up all the values on the variable for everyone in the sample and dividing this figure by the total number of people in the sample to get an "average" score. The median is sometimes preferred to the mean in expressing the typical value for interval- or ratio-level variables since the mean could be considerably skewed by cases with extreme values (outliers).

Mean estimates are not meaningful for nominal- and ordinal-level variables. It does not make sense, for example, to add up the ethnic statuses of people in the sample and divide the result by the number of people in the sample to get an average ethnicity. In contrast, one could speak of the modal category of ethnic status in the sample, that is, the largest ethnic group in the study. Ordinal-level measures do not make assumptions about the exact distance between points on a scale that simply ranks individuals on some characteristic of interest. Computing averages using ordinal-level variables would be much like calculating the heights of a group of students in inches by means of a ruler on which the distances between each of the "inch" markers were all a little different.

Measures of Dispersion

A second major category of univariate statistics useful for describing the basic sample is measures of dispersion, which summarize how much variation there is across people in the sample in the answers they provide to a given survey question. The main types of measures of dispersion are the *range, variance,* and *standard deviation.*

Range. The range is simply the difference between the highest (maximum) and lowest (minimum) values that appear on the frequency table. For example, in Table 15.2, in which the values extend from one to five, the range is four (that is, five minus one). The range may be expressed either by the actual difference (four) or by the two extreme scores (one to five). The computation of the range assumes at least an interval level of measurement. For nominal-level measures, a variation ratio can be computed, which is simply the percentage of people that are *not* in the modal category (60 percent in the example in Table 15.2). For ordinal-level variables, decile or interquartile ranges are used. These are based on dividing the distribution of cases into ten equal parts (deciles), each containing 10 percent of the cases, *or* into four equal parts (quartiles), each containing 25 percent of the cases. The decile or interquartile range is expressed as the values for the cases that define the cutoff for the highest and lowest deciles (10 percent) or quartiles (25 percent) of the distribution of cases (not shown in Table 15.2).

Variance and Standard Deviation. The measures used most often in reflecting the degree of variation for interval or ratio data are variance and standard deviation measures. These are ways of looking at how much the values for the respondents in the sample differ from the typical value (generally the mean) for the sample. The variance is computed by calculating the difference between the value for each case in the sample and the mean on the characteristic for the sample, squaring these differences (so that positive and negative values do not cancel one another), adding these squared values for all the cases in the sample, and then dividing this sum by the total number of cases in the sample less one ($n - 1$) or by the sample size itself (n) for larger samples (more than thirty cases). The standard deviation is the square root of the variance.

Using Bivariate Statistics to Test for Relationships Between Variables

After the basic composition of the sample has been described, the next step in analyzing most survey data is to look at the relationship between two or more variables. In simple cross-sectional descriptive studies, investigators may want to look at differences between subgroups on variables related to the principal study objectives. For example, in the case of the alternative designs for addressing different research questions related to high school seniors' smoking behavior (see Table 2.2 in Chapter Two), researchers might be interested in looking at the prevalence of smoking among seniors in different age, sex, and race groups as well as among seniors as a whole. Group-comparison studies explicitly build in primary comparisons between certain groups in the design of the samples and selection of the samples of individuals to be included in the survey. Longitudinal studies focus on comparisons between data gathered at more than one point in time. In panel-type longitudinal designs these comparisons involve data gathered from the same people at different points in time. Finally, analytical surveys are explicitly concerned with testing hypotheses about the relationship between at least one independent and one dependent variable by means of cross-sectional, prospective, or retrospective survey designs. Figures 15.1 and 15.2 provide a summary of different bivariate statistical procedures for looking at the relationship between two survey variables. (Figure 15.2 appears in the following section.)

Nonparametric Procedures

Nominal. As displayed in the first example in Figure 15.1, the simplest procedure for examining the relationship between two variables based on a nominal level of measurement is a cross-tabulation of the variables. A relationship between the variables is suggested by the fact that people in the sample cluster in systematic ways in certain cells of the table, as with the examples cited earlier in Chapter Four.

The Pearson chi-square is one test statistic used to examine the statistical significance of such a relationship for independent samples. It basically looks at the "goodness of fit" between the distribution that is *observed* in each of the cells compared with the distribution that would be *expected,* given the number of people in the sample with the respective characteristics (X and Y), and assuming the variables are not related. The less that the pattern observed in the table matches the expected distribution, as measured by the Pearson chi-square test statistic, the less support there is for the null hypothesis that there is no relationship between the variables in this particular sample. Fisher's exact test can be used for tables that have only two rows and two columns and in which the expected number of cases in some cells of the cross-classification table is less than five.

The McNemar test is designed for use with related samples or before and after experimental designs to detect any significant changes in the status of subjects over time, such as whether employees who formerly smoked quit smoking after a worksite health promotion campaign. One would expect to find a higher proportion of nonsmokers after the campaign than before it.

The Cochran Q-test is used when three or more related groups are compared on some dichotomous variable, such as the proportion of enrollees in a new prepaid dental plan who had been to the dentist at least twice during the year for a preventive visit, in a longitudinal panel study of people interviewed annually over a three-year period. The underlying objective might be to see if there is an increased tendency to seek preventive dental services over time as a function of enhanced plan coverage and patient education efforts.

A variety of measures of the strength of the association between variables, based on cross-tabulations between nominal variables, are available. Some are

FIGURE 15.1. USING NONPARAMETRIC BIVARIATE STATISTICS TO TEST FOR RELATIONSHIPS BETWEEN VARIABLES.

Type of Measurement	Example	Bivariate Statistics		Measures of Strength of Association Between Variables
		Tests of Association Between Variables		
		Independent Samples	Related Samples	
Nominal (cross-tabulation of dependent variable by independent variable)	Independent Variable (X) X = 1 X = 2 Dependent Variable (Y) Y = 1 / Y = 2	Fisher's exact test (2 × 2 table) Chi-square contingency table analysis	McNemar test for significance of changes (2 × 2 table) Cochran Q-test	Phi coefficient Yule's Q (2 × K table) Coefficient of contingency Cramer's V Lambda Odds ratio
Ordinal (association of ranks between two variables)	Ranks Case ID Variable X Variable Y 001 5 1 002 5 1 003 5 1 004 5 1 005 5 1	Chi-square contingency table analysis		Goodman and Kruskal's gamma Kendall's tau-a, tau-b, tau-c Somer's d Spearman rank order coefficient
Mixed (differences in ranks between groups)	Groups Group X = 1 Group X = 2 Variable Y 5 1 5 1 5 1 5 1 5 1	Median test Mann-Whitney U test Kolmogorov-Smirnov Wald-Wolfowitz runs test Kruskal-Wallis (3+ groups)	Sign test Wilcoxon matched-pairs signed ranks test Friedman two-way analysis of variance (3+ groups)	Lambda Uncertainty coefficient Goodman and Kruskal's gamma Somer's d Eta coefficient

based on modifications of the chi-square test statistic so that they range from 0 to 1, with 0 corresponding to no association and 1 to perfect association between the variables. The phi coefficient, Yule's Q, the coefficient of contingency, and Cramer's V are examples of chi-square-based measures of association.

Other measures of association based on cross-tabulations of nominal variables are termed *proportional reduction in error* (PRE) statistics. PRE measures are based on formulas for computing how well the value of a dependent variable (Y) can be predicted from knowing the value of an independent variable (X). These statistics basically compare (1) a situation where the value of the dependent variable (such as being insured versus being uninsured) for any given case in the sample is estimated simply by determining how many people there are in the sample in each group of the dependent variable with (2) a situation in which the information on the value of the independent variable (such as whether the person works or not) is also used in estimating the value of the dependent variable for that case.

Odds ratios for case-control studies (discussed in Chapter Four) and relative risk estimates for cohort designs are used in epidemiological studies in particular for summarizing the strength of a given risk factor (or exposure) as predictive of a particular disease outcome (Kleinbaum, Kupper, & Morgenstern, 1982).

Ordinal. The second major type of analysis procedure for examining the bivariate relationship between (two) variables or groups is one that assumes an ordinal level of measurement of the study variables. As shown in Figure 15.1 for the example relating to the bivariate analyses of ordinal variables, the variables X and Y take on values of one to five. A respondent (case ID 005) might, for example, say in Question 32 of the AIDS survey (Resource B) that he thought he was *extremely likely* to get AIDS—for a rank of five on that variable (X)—but indicate in Question 34 that he would *not be at all ashamed* to get it—for a rank of one on that indicator (Y). To calculate the overall correspondence between these two ordinal variables (fear and shame of the disease), the researcher would compare the differences and similarities in the rankings of the two variables for *all* the cases in the sample (Cases 001, 002, 003, 004, and 005 in the example in Figure 15.1). The more the rankings of these variables correspond (either in a perfectly positive or perfectly negative direction), the more likely these ordinal test statistics are to indicate that a direct or inverse relationship exists between the variables.

The investigator might also be interested in comparing two groups (homosexuals and heterosexuals) to see if they differ on an ordinal variable (level of fear of AIDS). In that case, mixed procedures, based on nominal-level classification of individuals into the groups being compared, would be appropriate. Chi-square procedures are also used with ordinal data, particularly if the variables being considered have a limited number of categories and if there is no particular concern with an ordinal interpretation of the values for each variable.

The use of related sample tests would be relevant if the study design called for certain observations to be paired, as in a study of a sample of patients before and after they were told they had AIDS to see how they would rate their fear of the illness. The paired comparisons of the rankings of the patient and control cases on this fear scale would help test a hypothesis about the fear-arousal consequences of being diagnosed as having AIDS.

Parametric Procedures

Parametric procedures are based on the assumption that the distribution of the dependent variable of interest (Y) in the population from which the sample was drawn follows a particular pattern, such as the *normal distribution* (see Figure 15.2).

Interval or Ratio. One of the most popular parametric procedures for independent and dependent variables that assume an interval level of measurement is regression analysis. This form of analysis looks at the extent to which an interval-level variable Y (such as blood cholesterol level) is predicted by another interval-level variable X (the average daily intake of grams of fat).

Regression coefficients are generated that estimate the change in the dependent variable Y (cholesterol level) that results from a change in the independent variable X (grams of fat). Underlying the computation of the regression coefficient is the assumption that the X and Y values for each case can be plotted on a graph and a line drawn through these points that minimizes the squared difference between each of the points and this line—referred to as the "least squares" line (see example in Figure 15.2). The hypothesis being tested is whether or not a linear relationship between the variables exists, based on how well this line fits the data. The *t*-test and F-test statistics are used to test the statistical significance of the hypothesized relationship.

The dependent variable used in regression analysis when the variables are based on samples that are *not* independent is a difference computed between measures at different points in time for the same people or between matched cases. Examples would be comparisons before and after an intervention for the same people or comparisons between matched cases and controls in matched case-control designs.

The Pearson correlation coefficient, which is a measure of the strength of association between the two variables, ranges between -1.0 and $+1.0$. These procedures are powerful and useful ones and can serve as the basis for more

FIGURE 15.2. USING PARAMETRIC BIVARIATE STATISTICS TO TEST FOR RELATIONSHIPS BETWEEN VARIABLES.

| | | Bivariate Statistics | | |
| | | Tests of Association Between Variables | | Measures of Strength of Association Between Variables |
Type of Measurement	Example	Independent Samples	Related Samples	
Interval or Ratio (extent to which Y has a linear relationship to X)	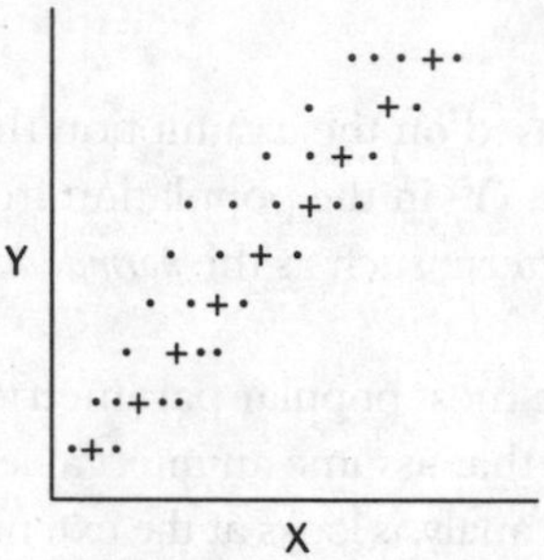 *(scatter plot of Y vs. X)*	Bivariate regression	Bivariate regression	Pearson correlation coefficient
Mixed (differences in means between groups)	*Variable X* *Mean of Y*	T-test of difference of means (2 groups)	Paired t-test of difference (2 groups)	Biserial correlation
				Point biserial correlation
Y = Interval or ratio X = Nominal	Group X = 1 $\bar{y}1$	One-way analysis of variance	One-way analysis of variance with repeated measures	
	Group X = 2 $\bar{y}2$			Eta coefficient
	Group X = 3 $\bar{y}3$			

sophisticated multivariate procedures (see Table 15.3 in the following section) that enable the impact of a number of other *control* variables also to be considered in the analyses.

Mixed. The final procedure reviewed in Figure 15.2 is a mixed one, where the dependent variable is an interval-level variable and the predictor variable is nominal. For example, one might be interested in looking at the level of blood cholesterol (Y) for African American and white children (X) and determining whether there are statistically significant differences between the two groups. This type of analysis can be conducted by using a *t*-test statistic of the difference between two means. Biserial or point biserial correlation coefficients can be computed to measure the association between the interval-level dependent variable and the dichotomous independent variable.

If there is interest in comparing means between more than two groups (African American, white, and Hispanic children, for example), then the one-way analysis of variance procedure, which uses the F-test statistic, is more appropriate. Analysis of variance will be discussed in more detail later in this chapter.

Using Multivariate Statistics to Explain Relationships Between Variables

The procedures summarized in Figure 15.3 and Table 15.3 are used when researchers want to add one or more additional variables to the analysis in an effort to further understand the relationship between two variables examined in the bivariate analyses. These procedures can be viewed as the statistical devices for actually carrying out the elaboration of the study hypotheses, which were discussed in Chapter Four and displayed in Figures 4.2 through 4.5.

Nonparametric Procedures

Nominal. The Pearson chi-square procedure could be expanded to include the analysis of a third nominal variable to see if the original relationship between X and Y holds when this control variable, expressed by an elaboration of the study hypotheses, is added. It may not be meaningful to expand the analysis in this way because the number of cases in some cells of the tables resulting from this cross-classification process may become very small. If more than 20 percent of the resulting cells have expected values of fewer than five cases, it is not meaningful to use the chi-square test statistic.

Loglinear analysis and weighted least squares (WLS) procedures are more appropriate procedures to use when all the predictors for a categoric dependent variable are also nominal-level variables. The Mantel-Haenszel procedure is used quite frequently in epidemiological analyses of dichotomous independent and dependent variables. It combines data from several 2 x 2 tables (resulting from cross-classifications of dichotomous variables) into a single estimate (expressed as an odds ratio) of the probability of having a disease (yes/no), based on the status of the respondents' exposure (yes/no) to a number of different risk conditions (Rosner, 1994).

Ordinal. The Kendall coefficient of concordance expresses the strength of association among three or more ordinal-level variables. Several procedures (previously

FIGURE 15.3. USING NONPARAMETRIC MULTIVARIATE STATISTICS TO EXPLAIN RELATIONSHIPS BETWEEN VARIABLES.

Type of Measurement	Example	Multivariate Statistics		
		Tests of Association Between Variables		Measures of Strength of Association Between Variables
		Independent Samples	Related Samples	
Nominal (cross-tabulation of dependent variable by independent variable by control variables)	*(see contingency tables below)*	Chi-square multidimensional contingency table analysis Loglinear analysis Weighted least squares Mantel-Haenszel chi-square	Cochran Q-test	Coefficient of contingency Cramer's V Lambda Symmetric lambda Odds ratio
Ordinal (association of ranks between three or more variables)	*(see Ranks table below)*	Chi-square multidimensional contingency table analysis		Kendall coefficient of concordance

Example (Nominal):

Z = 1

	X = 1	X = 2	X = 3
Y = 1			
Y = 2			

Z = 2

	X = 1	X = 2	X = 3
Y = 1			
Y = 2			

Example (Ordinal):

Ranks

Case ID	Variable X	Variable Y	Variable Z
001	1	5	3
002	2	4	2
003	3	3	1
004	4	2	5
005	5	1	4

listed as "mixed" procedures in Figure 15.1) are useful in comparing groups when the dependent variable does not meet the assumptions of interval- or ratio-level measurement. The Median and Kruskal-Wallis tests (for three or more groups) permit different groups, created by a cross-classification of the independent (X) and control (Z) variables, to be compared on an ordinal dependent variable (Y). The Friedman two-way analysis of variance procedure is used when the groups being compared are related.

Parametric Procedures

Interval or Ratio. Multiple regression procedures may be used when two or more interval-level measures serve as predictors of some normally distributed interval-level dependent variable (see Table 15.3). In this procedure the regression coefficient for any particular independent variable (X) represents the change in the dependent variable (Y) associated with a one-unit change in X, while the levels of the control variables (Z1, Z2, and so on) are held constant.

Mixed. Analysis of variance (ANOVA) procedures are based on the same underlying statistical model used in regression. In fact, ANOVA is similar to dummy variable regression, in which a series of dichotomous variables are used to represent the categories of a nominal variable. In contrast to regular regression procedures, analysis of variance focuses on comparing the means for cross-classifications of two or more groups of people, not on estimating coefficients that reflect the magnitude of change in the dependent variable associated with a unit change in the independent variables.

For example, one may want to look at the differences in the average cholesterol level for African American and white children (X), while controlling for whether the children are poor or not (Z) (referred to as two-way analysis of variance since the effects of two predictor variables are being examined). An F-test statistic can be used to summarize the difference in the variances between and within the resulting groups on the dependent variable (Y) of interest. The greater the variances *between* groups compared with the variance *within* groups, the more likely it is that the differences between the groups are significant. Analysis of variance can be used to test these relationships for independent and related samples as well as to compute a multiple correlation coefficient to measure the strength of the association between the dependent variable and a linear combination of the independent variables.

For analysis of covariance procedures, means on the dependent variable Y (cholesterol level) are compared for groups of individuals identified by a nominal variable X (African American versus white children), using some interval-level

TABLE 15.3. USING PARAMETRIC MULTIVARIATE STATISTICS TO EXPLAIN RELATIONSHIPS BETWEEN VARIABLES.

Type of Measurement	Example	Multivariate Statistics		
		Tests of Association Between Variables		Measures of Strength of Association Between Variables
		Independent Samples	Related Samples	
Interval or Ratio (extent to which Y has a linear relationship to X, Z, and so on)	$Y=a+b_1X+b_1Z_1+b_2Z_2+b_nZ_n+e$	Multiple regression	Multiple regression of difference scores	Multiple correlation coefficient
Mixed (differences in means between groups, controlling for other characteristics) Y=Interval or Ratio X=Nominal Z=Nominal	Variable X and Variable Z Mean of Y X=1 by Z=1 $\bar{y}11$ X=1 by Z=2 $\bar{y}12$ X=2 by Z=1 $\bar{y}21$ X=2 by Z=2 $\bar{y}22$	Analysis of variance	Analysis of variance with repeated measures	Multiple correlation coefficient
Y=Interval or Ratio X=Nominal Z=Interval	Variable X with Z X=1 with Z $\bar{y}1adjZ$ X=2 with Z $\bar{y}2adjZ$	Analysis of covariance	Analysis of covariance with repeated measures	Multiple correlation coefficient
(differences in percent between groups, controlling for other characteristics) Y=Dichotomy X=Nominal Z=Mixed	Variable X and Variable Z % of Y X=1 by Z=1 y11% X=1 by Z=2 y12% X=2 by Z=1 y21% X=2 by Z=2 y22%	Logistic regression	Logistic regression of change in status	Odds ratio

control variable Z. In the example just cited, an interval-level control variable Z (family income), rather than the nominal-level variable Z (poverty status), could be used. In that case, an analysis of covariance procedure would be more appropriate than an analysis of variance procedure. The analysis of covariance procedure then statistically controls or adjusts for the fact that the relation between the continuous dependent variable and race is also affected by this continuous control variable.

When the dependent variable of interest is *dichotomous* (whether the cholesterol reading is high or not, as determined by a normative cutoff point) rather than interval-level (the cholesterol reading itself), and a variety of nominal, interval, or ratio measures are used as independent or control variables, it is appropriate to use probit or logistic regression procedures (Hosmer & Lemeshow, 1989; Hosmer, Taber, & Lemeshow, 1991). The test statistics for these procedures do not assume the same underlying sampling distributions found in the multiple regression approach for analyzing continuous dependent variables (Cleary & Angel, 1984). The regression coefficients become estimates of odds ratios, which can be converted to estimates of the probability that a certain outcome (Y) will occur, based on its relationship to other variables (X, Z). A chi-square statistic can be used to test the statistical significance of these coefficients. Hanley (1983, p. 172) has argued that logistic regression "now stands in the same relation to binary (dichotomous) response data as classical regression does to continuous (interval) response data" in the analysis of epidemiological data.

Many other procedures are also available to researchers. Path analysis and LISREL *(LInear Structural RELations)* are, for example, powerful procedures for modeling the causal linkages between variables implied in complex conceptual frameworks and, in the instance of LISREL, for quantifying the validity and reliability of the variables used to measure the multidimensional constructs in these models (Jöreskog, 1993; Jöreskog & Sörbom, 1979). Multivariate analysis of variance (MANOVA) examines the relationship between multiple independent and dependent variables (such as several different measures of the health-related quality of life construct) (Neter, Wasserman, & Kutner, 1990).

Mapping Out the Analysis Plan

Constructing a measurement matrix and considering the relevance of alternative statistical procedures for measuring and modeling the study objectives sets the stage for the formulation of the analysis plan for the study (Fink, 1995a). A sample guide for this process, based on the dentists survey, appears in Table 15.4.

The first and primary reference point for developing the analysis plan is the study's research objectives (and hypotheses, if applicable). The objectives should

TABLE 15.4. MAPPING OUT THE ANALYSIS PLAN.

Study Objective	Number and Type of Variables		Analytic Procedures
	Independent Variable	Dependent Variable	
	One variable (neither independent or dependent)		
To describe the importance of technical, patient, and cost factors in influencing preferences for particular therapies.		Ordinal: ranking of factors as first, second, or third in importance	frequency, percent, mode, median
	One independent and one dependent variable		
To compare the importance of technical, patient, and cost factors in influencing preferences for particular therapies by dentists practicing in different countries.	Nominal (2 categories): Spokane versus other	Nominal: patient versus other factors as *most important*	chi-square; Fisher's exact test
		Ordinal: category ranking of factors as first, second, or third in importance	chi-square; median test; Mann-Whitney U-test; Kolmogorov-Smirnov; Wald-Wolfowitz runs test
		Interval (or Interval-like): mean rating of importance	t-test; one-way analysis of variance
	Nominal (3 + categories): Spokane, King, Pierce, Snohomish	Nominal: patient versus other factors as *most important*	chi-square
		Ordinal: category ranking of factors as first, second, or third in importance	chi-square; Kruskall-Wallis
		Interval (or Interval-like): mean rating of importance	one-way analysis of variance
	Two or more independent variables		
To analyze the relative importance of practice beliefs, practice characteristics and organization, and patient characteristics as predictors of the factors influencing dentists' preferences for particular therapies.	Nominal (all)	Nominal	chi-square; log linear analysis; weighted least squares; Mantel-Haenszel chi-square
	Nominal (all)	Interval (or Interval-like)	analysis of variance
	Nominal and interval	Interval (or Interval-like)	analysis of covariance
	Interval (or Interval-like)	Interval (or Interval-like)	multiple regression
	Interval (or Interval-like)	Nominal (dichotomy)	logistic regression; probit

clearly convey who and what represent the central focus of the study as well as the underlying study design with respect to the number of groups of interest and when (or how often) the data will be gathered. The study objectives for the dentists survey, as well as the others used as primary examples throughout the text, were displayed in Table 2.3 in Chapter Two.

Second, the number and types of variables used in addressing the study objectives must be considered. The measurement matrix (Table 15.1) serves as a useful reference for this step in the process. For descriptive purposes, discrete variables may be analyzed separately using simple univariate statistics. When two or more variables are used, independent and dependent variables should be distinguished in the analysis. In analytical and experimental studies, these should be clearly identified in the study hypothesis: the independent variable is hypothesized to cause or influence the occurrence of the dependent variable. With respect to descriptive studies, the designation of independent and dependent variables is relevant when there is a group-comparison or longitudinal aspect to the design. In those instances, the groups being compared or the passage of time can be viewed as independent variables that are assumed to be associated with or predictive of some other attribute or outcome (dependent variable).

The third and final step, based on the criteria reviewed earlier, is to choose the relevant analytic procedures that most appropriately mirror and model statistically what the study objectives are intended to convey substantively. The basic logic for formulating an analysis plan is illustrated in Table 15.4, drawing upon the dentists survey as an example.

As indicated earlier in this chapter (and summarized in Table 2.3), the first principal objective of the dentists survey was to describe the importance of different factors in influencing the preferences for selected therapies. The therapies of interest and the array of technical, patient, and cost factors that were thought likely to influence dentists' choosing one over the other are arrayed in Questions 1 through 16 of the survey questionnaire (Resource C). After reviewing each factor, dentists were asked to indicate which was the most, second most, and third most important factor influencing their choice of therapies (Questions 4, 8, 12, and 16). The frequency, percentages, mode, or median of the individual factors, as well as type of factor, cited in these respective ranks (as first, second, or third in importance) could be used to reflect their relative importance (Grembowski, Milgrom, & Fiset, 1988, 1989).

The second objective concerned comparing the importance of these factors for dentists practicing in different counties. The choice of a bivariate statistical procedure to address this objective would be influenced by the number of counties being compared (two versus three or more), as well as the form of the variable used for characterizing the importance rating assigned to the different factors. The analysis could, for example, focus on the *most* important (first) reason cited for a given therapy and categorize it as a technical, patient, or cost factor. The bivariate cross-tabulation would then display the distribution of these factors for dentists in the different counties and a chi-square or Fisher's exact test could be used to test for the significance of the difference between counties. (The Fisher's exact test would assume that only two counties were being compared and that the three categories of factors were collapsed into two—patient versus other factors, for example.)

Another measurement alternative is to assign an explicit rank (1, 2, 3) for each type of factor for each dentist, reflecting whether the dentist listed a factor as the most, second most, or third most important one in influencing the choice of treatment. The ranks for each of the factors could then be examined across dentists in the different counties using bivariate analytic procedures that assume an ordinal-level dependent variable (ranks for a given factor by county).

A third approach is to construct an interval (or interval-like) mean rating of importance through, for example, comparing the average rank (first, second, or third) or number of times a given type of factor (technical, patient, or cost) was listed as the most important one (first) for dentists in different counties, using either a t-test (two counties) or one-way analysis of variance (three or more counties).

Other approaches may also be relevant depending on the underlying research question and associated variables of interest.

An implicit analytic objective, particularly before proceeding with multivariate analysis procedures, may be to examine the bivariate correlations between potential predictor variables and the dependent variable to be considered in those analyses. This can serve as a basis for identifying and screening in (using) only those variables that are significantly correlated with the dependent variable into the multivariate stage of the analysis. An array of nominal- and ordinal-level correlational statistics are available (see Figures 15.1 and 15.2). The Pearson correlation coefficient is used with interval-level data.

The third major analytic objective of the dentists survey concerned the relative importance of practice beliefs, practice characteristics and organization, and patient characteristics as predictive of the factors influencing dentists' choice of therapies. As displayed in Table 15.4, different forms of the candidate independent and dependent variables would dictate the choice of different analytic procedures. Researchers in this study chose to focus on patient factors because they may be most reflective of the extent to which dentists practice patient-centered care. The investigators used multiple regression to examine the extent to which an array of characteristics influenced dentists' propensity to consider *patient* factors in their choice of therapies (Grembowski, Milgrom, & Fiset, 1988). Not all of the procedures displayed as examples in Table 15.4 would be executed in a single study.

Setting Up Mock Tables

Before considering any particular statistical approach to analyzing data, the researcher should give thought to the kinds of tables appropriate to displaying the data for purposes of addressing the study objectives or hypotheses. Constructing mock tables—tables formatted in the way that the data will eventually be reported but not filled in until the data are analyzed—forces the investigator to think concretely about how the information that is gathered in the study will actually be utilized. Running computer programs to conduct fancy statistical analyses without a clear idea of the specific relationships that need to be examined will waste the researcher's time and resources and most probably produce output that the investigator does not really know how to use or interpret anyway.

Sample mock tables were provided in Exhibit 4.1 (Chapter Four). Mock tables should be configured for the analysis to be used to address each study objective (Table 15.4). The table title and headings should clearly identify the study constructs and subgroups for which data are to be reported. The tables should also reflect intended transformations of the data, such as collapsing the original data into categories, constructing summary scales or indexes, or defining the meaning of the special coding of dichotomous variables (as 1 versus 0) in regression analysis (what the categories 1 and 0 represent, such as male versus female or smoker versus nonsmoker). As indicated in Chapter Four (Exhibit 4.1), for cross-sectional analytic designs, the percentages on the dependent variable (being a smoker or not) should sum to 100 percent *within* each category of the independent variable (friends' smoking behavior). The percentages could then be compared *across* groups to determine which group, if any, is more likely to fall into a certain category of the dependent variable.

In addition, at the bottom of each mock table, the investigator should indicate the statistical procedure to be used in carrying out the analysis reported in the table (such as frequencies, means, Pearson chi-square, *t*-test, analysis of variance, and so on), as well as the study objective or hypothesis the analysis is intended to address. Researchers are encouraged to review tables in the published literature in their field as a source of examples for how the data for their study would be reported.

Special Considerations for Special Populations

If certain groups are to be a special focus of the study, the implications need to be thought through up-front in planning the design analysis of the survey—not after the data are collected.

Selected Examples

The findings from the National Center for Health Statistics–National Health Interview Survey are routinely reported in Series 10 of the NCHS Vital and Health Statistics Series. Special topics are also addressed in periodic NCHS Advance Data Series publications, and trend analyses using NCHS–NHIS data appear in the annual publication *Health: United States*. These reports are primarily descriptive in nature. In addition, NCHS makes the data available for secondary analyses and contracts directly with academic investigators for a more analytic look at the rich array of data available through the NCHS–NHIS core survey and special supplements.

Analyses of the Chicago AIDS survey have focused on the predictors of knowledge, attitudes, and behaviors related to AIDS, with a special focus on minority populations (Albrecht, Levy, Sugrue, Prohaska, & Ostrow, 1989; Prohaska, Albrecht, Levy, Sugrue, & Kim, 1990). The descriptive data provided by this survey also offered useful baseline information for the design of an AIDS education program in that city.

The analytic focus of the dentists survey has received considerable attention in this chapter. This survey was, however, part of a larger and much more comprehensive project of research that linked the survey information gathered from dentists serving Washington Education Association members and their dependents to dental insurance claims data for patients seen by dentists participating in the survey. The purpose of this larger project was to examine the relative importance of the array of factors examined here on the actual rates and variations in patterns of utilization of different dental procedures and therapies (Grembowski, Milgrom, & Fiset, 1988, 1989, 1990a, 1990b, 1991). This study then serves to demonstrate the utility of linking survey and record data in addressing research questions by drawing upon the unique strengths of each data source.

Guidelines for Minimizing Survey Errors

Developing an analysis *plan* means just that! It pays many times over to start with a well-articulated approach for analyzing the data. Other ideas about how to analyze the data will, of course, occur once the data gathering process begins and the distributions on key variables of interest or the results of preliminary analyses are available. However, if one has a basic plan in mind, subsequent departures then can be a further exploration of a rich mine of information. If a plan is not formulated in advance, however, the process may be more like sifting through a mound of sand and rubble in hopes of finding some gems.

Supplementary Sources

Different statistics textbooks focus on the analysis of survey data from different disciplinary perspectives, including, for example, the social sciences (Bainbridge, 1989, 1992; Bohrnstedt & Knoke, 1994; Nachmias & Nachmias, 1992); biometry (Forthofer & Lee, 1995; Kitchens, 1987; Rosner, 1994); and epidemiology (Kahn & Sempos, 1989; Kleinbaum, Kupper, & Morgenstern, 1982). See Fink (1995a) for straightforward guidance regarding how to develop an approach to analyzing survey data in general.

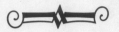

CHAPTER SIXTEEN

WRITING THE RESEARCH REPORT

Chapter Highlights

1. The following criteria should be considered in deciding what and how much to say in the final report: (1) the audience, (2) the mode of dissemination, and (3) the replicability of the study's methodology and results.

2. A comprehensive final research report should contain an executive summary, a statement of the problem or research question addressed in the study, a review of relevant literature, and a description of the study design and hypotheses. It should also include a discussion of the survey's methods, its findings, and the implications and relevance of these results. At times, it is appropriate to include a copy of the survey questionnaire as well as additional material on the methods used in conducting the study.

3. The researcher should provide an assessment of the overall strengths and limitations of the study when presenting the final survey results.

The final step in designing and conducting a survey is dissemination of the results to interested audiences. This chapter presents the criteria and guidelines for preparing a final report and points out material in the preceding chapters that will be useful to review when writing it.

Criteria for Writing Research Reports

Criteria for writing reports include (1) the intended audience for the report; (2) the appropriate scope and format of the report given the proposed method of disseminating the study results; and (3) the replicability of the study from the documentation provided on how it was designed and conducted.

Knowing exactly who the audience for the report will be provides an important point of reference in deciding what to emphasize and how much technical detail to include in the report. A project funder or a dissertation committee might want full documentation of the methods that were used in carrying out the study as well as a detailed exposition of what was learned. A hospital or health maintenance organization's board of directors might be more interested in a clear and interpretable presentation of the findings and less concerned about documentation of the methodologies used in carrying out the study. Professional colleagues might want to be given enough details about how the study was designed and conducted to enable them to replicate it or compare some aspects of it with research that they or others have conducted.

In any case, the researcher needs to communicate as clearly as possible the information desired by the respective audiences. Jargon and technical shorthand should be minimized. Examples are often more useful than are long technical descriptions in illustrating complex materials or abstract concepts. Also, failure to understand the material oneself shows in how a report is written.

It is useful to have a friend or colleague read an early draft. Even if she does not fully understand all the technical details of a study, she will be able to identify areas that seem unclear or poorly written. If what is written makes sense to the friend or colleague, the author can be assured that he or she is at least on the way to getting the material across to the audience for whom it is ultimately intended.

A second issue to consider before starting to write the report is the form in which the final results of the study will be disseminated. Table 16.1 presents a suggested outline for a final research report. Sections or appendixes of this kind of report will be more or less comprehensive, depending on whether the report is a thesis or dissertation, a formal project report to a funder, a research monograph, a book, a working paper, a journal article, a research note, or a nontechnical summary for a lay audience.

The form and format of a thesis or dissertation, a formal project report, or a research monograph generally permit comprehensive exposition and documentation of the study methodology. This means including the survey questionnaire and a detailed methodological appendix in the final research report. If the

TABLE 16.1. OUTLINE OF THE RESEARCH REPORT.

Sections	Chapter References
Executive Summary	16
I. Statement of the problem	2
II. Review of the literature	1
III. Methods	
A. Study design	2
B. Sample design	6, 7
C. Data collection	5, 13
D. Questionnaire design	8–12
E. Measurement	3
F. Data preparation	14
G. Analysis plan	4, 15
IV. Results	4, 15
V. Conclusions	16
Appendixes	
Methodological appendix	3–7, 13, 14
Survey questionnaire	8–12
References	16

results of the research are being prepared for publication as a book, some methodological detail will have to be eliminated depending on the projected length and audience for the book. Working papers and journal articles do not generally contain extensive appendix material. Although the basic outline for a research report can be used in drafting such papers, each section should be a much-reduced version of what would appear in a comprehensive final report. Working papers are sometimes considered early drafts of articles that will eventually be submitted for publication. Such papers can be circulated to colleagues for informal review and comment. This provides an opportunity to revise the manuscript before sending it to a journal for formal consideration for publication. Research notes generally report on a very limited aspect of a study's methodology or findings. Articles for a lay audience may focus on the study findings and their implications for issues of particular interest to that audience.

Researchers should also bear in mind that one of the best guarantees of a good final research report is a good initial research proposal. The outline in Table 16.1 can also be used as a guide for drafting either a prospectus or a full-blown research proposal for a project. As indicated throughout this book, thinking through the problem to be addressed in the study, identifying related studies and research, figuring out how to design the survey to address the study's main objectives or hypotheses, and specifying the precise methods and procedures for carrying out the study and analyzing the data—*before* beginning to collect them—are critical for ensuring that the study will be carried out as it should be.

Using the prospectus or proposal as a way to specify as many of these aspects as possible beforehand also provides a solid foundation for the first draft of the final report. Documentation of formal specifications for the final report (such as format requirements for theses or government reports) should be obtained before writing the proposal. The investigator will then already have in hand materials that match what should be included in the final report in both form *and* substance.

A third criterion to have in mind when deciding what to include in a final research report is whether other investigators will be able to replicate the methods and results of the study or compare them with those obtained in their own or others' research. Both applied and basic research are best served by building on and extending previous research in the field and by replicating or disconfirming results across studies—provided that there is always a clear understanding of the similarities and differences in the design and methods of the different studies. Of course, full research reports provide a better opportunity to include comprehensive detail on how a survey was carried out than do working papers, articles, or research notes. However, even a short report should contain a clear description of the study's methodology. A useful question to keep in mind throughout the course of study is the following: Can I document and defend not only what I did but also how and why it differs from what was done in similar studies?

Outline of the Research Report

A working outline for a research report, along with references to the chapters in this book that can be useful in preparing it, are presented in Table 16.1. An executive summary of the methods and major findings for the study should appear at the beginning of the report. This summary should be written after all the other sections of the report have been drafted and there has been an opportunity to reflect on and identify the major findings and implications of the study. The summary must be written in a clear and concise manner because many readers will rely either heavily or exclusively on it to get an idea of how the study was carried out and what was learned from it. Executive summaries for books or monographs may be two or three pages in length. For articles, working papers, or theses, these summaries may have to be limited to abstracts or no more than 125 to 250 words.

Section I of the main body of the report should contain the *statement of the problem* to be addressed in the study. Chapter Two provides guidelines for phrasing researchable questions that can serve as the basis for an inquiry into a problem of interest to the investigator. Stating the problem at the beginning of the report aids the reader in understanding why the study was undertaken and what the researchers hoped to learn from it. A clear and concise statement of the problem requires that survey designers identify and read related research on the issue and integrate it into their own inquiry. The study objectives and hypotheses would be stated in this section after a case is made for the importance of addressing the topic.

What has been learned from other studies can be summarized in a formal *review of the literature,* that is, Section II of the report. Chapter One and Resources D and E provide an overview of sources and examples of health surveys that might be useful in compiling such a review. This review should not try to cover everything that has been written about the topic but it should make clear the current state of the art of research—both methodological and substantive—on the issue and how the question posed in the current study will contribute to fuller understanding of the issue.

Section III of the report should contain a description of the *methods* for the investigation of the problem under study. Thus, the methods section should include a description of the study design, sample design, data collection methods, questionnaire design, variable definitions and related measurement issues, the procedures for preparing the data for analysis, and the proposed analysis plan. Chapters Two through Fifteen (and particularly the tables and figures in those chapters) provide useful guidance for what to include in this section of the report.

Chapter Two provides an overview of relevant survey designs. The subsection on *study design* should describe the design and why it is a fitting one for addressing the study's objectives and hypotheses. A discussion of the *sample design* for the study, for instance, should include a description of the target population, sample frame, and sampling elements for the survey; the type of sample and how it was selected, including any procedures for oversampling certain subgroups; the sample size; response rates; procedures for weighting the data; standard errors and design effects for major estimates; and, when appropriate, a discussion of the magnitude of biases due to the noncoverage or nonresponse of certain groups and how these biases were dealt with in the analyses.

Another important subsection of the methods section of the report is a description of the *data collection* procedures employed in the study. This should include an overview of the principal data collection method used (paper-and-pencil or computer-assisted personal, telephone, or self-administered approach or some combination of these methods) and the pros and cons of the method for this particular study. The procedures for the pilot study and pretests of the instrument, the results of these trial runs, and how the questionnaire was modified in response to what was learned from them could be summarized in this section. The criteria and procedures for hiring, training, and supervising interviewers or other data collection personnel and following up and monitoring the fieldwork for the study should also be summarized in this section of the report.

A discussion of the *questionnaire design* would describe the sources for the questions in the questionnaire and the principles used in modifying them or formulating new ones. A section on *measurement* could present the operational and variable definitions and related summary indicators or scales used in measuring the major concepts of interest in the study as well as how the validity and reliability of these measures were evaluated.

Another important aspect of the survey to document in this section of the final report is the process of *data preparation*, that is, the procedures for translating the data into numerical codes, entering them into a computerized medium, cleaning and correcting them, and imputing or estimating information on key study variables.

A final subsection of the methods section should include a review of the *analysis plan*, containing a description of the statistical procedures to be used in analyzing the data and why they are appropriate given the study design; the level of measurement of survey variables; and the research questions and hypotheses that were addressed in the study. Researchers may want to incorporate the survey questionnaire and more extensive information on the methods used in carrying out the study into appendixes at the end of the report.

Section IV, the discussion of the *results* of the study, should come next, and here the researchers would find it helpful to consult Chapters Four and Fifteen of this book. The order and presentation of the findings in this section should be clearly related to the study objectives and hypotheses presented in Section I. If mock tables were prepared in formulating the analysis plan for the study, they can serve as the basis for selecting the tables to produce and include in the final report. The titles and headings used for the tables should fully describe their content. Conventions for numbering, punctuating, capitalizing, and formatting table titles and headings should be consistent *across* tables. The data reported in the tables should be double-checked against the computer runs on which they are based.

The text should be written so that readers do not have to refer constantly to the tables to understand the findings. At the same time, however, it should be clear where the data cited in the text come from in the tables. Tables can be placed either in the body of the text or at the end of the sections of the text in which they are described. Their placement depends on which approach would be more convenient for the reader, and on any formal requirements for the format of the final report.

The presentation and discussion of the findings in Section IV of the report should focus principally on describing the empirical results of the study. In the *conclusions* section—Section V—the researcher can be more speculative in discussing what these findings *mean:* how they relate to or extend previous research in the area; what the limitations and contributions of this particular study are in advancing research on the topic; what further research seems warranted; and what the particular theoretical, policy, or programmatic implications of the study are.

A list of the references cited in the report should follow the appendixes. The format for these references should be based on requirements specified by the funder, publisher, or thesis committee, as appropriate. The author should double-check that all references cited in the text appear in the list of references and that the correct spelling of the authors' names and dates of publication are used when cited.

An Overview of Survey Errors

Finally, when interpreting and presenting the final results of their study, health survey researchers should evaluate its overall strengths and limitations through a systematic review of the errors in the survey.

In the discussion that follows, the systematic and random errors that can be made at each stage of designing and conducting a health survey—all addressed in previous chapters—are summarized in the context of a total survey error approach to evaluating the overall quality of the survey.

Study Design

Decisions regarding when, with whom, or where the study was done may have major implications for the accuracy and generalizability of study findings. Assessments of analytical and experimental designs should consider their internal and external validity in particular. Might factors other than those that were hypothesized or intended account for observed outcomes and to what extent might the selectivity or artificiality of the research environment itself limit the broader applicability of what was learned? Suggestions could be provided with respect to the types of studies that are needed to address identified weaknesses. These issues are discussed in Chapter Two of this volume in particular.

Sample Design

Variable errors are always part of the sampling process for surveys because only a random subset of the entire group of interest for the study is selected. Standard errors are used to estimate the amount of variable (or sampling) error associated with samples of a certain size chosen in particular ways. Biases or systematic errors in sampling result when the basis used for sampling (phone numbers in a telephone directory, for example) means that certain groups will be left out (people with unlisted numbers or new phones), so that the statistics based on the sample will always be different from the "true" picture for the population of interest (people with phones). These and other sources of errors during the sampling process, as well as the methods for dealing with them, are discussed in Chapters Six and Seven.

Estimates of the standard errors and design effects for the survey, as well as the basis for evaluating the statistical significance of study findings, should be reported. Any problems with noncoverage or nonresponse biases in the data should also be discussed. When possible, comparisons of the distributions should be made with other data sources to estimate the possible magnitude of these biases, and response-rate and poststratification weighting procedures should be applied.

Data Collection

Response effects are biases or variable errors that can result from the data collection tasks themselves (problems with the questionnaire or method of data collection chosen) or from certain behaviors on the part of the interviewer or respondent. For example, researchers may vary the phrasing of a question for different respondents or respondents may answer the question the way that they think the interviewer wants them to answer it. These and other errors that can occur during the data collection planning and implementation stages of a survey, as well as ways to minimize them, are discussed in Chapters Eight through Thirteen.

Researchers should report any problems encountered in carrying out the fieldwork for the study that could give rise to variable or systematic response effects in the data.

Measurement

The classic approaches to estimating a systematic and variable error in defining the variables used in a survey are validity and reliability analyses, respectively (see Chapter Three). Measures of validity or bias assume that there is a "true" value (medical records, for example) against which the estimates obtained through the survey (respondent reports of the numbers of visits they made to their physician in the year) can be compared. Indexes of variable error or reliability measure the correspondence between repeated measures of comparable questions or procedures.

It may be difficult in some instances to determine whether a particular type of error reflects a bias or a variable error or to estimate bias when it is not clear what the "true" answers to certain types of items, such as attitudinal questions, actually are. However, the final report of the study should contain some discussion of the reliability and validity of the data gathered in the survey.

Data Preparation

Sources of bias and variable errors during the coding and processing of survey data and the ways to reduce them are described in Chapter Fourteen. Random errors can be made when the data are assigned numerical codes or entered into the computer. The checking procedures used to identify and correct data entry errors should be described. Correspondingly, biases can result if large numbers of certain types of people—those with very low incomes, for example—refuse to report this information when asked. The data imputation procedures used to reduce these errors and the substantive impact of making up these data should also be reported.

Analysis

Finally, the capstone for the survey undertaking is whether the data that are ultimately gathered adequately and accurately answer the questions that motivated their collection. The study objectives and hypotheses serve as the compass and the analyses the anchor for a well-planned survey.

This book provides a map for undertaking the journey.

RESOURCE A

PERSONAL INTERVIEW SURVEY: NATIONAL CENTER FOR HEALTH STATISTICS HEALTH INTERVIEW SURVEY, 1995

Resource A begins on the next page. The research for Resource A was supported by the National Center for Health Statistics, Centers for Disease Control and Prevention, Department of Health and Human Services. The data were collected in 1995 under the auspices of the Division of Health Interview Statistics (DHIS), National Center for Health Statistics (Owen T. Thornberry, DHIS).

Book ___ of ___ books	Batch number 3-7	RT 10	Coder status 8

OMB No. 0920-0214: Approval Expires 09/30/96

Notice – Information contained on this form which would permit identification of any individual or establishment has been collected with a guarantee that it will be held in strict confidence, will be used only for purposes stated for this study, and will not be disclosed or released to others without the consent of the individual or the establishment in accordance with section 308(d) of the Public Health Service Act (42 USC 242m). Public reporting burden for this collection of information is estimated to average 30 minutes per response including the time for reviewing instructions, searching existing data sources, gathering and maintaining the data needed, and completing and reviewing the collection of information. Send comments regarding this burden estimate or any other aspect of this collection of information, including suggestions for reducing this burden, to PHS Reports Clearance Officer, ATTN: PRA (0920-0214); Hubert H. Humphrey Building, Room 737-F, 200 Independence Avenue, SW; Washington, DC 20201.

1. RO 9-10	2. Sample 11-13 Suffix 14	3. Week 15-16	4. Segment type 1 ☐ Area 2 ☐ Permit

FORM HIS-1 (1995) (5-1-95)

U.S. DEPARTMENT OF COMMERCE
BUREAU OF THE CENSUS
ACTING AS COLLECTING AGENT FOR THE
U.S. DEPARTMENT OF HEALTH AND HUMAN SERVICES
PUBLIC HEALTH SERVICE

5. Control number

PSU 17-21	Segment 22-25	Suffix 26-27	Serial 28-29	Suffix 30	Check digit 31

6. Screening status 1 ☐ S 2 ☐ I   32

NATIONAL HEALTH INTERVIEW SURVEY

RT 11 3 S.T. (Item 4)

7a. What is your exact address? *(Including House No., Apt. No., or other identification; county and ZIP Code)*   4-8

9-119

LISTING SHEET

Sheet _____

City	State	County	ZIP Code

Line No. _____

b. Is this your mailing address? *(Mark box or specify if different; include county and ZIP Code)*   RT 12 4-83

☐ Same as 7a

City	State	County	ZIP Code

c. GQ name   84-117   Sample unit No. _____   Type code 118-120

8. YEAR BUILT (Area segments only)

☐ Ask *(Except for group quarters, mobile homes, trailers, tents, boats, and other units not in structures.)*
☐ Do not ask

When was this structure originally built?

☐ Before 4-1-90 *(Continue interview)*
☐ After 4-1-90 *(Complete 9c when required; END interview)*

9. COVERAGE QUESTIONS

☐ Ask items that are marked
☐ Do not ask

a. ☐ Are there any other living quarters — either occupied or vacant — in this building?   ☐ Yes *(Fill Table X)* ☐ No

b. ☐ Are there any other living quarters — either occupied or vacant — on this floor?   ☐ Yes *(Fill Table X)* ☐ No

c. ☐ Is there any other building, mobile home, or trailer — either occupied or vacant — on this property for people to live in?   ☐ Yes *(Fill Table X)* ☐ No

10a. LAND USE   35

1 ☐ URBAN *(11)*
2 ☐ RURAL
  – Reg. units and G.Q. units coded 92-N or 93-N in 7c – Ask item 10b
  – GQ units not coded 92-N or 93-N in 7c – Mark "No" in item 10b without asking

b. During the past 12 months, did sales of crops, livestock, and other farm products from this place amount to $1,000 or more?

1 ☐ Yes *(11)*
2 ☐ No   34

11. CLASSIFICATION OF LIVING QUARTERS – Mark by observation

a. LOCATION of unit   35   **b. Access**   36

Unit is:

1 ☐ In Group Quarters – *Refer to GQ Table on pages 4-7 through 4-15 of the 11-8, FR Listing and Coverage Manual; then complete 11c or d*
2 ☐ NOT in Group Quarters *(11b)*

1 ☐ Direct *(11c)*
2 ☐ Through another unit – *Not a separate HU; combine with unit through which access is gained. (Apply merged unit procedures if additional living quarters space was listed separately.)*

c. HOUSING unit *(Mark one)*   37-38

01 ☐ House, apartment, flat
02 ☐ HU in nontransient hotel, motel, etc.
03 ☐ HU-permanent in transient hotel, motel, etc.
04 ☐ HU in rooming house
05 ☐ Mobile home or trailer with no permanent room added
06 ☐ Mobile home or trailer with one or more permanent rooms added
07 ☐ HU not specified above – *Describe*

d. GROUP QUARTERS (GQ) unit *(Mark one)*

08 ☐ Quarters not HU in rooming or boarding house
09 ☐ Unit not permanent in transient hotel, motel, etc.
10 ☐ Unoccupied site for mobile home, trailer, or tent
11 ☐ Student quarters in college dormitory
12 ☐ GQ unit not specified above – *Describe*

12a. What is the telephone number here?   39   Area code/number   40-49

☐ None

b. Is there any working telephone located INSIDE your home?   50   1 ☐ Yes 2 ☐ No

13. Interview observed?   51   1 ☐ Yes 2 ☐ No

14a. Field representative's name   Code 52-53

b. Language of interview   54
1 ☐ English 3 ☐ Both English and Spanish
2 ☐ Spanish 8 ☐ Other

---

15. Neighbor screening results *(Mark if "S" in item 6)*   55

0 ☐ Neighbors not contacted
1 ☐ Screened out by neighbors
2 ☐ Eligible per neighbor
3 ☐ Undetermined by neighbors

16. Noninterview reason   56-57 58

TYPE A

01 ☐ Refused
02 ☐ No one home, repeated calls
03 ☐ Temporarily absent
04 ☐ Language problem
05 ☐ Other *(Specify)*

Indicate best estimate of race/ethnicity for each Type A

1 ☐ Black/Hispanic
2 ☐ Not Black/Hispanic
3 ☐ Unknown

Fill items 1–7a, 8 and 10 as applicable; 11, 13–17.

TYPE B

06 ☐ Vacant, nonseasonal
07 ☐ Vacant, seasonal
08 ☐ Occupied entirely by URE
09 ☐ Occupied entirely by AF members
10 ☐ Occupied – screened out by household
11 ☐ Occupied – screened out by neighbors
12 ☐ Unfit or to be demolished
13 ☐ Under construction – not ready
14 ☐ Converted to temporary business or storage
15 ☐ Unoccupied site for mobile home, trailer, or tent
16 ☐ Permit granted – construction not started
17 ☐ Other *(Specify)*

Fill items 1–7a, 8–10 as applicable; 11, 13–17.

TYPE C

18 ☐ Unused line of listing sheet
19 ☐ Demolished
20 ☐ House or trailer moved
21 ☐ Outside segment boundaries
22 ☐ Converted to permanent business or storage
23 ☐ Merged
24 ☐ Condemned
25 ☐ Built after April 1, 1990
26 ☐ Other *(Specify)*

Fill items 1–7a, 9c if marked; 13–17, send inter-Comm.

RT 10   33

17. Record of calls   59-69

	Month	Date	Beginning time	Ending time	Completed Mark (X)
1		P	a.m. p.m.	a.m. p.m.	
		T			
2		P	a.m. p.m.	a.m. p.m.	
		T			
3		P	a.m. p.m.	a.m. p.m.	
		T			
4		P	a.m. p.m.	a.m. p.m.	
		T			
5		P	a.m. p.m.	a.m. p.m.	
		T			
6		P	a.m. p.m.	a.m. p.m.	
		T			

18. List column numbers of persons requiring callbacks, and indicate reason(s).   ☐ None   70-77

Person No.	S.S No.	Other	Person No.	S.S No.	Other

19. Record of additional contacts   78-81

	Month	Date	Beginning time	Ending time	Completed Person No.
1		P	a.m. p.m.	a.m. p.m.	
		T			
2		P	a.m. p.m.	a.m. p.m.	
		T			
3		P	a.m. p.m.	a.m. p.m.	
		T			
4		P	a.m. p.m.	a.m. p.m.	
		T			

☐ Old age ☐ Cov. ☐ In name

A. HOUSEHOLD COMPOSITION PAGE		**1**

1a. What are the names of all persons living or staying here? Start with the name of the person or one of the persons who owns or rents this home. Enter name in **REFERENCE PERSON** column.

1. First name | Mid. init. | Age
Last name | | Sex
| | 1 ☐ M
| | 2 ☐ F

b. What are the names of all other persons living or staying here? Enter names in columns.

If "Yes," enter names in columns

c. I have listed (read names). **Have I missed:**

	Yes	No
— any babies or small children?	☐	☐
— any lodgers, boarders, or persons you employ who live here?	☐	☐
— anyone who USUALLY lives here but is now away from home traveling or in a hospital?	☐	☐
— anyone else staying here?	☐	☐

2. Relationship **REFERENCE PERSON**

3. Date of birth
Month | Date | Year

HOSP.	WORK	RD	2-WK. DV
00 ☐ None	1 ☐ Wa	1 ☐ Yes	00 ☐ None
Number	2 ☐ Wb	2 ☐ No	Number

C1

d. Do all of the persons you have named usually live here? ☐ Yes (2)
☐ No (APPLY HOUSEHOLD MEMBERSHIP RULES. Delete nonhousehold members by an "X" from 1–C2 and enter reason.)

Probe if necessary:

C2

Does – – usually live somewhere else?

Ask for all persons beginning with column 2:

LA | RA | DV | INJ. | CL LTR | HS | COND.

2. What is – – relationship to (reference person)?

3. What is – – date of birth? (Enter date and age and mark sex.)

LA | RA | DV | INJ. | CL LTR | HS | COND.

REFERENCE PERIODS

LA | RA | DV | INJ. | CL LTR | HS | COND.

A1

2-WEEK PERIOD	LA RA DV INJ. CL LTR HS COND.
12-MONTH DATE	LA RA DV INJ. CL LTR HS COND.
13-MONTH HOSPITAL DATE	

A2 ASK CONDITION LIST _____ .

LA | RA | DV | INJ. | CL LTR | HS | COND.

A3 Refer to ages of all HH members.

A3 ☐ All persons 65 and over (5)
☐ Other (4a)

4a. Are any of the persons in this household now on full-time active duty with the armed forces?
☐ Yes (4b) ☐ No (5)

b. Who is this? Mark "AF member" box in person's column

4b. ☐ AF member

c. Anyone else?
☐ Yes (Reask 4b and c) ☐ No (4d)

Ask for each person with "AF member" box marked in 4b.

d. Where does – – usually live and sleep, here or somewhere else? Mark box in person's column.

4d. ☐ Living at home (Exclude from health questions)
☐ Not living at home (Delete from household by an "X" from 1–C2)

HAND CARD O.

5a. Are any of those groups – – National origin or ancestry? (Where did – – ancestors come from?)

5a. 1 ☐ Yes (5b)
2 ☐ No (NP)

b. Please give me the number of the group. Circle all that apply.

b.

1 – Puerto Rican	3 – Mexican/Mexicano	5 – Chicano	7 – Other Spanish
2 – Cuban	4 – Mexican American	6 – Other Latin American	

1 2 3 4 5 6 7

HAND CARD R. Ask first alternative for first person; ask second alternative for other persons.

6a. What is the number of the group or groups which represents – – race?]
[**What is – – race?**

Circle all that apply. ASIAN OR PACIFIC ISLANDER (API)

1 – White	4 – Eskimo	6 – Chinese	10 – Vietnamese	14 – Guamanian
2 – Black/African American	5 – Aleut	7 – Filipino	11 – Japanese	15 – Other API – Specify
3 – Indian (American)		8 – Hawaiian	12 – Asian Indian	16 – Other race – Specify
		9 – Korean	13 – Samoan	

6a. 1 2 3 4 5 6 7 8 9
10 11 12 13 14 15⤲ 16⤲

_____
(Specify)

Ask if multiple entries in 6a:

b. Which of those groups, that is, (entries in 6a) **would you say BEST represents – – race?**

b. 1 2 3 4 5 6 7 8 9
10 11 12 13 14 15⤲ 16⤲

_____
(Specify)

c. Mark observed race of respondent(s) only.

c. 1 ☐ W 2 ☐ B 3 ☐ O

A4 Refer to item 6 "Status" on the Household Page.

A4 ☐ G (Item A5)
☐ I (Next page)

A5 Refer to 5a and 6a above for all household members. Mark (X) first appropriate box.

A5 ☐ Any "Yes" in 5a (Next page)
☐ Any "2" in 6a (Next page)
☐ All others (7)

7. Enter person number of the respondent and then read:

Not every household in our survey is asked all questions. I have all the information about your household that I need at this time.

END INTERVIEW

Person number _____
Respondent _____

INTRODUCTION AND HOSPITAL PROBE

If related persons 17 and over are listed in addition to the respondent and are not present, say:
We would like to have all adult family members who are at home take part in the interview. Are *(names of persons 17 and over)* **at home now?** *If "Yes," ask:* **Could they join us?** *(Allow time)*

Read to respondent(s):   **This survey is being conducted to collect information on the nation's health. I will ask about hospitalizations, disability, visits to doctors, illness in the family, and other health related items.**

HOSPITAL PROBE

1a. Since *(13-month hospital date)* a year ago, was – – a patient in a hospital OVERNIGHT?	**1a.**	1 ☐ Yes *(1b)* 2 ☐ No *(Mark "HOSP." box, THEN NP)*
b. How many different times did – – stay in any hospital overnight or longer since *(13-month hospital date)* a year ago?	**b.**	_____ Number of times } *(Make entry in "HOSP." box THEN NP)*
Ask for each child under one: **2a.** Was – – born in a hospital?	**2a.**	1 ☐ Yes *(2b)* 2 ☐ No *(NP)*
Ask for mother and child: **b.** Have you included this hospitalization in the number you gave me for – –?	**b.**	1 ☐ Yes *(NP)* 2 ☐ No *(Correct 1 and "HOSP." box)*

FOOTNOTES

B. LIMITATION OF ACTIVITIES PAGE

B1	Refer to age.	**B1**	1 ☐ 18–69 (1) 2 ☐ Other (NP)
1.	**What was – – doing MOST OF THE PAST 12 MONTHS; working at a job or business, keeping house, going to school, or something else?** Priority if 2 or more activities reported: (1) Spent the most time doing; (2) Considers the most important.	**1.**	1 ☐ Working (2) 2 ☐ Keeping house (3) 3 ☐ Going to school (5) 4 ☐ Something else (5)
2a.	**Does any impairment or health problem NOW keep – – from working at a job or business?**	**2a.**	1 ☐ Yes (7) ☐ No
b.	**Is – – limited in the kind OR amount of work – – can do because of any impairment or health problem?**	**b.**	2 ☐ Yes (7) 3 ☐ No (6)
3a.	**Does any impairment or health problem NOW keep – – from doing any housework at all?**	**3a.**	4 ☐ Yes (4) ☐ No
b.	**Is – – limited in the kind OR amount of housework – – can do because of any impairment or health problem?**	**b.**	5 ☐ Yes (4) 6 ☐ No (5)
4a.	**What (other) condition causes this?** Ask if injury or operation: **When did [the** (injury) **occur?/ – – have the operation?]** Ask if operation over 3 months ago: **For what condition did – – have the operation?** If pregnancy/delivery or 0–3 months injury or operation – Reask question 3 where limitation reported, saying: **Except for – –** (condition), . . .? On reask 4b/c.	**4a.**	(Enter condition in C2, THEN 4b) 1 ☐ Old age (Mark "Old age" box, THEN 4c)
b.	**Besides** (condition) **is there any other condition that causes this limitation?**	**b.**	☐ Yes (Reask 4a and b) ☐ No (4d)
c.	**Is this limitation caused by any (other) specific condition?**	**c.**	☐ Yes (Reask 4a and b) ☐ No
	Mark box if only one condition.	**d.**	☐ Only 1 condition
d.	**Which of these conditions would you say is the MAIN cause of this limitation?**		_____ Main cause
5a.	**Does any impairment or health problem keep – – from working at a job or business?**	**5a.**	1 ☐ Yes (7) ☐ No
b.	**Is – – limited in the kind OR amount of work – – could do because of any impairment or health problem?**	**b.**	2 ☐ Yes (7) 3 ☐ No
B2	Refer to questions 3a and 3b.	**B2**	1 ☐ "Yes" in 3a or 3b (NP) 2 ☐ Other (6)
6a.	**Is – – limited in ANY WAY in any activities because of an impairment or health problem?**	**6a.**	1 ☐ Yes ☐ No (NP)
b.	**In what way is – – limited?** Record limitation, not condition.	**b.**	_____ Limitation
7a.	**What (other) condition causes this?** Ask if injury or operation: **When did [the** (injury) **occur?/ – – have the operation?]** Ask if operation over 3 months ago: **For what condition did – – have the operation?** If pregnancy/delivery or 0–3 months injury or operation – Reask question 2, 5, or 6 where limitation reported, saying: **Except for – –** (condition), . . .? OR reask 7b/c.	**7a.**	(Enter condition in C2, THEN 7b) 1 ☐ Old age (Mark "Old age" box, THEN 7c)
b.	**Besides** (condition) **is there any other condition that causes this limitation?**	**b.**	☐ Yes (Reask 7a and b) ☐ No (7d)
c.	**Is this limitation caused by any (other) specific condition?**	**c.**	☐ Yes (Reask 7a and b) ☐ No
	Mark box if only one condition.	**d.**	☐ Only 1 condition
d.	**Which of these conditions would you say is the MAIN cause of this limitation?**		_____ Main cause

B. LIMITATION OF ACTIVITIES PAGE, Continued

B3	*Refer to age.*	**B3**	0 ☐ Under 5 *(10)* 2 ☐ 18–69 *(NP)* 1 ☐ 5–17 *(11)* 3 ☐ 70 and over *(8)*

8. What was – – doing MOST OF THE PAST 12 MONTHS; working at a job or business, keeping house, going to school, or something else?
Priority if 2 or more activities reported: (1) Spent the most time doing; (2) Considers the most important.

8.
1 ☐ Working
2 ☐ Keeping house
3 ☐ Going to school
4 ☐ Something else

9a. Because of any impairment or health problem, does – – need the help of other persons with – – personal care needs, such as eating, bathing, dressing, or getting around this home?

9a. 1 ☐ Yes *(13)* ☐ No

b. Because of any impairment or health problem, does – – need the help of other persons in handling – – routine needs, such as everyday household chores, doing necessary business, shopping, or getting around for other purposes?

b. 2 ☐ Yes *(13)* 3 ☐ No *(12)*

10a. Is – – able to take part AT ALL in the usual kinds of play activities done by most children – – age?

10a. ☐ Yes 0 ☐ No *(13)*

b. Is – – limited in the kind OR amount of play activities – – can do because of any impairment or health problem?

b. 1 ☐ Yes *(13)* 2 ☐ No *(12)*

11a. Does any impairment or health problem NOW keep – – from attending school?

11a. 1 ☐ Yes *(13)* ☐ No

b. Does – – attend a special school or special classes because of any impairment or health problem?

b. 2 ☐ Yes *(13)* ☐ No

c. Does – – need to attend a special school or special classes because of any impairment or health problem?

c. 3 ☐ Yes *(13)* ☐ No

d. Is – – limited in school attendance because of – – health?

d. 4 ☐ Yes *(13)* 5 ☐ No

12a. Is – – limited in ANY WAY in any activities because of an impairment or health problem?

12a. 1 ☐ Yes 2 ☐ No *(NP)*

b. In what way is – – limited?   *Record limitation, not condition.*

b.
_____
Limitation

13a. What (other) condition causes this?
Ask if injury or operation: When did [the (injury) occur?/ – – have the operation?]
Ask if operation over 3 months ago: For what condition did – – have the operation?
If pregnancy/delivery or 0–3 months injury or operation —
  Reask question where limitation reported, saying: Except for – – (condition), . . .?
  OR reask 13b/c.

13a. *(Enter condition in C2, THEN 13b)*
1 ☐ Old age *(Mark "Old age" box, THEN 13c)*

b. Besides *(condition)* is there any other condition that causes this limitation?

b. ☐ Yes *(Reask 13a and b)*
☐ No *(13d)*

c. Is this limitation caused by any (other) specific condition?

c. ☐ Yes *(Reask 13a and b)*
☐ No

Mark box if only one condition.
d. Which of these conditions would you say is the MAIN cause of this limitation?

d. ☐ Only 1 condition
_____
Main cause

FOOTNOTES

FORM HIS-1 (5-1-95)

	B. LIMITATION OF ACTIVITIES PAGE, Continued		
B4	*Refer to age.*	**B4**	0 ☐ Under 5 *(NP)* 2 ☐ 60–69 *(14)* 1 ☐ 5–59 *(B5)* 3 ☐ 70 and over *(NP)*
B5	*Refer to "Old age" and "LA" boxes. Mark first appropriate box.*	**B5**	☐ "Old age" box marked *(14)* ☐ Entry in "LA" box *(14)* ☐ Other *(NP)*
14a.	**Because of any impairment or health problem, does – – need the help of other persons with – – personal care needs, such as eating, bathing, dressing, or getting around this home?** *If under 18, skip to next person; otherwise ask:*	**14a.**	1 ☐ Yes *(15)* ☐ No
b.	**Because of any impairment or health problem, does – – need the help of other persons in handling – – routine needs, such as everyday household chores, doing necessary business, shopping, or getting around for other purposes?**	**b.**	2 ☐ Yes *(15)* 3 ☐ No *(NP)*

15a.	**What (other) condition causes this?**
	Ask if injury or operation: **When did [the** *(injury)* **occur?/ – – have the operation?]**
	Ask if operation over 3 months ago: **For what condition did – – have the operation?**
	If pregnancy/delivery or 0–3 months injury or operation —
	   Reask question 14 where limitation reported, saying: **Except for – –** *(condition),* **. . .?**
	   OR reask 15b/c.
		15a.	*(Enter condition in C2, THEN 15b)*
			
			1 ☐ Old age *(Mark "Old age" box,
			THEN 15c)*

b.	**Besides** *(condition)* **is there any other condition that causes this limitation?**	**b.**	☐ Yes *(Reask 15a and b)* ☐ No *(15d)*
c.	**Is this limitation caused by any (other) specific condition?**	**c.**	☐ Yes *(Reask 15a and b)* ☐ No
d.	*Mark box if only one condition.* **Which of these conditions would you say is the MAIN cause of this limitation?**	**d.**	☐ Only 1 condition Main cause

FOOTNOTES

   FORM HIS 1 (5-1-95)

D. RESTRICTED ACTIVITY PAGE   PERSON 1

Hand calendar.

{The next questions refer to the 2 weeks outlined in red on that calendar, beginning Monday, *(date)* and ending this past Sunday *(date)*.}

D1 *Refer to age.*
☐ Under 5 *(4)*   ☐ 5–17 *(3)*   ☐ 18 and over *(1)*

1a. DURING THOSE 2 WEEKS, did – – work at any time at a job or business not counting work around the house? (Include unpaid work in the family [farm/business].)

1 ☐ Yes *(Mark "Wa" box, THEN 2)*   2 ☐ No

b. Even though – – did not work during those 2 weeks, did – – have a job or business?

1 ☐ Yes *(Mark "Wb" box, THEN 2)*   2 ☐ No *(4)*

2a. During those 2 weeks, did – – miss any time from a job or business because of illness or injury?

☐ Yes   00 ☐ No *(4)*

b. During that 2-week period, how many days did – – miss more than half of the day from – – job or business because of illness or injury?

00 ☐ None *(4)*   [No. of work-loss days]   *(4)*

3a. During those 2 weeks, did – – miss any time from school because of illness or injury?

☐ Yes   00 ☐ No *(4)*

b. During that 2-week period, how many days did – – miss more than half of the day from school because of illness or injury?

00 ☐ None   [No. of school-loss days]

4a. During those 2 weeks, did – – stay in bed because of illness or injury?

☐ Yes   00 ☐ No *(6)*

b. During that 2-week period, how many days did – – stay in bed more than half of the day because of illness or injury?

00 ☐ None *(6)*   [No. of bed days]   *(D2)*

D2 *Refer to 2b and 3b.*
☐ No days in 2b or 3b *(6)*
☐ 1 or more days in 2b or 3b *(5)*

5. On how many of the *(number in 2b or 3b)* days missed from [work/school] did – – stay in bed more than half of the day because of illness or injury?

00 ☐ None   _____
No. of days

Refer to 2b, 3b, and 4b.

6a. (Not counting the day(s) [missed from work / missed from school / (and) in bed] **),**

Was there any (OTHER) time during those 2 weeks that – – cut down on the things – – usually does because of illness or injury?

☐ Yes   00 ☐ No *(D3)*

b. (Again, not counting the day(s) [missed from work / missed from school / (and) in bed] **),**

During that period, how many (OTHER) days did – – cut down for more than half of the days because of illness or injury?

00 ☐ None   [No. of cut-down days]

D3 *Refer to 2–6.*
☐ No days in 2–6 *(Mark "No" in RD, THEN NP)*
☐ 1 or more days in 2–6 *(Mark "Yes" in RD, THEN 7)*

Refer to 2b, 3b, 4b, and 6b.

7a. What (other) condition caused – – to [miss work / miss school / (or) stay in bed / (or) cut down] **during those 2 weeks?**

(Enter condition in C2, THEN 7b)

b. Did any other condition cause – – to [miss work / miss school / (or) stay in bed / (or) cut down] **during that period?**

1 ☐ Yes *(Reask 7a and b)*   2 ☐ No

FOOTNOTES

     FORM HIS-1 (5-1-95)

E. 2-WEEK DOCTOR VISITS PROBE PAGE	
Read to respondent: **These next questions are about health care received during the 2 weeks outlined in red on that calendar.**	

E1	*Refer to age.*	**E1**	☐ Under 14 *(1b)* ☐ 14 and over *(1a)*
1a. During those 2 weeks, how many times did – – see or talk to a medical doctor? (Include all types of doctors, such as dermatologists, psychiatrists, and ophthalmologists, as well as general practitioners and osteopaths.) (Do not count times while an overnight patient in a hospital.) **b. During those 2 weeks, how many times did anyone see or talk to a medical doctor about – –? (Do not count times while an overnight patient in a hospital.)**		**1a. and b.**	00 ☐ None ┌────────┐ │ │ *(NP)* └────────┘ Number of times
2a. (Besides the time(s) you just told me about) During those 2 weeks, did anyone in the family receive health care at home or go to a doctor's office, clinic, hospital or some other place? Include care from a nurse or anyone working with or for a medical doctor. Do not count times while an overnight patient in a hospital. ☐ Yes ☐ No *(3a)*			
b. Who received this care? *Mark "DR Visit" box in person's column.*		**2b.**	☐ DR Visit
c. Anyone else? ☐ Yes *(Reask 2b and c)* ☐ No			
Ask for each person with "DR Visit" in 2b: **d. How many times did – – receive this care during that period?**		**d.**	┌────────┐ │ │ └────────┘ Number of times
3a. (Besides the time(s) you already told me about) During those 2 weeks, did anyone in the family get any medical advice, prescriptions or test results over the PHONE from a doctor, nurse, or anyone working with or for a medical doctor? ☐ Yes ☐ No *(E2)*			
b. Who was the phone call about? *Mark "Phone call" box in person's column.*		**3b.**	☐ Phone call
c. Were there any calls about anyone else? ☐ Yes *(Reask 3b and c)* ☐ No			
Ask for each person with "Phone call" in 3b: **d. How many telephone calls were made about – –?**		**d.**	┌────────┐ │ │ └────────┘ Number of calls

E2	*Add numbers in 1, 2d, and 3d for each person. Record total number of visits and calls in "2-WK. DV" box in Item C1.*

FOOTNOTES

F. 2-WEEK DOCTOR VISITS PAGE	DR VISIT 1

	Refer to C1, "2-WK. DV" box.		**PERSON NUMBER** _____
F1	*Refer to age.*	**F1**	☐ Under 14 *(1b)* ☐ 14 and over *(1a)*
1a.	On what (other) date(s) during those 2 weeks did -- see or talk to a medical doctor, nurse, or doctor's assistant?	**1a.** **and**	
b.	On what (other) date(s) during those 2 weeks did anyone see or talk to a medical doctor, nurse, or doctor's assistant about --?	**b.**	_____ _____ OR { 7777 ☐ Last week Month Date 8888 ☐ Week before
	Ask after last DR visit column for this person:		
c.	Were there any other visits or calls for -- during that period? *Make necessary correction to 2-Wk. DV box in C1.*	**c.**	1 ☐ Yes *(Reask 1a or b and c)* 2 ☐ No *(Ask 2-6 for each visit)*
2.	Where did -- receive health care on *(date in 1)*, at a doctor's office, clinic, hospital, some other place, or was this a telephone call?	**2.**	01 ☐ Telephone
			Not in hospital: **Hospital**
	If doctor's office: Was this office in a hospital? *If hospital:* Was it the outpatient clinic or the emergency room? *If clinic:* Was it a hospital outpatient clinic, a company clinic, a public health clinic, or some other kind of clinic? *If lab:* Was this lab in a hospital? What was done during this visit? *(Footnote)*		02 ☐ Home 08 ☐ O. P. clinic 03 ☐ Doctor's office 09 ☐ Emergency room 04 ☐ Co. or Ind. clinic 10 ☐ Doctor's office 05 ☐ Other clinic 11 ☐ Lab 06 ☐ Lab 12 ☐ Overnight patient *(6)* 07 ☐ Other *(Specify)* ↗ 88 ☐ Other *(Specify)* ↗
	Ask 3b if under 14.	**3a.** **and** **b.**	
3a.	Did -- actually talk to a medical doctor?		1 ☐ Yes *(3f)* 8 ☐ DK if M.D. *(3c)*
b.	Did anyone actually talk to a medical doctor about --?		2 ☐ No *(3c)* 9 ☐ DK who was seen *(3f)*
c.	What type of medical person or assistant was talked to?	**c.**	_____ 99 ☐ DK Type
d.	Does the *(entry in 3c)* work with or for ONE doctor or MORE than one doctor?	**d.**	1 ☐ One *(3f)* 2 ☐ More 3 ☐ None *(4)* 9 ☐ DK
e.	For this [visit/call] what kind of doctor was the *(entry in 3c)* working with or for — a general practitioner or specialist?	**e.** **and** **f.**	1 ☐ GP *(4)* 2 ☐ Specialist *(3g)* 9 ☐ DK *(4)*
f.	Is that doctor a general practitioner or a specialist?		
g.	What kind of specialist?	**g.**	_____ Kind of specialist
	Ask 4b if under 14.	**4a.** **and** **b.**	1 ☐ Condition *(Item C2, THEN 4g)* 2 ☐ Pregnancy *(4e)*
4a.	For what condition did -- see or talk to the [doctor/*(entry in 3c)*] on *(date in 1)*? *Mark first appropriate box.*		3 ☐ Test(s) or examination *(4c)* 8 ☐ Other *(Specify)* ↗
b.	For what condition did anyone see or talk to the [doctor/*(entry in 3c)*] about -- on *(date in 1)*? *Mark first appropriate box.*		_____ *(4g)*
c.	Was a condition found as a result of the [test(s)/examination]?	**c.**	☐ Yes *(4h)* ☐ No
d.	Was this [test/examination] because of a specific condition -- had?	**d.**	☐ Yes *(4h)* ☐ No *(4g)*
e.	During the past 2 weeks was -- sick because of her pregnancy?	**e.**	☐ Yes ☐ No *(4g)*
f.	What was the matter?	**f.**	_____ *(Item C2, THEN 4g)* Condition
g.	During this [visit/call] was the [doctor/*(entry in 3c)*] talked to about any (other) condition?	**g.**	☐ Yes ☐ No *(5)*
h.	What was the condition?	**h.**	☐ Pregnancy *(4e)* _____ *(Item C2, THEN 4g)* Condition
	Mark box if "Telephone" in 2.	**5a.**	0 ☐ Telephone in 2 1 ☐ Yes 2 ☐ No *(6)*
5a.	Did -- have any kind of surgery or operation during this visit, including bone settings and stitches?		*(Next Dr. visit)*
b.	What was the name of the surgery or operation? *If name of operation not known, describe what was done.*	**b.**	(1) _____ (2) _____
c.	Was there any other surgery or operation during this visit?	**c.**	☐ Yes *(Reask 5b and c)* ☐ No
	Go to next DV if "Home" in 2.	**6.**	City/County _____ / ___ State/ZIP Code _____ / ___
6.	In what city (town), county, and State is the *(place in 2)* located?		

G. HEALTH INDICATOR PAGE

1a. During the 2-week period outlined in red on that calendar, has anyone in the family had an injury from an accident or other cause that you have not yet told me about?

☐ Yes   ☐ No *(2)*

b. Who was this? *Mark "Injury" box in person's column.*

1b. ☐ Injury

c. What was – – injury?
Enter injury(ies) in person's column.

c.

_____
Injury

d. Did anyone have any other injuries during that period?

☐ Yes *(Reask 1b, c, and d)*   ☐ No

Ask for each injury in 1c:

e. As a result of the *(injury in 1c)* **did [– – /anyone] see or talk to a medical doctor or assistant (about – –) or did – – cut down on – – usual activities for more than half of a day?**

e. ☐ Yes *(Enter injury in C2, THEN 1e for next injury)*
☐ No *(1e for next injury)*

---

2. During the past 12 months, {that is, since *(12-month date)* **a year ago} ABOUT how many days did illness or injury keep – – in bed more than half of the day? (Include days while an overnight patient in a hospital.)**

2. 000 ☐ None

_____ No. of days

3a. During the past 12 months, ABOUT how many times did [– – /anyone] see or talk to a medical doctor or assistant (about – –)? (Do not count doctors seen while an overnight patient in a hospital.) (Include the *(number in 2-WK DV box)* **visit(s) you already told me about.)**

3a. 000 ☐ None *(3b)*
000 ☐ Only when overnight patient in hospital   } *(NP)*

_____ No. of visits

b. About how long has it been since [– – /anyone] last saw or talked to a medical doctor or assistant (about – –)? Include doctors seen while a patient in a hospital.

b. 1 ☐ Interview week *(Reask 3b)*
2 ☐ Less than 1 yr. *(Reask 3a)*
3 ☐ 1 yr., less than 2 yrs.
4 ☐ 2 yrs., less than 5 yrs.
5 ☐ 5 yrs. or more
0 ☐ Never

---

4. Would you say – – health in general is excellent, very good, good, fair, or poor?

4. 1 ☐ Excellent   4 ☐ Fair
2 ☐ Very good   5 ☐ Poor
3 ☐ Good

Mark box if under 18.
5a. About how tall is – – without shoes?

5a. ☐ Under 18 *(NP)*

_____ Feet _____ Inches

b. About how much does – – weigh without shoes?

b.

_____ Pounds

FOOTNOTES

H. CONDITION LISTS 1 AND 2

Read to respondent(s) and ask list specified in A2:
Now I am going to read a list of medical conditions. Tell me if anyone in the family has had any of these conditions, even if you have mentioned them before.

1a. Does anyone in the family *(read names)* **NOW HAVE —** *If "Yes," ask 1b and c.*	**2a. Does anyone in the family** *(read names)* **NOW HAVE —** *If "Yes," ask 2b and c.*
b. Who is this?	**b. Who is this?**
c. Does anyone else NOW have — *Enter condition and letter in appropriate person's column.*	**c. Does anyone else NOW have —** *Enter condition and letter in appropriate person's column.*

1

A. PERMANENT stiffness or any deformity of the foot, leg, fingers, arm, or back? *(Permanent stiffness — joints will not move at all.)*

B. Paralysis of any kind?

1d. DURING THE PAST 12 MONTHS, did anyone in the family have — *If "Yes," ask 1e and f.*

e. Who is this?

f. DURING THE PAST 12 MONTHS, did anyone else have —
Enter condition and letter in appropriate person's column.
C–L are conditions affecting the bone and muscle.
M–W are conditions affecting the skin.

	Reask 1d.
C. Arthritis of any kind or rheumatism?	**M. A tumor, cyst, or growth of the skin?**
D. Gout?	**N. Skin cancer?**
E. Lumbago?	**O. Eczema or Psoriasis?** (ek'sa-ma) or (so-rye'uh-sis)
F. Sciatica?	**P. TROUBLE with dry or itching skin?**
G. A bone cyst or bone spur?	**Q. TROUBLE with acne?**
H. Any other disease of the bone or cartilage?	**R. A skin ulcer?**
I. A slipped or ruptured disc?	**S. Any kind of skin allergy?**
J. REPEATED trouble with neck, back, or spine?	**T. Dermatitis or any other skin trouble?**
K. Bursitis?	**U. TROUBLE with ingrown toenails or fingernails?**
L. Any disease of the muscles or tendons?	**V. TROUBLE with bunions, corns, or calluses?**
	W. Any disease of the hair or scalp?

2

A–L are conditions affecting { Hearing / Vision / Speech }

Conditions M–AA are impairments.

	Reask 2a.
A. Deafness in one or both ears?	**O. A missing joint?**
B. Any other trouble hearing with one or both ears?	**P. A missing breast, kidney, or lung?**
C. Tinnitus or ringing in the ears?	**Q. Palsy or cerebral palsy? (ser'a-bral)**
D. Blindness in one or both eyes?	**R. Paralysis of any kind?**
E. Cataracts?	**S. Curvature of the spine?**
F. Glaucoma?	**T. REPEATED trouble with neck, back, or spine?**
G. Color blindness?	**U. Any TROUBLE with fallen arches or flatfeet?**
H. A detached retina or any other condition of the retina?	**V. A clubfoot?**
I. Any other trouble seeing with one or both eyes EVEN when wearing glasses?	**W. A trick knee?**
J. A cleft palate or harelip?	**X. PERMANENT stiffness or any deformity of the foot, leg, or back?** *(Permanent stiffness — joints will not move at all.)*
K. Stammering or stuttering?	**Y. PERMANENT stiffness or any deformity of the fingers, hand, or arm?**
L. Any other speech defect?	**Z. Mental retardation?**
M. Loss of taste or smell which has lasted 3 months or more?	**AA. Any condition caused by an accident or injury which happened more than 3 months ago?** *If " Yes," ask:* **What is the condition?**
N. A missing finger, hand, or arm; toe, foot, or leg?	

H. CONDITION LISTS 3 AND 4

Read to respondent(s) and ask list specified in A2:
Now I am going to read a list of medical conditions. Tell me if anyone in the family has had any of these conditions, even if you have mentioned them before.

3

3a. DURING THE PAST 12 MONTHS, did anyone in the family *(read names)* **have —** If **"Yes,"** ask 3b and c.

b. Who was this?

c. DURING THE PAST 12 MONTHS, did anyone else have —

Enter condition and letter in appropriate person's column.

Make no entry in item C2 for cold; flu; red, sore, or strep throat; or "virus" even if reported in this list.

Conditions affecting the digestive system.

A. Gallstones?	*Reask 3a.* N. Enteritis?
B. Any other gallbladder trouble?	O. Diverticulitis? (Dye-ver-tic-yoo-lye'tis)
C. Cirrhosis of the liver?	P. Colitis?
D. Fatty liver?	Q. A spastic colon?
E. Hepatitis?	R. FREQUENT constipation?
F. Yellow jaundice?	S. Any other bowel trouble?
G. Any other liver trouble?	T. Any other intestinal trouble?
H. An ulcer?	U. Cancer of the stomach, intestines, colon, or rectum?
I. A hernia or rupture?	
J. Any disease of the esophagus?	V. During the past 12 months, did anyone (else) in the family have any other condition of the digestive system?
K. Gastritis?	
L. FREQUENT indigestion?	*If "Yes," ask: Who was this? — What was the condition? Enter in item C2, THEN reask V.*
M. Any other stomach trouble?	

4

4a. DURING THE PAST 12 MONTHS, did anyone in the family *(read names)* **have —** If **"Yes,"** ask 4b and c.

b. Who was this?

c. DURING THE PAST 12 MONTHS, did anyone else have —

Enter condition and letter in appropriate person's column.

A–B are conditions affecting the glandular system.
C is a blood condition.
D–I are conditions affecting the nervous system.
J–Y are conditions affecting the genito-urinary system.

A. A goiter or other thyroid trouble?	*Reask 4a.* N. Any other kidney trouble?
B. Diabetes?	O. Bladder trouble?
C. Anemia of any kind?	P. Any disease of the genital organs?
D. Epilepsy?	Q. A missing breast?
E. REPEATED seizures, convulsions, or blackouts?	R. Breast cancer?
F. Multiple sclerosis?	S. * Cancer of the prostate?
G. Migraine?	T. * Any other prostate trouble?
H. FREQUENT headaches?	U. ** Trouble with menstruation?
I. Neuralgia or neuritis?	V. ** A hysterectomy? If "Yes," ask: For what condition did – – have a hysterectomy?
J. Nephritis?	W. ** A tumor, cyst, or growth of the uterus or ovaries?
K. Kidney stones?	X. ** Any other disease of the uterus or ovaries?
L. REPEATED kidney infections?	Y. **Any other female trouble?
M. A missing kidney?	*Ask only if males in family. **Ask only if females in family.

FORM HIS-1 (5-1-95)

H. CONDITION LISTS 5 AND 6

Read to respondent(s) and ask list specified in A2:
Now I am going to read a list of medical conditions. Tell me if anyone in the family has had any of these conditions, even if you have mentioned them before.

5

5a. Has anyone in the family *(read names)* **EVER had —**

If *"Yes,"* ask 5b and c.

b. Who was this?

c. Has anyone else EVER had —

Enter condition and letter in appropriate person's column.

Conditions affecting the heart and circulatory system.

A. Rheumatic fever?	**G. A stroke or a cerebrovascular accident? (ser'a-bro vas ku-lar)**
B. Rheumatic heart disease?	
C. Hardening of the arteries or arteriosclerosis?	**H. A hemorrhage of the brain?**
D. Congenital heart disease?	**I. Angina pectoris? (pek'to-ris)**
E. Coronary heart disease?	**J. A myocardial infarction?**
F. Hypertension, sometimes called high blood pressure?	**K. Any other heart attack?**

5d. DURING THE PAST 12 MONTHS, did anyone in the family have —

If *"Yes,"* ask 5e and f.

e. Who was this?

f. DURING THE PAST 12 MONTHS, did anyone else have —

Enter condition and letter in appropriate person's column.

Conditions affecting the heart and circulatory system.

L. Damaged heart valves?	**Q. Any blood clots?**
M. Tachycardia or rapid heart?	**R. Varicose veins?**
N. A heart murmur?	**S. Hemorrhoids or piles?**
O. Any other heart trouble?	**T. Phlebitis or thrombophlebitis?**
P. An aneurysm? (an yoo-rizm)	**U. Any other condition affecting blood circulation?**

6

6a. DURING THE PAST 12 MONTHS, did anyone in the family *(read names)* **have —**

If *"Yes,"* ask 6b and c.

b. Who was this?

c. DURING THE PAST 12 MONTHS, did anyone else have —

Enter condition and letter in appropriate person's column.

Make no entry in item C2 for cold; flu; red, sore, or strep throat; or "virus" even if reported in this list.

Conditions affecting the respiratory system.

	Reask 6a.
A. Bronchitis?	**K. A missing lung?**
B. Asthma?	**L. Lung cancer?**
C. Hay fever?	**M. Emphysema?**
D. Sinus trouble?	**N. Pleurisy?**
E. A nasal polyp?	**O. Tuberculosis?**
F. A deflected or deviated nasal septum?	**P. Any other work-related respiratory condition, such as dust on the lungs, silicosis, asbestosis, or pneu-mo-co-ni-o-sis?**
G. * Tonsilitis or enlargement of the tonsils or adenoids?	
H. * Laryngitis?	**Q. During the past 12 months did anyone (else) in the family have any other respiratory, lung, or pulmonary condition?** If *"Yes,"* ask: Who was this? — What was the condition? *Enter in item C2, THEN reask Q.*
I. A tumor or growth of the throat, larynx, or trachea?	
J. A tumor or growth of the bronchial tube or lung?	

*** If reported in this list only, ask:**

1. How many times did - - have *(condition)* **in the past 12 months?**

If 2 or more times, enter condition in item C2.

If only 1 time, ask:

2. How long did it last? *If 1 month or longer, enter in item C2.*

If less than 1 month, do not record.

If tonsils or adenoids were removed during past 12 months, enter the condition causing removal in item C2.

J. HOSPITAL PAGE	HOSPITAL STAY 1		
1. *Refer to C1, "HOSP." box.*	**1.** **PERSON NUMBER** _____		
2. **You said earlier that – – was a patient in the hospital since** *(13-month hospital date)* **a year ago. On what date did – – enter the hospital ([the last time/the time before that])?** *Record each entry date in a separate Hospital Stay column.*	**2.** Month	Date	Year 19 ___
3. **How many nights was – – in the hospital?**	**3.** 0000 ☐ None *(Next HS)* _____ Nights		
4. **For what condition did – – enter the hospital?** • *For delivery ask:* **Was this a normal delivery?** *If "No," ask:* **What was the matter?** • *For newborn ask:* **Was the baby normal at birth?** *If "No," ask:* **What was the matter?** • *For initial "No condition" ask:* **Why did – – enter the hospital?** • *For tests, ask:* **What were the results of the tests?** *If no results, ask:* **Why were the tests performed?**	**4.** 1 ☐ Normal delivery 2 ☐ Normal at birth 3 ☐ No condition ☐ Condition ↗ } (5) _____		
J1 *Refer to questions 2, 3, and 2-week reference period.*	**J1** ☐ At least one night in 2-week reference period *(Enter condition in C2, THEN 5)* ☐ No nights in 2-week reference period *(5)*		
5a. **Did – – have any kind of surgery or operation during this stay in the hospital, including bone settings and stitches?**	**5a.** 1 ☐ Yes 2 ☐ No *(6)*		
b. **What was the name of the surgery or operation?** *If name of operation not known, describe what was done.*	**b.** (1) _____ (2) _____ (3) _____		
c. **Was there any other surgery or operation during this stay?**	**c.** ☐ Yes *(Reask 5b and c)* ☐ No		
6. **What is the name and address of this hospital?**	**6.** Name Number and street City or County State		
FOOTNOTES			

FORM HIS-1 (5-1-95)

CONDITION 1	PERSON NO. ____

1. Name of condition

Mark "2-wk. ref. pd." box without asking if "DV" or "HS" in C2 as source.

2. When did [– –/anyone] last see or talk to a doctor or assistant about – – (condition)?

- 0 ☐ Interview week *(Reask 2)*
- 1 ☐ 2-wk. reference period
- 2 ☐ Over 2 weeks, less than 6 mos.
- 3 ☐ 6 mos., less than 1 yr.
- 4 ☐ 1 yr., less than 2 yrs.
- 5 ☐ 2 yrs., less than 5 yrs.
- 6 ☐ 5 yrs. or more
- 7 ☐ Dr. seen, DK when
- 8 ☐ DK if Dr. seen
- 9 ☐ Dr. never seen   } *(3b)*

3a. (Earlier you told me about – – (condition)) Did the doctor or assistant call the (condition) by a more technical or specific name?

- 1 ☐ Yes
- 2 ☐ No
- 9 ☐ DK

Ask 3b if "Yes" in 3a, otherwise transcribe condition name from item 1 without asking:

b. What did he or she call it? _____
(Specify)

- 1 ☐ Color Blindness *(NC)*
- 3 ☐ Normal pregnancy, normal delivery, vasectomy *(5)*
- 2 ☐ Cancer *(3e)*
- 4 ☐ Old age *(NC)*
- 8 ☐ Other *(3c)*

c. What was the cause of – – (condition in 3b)? *(Specify)* ↗

Mark box if accident or injury.   0 ☐ Accident/injury *(Probe, then 5)*

d. Did the (condition in 3b) result from an accident or injury?

Ask probes as necessary. Record responses in 3c:
- 1 ☐ Yes *(Probe, then 5)*   **(How did the accident happen?)**
- 2 ☐ No   **(What was – – doing at the time of the injury?)**

Ask 3e if the condition name in 3b includes any of the following words:

Ailment	Attack	Condition	Disease	Measles	Trouble
Anemia	Bad	Cyst	Disorder	Problem	Tumor
Asthma	Cancer	Defect	Growth	Rupture	Ulcer

e. What kind of (condition in 3b) is it? _____
(Specify)

Ask 3f only if allergy or stroke in 3b–e:

f. How does the [allergy/stroke] NOW affect – –? *(Specify)* ↗

For stroke, fill remainder of this condition page for the first present effect. Enter in item C2 and complete a separate condition page for each additional present effect.

Page 30

Ask 3g if there is an impairment (refer to Card CP2) or any of the following entries in 3b–f:

Abscess	Growth	Rupture
Ache (except head or ear)	Hemorrhage	Soreness)
Bleeding (except menstrual)	Infection	Stiff(ness)
Blood clot	Inflammation	Tumor
Boil	Neuralgia	Ulcer
Cancer	Neuritis	Varicose veins
Cramps (except menstrual)	Pain	Weak(ness)
Cyst	Palsy	
Damage	Paralysis	

g. What part of the body is affected? _____
(Specify)

Show the following detail:

Head	skull, scalp, face
Back/spine/vertebrae	upper, middle, lower
Side	left or right
Ear	inner or outer; left, right, or both
Eye	left, right, or both
Arm	shoulder, upper, elbow, lower or wrist; left, right, or both
Hand	entire hand or fingers only; left, right, or both
Leg	hip, upper, knee, lower, or ankle; left, right, or both
Foot	entire foot, arch, or toes only; left, right, or both

Except for eyes, ears, or internal organs, ask 3h if there are any of the following entries in 3b–f:

Infection	Sore	Soreness

h. What part of the (part of body in 3b–g) is affected by the [infection/sore/soreness] – the skin, muscle, bone, or some other part?

(Specify) _____

Ask if there are any of the following entries in 3b–f:

Tumor	Cyst	Growth

4. Is this [tumor/cyst/growth] malignant or benign?

- 1 ☐ Malignant
- 2 ☐ Benign
- 9 ☐ DK

5.
a. When was – – (condition in 3b/3f) first noticed?

b. When did – – (name of injury in 3b)?

- 1 ☐ 2-wk. ref. pd.
- 2 ☐ Over 2 weeks to 3 months
- 3 ☐ Over 3 months to 1 year
- 4 ☐ Over 1 year to 5 years
- 5 ☐ Over 5 years

Ask probes as necessary:

(Was it on or since (first date of 2-week ref. period) or was it before that date?)

(Was it less than 3 months or more than 3 months ago?)

(Was it less than 1 year or more than 1 year ago?)

(Was it less than 5 years or more than 5 years ago?)

K1

Refer to RD and C2.
1 ☐ "Yes" in "RD" box AND more than 1 condition in C2 *(6)*
8 ☐ Other *(K2)*

6a. **During the 2 weeks outlined in red on that calendar, did – –**
(condition) cause – – to cut down on the things – – usually does?

☐ Yes   ☐ No *(K2)*

b. **During that period, how many days did – – cut down for more**
than half of the day?

00 ☐ None *(K2)*   _____ Days

7. **During those 2 weeks, how many days did – – stay in bed for**
more than half of the day because of this condition?

00 ☐ None   _____ Days

Ask if "Wa/Wb" box marked in C1:
8. **During those 2 weeks, how many days did – – miss more than**
half of the day from – – job or business because of this condition?

00 ☐ None   _____ Days

Ask if age 5–17:
9. **During those 2 weeks, how many days did – – miss more than**
half of the day from school because of this condition?

00 ☐ None   _____ Days

K2

☐ Condition has "CL LTR" in C2 as source *(10)*
☐ Condition does not have "CL LTR" in C2 as source *(K4)*

10. **About how many days since (12-month date) a year ago, has this**
condition kept – – in bed more than half of the day? (Include
days while an overnight patient in a hospital.)

000 ☐ None   _____ Days

11. **Was – – ever hospitalized for – – (condition in 3b)?**

1 ☐ Yes   2 ☐ No

K3

☐ Missing extremity or organ *(K4)*
☐ Other *(12)*

12a. **Does – – still have this condition?**

1 ☐ Yes *(K4)*   2 ☐ No

b. **Is this condition completely cured or is it under control?**

2 ☐ Cured   8 ☐ Other *(Specify)* ↗
3 ☐ Under control *(K4)*

_____ *(K4)*

c. **About how long did – – have this condition before it was cured?**

000 ☐ Less than 1 month   **OR** _____   1 ☐ Months
                                    Number   2 ☐ Years

d. **Was this condition present at any time during the past 12 months?**

1 ☐ Yes   2 ☐ No

K4

0 ☐ Not an accident/injury *(NC)*
1 ☐ First accident/injury for this person *(14)*
8 ☐ Other *(13)*

13. **Is this (condition in 3b) the result of the same accident you**
already told me about?

☐ Yes *(Record condition page number where* → _____ *(NC)*
accident questions first completed.)   Page No.
☐ No

14. **Where did the accident happen?**

1 ☐ At home (inside house)
2 ☐ At home (adjacent premises)
3 ☐ Street and highway (includes roadway and public sidewalk)
4 ☐ Farm
5 ☐ Industrial place (includes premises) *(Specify)* _____
6 ☐ School (includes premises)
7 ☐ Place of recreation and sports, except at school
8 ☐ Other *(Specify)* ↗

Mark box if under 18.   ☐ Under 18 *(16)*

15a. **Was – – under 18 when the accident happened?**

1 ☐ Yes *(16)*   ☐ No

b. **Was – – in the Armed Forces when the accident happened?**

2 ☐ Yes *(16)*   ☐ No

c. **Was – – at work at – – job or business when the accident happened?**

3 ☐ Yes   4 ☐ No

16a. **Was a car, truck, bus, or other motor vehicle involved in the**
accident in any way?

1 ☐ Yes   2 ☐ No *(17)*

b. **Was more than one vehicle involved?**

1 ☐ Yes   2 ☐ No

c. **Was [it/either one] moving at the time?**

1 ☐ Yes   2 ☐ No

17a. **At the time of the accident what part of the body was hurt?**
What kind of injury was it?
Anything else?

Part(s) of body *	Kind of injury

Ask if box 3, 4, or 5 marked in Q. 5:
b. **What part of the body is affected now?**
How is – – (part of body) affected?
Is – – affected in any other way?

Part(s) of body *	Present effects **

* Enter part of body in same detail as for 3g.

** If multiple present effects, enter in C2 each one that is not the
same as 3b or C2 and complete a separate condition page for it.

L. DEMOGRAPHIC BACKGROUND PAGE

L1	Refer to age.	**L1**	☐ Under 5 *(NP)* ☐ 5–17 *(2)* ☐ 18 and over *(1)*
1a. Did – – EVER serve on active duty in the Armed Forces of the United States?		**1a.**	1 ☐ Yes *(1b)* 2 ☐ No *(2)*
b. When did – – serve? *Mark box in descending order of priority.* *Thus, if person served in Vietnam and in* *Korea mark VN.*	{ Vietnam Era (Aug. '64 to April '75) . . . . VN Korean War (June '50 to Jan. '55) . . . . KW World War II (Sept. '40 to July '47) . . . . WWII World War I (April '17 to Nov. '18) . . . . WWI Post Vietnam (May '75 to present) . . . . PVN Other Service (all other periods) . . . . OS	**b.**	1 ☐ VN 5 ☐ PVN 2 ☐ KW 8 ☐ OS 3 ☐ WWII 9 ☐ DK 4 ☐ WWI
c. Was – – **EVER an active member of a National Guard or military reserve unit?**		**c.**	☐ Yes 2 ☐ No *(2)* 7 ☐ DK *(2)*
d. Was ALL of – – **active duty service related to National Guard or military reserve training?**		**d.**	1 ☐ Yes 3 ☐ No 9 ☐ DK
2a. What is the highest grade or year of regular school – – **has ever attended?**		**2a.**	00 ☐ Never attended or kindergarten *(NP)* Elem: 1 2 3 4 5 6 7 8 High: 9 10 11 12 College: 1 2 3 4 5 6+
b. Did – – **finish the** <u>*(number in 2a)*</u> **[grade/year]?**		**b.**	1 ☐ Yes 2 ☐ No

FOOTNOTES

FORM HIS-1 (5-1-95)

L. DEMOGRAPHIC BACKGROUND PAGE, Continued

L2	*Refer to "Age" and "Wa/Wb" boxes in C1.*	**L2**	0 ☐ Under 18 *(NP)* 1 ☐ Wa box marked *(6a)* 2 ☐ Wb box marked *(5a)* 3 ☐ Neither box marked *(5b)*
5a.	**Earlier you said that – – has a job or business but did not work last week or the week before.** **Was – – looking for work or on layoff from a job during those 2 weeks?**	**5a.**	1 ☐ Yes *(5c)* 2 ☐ No *(6b)*
b.	**Earlier you said that – – didn't have a job or business last week or the week before.** **Was – – looking for work or on layoff from a job during those 2 weeks?**	**b.**	1 ☐ Yes 2 ☐ No *(NP)*
c.	**Which, looking for work or on layoff from a job?**	**c.**	1 ☐ Looking *(6c)* 3 ☐ Both *(6b)* 2 ☐ Layoff *(6b)*

6a.	**Earlier you said that – – worked last week or the week before.** *Ask 6b.*		
b.	**For whom did – – work?** *Enter name of company, business, organization, or other employer.*	**6b.** **and** **c.**	Employer ☐ NEV *(6g)* ☐ AF *(6e)*
c.	**For whom did – – work at – – last full-time job or business lasting 2 consecutive weeks or more?** *Enter name of company, business, organization, or other employer, or mark "NEV" or "AF" box in person's column.*		
d.	**What kind of business or industry is this?** *For example, TV and radio manufacturing, retail shoe store, State Labor Department, farm.*	**d.**	Industry
	If "AF" in 6b/c, mark "AF" box in person's column without asking.		Occupation ☐ AF *(NP)*
e.	**What kind of work was – – doing?** *For example, electrical engineer, stock clerk, typist, farmer.*	**e.**	
f.	**What were – – most important activities or duties at that job?** *For example, types, keeps account books, files, sells cars, operates printing press, finishes concrete.*	**f.**	Duties

	Complete from entries in 6b–f. If not clear, ask:		Class of worker
g.	**Was – –**	**g.**	1 ☐ P 5 ☐ I 2 ☐ F 6 ☐ SE 3 ☐ S 7 ☐ WP 4 ☐ L 8 ☐ NEV

Was – –

An employee of a PRIVATE company, business or individual for wages, salary, or commission?	**P**
A FEDERAL government employee?	**F**
A STATE government employee?	**S**
A LOCAL government employee?	**L**

Self-employed in OWN business, professional practice, or farm?	
Ask: Is the business incorporated?	
Yes	I
No	SE
Working WITHOUT PAY in family business or farm?	WP
— NEVER WORKED or never worked at a full-time job lasting 2 weeks or more	NEV

FOOTNOTES

L. DEMOGRAPHIC BACKGROUND PAGE, Continued

Mark box if under 14. If "Married" refer to household composition and mark accordingly.

7. Is -- now married, widowed, divorced, separated, or has -- never been married?

7.
- 0 ☐ Under 14
- 1 ☐ Married — spouse in HH
- 2 ☐ Married — spouse not in HH
- 3 ☐ Widowed
- 4 ☐ Divorced
- 5 ☐ Separated
- 6 ☐ Never married

8a. Was the total combined **FAMILY** income during the past 12 months — that is, yours, *(read names, including Armed Forces members living at home)* **more or less than $20,000?** Include money from jobs, social security, retirement income, unemployment payments, public assistance, and so forth. Also include income from interest, dividends, net income from business, farm, or rent, and any other money income received.

Read if necessary: **Income is important in analyzing the health information we collect. For example, this information helps us to learn whether persons in one income group use certain types of medical care services or have certain conditions more or less often than those in another group.**

8a.
- 1 ☐ $20,000 or more *(Hand Card I)*
- 2 ☐ Less than $20,000 *(Hand Card J)*

Read parenthetical phrase if Armed Forces member living at home or if necessary.

b. Of those income groups, which letter best represents the total combined **FAMILY** income during the past 12 months (that is, yours, *(read names, including Armed Forces members living at home)*)? Include wages, salaries, and other items we just talked about.

Read if necessary: **Income is important in analyzing the health information we collect. For example, this information helps us to learn whether persons in one income group use certain types of medical care services or have certain conditions more or less often than those in another group.**

b.

00 ☐ A	10 ☐ K	20 ☐ U
01 ☐ B	11 ☐ L	21 ☐ V
02 ☐ C	12 ☐ M	22 ☐ W
03 ☐ D	13 ☐ N	23 ☐ X
04 ☐ E	14 ☐ O	24 ☐ Y
05 ☐ F	15 ☐ P	25 ☐ Z
06 ☐ G	16 ☐ Q	26 ☐ ZZ
07 ☐ H	17 ☐ R	
08 ☐ I	18 ☐ S	
09 ☐ J	19 ☐ T	

R

a. *Mark first appropriate box.*

Ra.
- 1 ☐ Present for all questions
- 2 ☐ Present for some questions
- 3 ☐ Not present

b. *Enter person number of respondent.*

b.

_____
Person number(s) of respondent(s)

L3 *Enter person number of first parent listed or mark box.*

L3

_____
Person number of parent

00 ☐ None in household

L4 *Enter person number of spouse or mark box.*

L4

_____
Person number of spouse

00 ☐ None in household

FOOTNOTES

			RT 61
	L. DEMOGRAPHIC BACKGROUND PAGE, Continued		3–4

L5 | *Read to respondent:* **In order to determine how health practices and conditions are related to how long people live, we would like to refer to statistical records maintained by the National Center for Health Statistics.** | | |

L6 | *Enter date of birth from question 3 on Household Composition page.* | **L6** | **Date of birth**   5–11

       Month   Date   Year

9a. In what State or country was – – born?

Print the full name of the State or mark the appropriate box if the person was not born in the United States.

9a.

99 ☐ DK *(L7)*   12–13

_____ State

01 ☐ Puerto Rico   05 ☐ Cuba
02 ☐ Virgin Islands   06 ☐ Mexico
03 ☐ Guam   98 ☐ All other countries
04 ☐ Canada

If born in U.S., ask 9b only; if born in foreign country, ask 9c only.
b. Altogether, how many years has – – lived in *(State of present residence)***?**

b.   14

1 ☐ Less than 1 yr.
2 ☐ 1 yr., less than 5
3 ☐ 5 yrs., less than 10
4 ☐ 10 yrs., less than 15
5 ☐ 15 yrs. or more
9 ☐ DK

c. Altogether, how many years has – – lived in the United States?

c.   15

1 ☐ Less than 1 yr.
2 ☐ 1 yr., less than 5
3 ☐ 5 yrs., less than 10
4 ☐ 10 yrs., less than 15
5 ☐ 15 yrs. or more
9 ☐ DK

L7 | *Print full name, including middle initial, from question 1 on Household Composition page.* | **L7** | Last   16–35
First   36–50
Middle initial   51

Verify for males; ask for females.
10. What is – – father's LAST name? *Verify spelling. DO NOT write "Same".*

10. | Father's LAST name   52–71

Read to respondent: **We also need – – Social Security Number to link with vital statistics and other records of the Department of Health and Human Services to perform health-related research. Providing this information is voluntary and collected under the authority of the Public Health Service Act. There will be no effect on – – benefits if you do provide it and this number will not be given to any other government or nongovernment agency.**

Read if necessary: **The Public Health Service Act is title 42, United States Code, Section 242k.**

11. What is – – Social Security Number?

11.

999999999 ☐ DK   72–80

☐☐☐ – ☐☐ – ☐☐☐☐
Social Security Number

Mark if number obtained from   81

0 ☐ Does not have SSN
1 ☐ Memory
2 ☐ Records
7 ☐ Refused

L8 | *Mark box to indicate how Social Security number was or was not obtained.* | **L8** | 82

1 ☐ Self-personal
2 ☐ Self-telephone
3 ☐ Proxy-personal
4 ☐ Proxy-telephone

Page 50   FORM HIS-1 (5-1-95)

L. DEMOGRAPHIC BACKGROUND PAGE, Continued

Read to hhld. respondent: **The National Center for Health Statistics may wish to contact you again to obtain additional health related information. Please give me the name, address, and telephone number of a relative or friend who would know where you could be reached in case we have trouble reaching you. (Please give me the name of someone who is not currently living in the household.)** *Please print items 12–16.*

RT 62

12.	Contact Person name	3–4		25–39	40	14.	Area code/telephone number	97–106
	Last	5–24	First		Middle initial			

1 ☐ None
2 ☐ Refused
9 ☐ DK

107

13a. Address *(Number and street)*   41–65

b. City   66–85 State   86–87 ZIP Code   88–96

15. Relationship to household respondent   108–109

16. If you must be contacted again, what is the best time to call or visit?

FOOTNOTES

L. DEMOGRAPHIC BACKGROUND PAGE, Continued

17. **During the past 12 months, has your household been without telephone service for more than one week?** *If no phone, mark "Yes".*	110 1 ☐ Yes *(18)* 2 ☐ No ⎱ *(Supplement)* 9 ☐ DK ⎰
18. **For how long was your household without telephone service in the past 12 months?**	111-114 0123 ☐ Entire 12 months 0000 ☐ One week or less _____ ⎧ 1 ☐ Day(s) (Number) ⎨ 2 ☐ Week(s) ⎩ 3 ☐ Month(s) 9999 ☐ DK

FOOTNOTES

TABLE X – DETERMINING IF AN ADDITIONAL LIVING QUARTERS QUALIFIES AS AN EXTRA UNIT

ADDRESS OF ADDITIONAL LIVING QUARTERS	AREA SEGMENT		PERMIT SEGMENT	SEPARATENESS		NUMBER OF EXTRA UNITS
Check the listing sheet. Is the address already listed?	Are the additional living quarters within the area segment boundaries?	Are the additional living quarters in a Group Quarters (GQ)?	Are the additional living quarters within the same structure and within the same space occupied by the original sample unit? 1/	Do the occupants or intended occupants of the additional living quarters live and eat separately from all other persons on the property?	Do the occupants or intended occupants of the additional living quarters have direct access from the outside or through a common hall?	Have you found more than 3 EXTRA units?
(1)	(2)	(3)	(4)	(5)	(6)	(7)
☐ Yes - Enter sheet and line no.: Stop Table X Sheet ___ Line ___ ☐ No - Enter address or description, then go to column (2) or (4) depending on Seg.	☐ Yes - Go to column (3) ☐ No - Do not interview	☐ Yes - Do not interview ☐ No - Skip to column (5)	☐ Yes - Go to column (5) ☐ No - Do not interview	☐ Yes - Go to column (6) ☐ No - Not a separate unit. Stop Table X. Include quarters with original unit.	☐ Yes - An EXTRA unit. Go to column (7) ☐ No - Not a separate unit. Stop Table X. Include quarters with original unit.	☐ Yes - Call your office for instructions on which units to interview. 2/ ☐ No - Enter address on listing sheet. Interview parent and EXTRA units.
☐ Yes - Enter sheet and line no.: Stop Table X Sheet ___ Line ___ ☐ No - Enter address or description, then go to column (2) or (4) depending on Seg.	☐ Yes - Go to column (3) ☐ No - Do not interview	☐ Yes - Do not interview ☐ No - Skip to column (5)	☐ Yes - Go to column (5) ☐ No - Do not interview	☐ Yes - Go to column (6) ☐ No - Not a separate unit. Stop Table X. Include quarters with original unit.	☐ Yes - An EXTRA unit. Go to column (7) ☐ No - Not a separate unit. Stop Table X. Include quarters with original unit.	☐ Yes - Call your office for instructions on which units to interview. 2/ ☐ No - Enter address on listing sheet. Interview parent and EXTRA units.
☐ Yes - Enter sheet and line no.: Stop Table X Sheet ___ Line ___ ☐ No - Enter address or description, then go to column (2) or (4) depending on Seg.	☐ Yes - Go to column (3) ☐ No - Do not interview	☐ Yes - Do not interview ☐ No - Skip to column (5)	☐ Yes - Go to column (5) ☐ No - Do not interview	☐ Yes - Go to column (6) ☐ No - Not a separate unit. Stop Table X. Include quarters with original unit.	☐ Yes - An EXTRA unit. Go to column (7) ☐ No - Not a separate unit. Stop Table X. Include quarters with original unit.	2/ When your RO has determined which units to interview, enter the addresses on the listing sheets and proceed with the interviews.
FOOTNOTES			1/ Occupation of the same space occurs if a housing unit has been split into two or more separate housing units.			

☆U.S. GOVERNMENT PRINTING OFFICE: 1995-0-382-772

FORM HIS-1 (6-1-95)

OMB No. 0920-0214; Approval Expires 09/30/96

FORM HIS-3 (1995)
(5-1-95)

U.S. DEPARTMENT OF COMMERCE
BUREAU OF THE CENSUS
ACTING AS COLLECTING AGENT FOR THE
U.S. DEPARTMENT OF HEALTH AND HUMAN SERVICES
U.S. PUBLIC HEALTH SERVICE
CENTERS FOR DISEASE CONTROL
NATIONAL CENTER FOR HEALTH STATISTICS

NATIONAL HEALTH INTERVIEW SURVEY

1995 SUPPLEMENT BOOKLET

III. FAMILY RESOURCES

IV. YEAR 2000 OBJECTIVES

V. AIDS KNOWLEDGE AND ATTITUDES

NOTICE – Information contained on this form which would permit identification of any individual or establishment has been collected with a guarantee that it will be held in strict confidence, will be used only for purposes stated for this study, and will not be disclosed or released to others without the consent of the individual or the establishment in accordance with section 308(d) of the Public Health Service Act (42 USC 242m). Public reporting burden for this collection of information is estimated to average 45 minutes per response, including the time for reviewing instructions, searching existing data sources, gathering and maintaining the data needed, and completing and reviewing the collection of information. Send comments regarding this burden estimate or any other aspect of this collection of information, including suggestions for reducing this burden, to PHS Reports Clearance Officer; ATTN: PRA (0920-0214); Hubert H. Humphrey Building, Room 737-F, 200 Independence Avenue, SW; Washington, DC 20201.

1. RO	2. Sample	Suffix	3. Week	4. Book ____ of	RT 84
9-10	11-13	14	15-16	____ books	3-7
					8

5. Control number						6. Family number	32
PSU	Segment	Suffix	Serial	Suffix	Check digit		
17-21	22-25	26-27	28-29	30	31		

7. Field Representative's name	Code	33-35

8. Beginning time	36-39	40	9. Ending time	41-44	45
	1 ☐ a.m.			1 ☐ a.m.	
	2 ☐ p.m.			2 ☐ p.m.	

SAMPLE PERSON LIST

ITEM IV1	Are there any nondeleted persons 18+ years old in this family?	☐ Yes *(List by age, oldest to youngest)* ☐ No *(Section III)*

RT 85	3-4	5-6	7				8	9
Line No.	Person No.	Age	Sex	Last name	First name		SP	List No.
1			1 ☐ M 2 ☐ F				1 ☐	1
2			1 ☐ M 2 ☐ F				1 ☐	1
3			1 ☐ M 2 ☐ F				1 ☐	1
4			1 ☐ M 2 ☐ F				1 ☐	1
5			1 ☐ M 2 ☐ F				1 ☐	1
6			1 ☐ M 2 ☐ F				1 ☐	1
7			1 ☐ M 2 ☐ F				1 ☐	1
8			1 ☐ M 2 ☐ F				1 ☐	1
9			1 ☐ M 2 ☐ F				1 ☐	1

► *Refer to the 18+ part of the sample selection label and circle as applicable. Mark (X) the "SP" box in the column above for the selected sample person 18+. THEN, go to Section III.*

Notes

COMPLETE FINAL STATUS ITEMS ON BACK COVER

			RT 93
	Section IV – YEAR 2000 OBJECTIVES		3-4

			5
ITEM IV2	Refer to sample person selection label.	1 ☐ Y *(Item A1)* 2 ☐ A *(Section V, AIDS on page 59)*	

Part A – TOBACCO

ITEM A1	Adult SP status. *Begin here on Section IV callbacks.*	☐ Available *(1)* ☐ Callback required *(Item 18 on Household page of HIS-1)* ☐ Noninterview *(Response status on Back Cover)*	

			6
These next questions are about cigarette smoking. **1a. Have you smoked at least 100 cigarettes in your entire life?** *If asked: approximately 5 packs*		1 ☐ Yes *(1b)* 2 ☐ No 9 ☐ DK } *(Part B on page 51)*	

		7-8
b. How old were you when you first TRIED cigarettes?	_____ Age 99 ☐ DK	

		9-10
c. How old were you when you first started to smoke every day?	_____ Age 00 ☐ Never smoked every day 99 ☐ DK	

		11
2. Around this time LAST YEAR, were you smoking cigarettes everyday, some days, or not at all? *Mark (X) only one.*	1 ☐ Everyday 2 ☐ Some days 3 ☐ Not at all 9 ☐ DK	

		12
3a. Do you NOW smoke cigarettes everyday, some days, or not at all? *Mark (X) only one.*	1 ☐ Everyday *(4)* 2 ☐ Some days *(6)* 3 ☐ Not at all *(3b)* 9 ☐ DK *(6)*	

		13-15
b. How long has it been since you quit smoking cigarettes?	_____ { 1 ☐ Days (Number) { 2 ☐ Weeks { 3 ☐ Months } *(Part B on page 51)* { 4 ☐ Years 999 ☐ DK *(Part B on page 51)*	

		16-17
4. On the average, how many cigarettes do you now smoke a day?	_____ Cigarettes a day (Number) 99 ☐ DK	

		18
5. During the past 12 months, have you stopped smoking for one day or longer?	1 ☐ Yes 2 ☐ No } *(7)* 9 ☐ DK	

		19-20
6a. On how many of the past 30 days did you smoke cigarettes?	00 ☐ None *(7)* _____ Days (Number) } *(6b)* 99 ☐ DK	

		21-22
b. On the average, when you smoked DURING THE PAST 30 DAYS, about how many cigarettes did you smoke EACH day?	_____ Cigarettes a day (Number) 99 ☐ DK	

		23
7. Would you like to completely quit smoking cigarettes?	1 ☐ Yes 2 ☐ No 9 ☐ DK	

Notes

RT 94
3-4

Part B – NUTRITION	

5

1. Are you NOW trying to lose weight, gain weight, stay about the same, or are you not trying to do anything about your weight?

Mark (X) only one.

- 1 ☐ Lose weight *(2)*
- 2 ☐ Gain weight *(B1)*
- 3 ☐ Stay about the same *(2)*
- 4 ☐ Not trying to do anything *(B1)*

HAND CARD YB1. Read categories if telephone interview.

2. Are you currently doing any of these things to control your weight?

Mark (X) all that apply.

- 01 ☐ Joined a weight loss program — 6-7
- 02 ☐ Eating fewer calories — 8-9
- 03 ☐ Eating special products such as canned or powdered food supplements — 10-11
- 04 ☐ Exercising more — 12-13
- 05 ☐ Eating less fat — 14-15
- 06 ☐ Skipping meals — 16-17
- 07 ☐ Taking diet pills — 18-19
- 08 ☐ Taking laxatives — 20-21
- 09 ☐ Taking water pills or diuretics — 22-23
- 10 ☐ Vomiting — 24-25
- 11 ☐ Fasting for 24 hours or longer — 26-27
- 98 ☐ Something else – *Specify* 🗷 — 28-29

_____

- 00 ☐ Nothing — 30-31

32

ITEM B1

Refer to HIS-1.

- 1 ☐ SP was respondent for HIS-1 *(Transcribe question 5 from HIS-1, page 22–23, then ask 4a)*
- 2 ☐ SP was not respondent for HIS-1 *(3)*

3a. About how tall are you without shoes?

33-35

_____ _____
(Feet)   (Inches)

b. About how much do you weigh without shoes?

Read if SP is pregnant: **Please give your usual weight before becoming pregnant.**

36-38

_____
(Pounds)

The next questions are about salt in your diet.

4a. How often do you or the person who shops for your food buy items that are labeled "low salt", or "low sodium" — would you say always, often, sometimes, rarely or never?

Mark (X) only one.

39

- 0 ☐ Don't shop for food
- 1 ☐ Always
- 2 ☐ Often
- 3 ☐ Sometimes
- 4 ☐ Rarely
- 5 ☐ Never
- 9 ☐ DK

b. When you sit down at the table to eat, how often do you add salt to your food — would you say always, often, sometimes, rarely, or never? Do not include salt substitutes.

Mark (X) only one.

40

- 1 ☐ Always
- 2 ☐ Often
- 3 ☐ Sometimes
- 4 ☐ Rarely
- 5 ☐ Never
- 9 ☐ DK

5a. When you buy a food item for the first time, how often would you say you read the NUTRITIONAL INFORMATION about calories, fat and cholesterol sometimes listed on the label — would you say always, often, sometimes, rarely or never?

Mark (X) only one.

41

- 0 ☐ Don't buy food *(B2 on page 52)*
- 1 ☐ Always
- 2 ☐ Often
- 3 ☐ Sometimes ⎫
- 4 ☐ Rarely   ⎬ *(5b)*
- 5 ☐ Never   ⎭
- 9 ☐ DK

b. When you buy a food item for the first time, how often would you say you read the INGREDIENT list on the package — (would you say always, often, sometimes, rarely or never?)

Mark (X) only one.

42

- 0 ☐ Don't buy food
- 1 ☐ Always
- 2 ☐ Often
- 3 ☐ Sometimes
- 4 ☐ Rarely
- 5 ☐ Never
- 9 ☐ DK

Part B – NUTRITION – Continued		
ITEM B2 *Refer to age.*		1 ☐ 65+ *(6)* 2 ☐ Under 65 *(Part C on page 53)*	43

6a. Do you have meals delivered to your home by an agency or organization like Meals on Wheels?

1 ☐ Yes *(Part C on page 53)*
2 ☐ No ⎫
9 ☐ DK ⎭ *(6b)*

44

b. Do you NEED to have meals delivered to your home (by an agency or organization like Meals on Wheels)?

1 ☐ Yes
2 ☐ No
9 ☐ DK

45

7a. In the past 12 months, have you taken a class or attended a presentation on health topics?

1 ☐ Yes *(7b)*
2 ☐ No ⎫
9 ☐ DK ⎭ *(8)*

46

b. Where was the health class given — at a senior center, hospital, or some other place?

If multiple classes, probe for the location of the most recent.

Mark (X) only one.

1 ☐ Senior center
2 ☐ Hospital
3 ☐ Other place
9 ☐ DK

47

8a. In the past 12 months, did you participate in an exercise class or exercise program?

1 ☐ Yes *(8b)*
2 ☐ No ⎫
9 ☐ DK ⎭ *(Part C on page 53)*

48

b. Where was the exercise class given — at a senior center, hospital, or some other place?

If multiple classes, probe for the location of the most recent.

Mark (X) only one.

1 ☐ Senior center
2 ☐ Hospital
3 ☐ Other place
9 ☐ DK

49

Notes

Part C – CLINICAL PREVENTIVE SERVICES

The following questions are on immunizations.

| | | | 50 |

1. During the past 12 months, have you had a flu shot?

Read if necessary: **This vaccination is usually given in the Fall and protects against influenza for the flu season.**

1 ☐ Yes
2 ☐ No
9 ☐ DK

| | | 51 |

2. During the past TEN years, have you had a tetanus shot?

1 ☐ Yes
2 ☐ No
9 ☐ DK

| | | 52 |

3. Have you EVER had a pneumonia vaccination? This shot was first made available in 1977 and is usually given once in a person's lifetime.

1 ☐ Yes
2 ☐ No
9 ☐ DK

| | | 53 |

The following questions are about certain diseases and illnesses.

4. During the past 12 months, have you had diabetes?

(If appropriate, read: Do not include diabetes diagnosed ONLY during pregnancy.)

1 ☐ Yes
2 ☐ No
9 ☐ DK

| | | 54 |

5. (During the past 12 months, have you had) asthma, emphysema, chronic bronchitis, or tuberculosis?

1 ☐ Yes
2 ☐ No
9 ☐ DK

| | | 55 |

6. (During the past 12 months, have you had) any kind of chronic kidney disease?

1 ☐ Yes
2 ☐ No
9 ☐ DK

| | | 56 |

7. (During the past 12 months, have you had) liver disease, including cirrhosis?

1 ☐ Yes
2 ☐ No
9 ☐ DK

| | | 57 |

8. In the past 12 months, have you suffered from extreme fatigue lasting one month or longer?

1 ☐ Yes
2 ☐ No
9 ☐ DK

| | | 58 |

9. Are you currently being treated for any kind of cancer?

1 ☐ Yes
2 ☐ No
9 ☐ DK

| | | 59 |

10. Have you ever been told by a doctor that you have had a heart attack, heart failure, a chronic heart condition, or rheumatic heart disease?

1 ☐ Yes
2 ☐ No
9 ☐ DK

Notes

Part D – MENTAL HEALTH	

1a. During the past 2 weeks, would you say that you experienced a lot of stress, a moderate amount of stress, relatively little stress, or almost no stress at all?

Mark (X) only one.

	60
1 ☐ A lot	
2 ☐ Moderate ⎫	
3 ☐ Relatively little ⎬ *(1b)*	
4 ☐ Almost none ⎭	
5 ☐ DK what stress is *(4)*	
9 ☐ DK *(1b)*	

These next questions are about stress during the past 12 months.

	61

b. During the past 12 MONTHS, would you say that you experienced a lot of stress, a moderate amount of stress, relatively little stress, or almost no stress at all?

Mark (X) only one.

1 ☐ A lot
2 ☐ Moderate
3 ☐ Relatively little
4 ☐ Almost none
9 ☐ DK

2. During the past 12 months, how much effect has stress had on your health — a lot, some, hardly any, or none?

Mark (X) only one.

	62
1 ☐ A lot	
2 ☐ Some	
3 ☐ Hardly any or none	
9 ☐ DK	

3. (During the past 12 months), have you taken any steps to control or reduce stress in your life?

	63
1 ☐ Yes	
2 ☐ No	
9 ☐ DK	

4. (During the past 12 months), have you had any SERIOUS personal or emotional problems?

	64
1 ☐ Yes	
2 ☐ No	
9 ☐ DK	

5a. During the past 12 months, did you seek help from family or friends for ANY personal or emotional problems?

	65
1 ☐ Yes	
2 ☐ No	
9 ☐ DK	

b. (During the past 12 months), did you seek help from a therapist, counselor, or self-help group for ANY personal or emotional problems?

	66
1 ☐ Yes	
2 ☐ No	
9 ☐ DK	

c. (During the past 12 months), did you seek help from a priest, minister, rabbi, or other religious counselor for ANY personal or emotional problems?

	67
1 ☐ Yes	
2 ☐ No	
9 ☐ DK	

Notes

Part E – PHYSICAL ACTIVITY AND FITNESS

These next questions are about physical exercise.

| ITEM E1 | Mark from observation or previous information. | 1 ☐ SP is physically handicapped *(Describe in notes, THEN 1)* | 5 |
| | | 8 ☐ Other *(2 on page 57)* | |

HAND CALENDAR.		6
1a. In the past 2 weeks (outlined on that calendar), beginning Monday *(date)* and ending this past Sunday *(date)* , have you done any exercises, sports, or physically active hobbies?	1 ☐ Yes *(1b)* 2 ☐ No ⎫ 9 ☐ DK ⎭ *(3 on page 58)*	

b. What were they?

Record in 2a on page 57, THEN 1c.

c. Anything else?

☐ Yes *(Reask 1b and c)*
☐ No *(Mark "No" for all remaining activities in 2a, then go to 2b)*

Notes

Part E – PHYSICAL ACTIVITY AND FITNESS – Continued

NOTE: ASK ALL OF 2a BEFORE GOING TO 2b–d. | **NOTE:** ASK 2b–d FOR EACH ACTIVITY MARKED "YES" IN 2a.

HAND CALENDAR.

2a. In the past 2 weeks (outlined on that calendar), beginning Monday, *(date)*, and ending this past Sunday, *(date)*, have YOU done any of the following exercises, sports, or physically active hobbies —

b. How many times in the past 2 weeks did you [go/do] *(activity in 2a)*?

c. On the average, about how many minutes did you actually spend (doing) *(activity in 2a)* each time?

d. (What usually happened to your heart rate or breathing when you [did/went] *(activity in 2a)*)? Did you have a small, moderate, or large increase, or no increase at all in your heart rate or breathing?

	YES	NO	7	b.		8-9	c.		10-12	d.		13
(1) Walking for exercise?	1☐	2☐		(1) ____ Times			____ Minutes			1☐ Small 3☐ Large	2☐ Moderate 0☐ No inc.	9☐ DK
			14			15-16			17-19			20
(2) Gardening or yard work?	1☐	2☐		(2) ____ Times			____ Minutes			1☐ Small 3☐ Large	2☐ Moderate 0☐ No inc.	9☐ DK
			21			22-23			24-26			
(3) Stretching exercises?	1☐	2☐		(3) ____ Times			____ Minutes *(Next activity)*					
			27			28-29			30-32			33
(4) Weightlifting or other exercises to increase muscle strength?	1☐	2☐		(4) ____ Times			____ Minutes			1☐ Small 3☐ Large	2☐ Moderate 0☐ No inc.	9☐ DK
			34			35-36			37-39			40
(5) Jogging or running?	1☐	2☐		(5) ____ Times			____ Minutes			1☐ Small 3☐ Large	2☐ Moderate 0☐ No inc.	9☐ DK
			41			42-43			44-46			47
(6) Aerobics or aerobic dancing?	1☐	2☐		(6) ____ Times			____ Minutes			1☐ Small 3☐ Large	2☐ Moderate 0☐ No inc.	9☐ DK
			48			49-50			51-53			54
(7) Riding a bicycle or exercise bike?	1☐	2☐		(7) ____ Times			____ Minutes			1☐ Small 3☐ Large	2☐ Moderate 0☐ No inc.	9☐ DK
			55			56-57			58-60			61
(8) Stair climbing for exercise?	1☐	2☐		(8) ____ Times			____ Minutes			1☐ Small 3☐ Large	2☐ Moderate 0☐ No inc.	9☐ DK
			62			63-64			65-67			68
(9) Swimming for exercise?	1☐	2☐		(9) ____ Times			____ Minutes			1☐ Small 3☐ Large	2☐ Moderate 0☐ No inc.	9☐ DK
			69			70-71			72-74			75
(10) Playing tennis?	1☐	2☐		(10) ____ Times			____ Minutes			1☐ Small 3☐ Large	2☐ Moderate 0☐ No inc.	
			76			77-78						
(11) Playing golf?	1☐	2☐		(11) ____ Times *(Next activity)*								
			79			80-81						
(12) Bowling?	1☐	2☐		(12) ____ Times *(Next activity)*								
			82			83-84			85-87			88
(13) Playing baseball or softball?	1☐	2☐		(13) ____ Times			____ Minutes			1☐ Small 3☐ Large	2☐ Moderate 0☐ No inc.	9☐ DK
			89			90-91			92-94			95
(14) Playing handball, racquetball, or squash?	1☐	2☐		(14) ____ Times			____ Minutes			1☐ Small 3☐ Large	2☐ Moderate 0☐ No inc.	9☐ DK
(15) Skiing? ☐Yes ↗ ☐No *(16)*			96			97-98						
(a) Downhill?	1☐	2☐		(a) ____ Times *(Next activity)*								
			99			100-101			102-104			105
(b) Cross-country?	1☐	2☐		(b) ____ Times			____ Minutes			1☐ Small 3☐ Large	2☐ Moderate 0☐ No inc.	9☐ DK
			106			107-108						
(c) Water?	1☐	2☐	RT 96	(c) ____ Times *(Next activity)*								
	YES	NO	3-4			6-7			8-10			11
(16) Playing basketball?	1☐	2☐	5	(16) ____ Times			____ Minutes			1☐ Small 3☐ Large	2☐ Moderate 0☐ No inc.	9☐ DK
			12			13-14			15-17			18
(17) Playing volleyball?	1☐	2☐		(17) ____ Times			____ Minutes			1☐ Small 3☐ Large	2☐ Moderate 0☐ No inc.	9☐ DK
			19			20-21			22-24			25
(18) Playing soccer?	1☐	2☐		(18) ____ Times			____ Minutes			1☐ Small 3☐ Large	2☐ Moderate 0☐ No inc.	9☐ DK
			26			27-28			29-31			32
(19) Playing football?	1☐	2☐		(19) ____ Times			____ Minutes			1☐ Small 3☐ Large	2☐ Moderate 0☐ No inc.	9☐ DK

(20) Have you done any (other) exercises, sports, or physically active hobbies in the past 2 weeks?

1☐ Yes – **What were they?** 2☐ No   33
Anything else?

If activity listed above, mark "Yes" for it; otherwise, specify ↗

		34-35	(20a) ____ Times		36-37	____ Minutes		38-40	1☐ Small 3☐ Large	2☐ Moderate 0☐ No inc.	41 / 9☐ DK
(a) _____		42									
(b) _____		43-44	(20b) ____ Times		45-46	____ Minutes		47-49	1☐ Small 3☐ Large	2☐ Moderate 0☐ No inc.	50 / 9☐ DK

Part E – PHYSICAL ACTIVITY AND FITNESS – Continued	
3. About how long has it been since your last medical check-up? *Mark (X) only one.*	51 1 ☐ Less than 1 year *(4)* 2 ☐ 1 year, less than 2 years 3 ☐ 2 years, less than 3 years 4 ☐ 3 years, less than 4 years } *(END interview)* 5 ☐ 4+ years 6 ☐ Never had a check-up 9 ☐ DK *(4)*
4. During your last check-up, did the doctor recommend that you BEGIN or CONTINUE to do any type of exercise or physical activity? *If "Yes", ask:* **Was that begin or continue?**	52 1 ☐ Yes, to BEGIN 2 ☐ Yes, to CONTINUE 3 ☐ Yes, BOTH } *(END interview)* 4 ☐ No 9 ☐ DK

Notes

FORM HIS-3 (5-1-95)

RT 97
3-4

Section V – AIDS KNOWLEDGE AND ATTITUDES

ITEM V1	*Refer to sample person selection label.*	☐ A *(Item V2)* ☐ Y *(End Interview)*
ITEM V2	Adult SP status. *Begin here on Section V callbacks.*	☐ Available *(1)* ☐ Callback required *(Item 18 on Household page of HIS-1)* ☐ Noninterview *(Response status on Back Cover)*

These next questions are asked to determine what people know about the disease AIDS.   **5**

1. How much would you say you know about AIDS — a lot, some, a little, or nothing?

   1 ☐ A lot
   2 ☐ Some
   3 ☐ A little
   4 ☐ Nothing

2. In the past month, have you –   **6**

   a. seen any Public Service Announcements about AIDS on television?

   1 ☐ Yes
   2 ☐ No
   9 ☐ DK

   b. heard any Public Service Announcements about AIDS on the radio?   **7**

   1 ☐ Yes
   2 ☐ No
   9 ☐ DK

   c. received any brochures about AIDS from your workplace?   **8**

   Mark (X) only one.

   1 ☐ Yes
   2 ☐ No
   3 ☐ Not currently working
   4 ☐ Self employed
   9 ☐ DK

   d. received any brochures about AIDS from a church or religious organization?   **9**

   1 ☐ Yes
   2 ☐ No
   9 ☐ DK

   e. received any information about AIDS from the American Red Cross?   **10**

   1 ☐ Yes
   2 ☐ No
   9 ☐ DK

3. DO YOU THINK that doctors, nurses, dentists, and other health care workers should be allowed to REFUSE care to a person who has the AIDS virus?   **11**

   Mark (X) only one.

   1 ☐ Yes
   2 ☐ No
   3 ☐ It depends – *Specify* ⇗
   _____

   9 ☐ DK

4. I'm going to read some statements about AIDS. After I read each one, tell me whether you think it is true or false or if you don't know.

	True	False	Don't know
			12
a. The AIDS virus can be passed on through sexual intercourse between a man and a woman.	1 ☐	2 ☐	9 ☐
			13
b. A man with the AIDS virus can pass it on to another man through sexual intercourse.	1 ☐	2 ☐	9 ☐
			14
c. A pregnant woman who has the AIDS virus can give it to her baby.	1 ☐	2 ☐	9 ☐
			15
d. There is a vaccine available to the public that protects a person from getting the AIDS virus.	1 ☐	2 ☐	9 ☐
			16
e. A person who has the AIDS virus can look well and healthy.	1 ☐	2 ☐	9 ☐
			17
f. Oil-based lubricants, like vaseline, cause latex condoms to break.	1 ☐	2 ☐	9 ☐

Section V – AIDS KNOWLEDGE AND ATTITUDES – Continued

HAND CARD A1. Read introduction if telephone interview.

5. **(For the next statements, tell me if you think it is very likely, somewhat likely, somewhat unlikely, very unlikely, definitely not possible, or if you don't know how likely it is that a person will get the AIDS virus infection that way.)**

   (Now look at Card A1.) **In general, how likely do you think it is that a person will get AIDS or the AIDS virus from –**

	Very likely	Somewhat likely	Somewhat unlikely	Very unlikely	Def. not possible	Don't know
						18
a. using public toilets?	1 ☐	2 ☐	3 ☐	4 ☐	5 ☐	9 ☐
						19
b. working near or with someone who has the AIDS virus?	1 ☐	2 ☐	3 ☐	4 ☐	5 ☐	9 ☐
						20
c. sharing plates, forks, or glasses with someone who has the AIDS virus?	1 ☐	2 ☐	3 ☐	4 ☐	5 ☐	9 ☐
						21
d. sharing needles for drug use with someone who has the AIDS virus?	1 ☐	2 ☐	3 ☐	4 ☐	5 ☐	9 ☐
						22
e. being coughed or sneezed on by someone who has the AIDS virus?	1 ☐	2 ☐	3 ☐	4 ☐	5 ☐	9 ☐
						23
f. attending school with a child who has the AIDS virus?	1 ☐	2 ☐	3 ☐	4 ☐	5 ☐	9 ☐
						24

6. **How effective do you think the proper use of a condom is to prevent getting the AIDS virus through sexual activity? Would you say very effective, somewhat effective, not at all effective, or you don't know how effective it is?**

   Mark (X) only one.

   1 ☐ Very effective
   2 ☐ Somewhat effective
   3 ☐ Not at all effective
   4 ☐ Don't know how effective
   9 ☐ Don't know method

7. **Do you have any children aged 10 through 17?**   `25`

   1 ☐ Yes *(8)*
   2 ☐ No *(10)*

8. **Have you ever discussed AIDS with any of these children aged 10 through 17?**   `26`

   1 ☐ Yes
   2 ☐ No

9. **Have any of these children aged 10 through 17 had instruction at school about AIDS?**   `27`

   1 ☐ Yes
   2 ☐ No
   9 ☐ DK

10a. **Do you feel that information about AIDS should be taught in schools?**   `28`

   1 ☐ Yes *(10b)*
   2 ☐ No   } *(11)*
   9 ☐ DK

   b. **At what grade in school should AIDS education start?**   `29-30`

   Probe for EXACT grade if necessary

   Mark (X) only one.

   00 ☐ Kindergarten

Grade		Grade	
01 ☐ 1		08 ☐ 8	
02 ☐ 2		09 ☐ 9	
03 ☐ 3		10 ☐ 10	
04 ☐ 4		11 ☐ 11	
05 ☐ 5		12 ☐ 12	
06 ☐ 6		97 ☐ Refused	
07 ☐ 7		99 ☐ DK	

Notes

Section V – AIDS KNOWLEDGE AND ATTITUDES – Continued

11a. In the past 12 months, has your workplace offered an organized AIDS education program to its employees? Do not include merely distributing brochures as an organized education program.

Mark (X) only one.

| 31 |

1 ☐ Yes
2 ☐ No
3 ☐ Not currently working
4 ☐ Self employed
7 ☐ Refused
9 ☐ DK

HAND CARD A2. Read categories if telephone interview.

b. In the past 12 months, have you attended an organized AIDS education program at any of these places?

If "Yes," ask: **Which?**

Mark (X) all that apply.

1 ☐ A church or other religious organization — 32
2 ☐ A family planning clinic or STD clinic — 33
3 ☐ A hospital, HMO clinic or other health facility — 34
4 ☐ A school — 35
5 ☐ A social or civic club — 36
6 ☐ Your workplace — 37
7 ☐ Some other place – *Specify* ⟋ — 38

_____

8 ☐ Attended no programs — 39
9 ☐ DK — 40

Now, I am going to ask some questions about giving blood donations to a blood bank, such as the American Red Cross. But this does NOT include blood drawn at a doctor's office for laboratory analysis.

| 41 |

12. Have you ever given a blood donation?

1 ☐ Yes *(13a)*
2 ☐ No ⎫
9 ☐ DK ⎭ *(13c)*

13a. Have you given blood since March 1985?

| 42 |

1 ☐ Yes *(13b)*
2 ☐ *No* ⎫
9 ☐ *DK* ⎭ *(13c)*

b. In what month and year did you last give blood?

| 43-46 |

_____ / 19 _____
Month   Year

c. Do you expect to donate blood in the next 12 months?

| 47 |

1 ☐ Yes
2 ☐ No
9 ☐ DK

HAND CARD A1. Read categories if telephone interview

| 48 |

14. In general, while GIVING A BLOOD DONATION to a blood bank, how likely is it that a person will get the AIDS virus?

Mark (X) only one.

1 ☐ Very likely
2 ☐ Somewhat likely
3 ☐ Somewhat unlikely
4 ☐ Very unlikely
5 ☐ Definitely not possible
9 ☐ DK

The next questions are about the blood test for the AIDS virus infection. No questions will ask what the results are of any tests you may have had.

| 49 |

15a. (Except for tests you may have had as part of blood donations,) Have you ever had your blood tested for the AIDS virus infection?

1 ☐ Yes *(16)*
2 ☐ No *(15b)*
9 ☐ DK *(26 on page 63)*

b. Is there any particular reason why you have not been tested?

If "Yes," ask: **What is the reason?**

Any other?

Do not read list.

Mark (X) all that apply.

01 ☐ No reason — 50-51
02 ☐ Don't consider myself at risk of AIDS — 52-53
03 ☐ Doctor/HMO did not recommend it — 54-55
04 ☐ Don't believe test results are accurate — 56-57
05 ☐ Don't believe anything can be done if I am positive — 58-59
06 ☐ Don't like needles — 60-61
07 ☐ Don't trust results to be confidential — 62-63
08 ☐ Afraid of losing job, insurance, housing, friends, family, if people knew I was positive for AIDS infection — 64-65
09 ☐ Other – *Specify* ⟋ — 66-67

_____

99 ☐ DK — 68-69

(26 on page 63)

Section V – AIDS KNOWLEDGE AND ATTITUDES – Continued

16a. How many times have you had your blood tested for the AIDS virus infection (NOT including blood donations)?

01 ☐ One time *(16b)*

_____ Times ⎫ *(16c)*
(Number) ⎬

99 ☐ DK

`70-71`

b. Was it in the past 12 months?

1 ☐ Yes ⎫
2 ☐ No ⎬ *(17)*
9 ☐ DK ⎭

`72`

c. In the past 12 months, how many times have you had your blood tested for the AIDS virus infection (NOT including blood donations)?

00 ☐ None in past 12 months

_____ Times in past 12 months
(Number)

99 ☐ DK

`73-74`

17. In what month and year was your (last) blood test for the AIDS virus infection?

_____ / 19 _____
Month   Year

`75-78`

HAND CARD A3. Read categories if telephone interview.

18. Which of these would you say were the reasons for your (last) AIDS blood test (NOT including blood donations)? (Just tell me the numbers of your answers.)

(Anything else?)

Mark (X) all that apply.

01 ☐ Just to find out/Worried that you are infected
02 ☐ Because a doctor asked you to
03 ☐ Because the Health Department asked you to
04 ☐ Because a sex partner asked you to
05 ☐ For hospitalization or a surgical procedure
06 ☐ To apply for health or life insurance
07 ☐ To comply with guidelines for health workers
08 ☐ To apply for a new job
09 ☐ For military induction, separation or during military service
10 ☐ For immigration
11 ☐ For some other reason – *Specify* ⟍

`79-80`
`81-82`
`83-84`
`85-86`
`87-88`
`89-90`
`91-92`
`93-94`
`95-96`
`97-98`
`99-100`

97 ☐ Refused
99 ☐ DK

`101-102`
`103-104`

19. (Not including a blood donation) Where did you have your (last) blood test for the AIDS virus?

Mark (X) only one.

If "Clinic", Probe: **What kind of clinic is that?**

01 ☐ AIDS clinic/counselling/testing site
02 ☐ Community health clinic
03 ☐ Clinic run by employer
04 ☐ STD clinic   ⎫ *(20)*
05 ☐ Family planning/prenatal clinic
06 ☐ Other clinic

07 ☐ Doctor/HMO
08 ☐ Hospital/emergency room/outpatient clinic
09 ☐ Military induction, separation or military service site ⎫ *(22)*
10 ☐ Immigration site
11 ☐ At home/home visit by nurse/health worker
12 ☐ At home – self testing kit

13 ☐ Other location – *Specify* ⟍

_____ ⎫ *(20)*

97 ☐ Refused
99 ☐ DK

`105-106`

20. When your blood was (last) tested for the AIDS virus, were you REQUIRED to give your name?

1 ☐ Yes
2 ☐ No
7 ☐ Refused

`107`

21. (Again not including blood donations,) AT THE TIME they drew blood for your (last) test for the AIDS virus, did a health professional talk with you about the transmission, prevention or treatment of AIDS or about the meaning of the test?

1 ☐ Yes
2 ☐ No
9 ☐ DK

`108`

22. Did you get the results of your (last) blood test?

1 ☐ Yes *(23)*
2 ☐ No
3 ☐ Only notified if there ⎫ *(26 on page 63)*
was a problem   ⎬
9 ☐ DK

`109`

Section V – AIDS KNOWLEDGE AND ATTITUDES – Continued	

23. How long did you wait to get the results?

(Number) { 1 ☐ Days / 2 ☐ Weeks / 3 ☐ Months

999 ☐ DK

`110-112`

`RT 98`
`3-4`

24a. Did a health professional talk with you about AIDS when you were GIVEN THE RESULTS of your (last) test?

1 ☐ Yes *(24b)*
2 ☐ No ⎱ *(25)*
9 ☐ DK ⎰

`5`

HAND CARD A4. Read categories if telephone interview.

b. What kind of topics were covered in the discussion of AIDS? (Just tell me the numbers of your answers).

(Anything else?)

Mark (X) all that apply.

01 ☐ How AIDS is transmitted　`6-7`
02 ☐ How to prevent transmission　`8-9`
03 ☐ The correct use of condoms　`10-11`
04 ☐ Needle cleaning/using clean needles　`12-13`
05 ☐ Dangers of needle sharing　`14-15`
06 ☐ Abstinence from sex　`16-17`
07 ☐ Contraception　`18-19`
08 ☐ Safe sex practices　`20-21`
09 ☐ Other – *Specify* ⤵　`22-23`

99 ☐ DK/Don't remember　`24-25`

c. Did you ask questions about the information provided?

1 ☐ Yes
2 ☐ No
9 ☐ DK/Don't remember

`26`

d. Were you given any information that you did NOT understand?

1 ☐ Yes
2 ☐ No
9 ☐ DK/Don't remember

`27`

25. Were the results given to you in person, by telephone, by mail, or in some other way?

Mark (X) only one.

If more than one given, mark lowest numbered response.

1 ☐ In person
2 ☐ By telephone
3 ☐ By mail
4 ☐ In some other way
9 ☐ DK/Don't remember

`28`

26. Do you expect to have [a/another] blood test for the AIDS virus infection in the next 12 months, not including through blood donation?

1 ☐ Yes *(27)*
2 ☐ No ⎱ *(29 on page 64)*
9 ☐ DK ⎰

`29`

HAND CARD A5. Read intro and categories if telephone interview.

27. (I'm going to read some reasons people might have the blood test for the AIDS virus infection.)

Tell me which of these statements explain WHY YOU expect to have the blood test in the next 12 months. (Just tell me the numbers of your answers).

(Anything else?)

Mark (X) all that apply.

01 ☐ Because you want to find out if you are infected　`30-31`
02 ☐ Because it will be part of hospitalization or surgery you expect to have　`32-33`
03 ☐ Because you expect to apply for life or health insurance　`34-35`
04 ☐ Because you expect to apply for a job　`36-37`
05 ☐ Because you expect to join the military　`38-39`
06 ☐ Because of guidelines for health care workers　`40-41`
07 ☐ Because it will be a required part of some other activity that includes automatic AIDS testing　`42-43`
08 ☐ Because it is required in your non-health care employment　`44-45`
09 ☐ Because you plan to have/begin a sexual relationship　`46-47`
10 ☐ For some other reason – *Specify* ⤵　`48-49`

99 ☐ DK/Refused　`50-51`

28. Where will you have a blood test for the AIDS virus infection?

Mark (X) only one.

If "Clinic", Probe: **"What kind of clinic is that?"**

`52-53`

01 ☐ AIDS clinic/counselling/testing site
02 ☐ Community Health Clinic
03 ☐ Clinic run by employer
04 ☐ STD clinic
05 ☐ Family planning/prenatal clinic
06 ☐ Other clinic
07 ☐ Doctor/HMO
08 ☐ Hospital/emergency room/outpatient clinic
09 ☐ Military induction/separation or military service site
10 ☐ Red Cross/blood bank/blood drive
11 ☐ At home/in a visit by the nurse/health practitioner
12 ☐ At home – self testing kit
13 ☐ Other location – *Specify* ⤵

97 ☐ Refused
99 ☐ DK

Section V – AIDS KNOWLEDGE AND ATTITUDES – Continued	

29a. Have you ever known anyone personally who had AIDS or the AIDS virus?

- 1 ☐ Yes *(29b)*
- 2 ☐ No
- 7 ☐ Refused
- 9 ☐ Don't know if has/had AIDS or the AIDS virus } *(30)*

`54`

---

b. Who was that — a friend, relative, co-worker, or someone else?

Mark (X) all that apply.

- 1 ☐ Friend — `55`
- 2 ☐ Relative — `56`
- 3 ☐ Co-worker — `57`
- 4 ☐ Someone else – *Specify* ↗ — `58`

- 7 ☐ Refused — `59`
- 9 ☐ DK — `60`

---

30. What are your chances of GETTING the AIDS virus; would you say high, medium, low, or none?

Mark (X) only one.

- 1 ☐ High
- 2 ☐ Medium
- 3 ☐ Low
- 4 ☐ None
- 5 ☐ Already have AIDS or AIDS virus
- 7 ☐ Refused
- 9 ☐ DK

`61`

HAND CARD A6.

31. (I'm going to read five statements. AFTER I have read them all,) Tell me if ANY of these statements is true for YOU. Do NOT tell me WHICH statement or statements are true for you. Just IF ANY of them are.

Read statements only if telephone interview.

a. You have hemophilia and have received clotting factor concentrations.

b. You are a man who has had sex with another man at some time since 1980, even one time.

c. You have taken street drugs by needle at any time since 1980.

d. You have traded sex for money or drugs at any time since 1980.

e. Since 1980, you are or have been the sex partner of any person who would answer "Yes" to any of the items I have read.

- 1 ☐ Yes to at least one statement
- 2 ☐ No to all statements

`62`

The next questions are about Tuberculosis, or TB.

32. Are you worried about catching TB?

- 1 ☐ Yes *(33)*
- 2 ☐ No } *(34)*
- 9 ☐ DK

`63`

---

33. How worried are you about catching TB – a lot, some, a little, or not at all?

Mark (X) only one.

- 1 ☐ A lot
- 2 ☐ Some
- 3 ☐ A little
- 4 ☐ Not at all
- 9 ☐ DK

`64`

34a. How much would you say you know about Tuberculosis – a lot, some, a little, or nothing?

Mark (X) only one.

- 1 ☐ A lot
- 2 ☐ Some } *(34b)*
- 3 ☐ A little
- 4 ☐ Nothing *(V3 on page 65)*

`65`

---

b. Do you know how TB is spread from one person to another?

- 1 ☐ Yes *(34c)*
- 2 ☐ No *(V3 on page 65)*

`66`

HAND CARD A7. Read categories if telephone interview.

c. As you understand it, how is TB spread from one person to another?

(Any other way?)

Mark (X) all that apply.

- 1 ☐ Breathing the air around a person who is sick with TB — `67`
- 2 ☐ Through food and water — `68`
- 3 ☐ By sexual intercourse — `69`
- 4 ☐ It is inherited from parents — `70`
- 5 ☐ From mosquito or other insect bites — `71`
- 6 ☐ Other – *Specify* ↗ — `72`

- 9 ☐ DK — `73`

FORM HIS-2 (5-1-95)

Section V – AIDS KNOWLEDGE AND ATTITUDES – Continued

		74
ITEM V3	*Refer to age.*	₁ ☐ 59 or under *(35)* ₂ ☐ 60+ *(End Interview)*

		75
	HAND CARD A8. If telephone interview, end interview.	₀ ☐ Diaphragm
35.	**This card shows seven methods of birth control. Which of these do you think is the MOST effective for preventing pregnancy?** *Mark (X) only one.*	₁ ☐ Condom (rubber) ₂ ☐ IUD (loop, coil) ₃ ☐ Rhythm (safe period by calendar) ₄ ☐ Foam ₅ ☐ Pill ₆ ☐ Withdrawal (pulling out) ₇ ☐ DK methods ₉ ☐ DK

		76
	Refer to Card A8.	₀ ☐ Diaphragm
36.	**Which of these do you think is the MOST effective for preventing sexually transmitted diseases such as syphilis, gonorrhea or AIDS?** *Mark (X) only one.*	₁ ☐ Condom (rubber) ₂ ☐ IUD (loop, coil) ₃ ☐ Rhythm (safe period by calendar) ₄ ☐ Foam ₅ ☐ Pill ₆ ☐ Withdrawal (pulling out) ₇ ☐ DK methods ₉ ☐ DK

RECORD FINAL STATUS ON BACK COVER.

Notes

TELEPHONE INTERVIEW SURVEY: CHICAGO AREA GENERAL POPULATION SURVEY ON AIDS

Resource B begins on the next page. Pages 400–427 constitute the questionnaire portion. The interview manual is reprinted on pp. 428–441.

The research for Resource B was supported in part by the Centers for Disease Control and Prevention through the Comprehensive AIDS Prevention/ Education Program (CAPEP), City of Chicago, Department of Health, 1986 to 1987, and the University of Illinois, Chicago. The data were collected by the Survey Research Laboratory at the University of Illinois, Chicago (Study No. 606). Principal Questionnaire Developers: Gary L. Albrecht, Judith A. Levy, and Noreen M. Sugrue.

UNIVERSITY OF ILLINOIS
Survey Research Laboratory

Sequence Number	_____
Study #	606
Date of Interview	/ /
Interviewer ID	_____

Chicago Area
General Population Survey on AIDS

Screening Questionnaire
(Version 1)

Hello, my name is _____ , and I'm calling from the University of Illinois. Is this (*phone number*)? We are doing a study in the Chicago metropolitan area about people's opinions and behaviors related to health issues.

S1. In order to determine whom to interview, could you please tell me, of the adults 18 years of age or older currently living in your household, who had the most recent birthday? I don't mean who is the youngest, just who had a birthday last.

Informant *(Skip to Q.S4)* 1
Someone else *(Specify—Skip to Q.S3)* 2
_____
Don't know all birthdays, only some 3
Don't know any birthdays other than own
    (Skip to Q.S4) 4
Refused (Interview male head of household; if not
    available or none, interview female head of
    household. If this is the Informant, skip to Q.S4;
    otherwise, skip to Q.S3.) 9

(If Don't know all birthdays):
S2. Of the birthdays you <u>do</u> know, who had the most recent birthday?
Informant *(Skip to Q.S4)* 1
Someone else (Specify) 2
_____

S3. May I speak to that person? *(Repeat introduction.)*

S4. How old were you on your last birthday?
                    _____ years old

> *If* <u>R</u> *under 18 years, return to Q.S1.*
> *If* <u>R</u> *over 60 years, ask interview Q.1–Q.4 and end*
>   *interview.*

UNIVERSITY OF ILLINOIS
Survey Research Laboratory

Sequence Number	_____
Study #	___606___
Date of Interview	___/ /___
Interviewer ID	_____

Chicago Area
General Population Survey on AIDS

Screening Questionnaire
(Version 2)

Hello, my name is _____ , and I'm calling from the University of Illinois. Is this *(phone number)*? We are doing a study in the Chicago metropolitan area about people's opinions and behaviors related to health issues.

S1. In order to determine whom to interview, could you please tell me, of the adults 18 years of age or older currently living in your household, who had the most recent birthday? I don't mean who is the youngest, just who had a birthday last.

Informant *(Skip to Q.S4)* 1
Someone else *(Specify—Skip to Q.S3)* 2
_____
Don't know all birthdays, only some 3
Don't know any birthdays other than own
    (Skip to Q.S4) 4
*Refused (Interview male head of household; if not
    available or none, interview female head of
    household. If this is the Informant, skip to Q.S4;
    otherwise, skip to Q.S3.)* 9

(If Don't know all birthdays):
S2. Of the birthdays you <u>do</u> know, who had the most recent birthday?
Informant *(Skip to Q.S4)* 1
Someone else (Specify) 2
_____

S3. May I speak to that person? *(Repeat introduction.)*

S4. How old were you on your last birthday?
_____ years old

If <u>R</u> under 18 years, return to Q.S1. *If <u>R</u> over 60 years, ask interview Q.1–Q.4 and end interview.*

S5.   What is your racial background?

White *(Ask Q.1–Q.4 and end interview)* 1

Black...2

Asian *(Ask Q.1–Q.4 and end interview)* 3

Hispanic/Latino/Chicano *(Ask Q.1–Q.4 and end interview)* 4

Cuban *(Ask Q.1–Q.4 and end interview)*...............4

Mexican *(Ask Q.1–Q.4 and end interview)*..............4

Puerto Rican *(Ask Q.1-Q.4 and end interview)*.........4

Colombian *(Ask Q.1–Q.4 and end interview)*...........4

Argentinian *(Ask Q.1–Q.4 and end interview)*..........4

Other *(Specify—Ask Q.1–Q.4 and end interview)*.......5

Refused (Ask Q.1–Q.4 and end interview) 9

UNIVERSITY OF ILLINOIS
Survey Research Laboratory

Sequence Number	_____
Study #	606
Date of Interview	/ /
Interviewer ID	_____

Chicago Area
General Population Survey on AIDS

Screening Questionnaire
(Version 3)

Hello, my name is _____ , and I'm calling from the University of Illinois. Is this (*phone number*)? We are doing a study in the Chicago metropolitan area about people's opinions and behaviors related to health issues.

S1. In order to determine whom to interview, could you please tell me, of the adults 18 years of age or older currently living in your household, who had the most recent birthday? I don't mean who is the youngest, just who had a birthday last.

Informant *(Skip to Q.S4)* 1
Someone else *(Specify—Skip to Q.S3)*.................2

Don't know all birthdays, only some...............3
Don't know any birthdays other than own
    (Skip to Q.S4) 4
*Refused (Interview male head of household; if not
    available or none, interview female head of
    household. If this is the Informant, skip to Q.S4;
    otherwise, skip to Q.S3.)* 9

(If Don't know all birthdays):
S2. Of the birthdays you <u>do</u> know, who had the most recent birthday?
Informant *(Skip to Q.S4)* 1
Someone else (Specify) 2

S3. May I speak to that person? *(Repeat introduction.)*

S4. How old were you on your last birthday?
    _____ years old

> *If R under 18 years, return to Q.S1.*
> *If R over 60 years, ask interview Q.1–Q.4 and end
>   interview.*

S5. What is your racial background?

White *(Ask Q.1–Q.4 and end interview)* 1

Black *(Ask Q.1–Q.4 and end interview)*................2

Asian *(Ask Q.1–Q.4 and end interview)* 3

Hispanic/Latino/Chicano 4

Cuban 4

Mexican 4

Puerto Rican...4

Colombian 4

Argentinian 4

Other *(Specify—Ask Q.1–Q.4 and end interview)*.......5

_____

Refused (Ask Q.1–Q.4 and end interview) 9

UNIVERSITY OF ILLINOIS
Survey Research Laboratory

Chicago Area
General Population Survey on AIDS

Sequence Number	_____
Study #	606
Date of Interview	/ /
Interviewer ID	_____

*Time interview began (Use 24-hour clock):*_____

1. In general, would you say that your health is ...

    excellent...1
    good 2
    fair 3
    poor? 4
    Don't know..*8*
    Refused...*9*

2. How much do you worry about your health? Do you worry about it ...

    a great deal...1
    somewhat 2
    not at all?..3
    Don't know...*8*
    Refused..*9*

3a. Do you think the <u>media</u> present too much information, not enough information, or the right amount of information about health issues in general?

    Too much 1
    Not enough 2
    Right amount...3
    Don't know...*8*

b. Do you think the information is always accurate, sometimes accurate, or never accurate?

    Always...1
    Sometimes 2
    Never..3
    Don't know...*8*

4a. Do you think that <u>government officials</u> present too much information, not enough information, or the right amount of information about health issues in general?

    Too much 1
    Not enough 2
    Right amount...3
    Don't know...*8*

b.   Do you think the information is always accurate, sometimes accurate, or never accurate?

Always...1
Sometimes 2
Never 3
Don't know...8

5.   Who do you think should pay most of the costs for medical <u>treatment</u> for a person with a serious illness? Should <u>most</u> of the costs be paid by ... *(Circle one.)*

the person who is ill and his or her family..........1
the government...2
insurance companies...................................3
someone else? *(Specify)*.............................4

_____

Don't know...8

6.   How much have you heard or read about the health condition AIDS (Acquired Immune Deficiency Syndrome)? Have you heard or read a lot about AIDS, some, or nothing at all?

A lot 1
Some 2
Nothing at all *(Skip to Q.48, p. 29)* 3

7a. Where have you seen informa-   7b. Have you seen information or
     tion or heard about AIDS?   heard about AIDS from *(read*
     (Circle all that apply.)   *any categories not circled in Q.7a)?*

		Yes	No	*Don't know*
Television.....................01....		1	2	*8*
Radio ....02....		1	2	*8*
A newspaper ....03....		1	2	*8*
A magazine ....04....		1	2	*8*
A relative, friend, or neighbor..................05....		1	2	*8*
Your work ....06....		1	2	*8*
A school ....07....		1	2	*8*
An AIDS hotline.............08....		1	2	*8*
A clinic, doctor's office, or health center ....09....		1	2	*8*
Billboards, buses, or trains ..10....		1	2	*8*
Somewhere else *(Specify)*.....11....		1	2	*8*

_____   _____

Don't know *98*

8a.   In terms of <u>AIDS</u>, do you think the <u>media</u> present too much informa-
      tion, not enough information, or the right amount of information?

                    Too much 1
                    Not enough 2
                    Right amount..3
                    Don't know..*8*

 b.   Do you think the information is always accurate, sometimes accurate, or
      never accurate?

                    Always...1
                    Sometimes 2
                    Never...3
                    Don't know..*8*

9a.   In terms of <u>AIDS</u>, do you think <u>government</u> <u>officials</u> present too much
      information, not enough information, or the right amount of information?

                    Too much 1
                    Not enough 2
                    Right amount..3
                    Don't know..*8*

 b.   Do you think the information is always accurate, sometimes accurate, or
      never accurate?

                    Always...1
                    Sometimes 2
                    Never...3
                    Don't know..*8*

10.   Thinking about the next 5 years, do you think that the number of people
      in Illinois who get AIDS each year will. . .

                    increase greatly 1
                    increase somewhat 2
                    stay the same...3
                    decrease somewhat....................................4
                    decrease greatly? 5
                    Don't know..*8*

11. From what you have heard, how do people get infected with the AIDS virus? *(Probe with "What other ways?" until R says "None." Circle all that apply.)*

Receiving a blood transfusion......................01

Having sex with someone who has AIDS.........02

Having sex...03

Being homosexual 04

Using drugs..05

Sharing needles 06

Touching or contact with body fluids/saliva/
sweat/tears/urine.................................07

Other *(Specify)* 08

_____

_____

_____

Don't know 98

12. When a person gets AIDS, do you think this is <u>mainly</u> because of. . .

God's will 1

the person's bad luck...............................2

the person's behavior...............................3

something else? *(Specify)*...........................4

_____

Don't know..8

13. Compared to catching a cold, do you think it is easier, harder, or about the same to catch the AIDS virus?

Easier..1

Harder 2

Same 3

Don't know..8

14a. Is it possible or not possible for a pregnant woman to pass the AIDS virus to her unborn child?

Possible 1

Not possible..2

Don't know..8

b. Is it possible or not possible for a woman to become infected with the AIDS virus by having sex with a man who has AIDS?

Possible 1

Not possible..2

Don't know..8

c. Is it possible or not possible for a man to become infected with the AIDS virus by having sex with a woman who has AIDS?

    Possible 1
    Not possible...2
    Don't know...*8*

15. If a man uses a condom during sex, does this make getting AIDS through sexual activity less likely or not less likely?

    Less likely 1
    Not less likely 2
    Don't know...*8*

16. Do people infected with the AIDS virus develop AIDS ...

    always 1
    sometimes?...2
    Don't know...*8*

17. Is AIDS...

    always fatal...1
    sometimes fatal? 2
    Don't know...*8*

18a. Do you think that any of the people who have AIDS deserves to have the disease?

    Yes 1
    No *(Skip to Q.19a)*......................................2
    Don't know (Skip to Q.19a) *8*

    (If "Yes"):

b. Who? *(Circle all that apply.)*

    Homosexuals 1
    Drug users 2
    Other *(Specify)*..3

    _____

    _____

c. Why is that? *(Circle all that apply.)*

    Wrong/immoral behavior 1
    Illegal behavior 2
    Other *(Specify)*..3

    _____

    _____

19a.   Do you think that any of the people who have AIDS do <u>not</u> deserve to have the disease?

Yes 1
No *(Skip to Q.20a)* 2
Don't know (Skip to Q.20a) 8

(If "Yes"):

  b.   Who? *(Circle all that apply.)*

Children 1
People who get blood transfusions 2
Medical workers 3
Unaware sexual partner/spouse 4
Other *(Specify)* 5

_____

_____

  c.   Why is that? *(Circle all that apply.)*

Innocent victim 1
Other *(Specify)* 2

_____

_____

20a.   Have you personally ever known anyone diagnosed as having AIDS or as being infected with the AIDS virus?

Yes 1
No *(Skip to Q.21a)* 2
Don't know (Skip to Q.21a) 8
Refused (Skip to Q.21a) 9

  b.   Do you know one person or <u>more</u> than one person who has been diagnosed as having AIDS or as being infected with the AIDS virus?

One 1
More than one *(Skip to Q.20d)* 2

  c.   Is this person. . .

a family member 1
a close friend 2
someone you know, but do not know well? 3

┌─────────────────────┐
│   *Skip to Q.21a*   │
└─────────────────────┘

d.   Are any of these people. . .

		Yes	No
1)	family members	1	2
2)	close friends	1	2
3)	people you know, but do not know well?	1	2

21a. Some government health officials say that giving clean needles to users of illegal drugs would greatly reduce the spread of AIDS. Do you <u>favor</u> or <u>oppose</u> making clean needles available to people who use illegal drugs as a way to reduce the spread of AIDS?

Favor *(Skip to Q.22)* 1
Oppose. 2
Depends. 3
Don't know (Skip to Q.22) *8*

b.   Why is that? *(Circle all that apply.)*

Drugs are wrong/this would promote use. 1
Wouldn't help. 2
Government should do something else *(Specify)*. . . .3

_____

Other *(Specify)*. 4

_____

_____

22.   What steps do <u>you</u> think the <u>federal</u> government should take to control the spread of AIDS? *(Circle all that apply.)*

Education/information in media or in general . .01
Research/find cure 02
Condoms/condom ads. 03
Screen blood supply/test blood. 04
Set up clinics/provide treatment 05
Require testing of people 06
Isolate or quarantine people with AIDS 07
Nothing/nothing government can do. 08
Other *(Specify)* 09

_____

_____

_____

Don't know *98*

23a. Who do you think should pay most of the costs for medical <u>treatment</u> for a person with AIDS? Should <u>most</u> of the costs be paid by... *(Circle one.)*

the person who has AIDS and his or her family...1
the government...2
insurance companies...............................3
someone else? *(Specify)*..............................4

_____

Don't know...*8*

b. Who do you think should pay most of the costs for medical <u>research</u> about AIDS? Should <u>most</u> of the costs be paid by... *(Circle one.)*

private contributions 1
the government...2
insurance companies...............................3
someone else? *(Specify)*..............................4

_____

Don't know...*8*

24a. If a center to treat people with AIDS was going to be set up in your neighborhood, would you <u>favor</u> or <u>oppose</u> it?

Favor *(Skip to Q.25a)* 1
Oppose..*2*
Depends..*3*
Neither (Skip to Q.25a)..............................*4*
Don't know (Skip to Q.25a) *8*

(If "Oppose" or "Depends"):
b. Why is that?

_____

25a. If a person has a blood test that shows he or she was infected with the AIDS virus, should health officials tell the test results to anyone other than that person?

Yes...1
No *(Skip to Q.26)* 2
Don't know (Skip to Q.26) *8*

b. Who else should they tell? *(Circle all that apply.)*

Spouse..1
Person's sexual partner(s)/boyfriend/girlfriend....2
Person's family.......................................3
Person's employer 4
Other *(Specify)*......................................5

_____

Don't know...*8*

26. Many employers require medical tests as a condition of employment. Should an employer be allowed to require job applicants to be medically tested for. . .

		Yes	No	Depends on job	Don't know
a.	V.D. (venereal disease)? ...	1	2	7	8
b.	using illegal drugs?	1	2	7	8
c.	high blood pressure?	1	2	7	8
d.	having the AIDS virus? ...	1	2	7	8

27a. Should public schools teach students about AIDS?

Yes 1
No *(Skip to Q.28a)* 2

b. Beginning in what grade? _____

28a. Would you send your child to <u>elementary</u> school if a student in the school had AIDS?

Yes 1
No 2
Depends *3*
Don't know *8*

b. Would you send your child to <u>high school</u> if a student in the school had AIDS?

Yes 1
No 2
Depends *3*
Don't know *8*

29a. In terms of your own risk of getting AIDS, do you think you are. . .

at great risk 1
at some risk 2
at no risk for getting AIDS? 3
Don't know (Skip to Q.30a) *8*
Refused (Skip to Q.30a) *9*

b.   Why do you think you are *(Q.29a response)*? *(Probe with "What other reasons?"*
      until R says "None." Circle all that apply.)

                          Number of people date/have sexual contact
                              with..01
                          Knowledge of people date/have sexual contact
                              with..02
                          Blood transfusions 03
                          IV drug use/sharing needles.......................04
                          Specific sexual practices.............................05
                          Contact with blood/body fluids/person(s) with
                              AIDS..06
                          Other *(Specify)* 07

                          _____

                          _____

                          Don't know *98*

30a. Within the last year, how much would you say AIDS has caused you to
      change your lifestyle? Would you say AIDS has caused you to change your
      lifestyle a lot, some, or not at all?

                          A lot 1
                          Some 2
                          Not at all *(Skip to Q.31)* 3
                          Don't know (Skip to Q.31) *8*
                          Refused (Skip to Q.31) *9*

b.   What types of changes have you made in your lifestyle as a result of AIDS?
      (Probe with "What other changes?" until R replies "Nothing." Circle all that apply.)

                          Date or have sexual contact with fewer people...01
                          Know more about people I date or have sexual
                              contact with/am more selective..............02
                          Dating or sexual behavior, unspecified............03
                          Don't give blood 04
                          Don't have transfusions............................05
                          Other *(Specify)* 06

                          _____

                          _____

31.   In the next series of questions, I will ask you to answer by giving me a num-
      ber from 1 to 5. I will read you the same list of illnesses for each ques-
      tion. The first question is:

At one time or another, most of us have been afraid of becoming ill. Using a number between 1 and 5, where 1 means you are <u>not at all</u> afraid and 5 means you are <u>extremely</u> afraid, please tell me, how afraid are you of. . .

		Not at all afraid			Extremely afraid		*R has*	*DK*
a.	getting diabetes?...................	1	2	3	4	5	7	8
b.	getting cancer?....................	1	2	3	4	5	7	8
c.	getting AIDS?.....................	1	2	3	4	5	7	8
d.	getting a physically crippling disease?............................	1	2	3	4	5	7	8
e.	getting V.D. (venereal disease)? ...	1	2	3	4	5	7	8
f.	becoming mentally ill?............	1	2	3	4	5	7	8
g.	catching a common cold?.........	1	2	3	4	5	7	8

32. Now thinking about the future, indicate how <u>likely</u> you think it is that you will get the illness, where 1 means you are <u>not at all</u> likely to get the illness and 5 means you are <u>extremely</u> likely to get the illness. How likely are you to. . .

		Not at all likely			Extremely likely		*R has*	*DK*
a.	get diabetes?	1	2	3	4	5	7	8
b.	get cancer?	1	2	3	4	5	7	8
c.	get AIDS?..........................	1	2	3	4	5	7	8
d.	get a physically crippling disease?	1	2	3	4	5	7	8
e.	get V.D. (venereal disease)?	1	2	3	4	5	7	8
f.	become mentally ill?	1	2	3	4	5	7	8
g.	catch a common cold?	1	2	3	4	5	7	8

33. Please indicate how <u>serious</u> you think each illness is, where 1 means the illness is <u>not at all</u> serious and 5 means the illness is <u>extremely</u> serious. How serious is. . .

		Not at all serious			Extremely serious		*R has*	*DK*
a.	diabetes?	1	2	3	4	5	7	8
b.	cancer?	1	2	3	4	5	7	8
c.	AIDS?	1	2	3	4	5	7	8
d.	a physically crippling disease?	1	2	3	4	5	7	8
e.	V.D. (venereal disease)?............	1	2	3	4	5	7	8
f.	a mental illness?	1	2	3	4	5	7	8
g.	a common cold?	1	2	3	4	5	7	8

34. Some illnesses make people feel ashamed for having them and other ill-nesses do not. For this question, 1 means you would feel <u>not</u> at <u>all</u> ashamed of having the illness and 5 means you would feel <u>extremely</u> ashamed. How ashamed would you feel of. . .

		Not at all ashamed			Extremely ashamed		<u>R</u> has	DK
a.	having diabetes?	1	2	3	4	5	7	8
b.	having cancer?	1	2	3	4	5	7	8
c.	having AIDS?	1	2	3	4	5	7	8
d.	having a physically crippling disease?	1	2	3	4	5	7	8
e.	having V.D. (venereal disease)?	1	2	3	4	5	7	8
f.	being mentally ill?	1	2	3	4	5	7	8
g.	having a common cold?	1	2	3	4	5	7	8

35. Now please indicate how personally <u>responsible</u> you think a person is for having each illness, where 1 means a person is <u>not</u> at <u>all</u> responsible and 5 means a person is <u>completely</u> responsible. In general, how responsible do you think a person is for having. . .

		Not at all responsible			Completely responsible		<u>R</u> has	DK
a.	diabetes?	1	2	3	4	5	7	8
b.	cancer?	1	2	3	4	5	7	8
c.	AIDS?	1	2	3	4	5	7	8
d.	a physically crippling disease?	1	2	3	4	5	7	8
e.	V.D. (venereal disease)?	1	2	3	4	5	7	8
f.	a mental illness?	1	2	3	4	5	7	8
g.	a common cold?	1	2	3	4	5	7	8

36a. So that we can help prevent the spread of AIDS, we need to know more about the sexual practices and drug use patterns of the general public in the Chicago area. Some of these questions need to be rather detailed and personal. If you prefer not to answer a question, please tell me, and I will simply go on to the next question. We appreciate your cooperation in answering these questions.

b. Have you had sex with anyone in the past 5 years?

Yes 1
No *(Skip to Q.44a)* 2
Refused (Skip to Q.44a) 9

c. In the past 5 years, how many different people have you had as sexual partners?

_____

(If 2 or more, skip to Q.38)

Refused (Skip to Q.38)..................................99

37. Was that person a man or a woman?

Man...1

Woman 2

Refused...9

┌─────────────────────┐
│   *Skip to Q.39a*   │
└─────────────────────┘

38. Thinking about the past 5 years, has your sexual activity been. . .

with men 1

with women...2

with both men and women?.......................3

Refused...9

39a. How much do you know about the past sexual practices of your (partner/partners)? Do you know. . .

a lot 1

a little 2

nothing? 3

Refused...9

b. How much do you know about your sexual partners' past use of illegal drugs? Do you know. . .

a lot 1

a little 2

nothing? 3

No drug use...4

Refused...9

40a. People practice many different sexual activities, and some people practice things that other people do not. I am going to ask you about a few sexual activities that are important for us to learn about for this study. In some questions, I will give an explanation that you might or might not need. I must read each question the same way to everyone, so I appreciate your patience.

In the past 5 years, have you engaged in vaginal intercourse—that is, sexual intercourse involving the vagina (female sex organ)?

Yes 1
No *(Skip to Q.41a)* 2
Don't know (Skip to Q.41a) *8*
Refused (Skip to Q.41a) *9*

(Ask females only):

b. Did your (partner/partners) use a condom. . .

always 1
sometimes 2
never? 3
Refused *9*

(Ask males only):

c. Did you use a condom. . .

always 1
sometimes 2
never? 3
Refused *9*

41a. In the past 5 years, have you engaged in anal intercourse—that is, rectal intercourse?

Yes *(If female <u>R</u>, skip to Q.41e; if male <u>R</u>,*
    go to Q.41b) 1
No *(Skip to Q.42a)* 2
Don't know (Skip to Q.42a) *8*
Refused (Skip to Q.42a) *9*

(Ask males only):

b. We need to ask about both the active and the passive activities that are a part of anal intercourse. In the past 5 years, have you been the inserting (insertive), that is, the active partner?

Yes 1
No *(Skip to Q.41d)* 2
Don't know (Skip to Q.41d) *8*
Refused (Skip to Q.41d) *9*

(Ask males only):

c. Did you use a condom. . .

always 1
sometimes 2
never? 3
Refused *9*

(Ask males only):

d. In the past 5 years, have you been the receiving (receptive), that is, the passive partner?

Yes 1
No *(Skip to Q.42a)* 2
Don't know (Skip to Q.42a) *8*
Refused (Skip to Q.42a) *9*

(Ask males and females):

e. Did your (partner/partners) use a condom. . .

always 1
sometimes...2
never? 3
Refused *9*

42. To reduce the risk of getting AIDS, some people make sure they talk with their partners about sexual practices that help a person avoid getting AIDS.

(If R has had only 1 sex partner during past 5 years):

a. Have you talked about these matters with your sexual partner?

Yes 1
No 2

(If R has had 2 or more sex partners during past 5 years):

b. Have you talked about these matters with. . .

all 1
some...2
none of your sexual partners?.......................3
Refused *9*

43a. Now I am going to read you a list of changes   *(If Yes to Q.43a):*
that some people have made in their sexual   43b. Was this to
practices in order to reduce their risk of   reduce your
getting AIDS. Please tell me if you have   risk of
changed your behavior in any of these ways.   getting
In the past 12 months. . .   AIDS?

	Yes	No	*Not Applicable*		Yes	No
1. have you stopped having sex?	1	2	7		1	2
					(Skip to Q.44a)	
2. have you had sex with only one person?	1	2	7		1	2

3. have you had sex with fewer people than before hearing about AIDS?	1	2	7	1	2
4. have you stopped having certain kinds of sex?	1	2	7	1	2
5 have you used a condom or asked your partner to use a condom when having sex?	1	2	7	1	2
6. have you made any other changes in your sexual behavior? *(Specify)* .	1	2	7	1	2

_____

44a. Some people use needles when they take drugs. Do you personally know anyone who uses a needle to inject illegal drugs?

Yes 1
No *(Skip to Q.45a)* 2
Refused (Skip to Q.45a) 9

b. Do you know one person or <u>more</u> than one person who uses a needle to inject illegal drugs?

One.. 1
More than one *(Skip to Q.44d)* 2

c. Is this person. . .

a family member 1
a close friend... 2
someone you know, but do not know well?..........3

> *Skip to Q.45a*

d. Are any of these people. . .

		Yes	No
1.	family members?	1	2
2.	close friends?......................	1	2
3	people you know, but do not know well?	1	2

45a. In the past 5 years, have you used a needle to inject illegal drugs?

Yes 1

No *(Skip to Q.46a)* 2

Refused (Skip to Q.46a) 9

b. We need to know whether people share needles or do not share needles. In the past 5 years, have you ever shared a needle?

Yes 1

No *(Skip to Q.46a)* 2

Refused (Skip to Q.46a) 9

c. Have you shared a needle in the last month?

Yes 1

No 2

Refused 9

d. In the past 5 years, because of fear of AIDS, have you decided not to share needles for injecting drugs?

Yes 1

No 2

R quit using drugs 3

Refused 9

46a. Do you personally know or have you known anyone who is a homosexual male?

Yes 1

No *(Skip to Q.47)* 2

Don't know (Skip to Q.47) 8

Refused (Skip to Q.47) 9

b. Do you know one person or <u>more</u> than one person who is a homosexual male?

One 1

More than one *(Skip to Q.46d)* 2

c. Is this person. . .

a family member 1

a close friend 2

someone you know, but do not know well? 3

> *Skip to Q.47*

d.   Are any of these people...

		Yes	No
1.	family members?	1	2
2.	close friends?......................	1	2
3	people you know, but do not know well?	1	2

47.   For each of the statements I am going to read to you next, please tell me if you strongly agree, agree, disagree, or strongly disagree. *(Read a–e.)*

		strongly agree	agree	disagree	strongly disagree?	*R* *does not understand*
a.	Male homosexuals are disgusting. Do you ...	1	2	3	4	7
b.	Male homosexuality is a perversion. Do you	1	2	3	4	7
c.	Male homosexuality is a natural expression of sexuality in human men................	1	2	3	4	7
d.	Homosexual behavior between two men is just plain wrong	1	2	3	4	7
e.	Male homosexuality is merely a different kind of lifestyle that should not be condemned	1	2	3	4	7

48.   The following questions about you and your household are needed for statistical purposes only. What is the <u>highest</u> grade or year of school you have completed?

None 00
Elementary 01 02 03 04 05 06 07 08
High school.............................09 10 11 12
College...................................13 14 15 16
Some graduate school 17
Graduate or professional degree...................18
Trade school.......................................97
Don't know 98
Refused 99

49.   Are you currently. . .

married...1
not married but living with a sexual partner.......2
separated..3
divorced..4
widowed..5
never married?..6
Refused *9*

50.   Do you have any children age 17 or younger?

Yes..1
No 2
Don't know *8*
Refused *9*

51a. Are you currently employed?

Yes..1
No *(Skip to Q.51c)* 2

b.   Are you <u>self</u>-employed?

Yes *(Skip to Q.51d)*...................................1
No *(Skip to Q.51d)*...................................2

c.   Are you. . .

retired 1
disabled 2
a student *(Skip to Q.52a)* 3
keeping house *(Skip to Q.52a)* 4
temporarily unemployed...............................5
not looking for paid employment?
        (Skip to Q.52a)...................................6
Other (Specify—Skip to Q.52a) *7*

_____

d.   What (is/was) your job title? *(If respondent has/had more than one job, ask about the "main job.")*

_____

e.   What (are/were) your most important job activities or duties?

_____

f.   What kind of business or industry (is/was) this?

_____

g.   (Is/Was) this mainly. . .

                        manufacturing 1

                        wholesale trade 2

                        retail trade 3

                        some other area? *(Specify)* 4

52a.   What is your religious preference? Would you describe yourself as. . .

                        Protestant 1

                        Catholic *(Skip to Q.53)* 2

                        Jewish *(Skip to Q.53)* 3

                        something else? *(Specify—Skip to Q.53)* 4

                        No preference (Skip to Q.53) 7

                        Don't know (Skip to Q.53) 8

                        Refused (Skip to Q.53) 9

b.   Which Protestant denomination do you identify with?

                        Baptist 01

                        Congregationalist 02

                        Episcopalian, Anglican 03

                        Lutheran... 04

                        Methodist.. 05

                        Presbyterian 06

                        Other (Specify).. 07

                        None 97

                        Don't know 98

                        Refused... 99

53.   How important is religion in helping you cope with problems in your daily life? Is it. . .

                        very important... 1

                        somewhat important 2

                        not at all important? 3

                        Don't know 8

                        Refused 9

54.   Do you think of yourself as. . .

                        heterosexual 1

                        homosexual 2

                        bisexual? 3

                        Normal/straight.. 4

                        Other (Specify) 5

                        Don't understand terms 7

                        Don't know 8

                        Refused 9

55a.   What is your racial background? Are you. . .

White..1

Black 2

Asian *(Skip to Q.56a)* *3*

Something else? (Specify)

Hispanic/Latino/Chicano (Skip to Q.55c)............4

American Indian (Skip to Q.56a) 5

Other (Specify) 6

_____

Refused 9

b.   Are you of Hispanic origin?

Yes...1

No *(Skip to Q.56a)*..*2*

Refused 9

c.   Are you. . . *(Circle all that apply.)*

Mexican..1

Puerto Rican...2

Cuban 3

Something else? *(Specify)* 4

_____

Refused 9

56a.   For 1986, was your <u>total</u> <u>household</u> income from all sources before taxes. . .

less than $15,000..L

more than $15,000? *(Skip to Q.56d)* ....M

$15,000 exactly (Skip to Q.57)............................04

Don't know (Skip to Q.57)................................98

Refused (Skip to Q.57)...................................99

b.   Was it. . .

less than $10,000?

No *(Skip to Q.57)*.................................*03*

Yes...L

c.   Was it. . .

less than $5,000?

No *(Skip to Q.57)*.................................*02*

Yes *(Skip to Q.57)*................................*01*

Don't know (Skip to Q.57)................................98

Refused (Skip to Q.57)...................................99

d.   Was it. . .

less than $35,000?....................................L
more than $35,000? *(Skip to Q.56g)* ....M
($35,000 exactly) (Skip to Q.57).........................*07*
Don't know (Skip to Q.57)...............................*98*
Refused (Skip to Q.57)...................................*99*

e.   Was it. . .

less than $25,000?
No *(Skip to Q.57)*..................................06
Yes...L

f.   Was it. . .

less than $20,000?
No *(Skip to Q.57)*..................................05
Yes *(Skip to Q.57)*.................................04
Don't know (Skip to Q.57)...............................*98*
Refused (Skip to Q.57)...................................*99*

g.   Was it. . .

more than $50,000?
No...07
Yes..08
Don't know...*98*
Refused..*99*

57.   Do you live in the city of Chicago?
Yes...1
No *(Skip to Q.59)* 2
Don't know (Skip to Q.60) 8
Refused (Skip to Q.61) 9

58.   What is the name of the neighborhood where you live?

_____

┌─────────────────────┐
│   *Skip to Q.61*   │
└─────────────────────┘

59.   In what city or town do you live?

_____

60.   What is the name of the neighborhood where you live?

_____

61.   Finally, are there any other comments you would like to make about health issues in the Chicago metropolitan area?

_____

_____

_____

62.   Thank you very much for your cooperation.

63.   *(Do not ask.) Circle sex of respondent:*
                        Male *1*
                        Female *2*

64.   *Time interview ended (Use 24-hour clock):* _____

65.   *Interviewer comments:*
        _____
        _____
        _____
        _____

66.   *Interviewer: Did you edit?*
                        Yes *1*
                        No *2*

University of Illinois
SURVEY RESEARCH LABORATORY

Chicago Area
General Population Survey on AIDS
(SRL No. 606)

INTERVIEWER MANUAL

Purpose

This is a telephone survey of adults in the general population to learn people's opinions and behaviors related to important health issues.

Specifically, this is a Random Digit Dialing (RDD), non-CATI survey to learn about people's knowledge, attitudes, perceptions, and behaviors related to the health condition Acquired Immune Deficiency Syndrome, known as AIDS. AIDS is an infectious disease spread from one person to another by a virus. The virus is transmitted by intimate (usually sexual) contact and by the mixing of blood. Because of the ways in which the virus is transmitted, the prevention of AIDS requires that health officials know the extent to which people engage in certain sexual and drug-use practices. Based on results from a pilot study recently done at SRL, this survey includes questions about sensitive topics such as people's sexual and drug-use practices, in addition to questions about their knowledge and attitudes about AIDS and other health issues.

Sponsor

The study is sponsored by the U.S. Centers for Disease Control (CDC) and the Chicago Department of Public Health. The principal investigator for the survey is Dr. Gary Albrecht of the University of Illinois School of Public Health.

Assistance

If respondents have any questions about the survey, they should contact the project coordinator:

Patricia Murphy
996-5271
9:00 a.m. – 5:00 p.m.
Monday through Friday.

If respondents have any questions about AIDS, they should contact:

Illinois AIDS Hotline
1-800-AID-AIDS.

This is a toll-free call from anywhere in the state of Illinois.

Sample

The sampling unit for this survey is the telephone number. Telephone numbers in the six-county Chicago SMSA were chosen by RDD, that is, by adding selected digits to existing telephone exchanges (the first three digits of a phone number) to create complete 7-digit telephone numbers. For each sample telephone number, you will first determine if it is a household number. Then you will use a screening questionnaire to select the eligible respondent within the household.

Eligible Telephone Number

An eligible telephone number for this survey is the telephone number: (a) on an Interviewer Report Form (IRF), and (b) for a residence other than group quarters. Each of these criteria is explained below.

Telephone number on IRF. Only telephone numbers given to you on IRFs are eligible to be called. If you make contact with someone at a number other than the one on an IRF (as the result of misdialing, for example), *no one* at that number is to be interviewed. Similarly, if you dial the number on an IRF and learn from a recording that the sample telephone number has been changed, you should *not* call the new number.

Telephone number for residence. Only residential telephones are eligible for this survey. A residence is any place where people live on a permanent basis. A residential phone is a telephone located in a residence and used primarily for private, nonbusiness purposes.

Usually you will know when you have reached a business telephone by the way it is answered. That is, someone will answer by saying, for example, "Sears" or "Dr. Williams' office" or "Atlas Grocery." If such a clear indication is not given but you have some feeling that you might have reached a business telephone, you should probe to be sure. The screening questions to select a respondent will help you identify nonresidential telephones.

Telephone numbers for group quarters are not eligible. Group quarters consist of:

— 5 or more unrelated adults who are not related to the head of the household, or
— 6 or more unrelated adults in a household where no one is considered the head.

Examples of group quarters are nursing homes, dormitories, and fraternity houses. If you reach a telephone that serves *all* of the residents in a group quarters, the "household" living in the group quarters is *not* eligible for this survey. However, if you reach a telephone that is a private line in a group quarters, such as a private phone in a dorm room or in a nursing home room, the "household" living in that room is eligible for this survey.

As with business telephones, you usually will know when you have reached a group quarters telephone. The screening questions to identify a respondent also will help to identify group quarters.

Eligible Respondent

The eligible respondent in a household is the adult household member (male or female) age 18 years or older who has had the most recent birthday. A series of questions to determine which adult had the last birthday is asked in the screening questionnaire. If the adult household member having the last birthday is then determined to be over age 60, no interview will be conducted. In addition, some versions of the screening questionnaire include a question concerning the respondent's racial background.

Time Schedule

The time schedule for this study requires data collection to be completed by June 3, 1987. It is expected that you will complete at least 1,500 interviews with respondents.

Supervision

The supervisor for the survey is:

Betty Holman
996-9385

Gaining Cooperation and Establishing Rapport

An RDD sample means that respondents receive at least your initial call with no advance warning. Moreover, the topic of AIDS and the nature of the study means that you will be asking respondents to answer some questions that they might consider sensitive or threatening. Therefore, your ability to gain respondents' cooperation will be especially key to the success of this survey.

The respondent's cooperation depends, to a great extent, on your presentation and rapport. Emphasize the importance of participation by the selected respondent. If the respondent shows signs of being uncomfortable because he or she doesn't have much information or is afraid of saying the wrong things, reassure the person by emphasizing that:

1. We are not testing knowledge. What matters is what each person thinks about the various questions.
2. All the answers are kept confidential.

Special transition statements are included in the questionnaire to help reassure respondents. The most important assurance, however, will be your careful and confident way of asking the survey questions.

Answering Respondents' Questions

It is important that you are thoroughly familiar with this manual before you begin interviewing so that you can use appropriate information from it to respond to questions raised by respondents. In some instances, you will need to refer the respondent to another source for information; in other instances, you will need to answer the respondent's questions. Always respond in a clear, concise, and convincing manner, whether you are referring the person or answering the question.

Refer a respondent to Pat Murphy (996-5271), the project coordinator, if a question is about the survey in general and cannot be answered by the information in this manual. Such a question might be, "How much money is being spent on this study?" or "How can I learn the results of this survey?" Refer a respondent to the AIDS Hotline (1-800-AID-AIDS) for all information about AIDS. The information about AIDS that you are receiving in this manual and during the training is for your background only. You are *not* to use this information to explain survey questions for respondents or to answer questions they might raise about how AIDS is transmitted, how to get a blood test, and so forth.

Below are some questions that might be asked of you that you should practice answering so that you can do so easily. The questions will rarely be stated exactly as they are here. Be sure to listen carefully and understand what a person is asking, then answer briefly but directly to the point.

Is this a study of people with AIDS? No. This is a survey of people in the Chicago area to learn what the general public has heard or read and what people think about AIDS and other health problems. The people in our survey have been randomly selected for interviews.

How did you get my telephone number? Your number was randomly selected from among all of the possible telephone numbers in the Chicago area. We do not use mailing lists or telephone directories to identify telephone numbers.

Why talk to me? I don't know anything about AIDS. This is a study of the population in general, so we need to talk with people who do not know about AIDS, as well as people who do know about AIDS. We are interested in your opinions as well as your knowledge, and not every question in the survey is specifically about AIDS.

Why don't you call someone else? It is important that we talk to you because the procedures we used to select your telephone number and you individually do not allow us to replace you with someone else. Once a phone number and household member have been randomly selected, we must talk to that person. Otherwise, we would not get an accurate or scientific picture of the population.

How long will this take? I'm too busy. On the average, this interview takes about 30 minutes.

Why are you asking me such personal questions? To develop educational programs to help stop the spread of certain illnesses or viruses, we need to find out people's opinions and practices related to health issues. Your answers are completely confidential and you cannot be identified.

How can I get some information about AIDS? Where can people find out if they have AIDS? For anyone in the state of Illinois, there is a toll-free telephone number to call for information about AIDS and referral to AIDS-related services. The number is 1-800-AID-AIDS.

DATA COLLECTION FORMS AND PROCEDURES

For this study, you will be using an Interviewer Report Form (IRF), a Non-Interview Report Form (NIRF), a screening questionnaire, and the main questionnaire. There are three colors of IRFs: yellow, blue, and green. Depending on the color of the IRF, you will use one of three versions of the screening questionnaire. The screening questionnaires are also copied on yellow, blue, and green.

Interviewer Report Form (IRF)

The printed information on all three colors of IRFs is identical. A 5-digit sequential ID number and the full telephone number of each piece of sample will be written on the IRF, along with some other information that is needed by the Sampling Section. You will be concerned with only the case ID and telephone number.

A record of each attempt made to contact the sample telephone number is to be kept on the IRF. For each attempt, write the date, time, disposition code number, and your interviewer ID number. Also write, under "Appointments/Notes/Other" or "Interviewer Notes," an explanation of what happened during each contact attempt.

A maximum of 10 attempts is to be made on each telephone number for the purpose of completing an interview. Only one contact attempt should be made on a number during an interviewing shift, unless you obtain a busy signal or some indication that a respondent will be available later during the shift. For some disposition codes you must complete a Non-Interview Report Form (NIRF), which is discussed in the following section of this manual. On busy numbers, make a maximum of 3 tries about 3 minutes apart; record the attempts on a single line of the IRF.

When you assign a final disposition, check the line in the column headed "Final." Leave the line blank when the disposition is a pending one. In other words, each IRF will have only one line checked in the "Final" column.

Non-Interview Report Form (NIRF)

Please do a full NIRF as instructed in the manual information on disposition code definitions. Do not hesitate to report what you might consider an obvious situation or explanation. It is better to report too much information than too little. The information you provide is especially important for refusal conversion attempts.

SCREENING QUESTIONNAIRE

The screening questionnaire consists of 3 or 4 parts:
— an introduction, which includes verifying that the sample phone number was reached;
— questions for respondent selection that determine which adult member of the household had the last birthday; and
— a question to determine if the selected respondent is between 18 and 60 years of age.
— Some screeners also include a question to determine the respondent's racial background.

You must interview the individual whom you identify, by asking the screening questions, as the eligible respondent. The scientific validity of the survey requires that you interview *only* the person identified as the eligible respondent.

Introduction: Be sure to verify the phone number. If you have misdialed, dial the number again. If you again reach a number other than the one you dialed, do not try again; *notify your supervisor.*

Q.S1–S2   If informant will not provide name for "someone else," obtain a re-
           lationship or some other way to identify the person if a callback be-
           comes necessary.

Q.S3   If selected *R* is not available, schedule callback. Staple screener to IRF.

Q.S4   Follow the boxed instruction. This question is to ensure that the re-
           spondent is aged 18–60 years. Read the question only as it is written.

Q.S5   Notice that skip instructions are different on the blue and green ver-
           sions. Be sure to read carefully each time.

Disposition Codes

Disposition codes describe "what happened" as a result of each attempt. Be
sure to specify under "Appointments/Notes/Other" or on an NIRF, when appropriate, anything that will make it easier for someone to complete an interview or understand what happened during your contact attempt.

Following are the disposition and corresponding code numbers and definitions for this study:

PRE-RESPONDENT-SELECTION

Disposition	Code	Definition
Nonresidential	22	Telephone number reaches a nonresidence, i.e., business, professional office, nursing home, group quarters, etc. Final disposition.
Temporary disconnect	23	The number dialed has been temporarily disconnected. Pending disposition, or final after 2 attempts 1 week apart.
Other nonworking number	24	Includes all other nonworking numbers such as number changed, not in service, permanently disconnected, or not yet connected. Final disposition.
Initial refused screening	33	No one in the household is willing to give the information to select a respondent. Under "Appt/Other" and "Interviewer Notes," indicate exactly what the person said. Pending disposition.

Disposition	Code	Definition
Final refused screening	43	Informant refuses to complete screener in a refusal conversion attempt. Write a report of what happened in "Interviewer Notes." Final disposition.
Noncontact before screening	34	Use this code if no answer (NA), busy (after 3 tries), you reach an answering machine, no one in household is available to answer the screener questions, or the selected R cannot be interviewed at this time. Pending disposition, or final after 10 attempts.
Spanish-speaking household	36	Informant speaks Spanish but does not speak English. Pending disposition.
Other not screened	30	Some other situation not covered above. See supervisor before assigning this disposition. Pending or final disposition.

POST-RESPONDENT-SELECTION

Disposition	Code	Definition
Partial interview	11	Respondent terminated the interview part-way through it. Complete an NIRF and staple it to the back of the IRF. Pending disposition.
Completed interview	12	Interview is completed with selected respondent. Final disposition.
Initial refused interview	03	Selected respondent refuses to be interviewed or refuses to finish the entire interview. Complete an NIRF and staple it to the back of the IRF. Pending disposition.

Disposition	Code	Definition
Final refused interview	13	Selected *R* refuses to be interviewed in a refusal conversion attempt. Complete a second NIRF and staple it to the back of the IRF and initial NIRF. Final disposition.
Noncontact after screening	14	The selected respondent is not home (RHN) or not available (RNA) to complete the interview, or there is no answer (NA) or you reach an answering machine or the line is busy (after 3 tries). Pending disposition, or final after 10 attempts.
Unavailable for duration	15	*R* is selected, but is sick, on vacation, deaf, or cannot speak either English or Spanish and, therefore, is unavailable for the interview for the duration of this study. Complete an NIRF and attach it to the IRF. Final disposition.
Ineligible	21	There is no one currently living in the household who is 18 years or older; the selected *R* is over 60; or the selected *R* is ineligible according to the screening Q on racial background. Final disposition.
Other screened	20	Some other situation not covered by the above codes, for example, *R* requests male interviewer. See supervisor before assigning this disposition. Pending or final disposition.

MAIN QUESTIONNAIRE

General Instructions. Complete the questionnaire in black ink. Indicate any questions where the respondent expresses discomfort or confusion. Use the margins of the questionnaire to note the respondent's verbatim comments and any comments or observations you have.

After you finish each interview, complete the Interviewer Report Form and thoroughly edit the entire completed questionnaire. Edit in blue ink. Remember that the purpose of editing is not to change anything but to make your written record more complete and understandable to anyone reading it. Data reduction staff must be able to code what you have written. During editing you should do the following:

1. Make sure everything is clear and legible. Rewrite illegible words; write out all your abbreviations; make sure your circles are clear and do not run onto another answer code.
2. While the interview is still fresh in your mind, add any comments (in parentheses) in the left margin or at the end of the questionnaire. These comments should help anyone reading the questionnaire to understand the interview and to have a clearer picture of the whole interview situation.
3. Make sure that every appropriate question has an answer recorded or add an explanation (in parentheses) of why the question was not answered. Be sure to indicate probes with X, and always record the response to your probe.

During editing, you may discover an unanswered question or something else that may require a callback. Check with the supervisor to see if you should call back at this time. As an interviewer, you are responsible for making any error calls requested by the project team about your cases. A case is not completed until any errors have been corrected. Most of this can be eliminated by following correct skip patterns, probing for completeness and clarity, and by carefully editing each interview immediately after you have completed it.

Question by Question Instructions

Questions which require specific clarification are detailed below. It is important to be comfortable with these guidelines prior to actual interviewing.

Enter time interview began.

Q.3a   The "media" include television, radio, newspapers, magazines, and journals.

Q.5   Be sure to circle only *one* response. We want to know who should pay *most* of the costs.

Q.6   Note that page 29 is on pink paper.

Q.7a   Do *not* read the answer categories, and do *not* probe with "Where else?"

Q.7b   Read all categories that were not volunteered by *R* in Q.7a.

Q.10   Note that this asks about the number of people who *get* AIDS, not the number who have AIDS.

Q.11   Do not read answer categories. Record verbatim in "other" any answers given by *R* that are not listed. Use listed categories only when *R* gives exactly the response that appears.

Q.12   Probe to obtain the *one* mention *mainly* responsible.

Q.15   Synonyms for "condom" include "rubber," "prophylactic," and "boot." If *R* does not understand "condom," offer one of these synonyms, using "rubber" first.

Q.18b   Probe for types or groups of people—*not* for individual names.

Q.19b   Probe for types or groups of people—*not* for individual names. Probe for clarity.

Q.20a–d   If *R* indicates that the person is now deceased, rephrase the questions in the past tense.

Q.20c   Probe for the *single* answer that best reflects the relationship.

Q.21b   Be sure to probe responses that do not answer the question or are vague, such as "People who use illegal drugs could quit." Code answers that clearly fit the listed categories and write others verbatim under "other."

        A response that fits code 1 is, "Because it's encouraging drug addicts to continue using drugs." A response that fits code 2 is, "People who use other people's needles will continue to do that. This won't solve the problem." A response that fits code 3 is, "We should be spending the money for drug centers to help people get off drugs."

Q.22   Probe for specific answers. Use listed categories for responses that clearly fit, and write others verbatim in "other."

Q.23a–b   As in Q.5, be sure to circle only *one* response—who should pay *most* of the costs.

Q.24b   Probe for specific response. For example, if *R* opposes because "It's dangerous," probe for *what* the danger is and *who* is in danger.

Q.25b   Do not read categories.

Q.27b   Be sure to get a response that answers the question. Probe a response such as, "Before the 8th grade." Also be sure to get one specific grade. Probe a response like, "Grade 4 or 5."

Q.28a–b   Note that these questions say "if a student in the *school* had AIDS," not "if a student in the child's *class* had AIDS."

Q.29b   Do not read the list. Use listed categories only when *R* gives exact response. Record verbatim any answers given by *R* that are not listed.

Q.30a   "Lifestyle" is an intentionally broad term. It is not meant to cover only sexual practices. By "lifestyle," we mean *all* aspects of a person's life.

Q.30b   In addition to probing for completeness of response, probe as necessary for specific and clear responses. Do not use category 03 unless a response is unspecific even *after* you probe.

Q.31–35   If *R* volunteers that he or she has only one of the illnesses listed, circle code 7 and do not read the illness in subsequent questions in the series.

Q.36c   Probe for a specific number.

Q.39–41e   If the response to Q.36c was "1," use "partner" where applicable.

Q.39a–b   If *R* had more than 1 partner, we want an overall answer to these questions that considers all partners.

Q.40a   Synonyms for "vaginal intercourse" include "screwing" and "fucking." If *R* uses these synonyms, you can respond "That's another way to say it;" you are *not* to offer or use or repeat the synonyms.

Q.40b–c   Synonyms for "condom" include "rubber," "prophylactic," and "boot."

Q.41a   Synonyms for "anal intercourse" include "rectal intercourse," "sodomy," "butt fucking," "ass fucking," and "cornholing." If *R* uses those phrases, you can respond "That's another way to say it;" you are *not* to offer or use or repeat the synonyms.

Q.41b–d   If *R* seems uncertain about the terminology, you can explain that the *inserting* partner inserts his penis into the *receiving* partner's rectum.

Q.42a–b   Refer back to Q.36c to determine which question to ask.

Q.43a–f   We want to know if *R* changed any of the listed behaviors *to reduce his or her risk of getting AIDS*. If *R never engaged* in a particular activity, circle code 7. If the response to Q.43a is "Yes," ask Q.43b for that behavior before going on to the next listed behavior. If the *R* answers "Yes" to Q.43a for behavior 1, "stopped having sex," ask Q.43b and then skip to Q.44a *regardless* of whether the answer to Q.43b is "Yes" or "No."

Q.44c   Probe for the *single* answer that best reflects the relationship.

Q.46c   Probe for the *single* answer that best reflects the relationship.

Q.47   Use category 7 when the *R* does not understand a word or a phrase, so that he or she cannot respond to the question in terms of agreement or disagreement. Record a "Don't know" response only when the *R* understands the statement but cannot decide to what extent he or she agrees or disagrees with it.

Q.48   If *R* says "Trade school and high school," circle "trade school." If *R* says "Trade school and college," circle "college."

Q.49   You may circle more than one response if *R* volunteers more than one response.

Q.51c   Use category 5, "temporarily unemployed," for any *R* who is unemployed but job-hunting, regardless of the length of unemployment.

Q.51d   Get full job title. For example, if *R* says "engineer," probe for what kind.

Q.51e–f   Be sure to get specific and complete answers that can be used to code the occupation and industry. An activity of "office work" is not acceptable and must be probed. Similarly, "the government" is not a sufficient answer for the kind of business or industry.

Q.54   If *R* does not understand the answer categories, use code 7. Use code 8, "Don't know," only when *R* understands terms and does not know how to classify himself or herself. Use category 4 when the *R* volunteers one of the terms "normal" or "straight."

Q.55   Use "other," for example, for a response of "part white and part Asian." Record verbatim.

Q.56   Follow skip instructions very carefully. You have completed the question when you have circled a numbered category for the response.

Q.58–60   Confirm the spelling of any town or county that is not familiar to you.

Q.61   Do *not* probe for additional comments or clarification. Record verbatim the response given, whether one mention or more than one mention.

Q.63   Be sure to circle sex of *R*.

Q.64   Be sure to indicate the time the interview ended.

Q.65   Write any comments you have about the interview.

Q.66   In addition to editing, be sure to transfer the case Sequence Number from the IRF to the front of the questionnaire, and enter your ID number as well. Staple the IRF, Screener, and NIRF, if there is one, to the first page of the questionnaire.

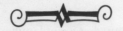

MAIL QUESTIONNAIRE SURVEY: WASHINGTON STATE STUDY OF DENTISTS' PREFERENCES IN PRESCRIBING DENTAL THERAPY

Resource C begins on the next page. Pages 443–456 constitute the questionnaire portion. Samples of cover letters and of a reminder postcard are reprinted on pp. 457–460.

The research for Resource C was supported by grant HS 05170 from the National Center for Health Services Research and Health Care Technology Assessment. The data were collected under the auspices of the Department of Community Dentistry, University of Washington, Seattle, 1987. Principal Investigator and Questionnaire Developer: David Grembowski.

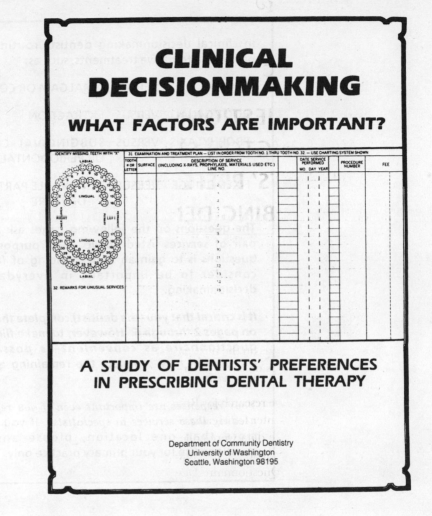

CLINICAL DECISIONMAKING

WHAT FACTORS ARE IMPORTANT?

A STUDY OF DENTISTS' PREFERENCES IN PRESCRIBING DENTAL THERAPY

Department of Community Dentistry
University of Washington
Seattle, Washington 98195

In clinical decisionmaking dentists routinely choose between alternative treatments, such as:

CROWN   VERSUS   AMALGAM OR COMPOSITE

ROOT CANAL   VERSUS   EXTRACTION

PROPHYLAXIS VERSUS   SUBGINGIVAL CURETTAGE
                                            OR PERIODONTAL SCALING

FIXED BRIDGE   VERSUS   REMOVABLE PARTIAL
                                            DENTURE

The questions on the following pages ask about each pair of services listed above. The purpose of these questions is to gain an understanding of factors YOU consider to be important in everyday clinical decisionmaking.

It is critical that you (the dentist) complete the questions on pages 2 through 6. However, to make filling out the questionnaire as convenient as possible, your receptionist may complete the remaining questions if you wish.

Your responses are important even if you refer patients needing these services to specialists. If you practice in more than one location, please answer this questionnaire for your primary practice only.

CROWN versus AMALGAM / COMPOSITE BUILDUP

Q-1 Listed below are some **PATIENT FACTORS** that may influence your decision to use either a crown OR an amalgam/composite buildup. Which of these factors are most important to YOU in making this choice? Although each clinical situation is somewhat different, please try to answer for the typical patient. (Please put the number in the appropriate box on the left. Answers may be explained in greater detail on the right.)

	RANK	FACTORS	COMMENTS
MOST IMPORTANT	☐	1 Age of patient 2 Caries rate 3 Medical history/conditions	
SECOND MOST IMPORTANT	☐	4 Patient's ability to tolerate procedure 5 Patient's oral hygiene status	
THIRD MOST IMPORTANT	☐	6 Patient's preference 7 Patient's previous experience with similar procedures 8 Other:_____	

Q-2 Listed below are some **TECHNICAL FACTORS** that may influence your choice of either a crown or an amalgam/composite buildup. Which of these factors are most important to YOU in making this choice?

	RANK	FACTORS	COMMENTS
MOST IMPORTANT	☐	9 Alignment/Tooth anatomy 10 Extent of tooth damage 11 Future plans for tooth	
SECOND MOST IMPORTANT	☐	12 My ability to do a good job (quality and efficiency) 13 Periodontal status	
THIRD MOST IMPORTANT	☐	14 Pulp status/Sensitivity 15 Other:_____	

Q-3 Listed below are some **COST FACTORS** that may influence your choice of these two services. Which of these factors are most important to YOU in making this choice?

	RANK	FACTORS	COMMENTS

MOST IMPORTANT	☐	16 Convenience to patient,
		  time in chair, number of
		  appointments	

SECOND MOST IMPORTANT	☐	17 Cost to Patient 18 Other:_____	

Q-4 Among ALL the factors listed above, from 1 to 18, which do you consider to be the MOST important in YOUR choice between these two services?

☐ MOST IMPORTANT   ☐ SECOND MOST   ☐ THIRD MOST
                               IMPORTANT   IMPORTANT

ROOT CANAL versus EXTRACTION

Q-5 Listed below are some **PATIENT FACTORS** that may influence your decision to use either an extraction OR a root canal (though an endodontist may actually perform the root canal). Which of these factors are most important to YOU in making this choice? (Please put the number of the appropriate box on the left. Answers may be explained in greater detail on the right.)

	RANK	FACTORS	COMMENTS
MOST IMPORTANT	☐	1 Age of Patient	
		2 Medical history/conditions	
		3 Number of missing teeth/caries teeth	
SECOND MOST IMPORTANT	☐	4 Oral hygiene status	
		5 Pain control demands of patient	
		6 Patient's ability to tolerate procedure	
THIRD MOST IMPORTANT	☐	7 Patient's preference	
		8 Patient's previous experience with similar procedures	
		9 Other:_____	

Q-6 Listed below are some **TECHNICAL FACTORS** that may influence your choice of the two services listed above. Which of these factors are most important to YOU in making this choice?

	RANK	FACTORS	COMMENTS
MOST IMPORTANT	☐	10 Difficulty of canals	
		11 Duration/extent of infection	
		12 Existing partial denture	
SECOND MOST IMPORTANT	☐	13 Extent of tooth damage	
		14 My ability to do a good job (quality and efficiency)	
THIRD MOST IMPORTANT	☐	15 Periodontal Status	
		16 Other:_____	

Q-7 Listed below are some **COST FACTORS** that may influence your choice of these two services. Which of these factors are most important to YOU in making this choice?

	RANK	FACTORS	COMMENTS
MOST IMPORTANT	☐	17 Convenience to patient, time in chair, number of appointments	
SECOND MOST IMPORTANT	☐	18 Cost to Patient	
		19 Other:_____	

Q-8 Among ALL the factors listed above, from 1 to 19, which do you consider to be the MOST important in YOUR choice between these two services?

☐ MOST IMPORTANT   ☐ SECOND MOST IMPORTANT   ☐ THIRD MOST IMPORTANT

FIXED BRIDGE versus REMOVABLE PARTIAL DENTURE

Q-9   Listed below are some **PATIENT FACTORS** that may influence your decision to use either a fixed bridge OR a removable partial denture <u>when both are possible</u>. Which of these factors are most important to YOU in making this choice? (Please put the number of the appropriate box on the left. Answers may be explained in greater detail on the right.)

	RANK	FACTORS		<u>COMMENTS</u>
MOST IMPORTANT	☐	1	Age of patient	
		2	Medical history/conditions	
		3	Number of missing teeth/caries teeth	
SECOND MOST IMPORTANT	☐	4	Oral hygiene status	
		5	Pain control demands of patient	
		6	Patient's ability to tolerate procedure	
THIRD MOST IMPORTANT	☐	7	Patient's preference	
		8	Patient's previous experience with procedure	
		9	Other:_____	

Q-10 Listed below are some **TECHNICAL FACTORS** that may influence your choice of these two services. Which of these factors are most important to YOU in making this choice?

	RANK	FACTORS		<u>COMMENTS</u>
MOST IMPORTANT	☐	10	Abutment contours/tipping	
		11	Extent of tooth damage	
		12	Length of edentulous span / abutment strength	
SECOND MOST IMPORTANT	☐	13	My ability to do a good job (quality, efficiency)	
		14	Periodontal status	
THIRD MOST IMPORTANT	☐	15	Soft tissue contours	
		16	Other:_____	

Q-11 Listed below are some **COST FACTORS** that may influence your choice of these two services. Which of these factors are most important to YOU in making this choice?

	RANK	FACTORS		<u>COMMENTS</u>
MOST IMPORTANT	☐	16	Convenience to patient, time in chair, number of appointments	
SECOND MOST IMPORTANT	☐	17	Cost to Patient	
		18	Other:_____	

Q-12 Among ALL the factors listed above, from 1 to 18, which do you consider to be the MOST important in YOUR choice between these two services?

☐ MOST IMPORTANT   ☐ SECOND MOST IMPORTANT   ☐ THIRD MOST IMPORTANT

PROPHYLAXIS versus SUBGINGIVAL
CURETTAGE/PERIODONTAL SCALING

Q-13 Listed below are some **PATIENT FACTORS** that may influence your decision to use either a prophylaxis OR subgingival curettage/periodontal scaling (though your hygienist or a periodontist may actually perform the service). Which of these factors are most important to YOU in making this choice? (Please put the number of the appropriate box on the left. Answers may be explained in greater detail on the right.)

	RANK	FACTORS	COMMENTS
MOST IMPORTANT	☐	1 Age of patient	
		2 Extent of calculus	
		3 Medical history/conditions	
SECOND MOST IMPORTANT	☐	4 Need for anesthesia	
		5 Oral hygiene status	
		6 Patient preference	
THIRD MOST IMPORTANT	☐	7 Patient's previous experience with similar procedures	
		8 Root caries	
		9 Tooth mobility	
		10 Other:_____	

Q-14 Listed below are some **TECHNICAL FACTORS** that may influence your choice of the two services listed above. Which of these factors are most important to YOU in making this choice?

	RANK	FACTORS	COMMENTS
MOST IMPORTANT	☐	11 My ability to do a good job	
		12 Periodontal/gingival status	
		13 Preparation for other perio/restorative procedures	
SECOND MOST IMPORTANT	☐	14 Other:_____	
THIRD MOST IMPORTANT	☐		

Q-15 Listed below are some **COST FACTORS** that may influence your choice of these two services. Which of these factors are most important to YOU in making this choice?

	RANK	FACTORS	COMMENTS
MOST IMPORTANT	☐	15 Convenience to patient, time in chair, number of appointments	
SECOND MOST IMPORTANT	☐	16 Cost to Patient	
		17 Other:_____	

Q-16 Among ALL the factors listed above, from 1 to 17, which do you consider to be the MOST important in YOUR choice between these two services?

☐ MOST IMPORTANT   ☐ SECOND MOST IMPORTANT   ☐ THIRD MOST IMPORTANT

PRACTICE BELIEFS

Q-17 To what extent do you AGREE or DISAGREE with each item below?
(Circle your answer)

		To what extent do you agree or disagree?		
a.	Plaque control programs are a prerequisite for dental treatment ..	STRONGLY AGREE	AGREE	DISAGREE	STRONGLY DISAGREE
b.	Dentists should present all treatment options to patients	STRONGLY AGREE	AGREE	DISAGREE	STRONGLY DISAGREE
c.	With dentist's advice, the patient should choose the service	STRONGLY AGREE	AGREE	DISAGREE	STRONGLY DISAGREE
d.	The primary focus of dentistry should be directed at controlling active disease rather than developing better preventive service	STRONGLY AGREE	AGREE	DISAGREE	STRONGLY DISAGREE
e.	If a patient opposes the dentist's recommended treatment, the dentist should try to convince the patient to accept it.	STRONGLY AGREE	AGREE	DISAGREE	STRONGLY DISAGREE
f.	If a patient does not accept the dentist's recommended treatment, the patient is dismissed from the practice.	STRONGLY AGREE	AGREE	DISAGREE	STRONGLY DISAGREE

Q-18 Which of the following best describes your entire practice during the past 12 months?
(Circle the number)

1   TOO BUSY TO TREAT ALL PEOPLE REQUESTING APPOINTMENTS

2   PROVIDED CARE TO ALL WHO REQUESTED APPOINTMENTS BUT THE PRACTICE WAS OVERWORKED

3   PROVIDED CARE TO ALL WHO REQUESTED APPOINTMENTS AND THE PRACTICE WAS NOT OVERWORKED

4   NOT BUSY ENOUGH - THE PRACTICE COULD HAVE TREATED MORE PATIENTS

To make filling out the questionnaire as convenient as possible, your receptionist may complete the remaining questions if you wish.

PRACTICE AND PATIENT CHARACTERISTICS

The questions below concern the most recent typical WEEK that you have worked. *YOU MAY WISH TO ASK YOUR RECEPTIONIST TO COMPLETE THE REST OF THE QUESTIONNAIRE FOR YOU.*

Q-19   During your most recent typical WEEK, how many patient visits were handled by the dentist and/or hygienist?

                                    _____ **VISITS**

Q-20   During the most recent typical WEEK, how much of the following types of care were provided in your practice? Please answer each question as indicated (Number of patients, number or teeth, etc.)

                                                              NUMBERS OF:

Oral diagnosis (initial and recall
    examinations) and x-rays .... _____ **PATIENTS**

Prophylaxis .... _____ **PATIENTS**

Fluoride treatments .... _____ **PATIENTS**

Sealants .... _____ **PATIENTS**

Operative Dentistry .... _____ **TEETH RESTORED**

Prosthodontics .... _____ **REMOVABLE APPLIANCES**

Crown and fixed bridge .... _____ **UNITS**

Oral surgery (number of oral surgery
    services and/or extractions) .... _____ **SERVICES OR EXTRACTIONS**

Periodontics (other than prophylaxis) .. _____ **PATIENTS**

Endodontics .... _____ **TEETH**

Orthodontics .... _____ **VISITS**

TMJ dysfunction .... _____ **VISITS**

Q-21   During your most recent typical WEEK, how far in advance did you have to schedule your average patient for the initial appointment of a treatment series (excluding emergency cases)?

   1   ONE OR TWO DAYS
   2   THREE DAYS TO A WEEK
   3   ONE OR TWO WEEKS
   4   TWO WEEKS TO A MONTH
   5   A MONTH OR MORE

Q-22   How long does the average patient have to wait to see the dentist AFTER the scheduled appointment?

   1   LESS THAN 5 MINUTES
   2   ABOUT 5-15 MINUTES
   3   ABOUT 16-30 MINUTES
   4   OVER 30 MINUTES

Q-23   Does your practice operate a patient recall system?

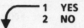

   1   YES
   2   NO

(If YES) Listed below are different recall practices. Please circle the number of all practices that you perform regularly.

   1   SCHEDULE 6-MONTH AND 1-YEAR CHECK-UPS AT CURRENT VISIT
   2   SEND PATIENT POSTCARD REMINDER TO MAKE AN APPOINTMENT FOR A CHECK-UP
   3   SEND PATIENT POSTCARD REMINDER A FEW DAYS BEFORE APPOINTMENT
   4   TELEPHONE PATIENT THE DAY BEFORE
   5   OTHER:_____

Q-24   Did you advertise the dental services of the practice during 1985 (through advertisements in the Yellow Pages, radio commercials, newspaper ads, direct mail or other means)?

   1   YES
   2   NO

Q-25   Excluding diagnostic and preventive services, do patients usually know how much their dental treatment will cost them, out-of-pocket, <u>before</u> treatment begins? (Circle your answer)

   1   MOST OF THE PATIENTS USUALLY KNOW
   2   SOME OF THE PATIENTS USUALLY KNOW
   3   ONLY A FEW OF THE PATIENTS USUALLY KNOW

The next set of questions deals with characteristics of all patients in your practice. We realize that some answers may be difficult to estimate, but please respond to the best of your ability.

Q-26   About what percent of the patients live in areas with fluoridated water?

_____ **PERCENT**

Q-27   Please estimate the percentage of patients in each of the following age groups:

AGE GROUPS

0-4	_____	PERCENT
5-18	_____	PERCENT
19-35	_____	PERCENT
36-65	_____	PERCENT
65 +	_____	PERCENT
	100%	

Q-28   To the best of your knowledge, about what percent of the patients are from households where the head of household is:

Unemployed	_____	PERCENT
Farm Worker	_____	PERCENT
Blue Collar Worker	_____	PERCENT
Clerical and Sale	_____	PERCENT
Professional, Manager, Owner	_____	PERCENT
	100%	

Q-29   About what percentage of your patients have each of the following categories of insurance?

No Insurance	_____	PERCENT
Private Dental Insurance or Pre-Payment	_____	PERCENT
Capitation	_____	PERCENT
Dental Public Assistance	_____	PERCENT
	100%	

PRACTICE ORGANIZATION

Q-30 Which ONE of the following BEST describes your (the dentist's) practice arrangement? For purposes of answering this questionnaire, "self employed" status includes one who is a shareholder in an incorporated practice. (Please circle the number)

    1 **EMPLOYED BY ANOTHER DENTIST**

    2 **SELF-EMPLOYED WITHOUT PARTNERS AND WITHOUT SHARING OF INCOME OR COSTS**

    3 **SELF-EMPLOYED WITHOUT PARTNERS BUT SHARING COSTS OF OFFICE AND/OR ASSISTANTS, ETC (BUT WITH NO INCOME-SHARING ARRANGEMENTS)**

    4 **SELF-EMPLOYED AS A PARTNER IN A COMPLETE PARTNERSHIP (BOTH INCOME AND EXPENSES SHARED)**
       Including the dentist to whom the questionnaire was sent, how many partners are there in the practice?_____PARTNERS

    5 **OTHER:_____**

Q-31 Which of the following categories best describes your private practice? (Circle the number.)

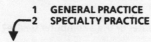

    1 **GENERAL PRACTICE**
    2 **SPECIALTY PRACTICE**

(If SPECIALTY PRACTICE) What area best describes your primary specialty?

    1 **ORAL SURGERY**

    2 **ORTHODONTICS**

    3 **PEDODONTICS**

    4 **PERIODONTICS**

    5 **PROSTHODONTICS**

    6 **ENDODONTICS**

Q-32 How many years have you been in this practice arrangement?
    _____ YEARS

Q-33 How many operatories do the dentist and hygienist use in this practice?
    _____ OPERATORIES

Q-34 How many full and part-time employees work in the practice? (Note: A secretary or receptionist who also provide chairside assistance at least 50% of the time should be counted as a chairside assistant.)

NUMBER OF EMPLOYEES

	Full-time	Part-time
Dental Hygienists	_____	_____
Chairside Assistants	_____	_____
Secretary/Receptionists	_____	_____

Q-35 What percent of your direct patient care time is spent in four-handed dentistry?

PERCENT OF TIME _____

Q-36 Does the dentist usually take time to explain complicated procedures to patients who are about to receive them? (Circle your answer)

     1   MOST OF THE TIME

     2   SOME OF THE TIME

     3   ALMOST NEVER

Q-37 Does your practice have a computer or use a computer service?

     1   NO

     2   YES - HAS ITS OWN COMPUTER

     3   YES - USES A COMPUTER SERVICE

(If YES) Which of the following tasks does the computer perform? (Circle all that apply.)

     1   PATIENT ACCOUNTING AND BILLING

     2   MAINTAINING EXPENSE RECORDS

     3   PROCESSING INSURANCE FORMS

     4   MAINTAINING TREATMENT RECORDS

     5   DIAGNOSIS AND MONITORING OF TREATMENT

     6   SCHEDULING PATIENTS

Q-38   Does the dentist do most of the practice's laboratory work or is a commercial dental laboratory used?

      1   DENTIST DOES MOST LAB WORK

      2   COMMERCIAL DENTAL LAB USED MOST OF THE TIME

Q-39   Please indicate the fees most often charged for the following procedures. For procedures that are not performed, write in "NA." If the procedure is performed free of charge, write in a zero.

Initial oral examination (excluding radiographs)	(0110)	$_____
Four Bitewing radiographs	(0270)	$_____
1-surface permanent amalgam	(2140)	$_____
2-surface permanent amalgam	(2150)	$_____
3-surface permanent amalgam	(2160)	$_____
Gold crown (full cast), single restoration	(2790)	$_____
Root canal therapy	(3310)	$_____
Periodontal scaling and root planing - entire mouth	(4340)	$_____
Complete upper denture	(5110)	$_____
Extraction, single tooth	(7110)	$_____

Q-40   From what dental school did the dentist receive the D.D.S. or D.M.D.?

_____

Q-41   When did the dentist receive the D.D.S. or D.M.D.?

      _____**YEAR RECEIVED DEGREE**

Q-42   About how many hours does the dentist usually work per week?

      _____**HOURS**

Q-43   Of the 52 weeks in 1985, about how many <u>weeks</u> did the dentist work in private practice?

      _____**WEEKS**

Is there anything we may have overlooked? Please use this space for any additional comments you would like to make about your dental practice.

_____

Your contribution to this effort is greatly appreciated. If you would like a summary of results, please print your name and address on the back of the return envelope. We will see that you receive it.

UNIVERSITY OF WASHINGTON
SEATTLE, WASHINGTON 98195

Department of Community Dentistry
School of Dentistry

[current date]

[name & address of dentist]

[Dear Dr. . . .]

I am writing to invite your participation in the Clinical Decisionmaking study
that we are conducting at the University of Washington. The purpose of the
study is to identify important factors that influence dentists' clinical decisions
and ultimately the demand for care among their patients.

In dentistry there are usually several different ways of treating a condition. For
example, dentists routinely choose between silver amalgams and cast crowns in
tooth restoration, between removable partial dentures and fixed bridges, and
between root canals and extractions, among other choices. Unfortunately, we
know very little about the practice patterns of dentists, and even less about
their reasons for preferring one treatment over another. The information from
this study may help dentists in prescribing therapy and may lead to improvements in the clinical education that dental students receive. Furthermore, the
more we can understand about the realities of clinical practice, the better we
can advise insurers on designs for plans which best meet patient needs. Study
results may also lead to future clinical studies investigating the effectiveness of
dental therapies in treating oral conditions.

We realize that dentists are extremely busy. A check for $10 is enclosed as an
expression of our appreciation for taking time to help with this important study.

Further details are presented in the enclosure. If you wish to participate in the
study, please complete and return the questionnaire in the enclosed, postage-
paid envelope. If you prefer not to participate, please send the questionnaire
back blank.

Thank you very much for your assistance!

Sincerely,

David Grembowski, Ph.D.
Research Assistant Professor

B 509 Health Sciences Building, SM-35 / Telephone: (206) 543-2034

INFORMATION SHEET
CLINICAL DECISIONMAKING STUDY
University of Washington
Department of Community Dentistry, SM-35
Seattle, Washington 98195

This is to invite your participation in our study of clinical decisionmaking in dentistry. The purpose of the study is to identify important factors that influence dentists' clinical decisions and ultimately the demand for care among their patients. The study is being conducted with the cooperation of the Washington Education Association (WEA) and the Washington Dental Service (WDS), and it is being funded by a grant from the National Center for Health Services Research in Washington, D.C.

This invitation is being sent to all dentists in your area that have a large number of WEA patients, as identified through WDS records. The questionnaire will take about 20 minutes to complete.

Your answers to all questions will be kept confidential and will be used only for statistical purposes. Only members of our research staff at the University of Washington will have access to the questionnaire. The questionnaire has an identification number so that we may check your name off our mailing list when we receive it.

The results of this study will be published in a professional dental journal, such as the Journal of the American Dental Association. Results will be presented in the form of tables showing averages, frequency distributions and other statistics to preserve confidentiality. Your name will never appear in any future article.

Although we hope you will participate in this study, it is entirely voluntary. You are free not to answer questions if you wish, but complete answers would be appreciated. You may refuse to participate and may withdraw from the study at any time. Your participation will not affect your relations with the WDS in any way. I WOULD BE HAPPY TO ANSWER ANY QUESTIONS YOU MIGHT HAVE NOW OR IN THE FUTURE. PLEASE WRITE OR CALL COLLECT (206) 543-2034.

You may receive a summary of results by writing "copy of results requested" on the back of the return envelope, and printing your name and address below it. Please *do not* put this information on the questionnaire itself.

Your cooperation is greatly appreciated!

Postcard follow-up mailed 1 week after first mailing to all dentists.

Recently, we sent you a questionnaire about clinical decisionmaking. If you have already returned the questionnaire, please accept our sincere thanks. If you have not responded and you have some questions about the study, you may call me collect, (206) 543-2034. If by some chance you did not receive the questionnaire or it was misplaced, please call collect, and I will get another one in the mail to you today.

Sincerely,

David Grembowski, Ph.D.
Research Assistant Professor

UNIVERSITY OF WASHINGTON
SEATTLE, WASHINGTON 98195

Department of Community Dentistry
School of Dentistry

[current date]

[name & address of dentist]

[Dear Dr. . . .]

About three weeks ago I wrote to you seeking your views on clinical decision-making. As of today we have not received your questionnaire.

I am writing to you again because of the importance each questionnaire has to the usefulness of this study. The purpose of the study is to identify important factors that influence dentists' clinical decisions and ultimately the demand for care among their patients. Usually, there are several different ways of treating a dental condition. Unfortunately, we know very little about dentists' preferences in prescribing therapy to their patients. The information from this study may help dentists in clinical decisionmaking and may lead to improvements in the clinical education that dental students receive. In addition, the more we can understand about the realities of clinical practice, the better we can advise insurers on designs for plans which best meet patient needs. The study's results may also lead to future clinical studies investigating the effectiveness of dental therapies in treating oral conditions. Further details are presented in the enclosure.

If you wish to participate in the study, please complete and return the questionnaire in the enclosed, postage-paid envelope.

Thanks for your help!

Sincerely,

David Grembowski, Ph.D.
Research Assistant Professor

B 509 Health Sciences Building, SM-35 / Telephone: (206) 543-2034

RESOURCE D

SELECTED SOURCES
ON HEALTH SURVEYS

Journals such as the *American Journal of Epidemiology,* the *American Journal of Public Health,* the *Journal of Health and Social Behavior,* and *Medical Care* routinely publish research articles based on data collected from health surveys. A number of journals published in the United States and elsewhere also report studies of methodological research on surveys in general and health surveys in particular. These include the *International Journal of Public Opinion Research,* the *Journal of the American Statistical Association,* the *Journal of Marketing Research,* the *Journal of Official Statistics, Public Opinion Quarterly,* and *Survey Methodology.*

The advent of indexes of periodical literature in a variety of areas and the computerization of databases of this literature have greatly facilitated researchers' access to previous studies in these areas (National Library of Medicine, 1992). These databases are generally available at research and university libraries through on-line access or CD-ROM disks. The databases produced by the National Library of Medicine (NLM), known as MEDLARS (Medical Literature Analysis and Retrieval System), are based on indexes to literature in medicine and the health professions (see selected list that follows). They are a particularly valuable source of bibliographical information on health survey methods and applications. MEDLINE, the international biomedical literature component of MEDLARS, is a widely utilized source for identifying relevant literature. Terms that might be used in combination with other descriptors for identifying health-related surveys in MEDLINE include *data collection, dental health surveys, diet surveys, health surveys, interviews, questionnaires,* and *sampling studies.* The NLM databases also include inventories of ongoing research projects in health services research (HSRPROJ) or dentistry (DENTALPROJ), for which published results are not yet available. Databases in related fields (nursing and allied health, education, psychology, and sociology) are also useful sources of information on methodological research or applications of surveys on related topics.

The information highway that has been opened up through the Internet provides a wide network of places to search for information on health surveys (Smith, 1995). World Wide Web addresses for selected agencies or sources are provided later in this resource. The POLL database produced by the nonprofit Roper Center for Public Opinion Research at the University of Connecticut provides the full text of surveys conducted by major U.S. polling firms such as Gallup, Harris, and Roper, among others (Snow, 1992). Public Opinion Research (por@unc.edu) is an on-line discussion group for academics and professionals interested in public opinion research.

The American Statistical Association, the Agency for Health Care Policy and Research (formerly the National Center for Health Services Research), the National Center for Health Statistics, and the U.S. Bureau of the Census also periodically hold conferences or proceedings devoted to methodological issues in the design and conduct of surveys. Many of the papers or presentations at those conferences report on studies of techniques developed and tested in health surveys, which can be used to guide decision making about the utility of these or related approaches. The Office of Management and Budget also periodically publishes instructive papers on survey methodology, with particular reference to federally sponsored surveys, in its Statistical Policy Working Paper Series.

University-based and other private and public data archives contain extensive data sets from national, state, and local health surveys. A selected list of these data archives also appears at the end of this resource. The Area Resource File, compiled by the Bureau of Health Professions in the U.S. Department of Health Resources and Services Administration, is a rich source of information on health care services and resources from surveys for each county in the United States. CDC WONDER, a menu-driven on-line program available from the Centers for Disease Control and Prevention (CDC), provides access to CDC reports and data sets. A number of schools of public health also serve as repositories for National Center for Health Statistics data disks and tapes. Potential users may request catalogues of the data sets available in these or other national or regional archives or consult university-based survey research organizations in their areas about health surveys that they have conducted.

Selected Sources on Health Surveys

I. Journals
   A. Studies using health surveys

American Journal of Clinical Nutrition
American Journal of Epidemiology
American Journal of Public Health
Annual Review of Public Health
Epidemiologic Reviews
Evaluation and the Health Professions
Health Affairs
Health Care Financing Review
Health Care Management Review
Health Education Quarterly
Health Marketing Quarterly
Health Services Research
Hospitals
Inquiry
International Journal of Epidemiology
International Journal of Health Services
Journal of Chronic Diseases
Journal of Community Health
Journal of Epidemiology and Community Health
Journal of Health Administration Education
Journal of Health Care Marketing
Journal of Health Politics, Policy, and Law
Journal of Health and Social Behavior
Journal of Public Health Policy
Medical Care
Medical Care Research and Review
Milbank Memorial Fund Quarterly
New England Journal of Medicine
Nursing Research
Public Health Nursing
Public Health Reports
Quality Review Bulletin
Social Science and Medicine
World Health Statistics Quarterly

B. Methodological studies on surveys

Advances in Consumer Research

Annual Review of Sociology

Applied Cognitive Psychology

Behavior Research Methods, Instruments, and Computers

Evaluation Review

International Journal of Public Opinion Research

Journal of the American Statistical Association

Journal of Economic and Social Measurement

Journal of Marketing Research

Journal of Official Statistics

Public Opinion Quarterly

Quantity and Quality

Sociological Methods and Research

Survey Methodology

II. Computerized bibliographic databases

A. MEDLARS (*MED*ical *L*iterature *A*nalysis *a*nd *R*etrieval *S*ystem)

- AIDSLINE (AIDS information onLINE)
- BIOETHICSLINE (BIOETHICS onLINE)
- CANCERLIT (CANCER LITerature)
- CATLINE (CATalog on LINE)
- DENTALPROJ (DENTAL research PROJects)
- DIRLINE (Directory of Information Sources onLINE)
- HealthSTAR (Health Services/Technology Assessment Research)
- HSTAT (Health Services/Technology Assessment Text)
- HSRPROJ (Health Services Research PROJects in progress)
- MEDLINE (MEDlars onLINE)
- POPLINE (POPulation information onLINE)

B. CINAHL (Cumulative Index to Nursing and Allied Health Literature)

C. ERIC (Educational Resources Information Center)

D. PSYCINFO (PSYChological literature INFOrmation database)

E. SSCI (Social Sciences Citation Index)

III. Internet information sources (Internet address: http://. . .)

Agency for Health Care Policy and Research

(. . .www.ahcpr.gov/)

Centers for Disease Control (. . .www.cdc.gov/)

Government Information Exchange (. . .www.info.gov/)

National Center for Health Statistics

(. . .www.cdc.gov/nchswww/nchshome.htm)

National Institutes of Health (. . .www.nih.gov)

National Library of Medicine (. . .www.nlm.nih.gov/)

U.S. Department of Health and Human Services (. . .www.os.dhhs.gov/)

World Health Organization (. . .www.who.ch/)

IV. Conference proceedings

American Statistical Association

- Section on Social Statistics
- Section on Survey Research Methods

Agency for Health Care Policy and Research (formerly the National Center for Health Services Research) and National Center for Health Statistics

- Conferences on Health Survey Research Methods

National Center for Health Statistics

- Conferences on Public Health Records and Statistics

U.S. Bureau of the Census

- Annual Research Conferences

V. Data Archives

Agency for Health Care Policy and Research

Executive Office Center

2101 East Jefferson Street, Suite 501

Rockville, MD 20852

(301) 594–1364

CDC WONDER

USD, Incorporated

2075-A West Park Place

Stone Mountain, GA 30087

(770) 469–4098

Inter-University Consortium for Political & Social Research

Institute for Social Research

University of Michigan

P.O. Box 1248

Ann Arbor, MI 48106

(313) 763–5010

Lou Harris Data Center (and) Social Science Data Library

Institute for Research in Social Science

Room 10, Manning Hall 026A

University of North Carolina

Chapel Hill, NC 27514

(919) 966–3346

National Archives and Records Administration
Center for Electronic Records
8601 Adelphi Road
College Park, MD 20740
(301) 713–6640

National Center for Health Statistics
Metro III Building
6525 Belcrest Road
Hyattsville, MD 20782
(301) 436–8500

National Opinion Research Center
University of Chicago
1155 East 60th Street
Chicago, IL 60637
(312) 753–7500

National Technical Information Service
U.S. Department of Commerce
Springfield, VA 22161
(703) 487–4650

RAND Corporation
Computer Services Department Data Facility
P.O. Box 202138
Santa Monica, CA 90407
(310) 393–0411, Ext. 7351

Roper Center User Services
The Roper Center for Public Opinion Research
Montieth Building, Room 421
University of Connecticut
341 Mansfield Road
Storrs, CT 06268–1164
(203) 486–4440

RESOURCE E

SELECTED EXAMPLES OF HEALTH SURVEYS

Selected examples of international, national, state, and local surveys are described here and in the table at the end of this resource.

International

The World Health Organization (WHO) has had a major role in encouraging cross-national comparative surveys in both developed and Third World countries. The WHO International Collaborative Study of Medical Care Utilization (Kohn & White, 1976) and the International Study of Dental Manpower Systems in Relation to Oral Health Status (Arnljot, Barmes, Cohen, Hunter, & Ship, 1985) carried out surveys in a number of different countries to gather data on the health care systems in those countries and the impact of medical care and dental care delivery systems on the population's health status and utilization. A follow-up study of the Dental Manpower Systems in Relation to Oral Health Status has been conducted under the auspices of WHO, the National Institute of Dental Research, and the Center for Health Administration Studies at the University of Chicago (Chen, Andersen, Barmes, Leclercq, & Lyttle, 1995).

WHO has also encouraged nations throughout the world to develop their own national health survey capacities. WHO conducted the World Fertility Survey (WFS) program from 1972 to 1984. Through that program WHO provided a core questionnaire and technical assistance for both developing and developed countries to collect data on fertility and family-planning practices (Cornelius, 1985). The Demographic and Health Surveys (DHS) program, funded by the U.S. Agency for International Development (AID), was initiated in 1984 as a follow-up to the WFS. That program provided financial and technical assistance for national sample surveys on population and maternal and child health in developing countries (Lapham & Westoff, 1986).

In 1979 WHO developed a National Household Survey Capability Programme to assist and encourage developing countries to undertake household surveys that would gather information on indicators needed for planning health care services (Carlson, 1985). WHO has also designed sampling methodologies to make it easier to estimate levels of immunization coverage through its Expanded Programme on Immunization (Bennett, Woods, Liyanage, & Smith, 1991; Lemeshow & Robinson, 1985). In 1982 a "rapid epidemiological assessment" program was initiated to encourage the design and implementation of surveys to gather needed health and health care information in developing countries more quickly and inexpensively (Smith & Olson, 1987).

Many developing countries have conducted their own health surveys on a range of topics (Kroeger, 1983; Ross & Vaughan, 1986). Normal problems of data comparability, collection, and quality in health surveys become even more of an issue in trying to carry out surveys in developing countries or in comparing data from countries with widely varying political, cultural, social, economic, and physical environments.

National: Other Countries

As already mentioned, WHO has provided support for carrying out health surveys in many developing and developed countries. Canada, Great Britain, and Switzerland, among other countries, have conducted their own surveys to measure their populations' health and health care practices (Catlin & Lussier, 1993; de Heer & Israëls, 1992). The North Karelia Project in Finland involved surveys of cohorts of residents in the North Karelia region to evaluate the impact of a major community-based campaign to prevent cardiovascular disease (Puska, et al., 1985). It paralleled comparable community-based cardiovascular risk intervention programs conducted in the United States in the Stanford Three-Community Study (Farquhar, et al., 1977) and the Minnesota Heart Health Study (Jacobs, et al., 1986). The SENECA study was a collaborative project among researchers throughout the European community to study the dietary intake, nutritional status, physical activity, lifestyle, and health of a cohort of elderly individuals in around twenty European towns and communities (Euronut SENECA Investigators, 1991).

National: United States

The American Hospital Association and the American Medical Association routinely gather information on U.S. hospitals and physicians, respectively (American Hospital Association, 1995; American Medical Association, 1995). Similarly, professional associations of physician specialty groups, dentists, nurses, and so on periodically survey their members to gather a variety of demographic and practice data (National Library of Medicine, 1992).

The Center for Health Administration Studies at the University of Chicago conducted a series of cross-sectional national surveys of health care utilization, expenditures, and access in 1953, 1958, 1963, 1970, 1976, and 1982 that provided a wealth of information on the impact on the American people of major changes in the organization and financing of health care (Aday & Andersen, 1975; Aday, Andersen, & Fleming, 1980; Aday, Fleming, & Andersen, 1984). The Robert Wood Johnson Foundation (RWJF) has continued this tradition through national surveys of the U.S. population's access to medical care in 1986 and 1994 (Berk, Schur, & Cantor, 1995; Freeman, Blendon, Aiken, Sudman, Mullinix, & Corey, 1987). The 1993 National Health Interview Survey was used to identify respondents for the 1994 RWJF survey to permit a more intensive follow-up of individuals with poor access or selected chronic conditions.

The National Center for Health Statistics (NCHS) is the major health survey data gathering agency of the U.S. government. It conducts its National Health Interview Survey continuously to gather (1) a core set of data on the health status and health care utilization of the American people each year and (2) supplementary information on a variable set of topics (such as smoking behavior, vitamin use, exercise patterns, knowledge and attitudes regarding AIDS) in selected years (NCHS, 1989b, 1990b, 1993e). The National Health and Nutrition Examination Survey (NHANES) program of NCHS and the Hispanic NHANES (HHANES) study of Hispanics in selected states collect direct clinical examination and laboratory data on study participants (NCHS, 1985b, 1992e, 1994e).

NCHS has drawn subsamples from selected National Health Interview Survey samples, as well as NHANES samples, to facilitate a Longitudinal Study of Aging (NCHS, 1987b; 1992f) and an Epidemiological Follow-Up Study (Cornoni-Huntley, et al., 1983; NCHS, 1990a, 1992c) so that more can be learned about changes in the health of the American public through use of prospective research designs.

NCHS has conducted several special surveys to describe the health practices of the U.S. population (1979–80 National Survey of Personal Health Practices and Consequences) (National Center for Health Statistics, 1981a, 1981c; Wilson & Elinson, 1981) or to monitor the nation's progress toward the U.S. Public Health Service's Objectives for Promoting Health and Preventing Disease (1985

National Health Promotion and Disease Prevention Survey) (National Center for Health Statistics, 1988a; Thornberry, Wilson, & Golden, 1986). Components of these surveys were subsequently incorporated into periodic supplements to the National Health Interview Survey.

The National Survey of Family Growth provides data on the fertility and family-planning characteristics of women in the childbearing years (National Center for Health Statistics, 1991b, 1993c). The NCHS National Maternal and Infant Health Survey and National Mortality Followback Surveys on samples of birth and death records provide a variety of information on the care surrounding births and deaths in this country (National Center for Health Statistics, 1993a; Sanderson, Placek, & Keppel, 1991). The National Immunization Survey (NIS) is a joint project of NCHS and the Centers for Disease Control and Prevention National Immunization Program to gather data on the immunization coverage of children nineteen months to thirty-five months of age (NCHS, 1994d).

Based on the recommendations of an Institute of Medicine Panel, in the early 1990s four NCHS record-based surveys (the National Hospital Discharge Survey, National Ambulatory Medical Care Survey, National Nursing Home Survey, and National Health Provider Inventory) were merged and expanded into one integrated survey of health care providers—the National Health Care Survey (NHCS). The National Nursing Home Follow-Up Survey follows a cohort of surviving residents sampled in the 1985 National Nursing Home Survey. In addition, three new surveys were added and incorporated into the NHCS—the National Survey of Ambulatory Surgery, National Hospital Ambulatory Medical Care Survey, and the National Home and Hospice Care Survey. This series of NHCS surveys gather data on the characteristics of the patients seen and services provided in the respective health care settings (Lipkind, 1995; NCHS, 1988b, 1993b, 1993d, 1994b; Wunderlich, 1992).

NCHS has also sponsored several special studies of health care coverage and expenditures. For example, the 1980 National Medical Care Utilization and Expenditure Survey, conducted in collaboration with the Health Care Financing Administration, collected data on the health care utilization and expenditures of a sample of the U.S. population, as well as samples of Medicaid beneficiaries in four states—California, New York, Michigan, and Texas (NCHS, 1983). The NCHS National Employer Health Insurance Survey, launched in 1994, is a national survey of businesses in both the private and public sector regarding employer provision of health insurance and spending for health care.

The Agency for Health Care Policy and Research (formerly the National Center for Health Services Research) has funded a number of surveys on the health care utilization and expenditures of the American public. That agency conducted the large-scale National Medical Care Expenditure Survey (NMCES) in 1977 (National Center for Health Services Research, 1981b) and launched an even more comprehensive study that oversampled a number of policy-relevant subgroups of interest (the poor, elderly, disabled, and others) in the 1987 National Medical Expenditure Survey (NMES) (National Center for Health Services Research, 1987). The 1996 Medical Expenditure Panel Survey (MEPS) was designed to gather data on the health care coverage and expenditures of the U.S. population that could be used directly in formulating health policy in this area. The sampling design for the MEPS was linked to the NHIS surveys, to economize on data collection costs and enhance the possibilities for integrating the data from these two major federally sponsored national surveys. The Medicare Current Beneficiary Survey (MCBS), developed by the Health Care Financing Administration, gathers data on health care utilization and expenditures from a representative panel of Medicare enrollees (Edwards, Sperry, & Edwards, 1992).

The Current Population Survey (CPS), a monthly survey of approximately 60,000 households conducted by the U.S. Bureau of the Census for the Bureau of Labor Statistics, and the Survey of Income and Program Participation (SIPP), a panel study carried out on a continuing basis by the U.S. Bureau of the Census since 1983, provide longitudinal data on health insurance coverage, disability, and utilization. They can supplement the data obtained by the large and complex NMCES and NMES surveys conducted every ten years and the data obtained by the National Health Interview Survey, which is conducted annually on different cross-sectional samples of the U.S. population (Cohany, Polivka, & Rothgeb, 1994; David, 1985; Kasprzyk, 1988; Wilensky, 1985).

A variety of other surveys are conducted by other federal agencies on health or health-related topics, such as smoking (Massey, Boyd, Mattson, & Feinleib, 1987), alcohol and drug use (National Institute on Drug Abuse, 1991), nutrition and food consumption practices (Brandt & McGinnis, 1984), and leisure-time physical activity (Stephens, Jacobs, & White, 1985; Brandt & McGinnis, 1985), among others.

A number of federal agencies periodically collect survey data or sponsor surveys on health-related topics. These include the Bureau of Labor Statistics, the Centers for Disease Control and Prevention, the Census Bureau, the Health Care Financing Administration, the National Cancer Institute, the National Institute of Mental Health, the National Institute on Drug Abuse, the Social Security Administration, and the Veterans Administration (Wunderlich, 1992).

In addition to the Robert Wood Johnson Foundation, the Commonwealth Fund, the Kaiser Family Foundation, the Flinn Foundation, and other private philanthropies have sponsored national or statewide surveys dealing with various aspects of health and health care system performance. Polls conducted by the major polling organizations (such as Gallup, Harris, and Roper) provide a timely reading of the pulse of the American public on an array of health policy issues (Blendon, Brodie, & Benson, 1995). The national survey of sexual practices in the United States, dealing with very sensitive topics, was made possible by a consortium of public and private funding sources (Laumann, Gagnon, Michael, & Michaels, 1994).

States: United States

Concerns with the growing numbers of uninsured in many states, as well as the dominance of managed care arrangements in both the private and public sectors, have given rise to an array of studies to assess the impact of these emerging trends and innovations (Gold, et al., 1995; Hurley, Freund, & Paul, 1993). Since 1981, the Centers for Disease Control and Prevention have sponsored Behavioral Risk Factor Surveys, using telephone interview designs in almost all the states and the District of Columbia to gather information on residents' health practices that could put them at risk of developing serious illness (such as obesity, lack of exercise, uncontrolled hypertension, smoking, heavy drinking) (Remington, et al., 1988). The Pregnancy Risk Assessment Monitoring System (PRAMS) involves surveys of new mothers sampled from birth certificates in participating states to obtain supplementary information on maternal behaviors during pregnancy and the early infancy of the child (Adams, et al., 1991).

Local: United States

A variety of health surveys have been conducted in U.S. communities. The Alameda County Human Population Laboratory Study, which examined the relationship of selected lifestyle and health practices to mortality and morbidity from 1965 to 1974 for a sample of residents of Alameda County, California, was a precursor to the national surveys of the consequences of personal health practices (Berkman & Breslow, 1983).

Health Hazard Appraisal (HHA) and Health Risk Appraisal (HRA) instruments have been developed and applied in a variety of work sites, universities, community wellness programs, health fairs, schools, and health care organizations. These appraisals generally involve a self-administered questionnaire and a physical exam in which minimal physical status data are collected (height, weight, blood pressure). Actuarial tables are then applied to estimate the years of life that can be gained by changing certain risky health behaviors or physical parameters. (See the October 1987 issue of *Health Services Research* for a series of articles on health risk assessment methods.)

The Community Hospital Program Access Impact Evaluation Surveys examined the impact of community hospital-sponsored group practices on the communities that they served (Aday, Andersen, Loevy, & Kremer, 1985). Comparable evaluations of rural practice models of primary care delivery (Sheps, et al., 1983) and of municipal hospital-sponsored primary care clinics for inner-city residents

(Fleming & Andersen, 1986) have similarly relied on health surveys to evaluate the impact of these programs on the populations that they were intended to serve.

The Framingham study was one of the first and best-designed prospective studies to examine the incidence of heart disease in a community (Dawber, 1980). Begun in 1947, the study collected a wealth of health interview survey and examination data on a cohort of residents of the town of Framingham, Massachusetts, over some forty years. The Framingham study served as the model for community-based cohort studies of cardiovascular disease in Tecumseh, Michigan (Epstein, et al., 1970) and Evans County, Georgia (Cassel, 1971).

The National Institute of Mental Health (NIMH) initiated surveys of residents of five urban areas, along with samples of residents of mental institutions in those areas, to estimate the incidence and prevalence of mental disorders, explore the causes of these diseases, and contribute to the planning of community mental health services (Regier, et al., 1984; Robins & Regier, 1991). This study was in particular concerned with testing the NIMH Diagnostic Interview Schedule, which was originally developed for clinical assessments of mental illness, in field survey settings. This NIMH Epidemiological Catchment Area study contributed greatly to the advancement of survey-based studies of mental illness in communities.

The RAND Corporation has been involved in several large-scale studies that have contributed to the development of survey measures of physical, mental, and social health and well-being. The RAND Health Insurance Experiment surveys involved interviews, self-administered questionnaires, and clinical examinations of individuals experimentally assigned to different health insurance plans. Its purpose was to examine the impact of varying levels of coverage on enrollees' health status, utilization, and expenditures (Brook, et al., 1984). The RAND Medical Outcomes Study attempted to trace the patterns of care and outcomes for individuals with particular types of chronic illness who were treated in different systems of medical care by different physician specialists (Stewart & Ware, 1992). The HIV Cost and Services Utilization Study (HCSUS) and its predecessor, the AIDS Cost and Services Utilization Survey (ACSUS), analyzed the utilization and costs of services provided to persons with HIV/AIDS.

The Patient Outcomes Research Teams (PORTS), funded by the Agency for Health Care Policy and Research, along with related outcomes assessment studies, have made extensive use of surveys to obtain patient-centered evaluations of functional capacity or quality of life associated with different treatment alternatives.

The growth of the managed care industry in health care has been accompanied by a growing interest in finding out from consumers what they want and how satisfied they are with the care they receive. Patient surveys are an important component of the resultant report cards issued on plan performance (National Committee for Quality Assurance, 1993, 1995a, 1995b).

TABLE E.1. SELECTED EXAMPLES OF HEALTH SURVEYS.

Study, Years (References)	Topics	Research Design	Population/Samples	Data Collection
International				
World Health Organization International Collaborative Study of Medical Care Utilization, 1967–1974 (Kohn & White, 1976)	Health care system Population Health status Utilization Satisfaction	Group-comparison	12 study areas in 7 countries/variable sample designs in 15,000 households with 47,648 individuals	Personal interviews
World Health Organization International Collaborative Study of Dental Manpower Systems in Relation to Oral Health Status, 1973–1981 (Arnljot, et al., 1985);	Health care system Population Health status Utilization Expenditures	Group-comparison	12 study areas in 10 countries/ variable sample designs of households and providers	Personal interviews, clinical exams, provider interviews
1988–1992 (Chen, Andersen, Barmes, Leclerq, & Lyttle, 1995)	Health care system Population Health status Utilization Expenditures	Group-comparison	7 study areas in 5 countries/variable sample designs of households and providers	Personal interviews, clinical exams, provider interviews
National—Other Countries				
Canadian National Population Health Survey, biennial survey, 1994–present (Catlin & Lussier, 1993)	Population Health status Utilization	Longitudinal—trend and panel	Sample of Canadian households and individuals	Personal interviews, telephone interviews
North Karelia Project (Finland), 1972–1982 (Puska, et al., 1985)	Health care system Population Health status Utilization	Longitudinal—cohort (prospective)	Independent random samples of age cohorts in North Karelia, Finland, in 1972, 1977, 1982	Personal interviews, clinical exams
SENECA Project (Euronut SENECA Investigators, 1991)	Population Health status	Longitudinal—cohort	Samples of cohorts born 1913–1918 in 19 towns in 12 countries	Personal interviews
National—United States				
American Hospital Association Annual Survey of Hospitals, 1946–present (AHA, 1995)	Health care system— hospitals	Longitudinal—trend	Sample of all (7,000) U.S. hospitals	Mail questionnaires
American Medical Association Periodic Survey of Physicians, 1966–present (AMA, 1995)	Health care system— physicians	Longitudinal—trend	Sample of all (500,000) U.S. physicians	Mail questionnaires

Survey	Content	Design	Sample	Data Collection
Center for Health Administration Studies National Surveys, 1953, 1958, 1963, 1970, 1976, 1982 (Aday & Andersen, 1975; Aday, Andersen, & Fleming, 1980; Aday, Fleming, & Andersen, 1984)	Population Health status Utilization Expenditures Satisfaction	Cross-sectional	Sample of U.S. population with some special oversamples: for example, poor, Hispanics, rural blacks	Personal interviews, telephone interviews (1982 only)
Health Care Financing Administration • Medicare Current Beneficiary Survey, 1991–present (Edwards, Sperry, & Edwards, 1992)	Population Health status Utilization Expenditures	Longitudinal—panel	Sample of Medicare population	Personal interviews
National Center for Health Statistics (NCHS) Periodic Population Surveys • Health Interview Survey (HIS), 1957–present (NCHS, 1985c, 1989b, 1990b, 1993e)	Population Health status Utilization Expenditures	Longitudinal—trend	Sample of U.S. households and individuals	Personal interviews
• National Health and Nutrition Examination Survey (NHANES), 1970–1975, 1976–1980, 1988–91, 1991–94 (NCHS, 1992e, 1994e)	Population Health status Utilization	Cross-sectional	Sample of U.S. households and individuals 1 month–74 years	Personal interviews, clinical exams
• Hispanic Health and Nutrition Examination Survey (HHANES), 1982–1984 (NCHS, 1985b)	Population Health status Utilization	Cross-sectional	Sample of Mexican-Americans in Southwestern states; Puerto Ricans in N.J., N.Y., and Conn.; Cubans in Dade Co., Fla., 6 months–74 years	Personal interviews, clinical exams
• National Immunization Survey, 1995–present (NCHS, 1994d)	Population Health status Utilization	Longitudinal—trend	Sample of children 19–35 months in U.S. households and selected states and local areas with phones	Telephone interviews
National Center for Health Statistics (NCHS) Special Population Surveys • National Medical Care Utilization and Expenditure Survey (NMCUES), 1980 (NCHS, 1983)	Population Health status Utilization Expenditures	Longitudinal—panel	Sample of 6,000 U.S. households; samples of 1,000 households with Medicaid beneficiaries in Calif., N.Y., Mich., and Tex.: Medicare and Medicaid Administrative Records Survey	Personal interviews, telephone interviews
• National Survey of Personal Health Practices and Consequences, 1979–1980 (NCHS, 1981a, 1981c)	Population Health status Utilization	Longitudinal—panel	Sample of all persons 20–64 years in U.S. households with phones	Telephone interviews

TABLE E.1. SELECTED EXAMPLES OF HEALTH SURVEYS, cont'd.

Study, Years (References)	Topics	Research Design	Population/Samples	Data Collection
• National Health Promotion and Disease Prevention Survey, 1985 (NCHS, 1985a, 1988a)	Population Health status Utilization	Cross-sectional	Sample of adults 18+ from 1985 NCHS–NHIS	Personal interviews
National Center for Health Statistics (NCHS) National Health Care Survey (NHCS) • National Hospital Discharge Survey, 1964–present (NCHS, 1981b, 1993b)	Health care system Population Health status Utilization	Longitudinal—trend	Sample of discharges from U.S. hospitals	Record abstraction
• National Ambulatory Medical Care Survey, 1973–present (NCHS, 1988b)	Health care system Population Health status Utilization	Longitudinal—trend	Sample of visits to office-based physicians	Patient log, patient record forms
• National Nursing Home Survey, 1973–1974, 1977, 1985, 1995 (NCHS, 1993d)	Health care system Population Health status Utilization Expenditures	Longitudinal—trend	Sample of U.S. nursing homes, staffs, and residents	Personal interviews, self-administered questionnaires
• National Survey of Ambulatory Surgery, 1994–present	Health care system Population Health status Utilization Expenditures	Longitudinal—trend	Sample of visits to U.S. free-standing and ambulatory surgery centers	Record abstraction
• National Hospital Ambulatory Medical Care Survey, 1992–present (Lipkind, 1995)	Health care system Population Health status Utilization Expenditures	Longitudinal—trend	Sample of visits to U.S. hospital emergency rooms and outpatient departments	Record abstraction
• National Home and Hospice Care Survey, 1992–present (NCHS, 1994b)	Health care system Population Health status Utilization Expenditures	Longitudinal—trend	Sample of U.S. home health agencies and hospices and their current patients and discharges	Personal interviews

Survey	Categories	Design	Sample	Data Collection
National Center for Health Statistics (NCHS) Vital Statistics Surveys • National Mortality Followback Survey, Selected Years: 1961–present (NCHS, 1993a)	Population Health status Utilization	Longitudinal—trend	Sample of death records representative of all deaths in U.S. in study period	Mail questionnaires
• National Survey of Family Growth, 1973, 1976, 1982, 1988, 1990 (NCHS, 1991b, 1993c)	Population Health status Utilization	Longitudinal—trend	Sample of women in U.S. of childbearing ages 15–44	Personal interviews, telephone interviews
• National Maternal and Infant Health Survey, 1988, 1991 (Sanderson, Placek, & Keppel, 1991)	Population Health status Utilization	Longitudinal—trend	Sample of U.S. live births, fetal deaths and infant deaths and associated providers	Mail questionnaires, personal interviews, telephone interviews
National Center for Health Services Research/Agency for Health Care Policy and Research (NCHSR/AHCPR) • National Medical Care Expenditure Survey (NMCES), 1977–1979 (NCHSR, 1981b)	Health system Population Health status Utilization Expenditures	Longitudinal—panel	Sample of U.S. population with 14,000 individuals; surveys of physicians, health facilities, and employers providing care or coverage	Personal interviews, diaries, mail questionnaires
• National Medical Expenditure Survey (NMES), 1987 (NCHSR, 1987)	Health system Population Health status Utilization Expenditures	Longitudinal—panel	Sample of U.S. population with 14,000 households, including oversamples of blacks, Hispanics, poor, elderly, disabled; Survey of American Indians and Alaska Natives; Medical Provider Surveys; Health Insurance Plans Survey; Institutional Population Survey; Medicare Records Survey	Personal interviews, diaries, mail questionnaires, telephone interviews
U.S. Department of Agriculture (USDA) • Continuing Survey of Food Intake by Individuals (CSFII), annual survey (Rizek & Pao, 1990)	Population Health status	Longitudinal—panel	Sample of U.S. population with special samples of age–sex and income subgroups	Personal interviews, telephone interviews

TABLE E.1. SELECTED EXAMPLES OF HEALTH SURVEYS, cont'd.

Study, Years (References)	Topics	Research Design	Population/Samples	Data Collection
States—United States				
Centers for Disease Control Behavioral Risk Factor Surveys, 1981–present (Remington, et al., 1988)	Population Health status	Cross-sectional	Samples of populations in the states and District of Columbia with telephones	Telephone interviews
Pregnancy Risk Assessment Monitoring System, selected years, 1988–present (Adams, et al., 1991)	Population Health status Utilization	Cross-sectional	Sample of new mothers from birth certificates in selected states	Mail questionnaire, telephone interviews
Local—United States				
Alameda Co. Human Population Laboratory Study, 1965–1974 (Berkman & Breslow, 1983)	Population Health status Utilization	Longitudinal—panel (prospective)	Samples of residents of Alameda Co., Calif., in 1965 and 1974	Self-administered questionnaires, personal interviews
Community Hospital Program (CHP) Access Impact Evaluation Surveys, 1980–1982 (Aday, Andersen, Loevy, & Kremer, 1985)	Health care system Population Health status Utilization	Quasi-experimental (program evaluation)	Samples of residents in service areas and patients of 12 study sites	Personal interviews
Framingham Study (Dawber, 1980)	Population Health status Utilization	Longitudinal—panel (prospective)	Samples of residents of Framingham, Mass., and their descendants	Personal interviews, self-administered questionnaires, clinical exams
National Institute of Mental Health (NIMH) Epidemiological Catchment Area Surveys, 1981–1982 (Robins & Regier, 1991)	Population Health status Utilization	Longitudinal—panel (prospective)	Samples of residents of 5 urban areas; residents of institutions	Personal interviews
RAND Health Insurance Experiment surveys, 1974–1984 (Brook, et al., 1984)	Health care system Population Health status Utilization Expenditures	Experimental design	Sample of 8,000 people in 2,750 families enrolled in different insurance plans in six sites across U.S.; claims and coverage data from insurers and providers	Personal interviews, self-administered questionnaires, clinical exams

Study	Focus	Design	Sample	Method
RAND Medical Outcomes Study, 1986–1989 (Stewart & Ware, 1992)	Health care system Population Health status Utilization	Comparative; longitudinal—panel	Sample of 700 physicians in four regions of U.S.: universe of patients seen by providers in 5 day screening period plus panel of 3,600 patients with selected tracer conditions	Self-administered questionnaires, telephone interviews, health care visit forms, patient diaries
Chicago Area General Population Survey on AIDS (Albrecht, Levy, Sugrue, Prohaska, & Ostrow, 1989)	Population Health status Utilization	Quasi-experimental (program evaluation baseline survey)	Sample of 1,540 from general adult population 18+ in Chicago metropolitan area, including oversampling of blacks, Hispanics	Telephone interviews
Washington State Study of Dentists' Preferences in Prescribing Dental Therapy (Grembowski, Milgrom, & Fiset, 1988)	Health care system	Cross-sectional	Sample of 200 generalist dentists in four counties of Washington State who provided services to Washington Education Association members and their dependents	Mail questionnaires

REFERENCES

Aaronson, N. K. (1989). Quality of life assessment in clinical trials: Methodologic issues. *Controlled Clinical Trials, 10* (Suppl. 4), 195S-208S.

Abramson, J. H. (1990). *Survey methods in community medicine* (4th ed.). Edinburgh: Churchill Livingstone.

Adams, M. M., Shulman, H. B., Bruce, C., Hogue, C., Brogan, D., & the PRAMS Working Group. (1991). The Pregnancy Risk Assessment Monitoring System: Design, questionnaire, data collection and response rates. *Paediatric and Perinatal Epidemiology, 5,* 333–346.

Adams-Esquivel, H., & Lang, D. A. (1987). The reliability of telephone penetration estimates in specialized target groups: The Hispanic case. *Journal of Data Collection, 27,* 35–39.

Adang, R. P., Vismans, F.-J. F. E., Ambergen, A. W., Talmon, J. L., Hasman, A., & Flendrig, J. A. (1991). Evaluation of computerized questionnaires designed for patients referred for gastrointestinal endoscopy. *International Journal of Biomedical Computing, 29,* 31–44.

Aday, L. A. (1993a). *At risk in America: The health and health care needs of vulnerable populations in the United States.* San Francisco: Jossey-Bass.

Aday, L. A. (1993b). Indicators and predictors of health services utilization. In S. J. Williams and P. R. Torrens (Eds.), *Introduction to health services* (4th ed., pp. 46–70). Albany, NY: Delmar Publishers.

Aday, L. A., Aitken, M. J., & Wegener, D. H. (1988). *Pediatric home care: Results of a national evaluation of programs for ventilator-assisted children.* Chicago: Pluribus Press.

Aday, L. A., & Andersen, R. (1975). *Development of indices of access to medical care.* Ann Arbor, MI: Health Administration Press.

Aday, L. A., Andersen, R., & Fleming, G. V. (1980). *Health care in the United States: Equitable for whom?* Thousand Oaks, CA: Sage.

Aday, L. A., Andersen, R., Loevy, S. S., & Kremer, B. (1985). *Hospital-physician sponsored primary care: Marketing and impact.* Ann Arbor, MI: Health Administration Press.

Aday, L. A., Chiu, G. Y., & Andersen, R. (1980). Methodological issues in health care surveys of the Spanish heritage population. *American Journal of Public Health, 70,* 367–374.

Aday, L. A., Fleming, G. V., & Andersen, R. (1984). *Access to medical care in the U.S.: Who has it, who doesn't.* Chicago: Pluribus Press.

Aday, L. A., Sellers, C., & Andersen, R. (1981). Potentials of local health surveys: A state-of-the-art summary. *American Journal of Public Health, 71,* 835–840.

Agency for Health Care Policy and Research. (1995). *Consumer survey information in a reforming health care system.* (Report No. AHCPR Pub. No. 95–0083). Rockville, MD: Author.

Albrecht, G. L. (1985). Videotape safaris: Entering the field with a camera. *Qualitative Sociology, 8,* 325–344.

Albrecht, G. L. (1989). The intelligent design of AIDS research strategies. In L. Sechrest, H. Freeman, & A. Mulley (Eds.), *Conference proceedings: Health services methodology: A focus on AIDS* (Report No. DHHS Pub. No. [PHS] 89–3439, pp. 67–74). Washington, DC: U.S. Government Printing Office.

Albrecht, G. L. (1993, May 3). *A Sociological Evaluation of Our Experience with AIDS: Research and Policy.* Paper presented at the American Sociological Association, Sydney A. Spivack Program in Applied Social Research and Social Policy and a Congressional Briefing, Washington, DC.

Albrecht, G. L., Levy, J. A., Sugrue, N. M., Prohaska, T. R., & Ostrow, D. G. (1989). Who hasn't heard about AIDS? *AIDS Education and Prevention, 1,* 261–267.

Albrecht, G. L., & Zimmerman, R. (1993). What does AIDS teach us about social science? *Advances in Medical Sociology, 3,* 1–18.

Allen, H. M., Jr., Darling, H., McNeill, D. N., & Bastien, F. (1994). The employee health care value survey: Round one. *Health Affairs, 13* (4), 25–41.

Alonso, J., Anto, J. M., & Moreno, C. (1990). Spanish version of the Nottingham Health Profile: Translation and preliminary validity. *American Journal of Public Health, 80,* 704–708.

Alwin, D. F. (1989). Problems in the estimation and interpretation of the reliability of survey data. *Quality & Quantity, 23,* 277–331.

Alwin, D. F., & Krosnick, J. A. (1985). The measurement of values in surveys: A comparison of ratings and rankings. *Public Opinion Quarterly, 49,* 535–552.

Alwin, D. F., & Krosnick, J. A. (1991). The reliability of survey attitude measurement: The influence of question and respondent attributes. *Sociological Methods & Research, 20,* 139–181.

American Hospital Association. (1995). *Hospital statistics.* Chicago: Author.

American Medical Association. (1995). *Physician characteristics and distribution in the United States.* Chicago: Author.

American Psychiatric Association. (1995). *Diagnostic and statistical manual of mental disorders* (4th ed.). Washington, DC: Author.

American Psychological Association. (1985). *Standards for educational and psychological testing.* Washington, DC: Author.

American Statistical Association. (1995). *What is a survey?* [brochure]. Washington, DC: Author.

Andersen, R. M., Aday, L. A., Lyttle, C. S., Cornelius, L. J., & Chen, M.-S. (1987). *Ambulatory care and insurance coverage in an era of constraint.* Chicago: Pluribus Press.

Andersen, R. M., Kasper, J., Frankel, M. R., & Associates. (1979). *Total survey error: Applications to improve health surveys.* San Francisco: Jossey-Bass.

Anderson, A. B., Basilevsky, A., & Hum, D. P. (1983). Missing data: A review of the literature. In P. H. Rossi, J. D. Wright, & A. B. Anderson (Eds.), *Handbook of survey research* (pp. 415–494). San Diego, CA: Academic Press.

Andrews, F. M. (1984). Construct validity and error components of survey measures: A structural modeling approach. *Public Opinion Quarterly, 48,* 409–442.

Andrich, D. (1988). *Rasch models for measurement.* Thousand Oaks, CA: Sage.

Aneshensel, C. S., Becerra, R. M., Fielder, E. P., & Schuler, R. H. (1989). Participation of Mexican American female adolescents in a longitudinal panel survey. *Public Opinion Quarterly, 53,* 548–562.

Aneshensel, C. S., Frerichs, R. R., Clark, V. A., & Yokopenic, P. A. (1982). Measuring depression in the community: A comparison of telephone and personal interviews. *Public Opinion Quarterly, 46,* 110–121.

Appel, M. V., & Nicholls, W. L., II (1993). New CASIC technologies at the U.S. Census Bureau. *Proceedings of the American Statistical Association, Section on Survey Research Methods, Vol. II,* 1079–1084.

Aquilino, W. S. (1994). Interview mode effects in surveys of drug and alcohol use: A field experiment. *Public Opinion Quarterly, 58,* 210–240.

Aquilino, W. S., & Lo Sciuto, L. A. (1990). Effects of interview mode on self-reported drug use. *Public Opinion Quarterly, 54,* 362–395.

Armenian, H. K. (Ed.). (1994). Applications of the case-control method. *Epidemiologic Reviews, 16* (1).

Armstrong, J. S., & Lusk, E. J. (1987). Return postage in mail surveys: A meta-analysis. *Public Opinion Quarterly, 51,* 233–248.

Arnljot, H. A., Barmes, D. E., Cohen, L. K., Hunter, P.B.V., & Ship, I. I. (1985). *Oral health care systems.* Lombard, IL: Quintessence.

Axinn, W. G., Fricke, T. E., & Thornton, A. (1991). The microdemographic community-study approach: Improving survey data by integrating the ethnographic method. *Sociological Methods & Research, 20,* 187–217.

Ayidiya, S. A., & McClendon, M. J. (1990). Response effects in mail surveys. *Public Opinion Quarterly, 54,* 229–247.

Babbie, E. (1990). *Survey research methods* (2nd ed.). Belmont, CA: Wadsworth.

Bachman, J. G., & O'Malley, P. M. (1984). Yea-saying, nay-saying, and going to extremes: Black-white differences in response styles. *Public Opinion Quarterly, 48,* 491–509.

Badia, X., & Alonso, J. (1995). Re-scaling the Spanish version of the Sickness Health Profile: An opportunity for the assessment of cross-cultural equivalence. *Journal of Clinical Epidemiology, 48,* 949–957.

Bailar, B. A., & Lanphier, C. M. (1978). *Development of survey methods to assess survey practices.* Washington, DC: American Statistical Association.

Bainbridge, W. S. (1989). *Survey research: A computer-assisted introduction.* Belmont, CA: Wadsworth.

Bainbridge, W. S. (1992). *Social research methods and statistics: A computer-assisted introduction.* Belmont, CA: Wadsworth.

Balas, E. A., Austin, S. M., Ewigman, B. G., Brown, G. D., & Mitchell, J. A. (1995). Methods of randomized controlled clinical trials in health services research. *Medical Care, 33,* 687–699.

Basch, C. E. (1987). Focus group interview: An underutilized research technique for improving theory and practice in health education. *Health Education Quarterly, 14,* 411–448.

Bauman, L. J., & Adair, E. G. (1992). The use of ethnographic interviewing to inform questionnaire construction. *Health Education Quarterly, 19,* 9–23.

Beatty, P. (1994). *NASA questionnaire development project: Developing an employee health survey from secondary sources.* (Report No. 13, National Center for Health Statistics, Cognitive Methods Staff Working Paper Series). Hyattsville, MD: National Center for Health Statistics.

Beatty, P. (1995). Understanding the standardized/nonstandardized interviewing controversy. *Journal of Official Statistics, 11,* 147–160.

Beaufait, D. W., Nelson, E. C., Landgraf, J. M., Hays, R. D., Kirk, J. W., Wasson, J. H., & Keller, A. (1991). COOP measures of functional status. In M. Stewart, F. Tudiver, M. J. Bass, E. V. Dunn, & P. G. Norton (Eds.), *Tools for primary care research* (pp. 151–167). Thousand Oaks, CA: Sage.

Becker, M. H. (1974). *The health belief model and personal health behavior.* Thorofare, NJ: Slack.

Beldt, S. F., Daniel, W. W., & Garcha, B. S. (1982). The Takahasi-Sakasegawa randomized response technique: A field test. *Sociological Methods and Research, 11,* 101–111.

Belson, W. (1981). *The design and understanding of survey questions.* Aldershot, England: Gower.

Belson, W. (1986). *Validity in survey research.* Brookfield, VT: Gower.

Bennett, S., Woods, T., Liyanage, W. M., & Smith, D. L. (1991). A simplified general method for cluster-sample surveys of health in developing countries. *World Health Statistics Quarterly, 44,* 98–106.

Bergner, M. (1985). Measurement of health status. *Medical Care, 23,* 696–704.

Bergner, M., Bobbitt, R. A., Carter, W. B., & Gilson, B. S. (1981). The Sickness Impact Profile: Development and final revision of a health status measure. *Medical Care, 19,* 787–805.

Bergner, M., Bobbitt, R. A., Kressel, S., Pollard, W. E., Gilson, B. S., & Morris, J. R. (1976). The Sickness Impact Profile: Conceptual formulation and methodology for the development of a health status measure. *International Journal of Health Services, 6,* 393–415.

Bergner, M., & Rothman, M. L. (1987). Health status measures: An overview and guide for selection. *Annual Review of Public Health, 8,* 191–210.

Berk, M. L., & Bernstein, A. B. (1988). Interviewer characteristics and performance on a complex health survey. *Social Science Research, 17,* 239–251.

Berk, M. L., Schur, C. L., & Cantor, J. C. (1995). Ability to obtain health care: Recent estimates from the Robert Wood Johnson Foundation national access to care survey. *Health Affairs, 14* (3), 139–146.

Berk, M. L., Wilensky, G. R., & Cohen, S. B. (1984). Methodological issues in health surveys: An evaluation of procedures used in the National Medical Care Expenditure Survey. *Evaluation Review, 8,* 307–326.

Berkanovic, E. (1980). The effect of inadequate language translation on Hispanics' response to health surveys. *American Journal of Public Health, 70,* 1273–1276.

Berkman, L. F., & Breslow, L. (1983). *Health and ways of living.* New York: Oxford University Press.

Berry, S. H., & Kanouse, D. E. (1987). Physician response to a mailed survey: An experiment in timing of payment. *Public Opinion Quarterly, 51,* 102–114.

Bethlehem, J. G., & Keller, W. J. (1991). The Blaise system for integrated survey processing. *Survey Methodology, 17,* 43–56.

Bickart, B. A., Blair, J., Menon, G., & Sudman, S. (1990). Cognitive aspects of proxy reporting of behavior. *Advances in Consumer Research, 17,* 198–206.

Bickart, B., Menon, G., Sudman, S., & Blair, J. (1992). Context effects in proxy judgments. *Advances in Consumer Research, 19,* 64–71.

Biemer, P., & Caspar R. (1994). Continuous quality improvement for survey operations: Some general principles and applications. *Journal of Official Statistics, 10,* 307–326.

Bicmcr, P. P., Groves, R. M., Lyberg, L. E., Mathiowetz, N. A., & Sudman, S. (Eds.). (1991). *Measurement errors in surveys.* New York: Wiley.

Billiet, J., & Loosveldt, G. (1988). Improvement of the quality of responses to factual survey questions by interviewer training. *Public Opinion Quarterly, 52,* 190–211.

Binson, D., Murphy, P. A., & Keer, D. (1987, May). *Threatening questions for the public in a survey about AIDS*. Paper presented at the annual meeting of the American Association for Public Opinion Research, Hershey, PA.

Bishop, G. F. (1987). Experiments with the middle response alternative in survey questions. *Public Opinion Quarterly, 51,* 220–232.

Bishop, G. F. (1990). Issue involvement and response effects in public opinion surveys. *Public Opinion Quarterly, 54,* 209–218.

Bishop, G. F., Oldendick, R. W., & Tuchfarber, A. J. (1982). Effects of presenting one versus two sides of an issue in survey questions. *Public Opinion Quarterly, 46,* 69–85.

Bishop, G. F., Tuchfarber, A. J., & Oldendick, R. W. (1986). Opinions on fictitious issues: The pressure to answer survey questions. *Public Opinion Quarterly, 50,* 240–250.

Blair, E. A., & Burton, S. (1987). Cognitive processes used by survey respondents to answer behavioral frequency questions. *Journal of Consumer Research, 14,* 280–288.

Blair, E. A., & Ganesh, G. K. (1991). Characteristics of interval-based estimates of autobiographical frequencies. *Applied Cognitive Psychology, 5,* 237–250.

Blair, J., Binson, D., & Murphy, P. (1992). Cognitive assessment of survey instruments and procedures for rare populations: IV drug users and the National Household Seroprevalence Survey. *Proceedings of the American Statistical Association, Section on Survey Research Methods,* pp. 770–775.

Blair, J., & Czaja, R. (1982). Locating a special population using random digit dialing. *Public Opinion Quarterly, 46,* 585–590.

Blendon, R. J., Brodie, M., & Benson, J. (1995). What happened to Americans' support for the Clinton health plan? *Health Affairs, 14* (2), 7–23.

Bless, H., Bohner, G., Hild, T., & Schwarz, N. (1992). Asking difficult questions: Task complexity increases the impact of response alternatives. *European Journal of Social Psychology, 22,* 309–312.

Blixt, S., & Dykema, J. (1993). Before the pretest: Question development strategies. *Proceedings of the American Statistical Association, Section on Survey Research Methods, Vol. II,* 1142–1147.

Blyth, B., & Piper, H. (1994). Speech recognition—A new dimension in survey research. *Journal of the Market Research Society, 36,* 183–203.

Bohrnstedt, G. W., & Knoke, D. (1994). *Statistics for social data analysis* (3rd ed.). Itasca, IL: F. E. Peacock.

Borenstein, M., & Cohen, J. (1988). *Statistical power analysis: A computer program.* Hillsdale, NJ: Erlbaum.

Bourque, L. B., & Clark, V. A. (1992). *Processing data: The survey example.* Thousand Oaks, CA: Sage.

Bourque, L. B., & Fielder, E. P. (1995). *How to conduct self-administered and mail surveys.* Thousand Oaks, CA: Sage.

Bowling, A. (1991). *Measuring health: A review of quality of life measurement scales.* Philadelphia: Open University Press.

Bowman, J. A., Redman, S., Dickinson, J. A., Gibberd, R., & Sanson-Fisher, R. W. (1991). The accuracy of pap smear utilization self-report: A methodological consideration in cervical screening research. *Health Services Research, 26,* 97–107.

Boyle, M. H., Furlong, W., Feeny, D., Torrance, G. W., & Hatcher, J. (1995). Reliability of the Health Utilities Index—Mark III used in the 1991 cycle 6 Canadian General Social Survey Health Questionnaire. *Quality of Life Research, 4,* 249–257.

Bradburn, N. M. (1982). Question-wording effects in surveys. In R. M. Hogarth (Ed.), *Question framing and response consistency* (pp. 65–76). New Directions for Methodology of Social and Behavioral Science, no. 1. San Francisco: Jossey-Bass.

Bradburn, N. M. (1983). Response effects. In P. Rossi, J. D. Wright, & A. B. Anderson (Eds.), *Handbook of survey research* (pp. 289–328). San Diego, CA: Academic Press.

Bradburn, N. M., & Danis, C. (1984). Potential contributions of cognitive research to survey questionnaire design. In T. B. Jabine, M. L. Straf, J. M. Tanur, & R. Tourangeau (Eds.), *Cognitive aspects of survey methodology: Building a bridge between disciplines* (pp. 101–129). Washington, DC: National Academy Press.

Bradburn, N. M., Rips, L. J., & Shevell, S. K. (1987). Answering autobiographical questions: The impact of memory and inference on surveys. *Science, 236,* 157–161.

Bradburn, N. M., & Sudman, S. (1988). *Polls and surveys: Understanding what they tell us.* San Francisco: Jossey-Bass.

Bradburn, N. M., Sudman, S., & Associates. (1979). *Improving interview method and questionnaire design: Response effects to threatening questions in survey research.* San Francisco: Jossey-Bass.

Braden, J. J., & Cohen, S. B. (1992). An application of small area estimation techniques to derive state estimates of insurance coverage from the 1987 NMES. *Proceedings of the American Statistical Association, Section on Survey Research Methods,* pp. 888–893.

Brandt, E. N., Jr., & McGinnis, J. M. (1984). Nutrition monitoring and research in the Department of Health and Human Services. *Public Health Reports, 99,* 544–549.

Brandt, E. N., Jr., & McGinnis, J. M. (1985). National Children and Youth Fitness Study: Its contribution to our national objectives. *Public Health Reports, 100,* 1–3.

Breslow, L. (1989). Health status measurement in the evaluation of health promotion. *Medical Care, 27* (Suppl. 3), S205–S216.

Brick, J. M., & Waksberg, J. (1991). Avoiding sequential sampling with random digit dialing. *Survey Methodology, 17,* 27–41.

Brick, J. M., Waksberg, J., Kulp, D., & Starer, A. (1995). Bias in list-assisted telephone samples. *Public Opinion Quarterly, 59,* 218–235.

Brook, R. H., Ware, J. E., Jr., Davies-Avery, A., Stewart, A. L., Donald, C. A., Rogers, W. H., Williams, K. N., & Johnston, S. A. (1979). Overview of adult health status measures fielded in Rand's Health Insurance Study [Entire issue]. *Medical Care, 17* (Suppl. 7).

Brook, R. H., Ware, Jr., J. E., Rogers, W. H., Keeler, E. B., Davies, A. R., Sherbourne, C. A., Goldberg, G. A., Lohr, K. N., Camp, P., & Newhouse, J. P. (1984). *The effect of coinsurance on the health of adults.* Santa Monica, CA: RAND Corporation.

Burchell, B., & Marsh, C. (1992). The effect of questionnaire length on survey response. *Quality & Quantity, 26,* 233–244.

Burgess, M. J., & Paton, D. (1993). Coding of respondent behaviour by interviewers to test questionnaire wording. *Proceedings of the American Statistical Association, Section on Survey Research Methods, Vol. I,* 392–397.

Burnam, M. A., & Koegel, P. (1988). Methodology for obtaining a representative sample of homeless persons: The Los Angeles Skid Row Study. *Evaluation Review, 12,* 117–152.

Burstein, L., Freeman, H. E., Sirotnik, K. A., Delandshere, G., & Hollis, M. (1985). Data collection: The Achilles heel of evaluation research. *Sociological Methods & Research,* 14, 65–80.

Burt, V. L., & Cohen, S. B. (1984). A comparison of methods to approximate standard errors for complex survey data. *Review of Public Data Use, 12,* 159–168.

Burton, S., & Blair, E. A. (1991). Task conditions, response formulation processes, and response accuracy for behavioral frequency questions in surveys. *Public Opinion Quarterly, 55,* 50–79.

Bush, J. W. (1984). General Health Policy Model/Quality of Well-Being (QWB) scale. In N. K. Wenger, M. E. Mattson, C. D. Furberg, & J. Elinson (Eds.), *Assessment of quality of life in clinical trials of cardiovascular therapies* (pp. 189–199). New York: LeJacq.

Buzzard, I. M., & Sievert, Y. A. (1994). Research priorities and recommendations for dietary assessment methodology. *American Journal of Clinical Nutrition, 59* (Suppl.), 275S–280S.

Camburn, D., & Cynamon, M. L. (1993). Observations of new technology and family dynamics in a survey of youth. *Proceedings of the American Statistical Association, Section on Social Statistics,* pp. 494–502.

Campbell, B. A. (1981). Race-of-interviewer effects among Southern adolescents. *Public Opinion Quarterly, 45,* 231–244.

Campbell, D. T., & Fiske, D. W. (1959). Convergent and discriminant validation by the multitrait-multimethod matrix. *Psychological Bulletin, 56,* 85–105.

Campbell, D. T., & Stanley, J. C. (1963). *Experimental and quasi-experimental designs for research.* Skokie, IL: Rand McNally.

Cannell, C., Miller, P. V., & Oksenberg, L. (1982). Research on interviewing techniques. In S. Leinhardt (Ed.), *Sociological methodology 1982* (pp. 389–437). San Francisco: Jossey-Bass.

Carlson, B. A. (1985). The potential of National Household Survey Programmes for monitoring and evaluating primary health care in developing countries. *World Health Statistics Quarterly, 38,* 38–64.

Carlson, B. L., & Cohen, S. B. (1991). Evaluation of the efficiency of using personal computers for regression analysis on complex survey data. *Proceedings of the American Statistical Association, Section on Survey Research Methods,* pp. 746–751.

Carlson, B. L., Cohen, S. B., & Monheit, A. C. (1992). Alternatives to costly mainframe logistic regression adjusting for complex survey design. *Proceedings of the American Statistical Association, Section on Survey Research Methods,* pp. 882–887.

Carlson, B. L., Johnson, A. E., & Cohen, S. B. (1990). An evaluation of the use of personal computers for variance estimation with complex survey data. *Proceedings of the American Statistical Association, Section on Survey Research Methods,* pp. 724–729.

Carmines, E. G., & Zeller, R. A. (1979). *Reliability and validity assessment.* Thousand Oaks, CA: Sage.

Cartwright, A. (1983). *Health surveys in practice and in potential.* London: King's Fund Publishing Office.

Casady, R. J., & Lepkowski, J. M. (1991). Optimal allocation for stratified telephone survey designs. *Proceedings of the American Statistical Association, Section on Survey Research Methods,* pp. 111–116.

Cassel, J. C. (Ed.). (1971). Evans County Cardiovascular and Cerebrovascular Epidemiologic Study. *Archives of Internal Medicine, 128,* 883–986.

Cassidy, C. M. (1994). Walk a mile in my shoes: Culturally sensitive food-habit research. *American Journal of Clinical Nutrition, 59* (Suppl.), 190S–197S.

Catlin, G., & Lussier, R. (1993). The development of Canada's national population health survey. *Proceedings of the American Statistical Association, Section on Social Statistics,* pp. 167–170.

Cella, D. F. (1995). Methods and problems in measuring quality of life. *Support Care Cancer, 3,* 11–22.

Chen, M., Andersen, R. M., Barmes, D. E., Leclercq, M.-H., & Lyttle, C. S. (Eds.). (1995). *Comparing oral health care systems: A second international collaborative study.* Manuscript submitted for publication.

Church, A. H. (1993). Estimating the effect of incentives on mail survey response rates: A meta-analysis. *Public Opinion Quarterly, 57,* 62–79.

Cleary, P. D., & Angel, R. (1984). The analysis of relationships involving dichotomous dependent variables. *Journal of Health and Social Behavior, 25,* 334–348.

Cleary, P. D., & McNeil, B. J. (1988). Patient satisfaction as an indicator of quality care. *Inquiry, 25,* 25–36.

Cockburn, J., Hill, D., Irwig, L., DeLuise, T., Turnbull, D., & Schofield, P. (1991). Development and validation of an instrument to measure satisfaction of participants at breast screening programmes. *European Journal of Cancer, 27,* 827–831.

Coffey, C. M. (1992). Multi-lingual, multi-cultural interviewing. *Proceedings of the Sawtooth Software Conference* (pp. 67–83). Ketchum, ID.

Cohany, S. R., Polivka, A. E., & Rothgeb, J. M. (1994). Revisions in the Current Population Survey effective January 1994. *Employment and Earnings, 41* (2), 13–37.

Cohen, J. (1988). *Statistical power analysis for the behavioral sciences* (2nd ed.). Hillsdale, NJ: Erlbaum.

Cohen, S. B., Burt, V. L., & Jones, G. K. (1986). Efficiencies in variance estimation for complex survey data. *American Statistician, 40,* 157–164.

Cohen, S. B., Xanthopoulos, J. A., & Jones, G. K. (1988). An evaluation of statistical software procedures appropriate for the regression analysis of complex survey data. *Journal of Official Statistics, 4,* 17–34.

Colombotos, J. (1969). Personal versus telephone interviews: Effect on responses. *Public Health Reports, 84,* 773–782.

Connell, F. A., Diehr, P., & Hart, L. G. (1987). The use of large databases in health care studies. *Annual Review of Public Health, 8,* 51–74.

Conover, W. J. (1980). *Practical nonparametric statistics* (2nd ed.). New York: Wiley.

Converse, J. (1987). *Survey research in the United States: Roots and emergence 1890–1960.* Berkeley: University of California Press.

Converse, J. M., & Presser, S. (1986). *Survey questions: Handcrafting the standardized questionnaire.* Thousand Oaks, CA: Sage.

Cook, T. D., & Campbell, D. T. (1979). *Quasi-experimentation: Design and analysis issues.* Boston: Houghton Mifflin.

Corey, C. R., & Freeman, H. E. (1990). Use of telephone interviewing in health care research. *Health Services Research, 25,* 129–144.

Cornelius, R. M. (1985). The World Fertility Survey and its implications for future surveys. *Journal of Official Statistics, 1,* 427–433.

Cornoni-Huntley, J., Barbano, H. E., Brody, J. A., Cohen, B., Feldman, J. J., Kleinman, J. C., & Madans, J. (1983). National Health and Nutrition Examination I—Epidemiologic Follow-Up Survey. *Public Health Reports, 98,* 245–251.

Corrigan, J. M. (1995). How do purchasers develop and use performance measures? *Medical Care, 33* (Suppl. 1), JS18–JS24.

Cotter, P. R., Cohen, J., & Coulter, P. B. (1982). Race-of-interviewer effects in telephone surveys. *Public Opinion Quarterly, 46,* 278–284.

Couper, M. P., & Burt, G. (1993). The impact of computer-assisted personal interviewing (CAPI) on interviewer performance: The CPS experience. *Proceedings of the American Statistical Association, Section on Survey Research Methods, Vol. I,* 189–193.

Couper, M. P., & Groves, R. M. (1992a). Interviewer reactions to alternative hardware for computer-assisted personal interviewing. *Journal of Official Statistics, 8,* 201–210.

Couper, M. P., & Groves, R. M. (1992b). The role of the interviewer in survey participation. *Survey Methodology, 18,* 263–277.

Cox, B. G., Binder, D. A., Chinnappa, B. N., Christianson, A., Colledge, M. J., & Kott, P. S. (Eds.). (1995). *Business Survey Methods.* New York: Wiley.

Cox, B. G., & Cohen, S. B. (1985). *Methodological issues for health care surveys.* New York: Marcel Dekker.

Creswell, J. W. (1994). *Research design: Qualitative and quantitative approaches.* Thousand Oaks, CA: Sage.

Crocker, L., & Algina, J. (1986). *Introduction to classical and modern test theory.* San Diego, CA: Harcourt Brace Jovanovich College Division.

Cronbach, L. J. (1951). Coefficient Alpha and the internal structure of tests. *Psychometrika, 16,* 297–334.

Crowne, D. P., & Marlowe, D. (1960). A new scale of social desirability independent of psychopathology. *Journal of Consulting Psychology, 24,* 349–354.

Currie, S., Li, L., & Wall, D. (1993). Emerging applications of GIS in survey processes. *Proceedings of the Annual Research Conference of the U.S. Bureau of the Census* (pp. 383–392).

Czaja, R. (1987–1988). Asking sensitive behavioral questions in telephone interviews. *International Quarterly of Community Health Education, 8,* 23–31.

Czaja, R., & Blair, J. (1990). Using network sampling in crime victimization surveys. *Journal of Quantitative Criminology, 6,* 185–206.

Czaja, R., & Blair, J. (1996). *Designing surveys: A guide to decisions and procedures.* Thousand Oaks, CA: Pine Forge Press.

Czaja, R., Blair, J., Bickart, B., & Eastman, E. (1994). Respondent strategies for recall of crime victimization incidents. *Journal of Official Statistics, 10,* 257–276.

Czaja, R., Blair, J., & Sebestik, J. P. (1982). Respondent selection in a telephone survey: A comparison of three techniques. *Journal of Marketing Research, 21,* 381–385.

Czaja, R. F., Snowden, C. B., & Casady, R. J. (1986). Reporting bias and sampling errors in a survey of a rare population using multiplicity counting rules. *Journal of the American Statistical Association, 81,* 411–419.

Czaja, R. F., Trunzo, D. H., & Royston, P. N. (1992). Response effects in a network survey. *Sociological Methods & Research, 20,* 340–366.

Czaja, R., Warnecke, R. B., Eastman, E., Royston, P., Sirken, M., & Tuteur, D. (1984). Locating patients with rare diseases using network sampling: Frequency and quality of reporting. In National Center for Health Services Research, *Health survey research methods: Proceedings of the fourth conference on health survey research methods.* (Report No. DHHS Publication No. [PHS] 84–3346, pp. 311–324). NCHSR Proceedings Series. Washington, DC: U.S. Government Printing Office.

David, M. (1985). Introduction: The design and development of SIPP. *Journal of Economic and Social Measurement, 13,* 215–224.

Davies, A. R., & Ware, J. E., Jr. (1988a). *GHAA's consumer satisfaction survey and user's manual.* Washington, DC: Group Health Association of America, Inc.

Davies, A. R., & Ware, J. E., Jr. (1988b). Involving consumers in quality of care assessment. *Health Affairs, 7* (1), 33–48.

Davies, A. R., & Ware, J. E., Jr. (1991). *GHAA's consumer satisfaction survey and user's manual.* Washington, DC: Group Health Association of America.

Davies, A. R., Ware, J. E., Jr., Brook, R. H., Peterson, J. R., & Newhouse, J. P. (1986). Consumer acceptance of prepaid and fee-for-service medical care: Results from a randomized controlled trial. *Health Services Research, 21,* 429–452.

Davies, A. R., Ware, J. E., Jr., & Kosinski, M. (1995). Standardizing health care evaluations. *Medical Outcomes Trust Bulletin, 3* (4), 2–3.

Davis, W. L., & DeMaio, T. J. (1993). Comparing the think–aloud interviewing technique with standard interviewing in the redesign of a dietary recall questionnaire. *Proceedings of the American Statistical Association, Section on Survey Research Methods, Vol. I,* 565–570.

Dawber, T. R. (1980). *The Framingham Study.* Cambridge, MA: Harvard University Press.

Dean, A. G., Dean, J. A., Coulombier, D., Brendel, K. A., Smith, D. C., Burton, A. H., Dicker, R. C., Sullivan, K., Fagan, R. F., & Arner, T. G. (1994). *Epi Info, Version 6.* Atlanta, GA: Centers for Disease Control and Prevention.

de Heer, W. F., & Israëls, A. Z. (1992). Response trends in Europe. *Proceedings of the American Statistical Association, Section on Survey Research Methods,* pp. 92– 101.

DeFriese, G. H. (1991). The secondary data bases of health services research: Need for a national inventory. *Health Services Research, 25,* 829–830.

Delbanco, T. L. (1992). Enriching the doctor-patient relationship by inviting the patient's perspective. *Annals of Internal Medicine, 116,* 414–418.

DeLeeuw, E. D., & Hox, J. J. (1988). The effects of response-stimulating factors on response rates and data quality in mail surveys: A test of Dillman's Total Design Method. *Journal of Official Statistics, 4,* 241–249.

Delgado, J. L., & Estrada, L. (1993). Improving data collection strategies. *Public Health Reports, 108,* 540–545.

DeMaio, T. J. (Ed.). (1983). *Approaches to developing questionnaires.* (Report No. 10, Statistical Policy Working Paper). Washington, DC: Office of Management and Budget.

Desvousges, W. H., & Frey, J. H. (1989). Integrating focus groups and surveys: Examples from environmental risk studies. *Journal of Official Statistics, 5,* 349–363.

deVaus, D. A. (1991). *Surveys in social research* (3rd ed.). London: Allen & Unwin.

DeVellis, R. F. (1991). *Scale development: Theory and applications.* Thousand Oaks, CA: Sage.

DiClemente, R. J., Zorn, J., & Temoshok, L. (1986). Adolescents and AIDS: A survey of knowledge, attitudes, and beliefs about AIDS in San Francisco. *American Journal of Public Health, 76,* 1443–1445.

Dielman, T. E., & Couper, M. P. (1995). Data quality in a CAPI survey: Keying errors. *Journal of Official Statistics, 11,* 141–146.

Dijkstra, N., & Van der Zouwen, J. (Eds.). (1982). *Response behavior in the survey interview.* London: Academic Press.

Dillman, D. A. (1978). *Mail and telephone surveys: The total design method.* New York: Wiley.

Dillman, D. A. (1983). Mail and other self-administered questionnaires. In P. H. Rossi, J. D. Wright, & A. B. Anderson (Eds.), *Handbook of survey research* (pp. 359–377). San Diego, CA: Academic Press.

Dillman, D. A. (1991). The design and administration of mail surveys. *Annual Review of Sociology, 17,* 225–249.

Dillman, D. A., & Sangster, R. L. (1991). *Mail surveys: A comprehensive bibliography, 1974–1989.* Chicago: Council of Planning Librarians.

Dillman, D. A., Sinclair, M. D., & Clark, J. R. (1993). Effects of questionnaire length, respondent-friendly design, and a difficult question on response rates for occupant-addressed census mail surveys. *Public Opinion Quarterly, 57,* 289–304.

Doyle, B. J., & Ware, J. E., Jr. (1977). Physician conduct and other factors that affect consumer satisfaction with medical care. *Journal of Medical Education, 52,* 793–801.

Dull, V. T. (1990). Interviewing special populations by telephone: A discussion. *ISSR Quarterly, 5,* 12–15.

Edgell, S. E., Himmelfarb, S., & Duchan, K. L. (1982). Validity of forced responses in a randomized response model. *Sociological Methods and Research, 11,* 89–100.

Edwards, B., Bittner, D., Edwards, W. S., & Sperry, S. (1993). CAPI effects on interviewers: A report from two major surveys. *Proceedings of the Annual Research Conference of the U.S. Bureau of the Census*, pp. 411–428.

Edwards, S., Slattery, M. L., Mori, M., Berry, T. D., Caan, B. J., Palmer, P., & Potter, J. D. (1994). Objective system for interviewer performance evaluation for use in epidemiologic studies. *American Journal of Epidemiology, 140*, 1020–1028.

Edwards, W. S., Sperry, S., & Edwards, B. (1992). Using CAPI in a longitudinal survey: A report from the Medicare Current Beneficiary Survey. *Proceedings of Statistics Canada Symposium 92: Design and Analysis of Longitudinal Surveys*, pp. 21–30.

Elbeck, M. (1992). Patient contribution to the design and meaning of patient satisfaction for quality assurance purposes: The psychiatric case. *Health Care Management Review, 17*, 91–95.

Elbeck, M., & Fecteau, G. (1990). Improving the validity of measures of patient satisfaction with psychiatric care and treatment. *Hospital and Community Psychiatry, 41*, 998–1001.

Elinson, J., & Siegmann, A. E. (1979). *Sociomedical health indicators.* Farmingdale, NY: Baywood.

Epstein, F. H., Napier, J. A., Block, W. D., Hayner, N. S., Higgins, M. P., Johnson, B. C., Keller, J. B., Metzner, H. L., Montoye, H. J., Ostrander, L. D., Jr., & Ullman, B. M. (1970). The Tecumseh Study. *Archives of Environmental Health, 21*, 402–407.

Ericsson, K. A., & Simon, H. A. (1993). *Protocol analysis: Verbal reports as data.* Cambridge, MA: MIT Press.

Euronut SENECA investigators. (1991). Design, methods, and participation. *European Journal of Clinical Nutrition, 45*, 5–22.

EuroQol Group. (1990). EuroQol—A new facility for the measurement of health-related quality of life. *Health Policy, 16*, 199–208.

Evans, R. G., Barer, M. L., & Marmor, T. R. (Eds.). (1994). *Why are some people healthy and others not? The determinants of health of populations.* Hawthorne, NY: Aldine.

Evans, R. G., & Stoddart, G. L. (1990). Producing health, consuming health care. *Social Science and Medicine, 31*, 1347–1363.

Ezzati-Rice, T. M., Fahimi, M., Judkins, D., & Khare, M. (1993). Serial imputation of NHANES III with mixed regression and hot-deck techniques. *Proceedings of the American Statistical Association, Section on Survey Research Methods, Vol. I*, 292–296.

Ezzati-Rice, T. M., Khare, M., Rubin, D. B., Little, R.J.A., & Schafer, J. L. (1993). A comparison of imputation techniques in the third National Health and Nutrition Examination survey. *Proceedings of the American Statistical Association, Section on Survey Research Methods, Vol. I*, 303–308.

Farquhar, J., Wood, P. D., Breitrose, H., Haskell, W. L., Meyer, A. J., Maccoby, N., Alexander, J. K., Brown, B. W., Jr., McAlister, A. L., Nash, J. D., & Stern, M. P. (1977). Community education for cardiovascular disease. *Lancet, 1*, 1192–1195.

Fecso, R. (1989). What is survey quality: Back to the future. *Proceedings of the American Statistical Association, Section on Survey Research Methods*, pp. 88–96.

Feeny, D. H., & Torrance, G. W. (1989). Incorporating utility-based quality-of-life assessment measures in clinical trials. *Medical Care, 27* (Suppl. 3), S190–S204.

Feeny, D. H., Torrance, G. W., Goldsmith, C. H., Furlong, W., & Boyle, M. (1993). A multi-attribute approach to population health status. *Proceedings of the American Statistical Association, Section on Social Statistics*, pp. 161–166.

Feinstein, A. R. (1987). *Clinimetrics.* New Haven: Yale University Press.

Feinstein, A. R. (1992). Benefits and obstacles for development of health status assessment measures in clinical settings. *Medical Care, 30* (Suppl. 5), MS50–MS56.

Fendrich, M., & Vaughn, C. M. (1994). Diminished lifetime substance use over time: An inquiry into differential underreporting. *Public Opinion Quarterly, 58,* 96–123.

Fern, E. F., Monroe, K. B., & Avila, R. A. (1986). Effectiveness of multiple request strategies: A synthesis of research results. *Journal of Marketing Research, 23,* 144–152.

Fienberg, S. E., Loftus, E. F., & Tanur, J. M. (1985). Cognitive aspects of health survey methodology: An Overview. *Milbank Memorial Fund Quarterly: Health and Society, 63,* 547–564.

Fienberg, S. E., & Tanur, J. M. (1989). Combining cognitive and statistical approaches to survey design. *Science, 243,* 1017–1022.

Fienberg, S. E., & Tanur, J. M. (1990). A historical perspective on the institutional bases for survey research in the United States. *Survey Methodology, 16,* 31–50.

Fink, A. (1995a). *How to analyze survey data.* Thousand Oaks, CA: Sage.

Fink, A. (1995b). *How to sample in surveys.* Thousand Oaks, CA: Sage.

Fink, J. C. (1983). CATI's first decade: The Chilton experience. *Sociological Methods & Research, 12,* 153–168.

Fitzpatrick, R. (1991a). Surveys of patient satisfaction: I. Important general considerations. *British Medical Journal, 302,* 887–889.

Fitzpatrick, R. (1991b). Surveys of patient satisfaction: II. Designing a questionnaire and conducting a survey. *British Medical Journal, 302,* 1129–1132.

Fleming, G. V., & Andersen, R. (1986). *Can access be improved while controlling costs?* Chicago: Pluribus Press.

Foddy, W. (1993). *Constructing questions for interviews and questionnaires: Theory and practice in social research.* Cambridge, England: Cambridge University Press.

Ford, K., & Norris, A. (1991). Methodological considerations for survey research on sexual behavior: Urban African American and Hispanic youth. *The Journal of Sex Research, 28,* 539–555.

Forsman, G. (1993). Sampling individuals within households in telephone surveys. *Proceedings of the American Statistical Association, Section on Survey Research Methods, Vol. II,* 1113–1118.

Forsyth, B. H., & Lessler, J. T. (1991). Cognitive laboratory methods: A taxonomy. In P. P. Biemer, R. M. Groves, L. E. Lyberg, N. A. Mathiowetz, & S. Sudman (Eds.), *Measurement errors in surveys* (pp. 393–418). New York: Wiley.

Forthofer, R. N., & Lee, E. S. (1995). *Introduction to biostatistics: A guide to design, analysis, and discovery.* San Diego: Academic Press.

Fowler, F. J., Jr. (1989a). Coding behavior in pretests to identify unclear questions. In F. J. Fowler, Jr. (Ed.). *Conference proceedings: Health survey research methods* (Report No. DHHS Publication No. [PHS] 89–3447, pp. 8–12). Washington DC: U.S. Government Printing Office.

Fowler, F. J., Jr. (Ed.). (1989b). *Conference proceedings: Health survey research methods.* (Report No. DHHS Publication No. [PHS] 89–3447). Washington, DC: U.S. Government Printing Office.

Fowler, F. J., Jr. (1992). How unclear terms affect survey data. *Public Opinion Quarterly, 56,* 218–231.

Fowler, F. J., Jr. (1993). *Survey research methods* (2nd ed.). Thousand Oaks, CA: Sage.

Fowler, F. J., Jr. (1995). *Improving survey questions: Design and evaluation.* Thousand Oaks, CA: Sage.

Fowler, F. J., Jr., Cleary, P. D., Magaziner, J., Patrick, D. L., & Benjamin, K. L. (1994). Methodological issues in measuring patient-reported outcomes: The agenda of the work group on outcomes assessment. *Medical Care, 32* (Suppl. 7), JS65–JS76.

Fowler, F. J., Jr., & Mangione, T. W. (1990). *Standardized survey interviewing: Minimizing interviewer related error.* Thousand Oaks, CA: Sage.

Fowler, F. J., Jr., Roman, A. M., & Di, Z. X. (1993). Mode effects in a survey of Medicare prostate surgery patients. *Proceedings of the American Statistical Association, Section on Survey Research Methods, Vol. II,* 730–735.

Fox, J. A., & Tracy, P. E. (1986). *Randomized response: A method for sensitive surveys.* Thousand Oaks, CA: Sage.

Freeman, H. E. (1983). Research opportunities related to CATI. *Sociological Methods & Research, 12,* 143–152.

Freeman, H. E., Blendon, R. J., Aiken, L. H., Sudman, S., Mullinix, C. F., & Corey, C. R. (1987). Americans report on their access to health care. *Health Affairs, 6* (1), 6–18.

Freeman, H. E., Kiecolt, K. J., Nicholls, W. L., II, & Shanks, J. M. (1982). Telephone sampling bias in surveying disability. *Public Opinion Quarterly, 46,* 392–407.

Freeman, H. E., and Shanks, J. M. (1983). Foreword: Special issue on the emergence of computer-assisted survey research. *Sociological Methods & Research, 12,* 115–118.

Freidenberg, J., Mulvihill, M., & Caraballo, L. R. (1993). From ethnography to survey: Some methodological issues in research on health seeking in East Harlem. *Human Organization, 52,* 151–161.

Frey, J. H., & Fontana, A. (1991). The group interview in social research. *The Social Science Journal, 28,* 175–187.

Frey, J. H., & Oishi, S. M. (1995). *How to conduct interviews by telephone and in person.* Thousand Oaks, CA: Sage.

Froberg, D. G., & Kane, R. L. (1989a). Methodology for measuring health-state preferences—I: Measurement strategies. *Journal of Clinical Epidemiology, 42,* 345–354.

Froberg, D. G., & Kane, R. L. (1989b). Methodology for measuring health-state preferences—II: Scaling methods. *Journal of Clinical Epidemiology, 42,* 459–471.

Froberg, D. G., & Kane, R. L. (1989c). Methodology for measuring health-state preferences—III: Population and context effects. *Journal of Clinical Epidemiology, 42,* 585–592.

Froberg, D. G., & Kane, R. L. (1989d). Methodology for measuring health—state preferences—IV: Progress and a research agenda. *Journal of Clinical Epidemiology, 42,* 675–685.

Furse, D. H., & Stewart, D. W. (1982). Monetary incentives versus promised contribution to charity: New evidence on mail survey response. *Journal of Marketing Research, 19,* 375–380.

Furse, D. H., Stewart, D. W., & Rados, D. L. (1981). Effects of foot-in-the-door, cash incentives, and follow-ups on survey response. *Journal of Marketing Research, 18,* 473–478.

Gardenier, J. S. (1991). Large surveys on small computers: NCHS's CAPI system. *Proceedings of the American Statistical Association, Section on Survey Research Methods,* pp. 141–145.

Gardenier, J. S. (1993). Three aspects of CLASIC. *Proceedings of the American Statistical Association, Section on Survey Research Methods, Vol. I,* 173–176.

Gaskell, G. D., O'Muircheartaigh, C. A., & Wright, D. B. (1994). Survey questions about the frequency of vaguely defined events: The effects of response alternatives. *Public Opinion Quarterly, 58,* 241–254.

Geer, J. G. (1991). Do open-ended questions measure "salient" issues? *Public Opinion Quarterly, 55,* 360–370.

General Accounting Office. (1994). *Health care reform: "Report cards" are useful but significant issues need to be addressed.* (Report No. GAO/HEHS–94–219). Washington, DC: U.S. Government Printing Office.

Gerteis, M., Edgman-Levitan, S., Daley, J., & Delbanco, T. L. (Eds.). (1993). *Through the patient's eyes: Understanding and promoting patient-centered care.* San Francisco: Jossey-Bass.

Gill, T. M., & Feinstein, A. R. (1994). A critical appraisal of the quality of quality-of-life measurements. *Journal of the American Medical Association, 272,* 619–626.

Gilljam, M., & Granberg, D. (1993). Should we take don't know for an answer? *Public Opinion Quarterly, 57,* 348–357.

Gold, M., Hadley, J., Eisenhower, D., Hall, J., Metcalf, C., Nelson, L., Chu, K., Strouse, R., & Colby, D. (1995). Design and feasibility of a national Medicaid access survey with state-specific estimates. *Medical Care Research and Review, 52,* 409–430.

Gold, M., & Wooldridge, J. (1995). Plan-based surveys of satisfaction with access and quality of care: Review and critique. In Agency for Health Care Policy and Research, *Consumer survey information in a reforming health care system* (Report No. AHCPR Pub. No. 95–0083, pp. 75–109). Rockville, MD: Agency for Health Care Policy and Research.

Goldberg, H. I., & Cummings, M. A. (1994). Conducting medical effectiveness research: A report from the Inter-PORT work groups [Entire issue]. *Medical Care, 32* (Suppl. 7).

Gower, A. R. (1994). Questionnaire design for business surveys. *Survey Methodology, 20,* 125–136.

Goyder, J. (1985). Face-to-face interviews and mailed questionnaires: The net difference in response rate. *Public Opinion Quarterly, 49,* 234–252.

Grady, K. E., & Wallston, B. S. (1988). *Research in health care settings.* Thousand Oaks, CA: Sage.

Grammatik IV. (1991). *The easiest way to improve your writing.* [Computer software program]. San Francisco: Reference Software.

Greenfield, S., & Nelson, E. C. (1992). Recent developments and future issues in the use of health status assessment measures in clinical settings. *Medical Care, 30* (Suppl. 5), MS23–MS41.

Grembowski, D., Milgrom, P., & Fiset, L. (1988). Factors influencing dental decision making. *Journal of Public Health Dentistry, 48,* 159–167.

Grembowski, D., Milgrom, P., & Fiset, L. (1989). Clinical decision making among dental students and general practitioners. *Journal of Dental Education, 53,* 189–192.

Grembowski, D., Milgrom, P., & Fiset, L. (1990a). Factors influencing variation in dentist service rates. *Journal of Public Health Dentistry, 50,* 244–250.

Grembowski, D., Milgrom, P., & Fiset, L. (1990b). Variation in dentist service rates in a homogeneous patient population. *Journal of Public Health Dentistry, 50,* 235–243.

Grembowski, D., Milgrom, P., & Fiset, L. (1991). Dental decision making and variation in dentist service rates. *Social Science and Medicine, 32,* 287–294.

Grembowski, D., Patrick, D., Diehr, P., Durham, M., Beresford, S., Kay, E., & Hecht, J. (1993). Self-efficacy and health behavior among older adults. *Journal of Health and Social Behavior, 34,* 89–104.

Groves, R. M. (1983). Implications of CATI. *Sociological Methods & Research, 12,* 199–215.

Groves, R. M. (1987). Research on survey data quality. *Public Opinion Quarterly, 51,* S156–S172.

Groves, R. M. (1989). *Survey errors and survey costs.* New York: Wiley.

Groves, R. M. (1990a). On the path to quality improvement in social measurement: Developing indicators of survey errors and survey costs. *Proceedings of the American Statistical Association, Section on Survey Research Methods,* pp. 1–10.

Groves, R. M. (1990b). Theories and methods of telephone surveys. *Annual Review of Sociology, 16,* 221–240.

Groves, R. M., Biemer, P. P., Lyberg, L. E., Massey, J. T., Nicholls, W. L., II, & Waksberg, J. (1988). *Telephone survey methodology.* New York: Wiley.

Groves, R. M., Cialdini, R. B., & Couper, M. P. (1992). Understanding the decision to participate in a survey. *Public Opinion Quarterly, 56,* 475–495.

Groves, R. M., & Fultz, N. H. (1985). Gender effects among telephone interviewers in a survey of economic attitudes. *Sociological Methods & Research, 14,* 31–52.

Groves, R. M., & Kahn, R. L. (1979). *Surveys by telephone: A national comparison with personal interviews.* San Diego: Academic Press.

Groves, R. M., & Magilavy, L. J. (1981). Increasing response rates to telephone surveys: A door in the face for foot-in-the-door? *Public Opinion Quarterly, 45,* 346–358.

Groves, R. M., & Mathiowetz, N. A. (1984). Computer-assisted telephone interviewing: Effects on interviewers and respondents. *Public Opinion Quarterly, 48,* 356–369.

Groves, R. M., & Nicholls, W. L., II. (1986). The status of computer-assisted telephone interviewing: Part II—Data quality issues. *Journal of Official Statistics, 2,* 117–134.

Gunn, W. J., & Rhodes, I. N. (1981). Physician response rates to a telephone survey: Effects of monetary incentive level. *Public Opinion Quarterly, 45,* 109–115.

Guyatt, G. H., Deyo, R. A., Charlson, M., Levine, M. N., & Mitchell, A. (1989). Responsiveness and validity in health status measurement: A clarification. *Journal of Clinical Epidemiology, 42,* 403–408.

Hadorn, D. C., Sorensen, J., & Holte, J. (1995). Large-scale health outcomes evaluation: How should quality of life be measured? Part II—Questionnaire validation in a cohort of patients with advanced cancer. *Journal of Clinical Epidemiology, 48,* 619–629.

Hadorn, D. C., & Uebersax, J. (1995). Large-scale health outcomes evaluation: How should quality of life be measured? Part I—Calibration of a brief questionnaire and a search for preference subgroups. *Journal of Clinical Epidemiology, 48,* 607–618.

Hagan, D. E., & Collier, C. M. (1983). Must respondent selection procedures for telephone surveys be invasive? *Public Opinion Quarterly, 47,* 547–556.

Hakim, C. (1982). *Secondary analysis in social research.* London: Allen & Unwin.

Haley, S. M., McHorney, C. A., & Ware, J. E., Jr. (1994). Evaluation of the MOS SF–36 physical functioning scale (PF–10): I. Unidimensionality and reproducibility of the Rasch Item Scale. *Journal of Clinical Epidemiology, 47,* 671–684.

Hall, J. A., & Dornan, M. C. (1988). Meta-analysis of satisfaction with medical care: Description of research domain and analysis of overall satisfaction levels. *Social Science and Medicine, 27,* 637–644.

Hall, J. A., Epstein, A. M., & McNeil, B. J. (1989). Multidimensionality of health status in an elderly population. *Medical Care, 27* (Suppl. 3), S168–S177.

Hall, J. A., Milburn, M. A., & Epstein, A. M. (1993). A causal model of health status and satisfaction with medical care. *Medical Care, 31,* 84–94.

Hambleton, R. K., Swaminathan H., & Rogers, H. J. (1991). *Fundamentals of item response theory.* Thousand Oaks, CA: Sage.

Hanley, J. A. (1983). Appropriate uses of multivariate analysis. *Annual Review of Public Health, 4,* 155–180.

Hansluwka, H. E. (1985). Measuring the health of populations: Indicators and interpretations. *Social Science and Medicine, 20,* 1207–1224.

Hansson, L., Björkman, T., & Berglund, I. (1993). What is important in psychiatric inpatient care? Quality of care from the patient's perspective. *Quality Assurance in Health Care, 5,* 41–47.

Hay, D. A. (1990). Does the method matter on sensitive survey topics? *Survey Methodology, 16,* 131–136.

Hayes-Bautista, D. E. (1983). On comparing studies of different Raza populations. *American Journal of Public Health, 73,* 274–276.

Hayes-Bautista, D. E., & Chapa, J. (1987). Latino terminology: Conceptual bases for standardized terminology. *American Journal of Public Health, 77,* 61–68.

Hays, R. D., Larson, C., Nelson, E. C., & Batalden, P. B. (1991). Hospital quality trends: A short-form patient-based measure. *Medical Care, 29,* 661–668.

Heberlein, T. A., & Baumgartner, R. (1981). Is a questionnaire necessary in a second mailing? *Public Opinion Quarterly, 45,* 102–108.

Hendershot, G. E. (1990, November). *National Health Interview Survey: Capabilities and constraints.* Paper presented at the meeting on the technical feasibility of a national health interview survey on disability, National Center for Health Statistics, Hyattsville, MD.

Hennekens, C. H., & Buring, J. E. (1987). *Epidemiology in medicine.* Boston: Little, Brown.

Henry, G. T. (1990). *Practical sampling.* Thousand Oaks, CA: Sage.

Herrmann, D. (1994). *The contributions of the NCHS Collaborative Research Program to memory research.* (Report No. 14, National Center for Health Statistics, Cognitive Methods Staff Working Paper Series). Hyattsville, MD: National Center for Health Statistics.

Herzog, A. R., & Rodgers, W. L. (1988). Interviewing older adults: Mode comparison using data from a face-to-face survey and a telephone resurvey. *Public Opinion Quarterly, 52,* 84–99.

Herzog, A. R., & Rodgers, W. L. (1989). Age differences in memory performance and memory ratings as measured in a sample survey. *Psychology and Aging, 4,* 173–182.

Hidiroglou, M. A., Drew, J. D., & Gray, G. B. (1993). A framework for measuring and reducing nonresponse in surveys. *Survey Methodology, 19,* 81–94.

Hippler, H.-J., & Hippler, G. (1986). Reducing refusal rates in the case of threatening questions: The 'door-in-the-face' technique. *Journal of Official Statistics, 2,* 25–33.

Hippler, H.-J., & Schwarz, N. (1986). Not forbidding isn't allowing: The cognitive basis of the forbid-allow asymmetry. *Public Opinion Quarterly, 50,* 87–96.

Hippler, H.-J., & Schwarz, N. (1989). 'No opinion'-filters: A cognitive perspective. *International Journal of Public Opinion Research, 1,* 77–87.

Hippler, H.-J., Schwarz, N., & Sudman, S. (Eds.). (1987). *Social information processing and survey methodology.* New York: Springer.

Hirschi, T., & Selvin, H. (1967). *Delinquency research: An appraisal of analytic methods.* New York: Free Press.

Hochstim, J. R. (1967). A critical comparison of three strategies of collecting data from households. *Journal of the American Statistical Association, 62,* 976–989.

Hofman, L.P.M.B., & Keller, W. J. (1991). Design and management of computer assisted interviews in The Netherlands. *Proceedings of the American Statistical Association, Section on Social Statistics,* pp. 306–311.

Hornik, J., Zaig, T., Shadmon, D., & Barbash, G. I. (1990). Comparison of three inducement techniques to improve compliance in a health survey conducted by telephone. *Public Health Reports, 105,* 524–529.

Hosmer, D. W., Jr., & Lemeshow, S. (1989). *Applied logistic regression.* New York: Wiley.

Hosmer, D. W., Jr., Taber, S., & Lemeshow, S. (1991). The importance of assessing the fit of logistic regression models: A case study. *American Journal of Public Health, 81,* 1630–1635.

House, C. C. (1985). Questionnaire design with computer-assisted telephone interviewing. *Journal of Official Statistics, 1,* 209–219.

House, C. C., & Nicholls, W. L., II. (1988). Questionnaire design for CATI: Design objectives and methods. In R. M. Groves, P. P. Biemer, L. E. Lyberg, J. T. Massey, W. L. Nicholls, II, & J. Waksberg (Eds.), *Telephone survey methodology.* New York: Wiley.

Hubbard, R., & Little, E. L. (1988). Promised contributions to charity and mail survey responses: Replication with extension. *Public Opinion Quarterly, 52,* 223–230.

Hulka, B. S., Kupper, L. L., Daly, M. B., Cassel, J. C., & Schoen, F. (1975). Correlates of satisfaction and dissatisfaction with medical care: A community perspective. *Medical Care, 13,* 648–658.

Hulka, B. S., Zyzanski, S. J., Cassel, J. C., & Thompson, S. J. (1970). Scale for the measurement of attitudes toward physicians and primary medical care. *Medical Care, 8,* 429–435.

Hulley, S. B., & Cummings, S. R. (1988). *Designing clinical research: An epidemiologic approach.* Baltimore, MD: Williams & Wilkins.

Hunt, S. D., Sparkman, R. D., Jr., & Wilcox, J. B. (1982). The pretest in survey research: Issues and preliminary findings. *Journal of Marketing Research, 19,* 269–273.

Hunt, S. M., & McEwen, J. (1980). The development of a subjective health indicator. *Sociology of Health and Illness, 2,* 231–246.

Hunt, S. M., McKenna, S. P., McEwen, J., Williams, J., & Papp, E. (1981). The Nottingham Health Profile: Subjective health status and medical consultations. *Social Science and Medicine, 15A,* 221–229.

Hurley, R. E., Freund, D. A., & Paul, J. E. (1993). *Managed care in Medicaid: Lessons for policy and program design.* Ann Arbor, MI: Health Administration Press.

Huttenlocher, J., Hedges, L. V., & Bradburn, N. M. (1990). Reports of elapsed time: Bounding and rounding processes in estimation. *Journal of Experimental Psychology: Learning, Memory and Cognition, 16,* 196–213.

Hyman, H. (1955). *Survey design and analysis.* New York: Free Press.

Institute of Medicine. (1991). *Disability in America: Toward a national agenda for prevention.* Washington, DC: National Academy Press.

Jabine, T. B., Straf, M. L., Tanur, J. M., & Tourangeau, R. (1984). *Cognitive aspects of survey methodology: Building a bridge between disciplines.* Washington, DC: National Academy Press.

Jacobs, D. R., Jr., Luepker, R. V., Mittelmark, M. B., Folsom, A. R., Pirie, P. L., Mascioli, S. R., Hannan, P. J., Pechacek, T. F., Bracht, N. F., Carlaw, R. W., Kline, F. G., & Blackburn, H. (1986). Community-wide prevention strategies: Evaluation design of the Minnesota Heart Health Program. *Journal of Chronic Diseases, 39,* 775–788.

Jacobs, M., Cross, J., & Smailes, E. (1994). CIM: Computer interviewing by mail: Feasibility, advantages, disadvantages and costs. *Quality & Quantity, 28,* 137–150.

James, J. M., & Bolstein, R. (1990). The effect of monetary incentives and follow-up mailings on the response rate and response quality in mail surveys. *Public Opinion Quarterly, 54,* 346–361.

Jobe, J. B., & Mingay, D. J. (1989). Cognitive research improves questionnaires. *American Journal of Public Health, 79,* 1053–1055.

Jobe, J. B., & Mingay, D. J. (1990). Cognitive laboratory approach to designing questionnaires for surveys of the elderly. *Public Health Reports, 105,* 518–524.

Jobe, J. B., & Mingay, D. J. (1991). Cognition and survey measurement: History and overview. *Applied Cognitive Psychology, 5,* 175–192.

Jobe, J. B., Tourangeau, R., & Smith, A. F. (1993). Contributions of survey research to the understanding of memory. *Applied Cognitive Psychology, 7,* 567–584.

Jobe, J. B., White, A. A., Kelley, C. L., Mingay, D. J., Sanchez, M. J., & Loftus, E. F. (1990). Recall strategies and memory for health-care visits. *The Milbank Quarterly, 68,* 171–189.

Johnson, A. E. (1993). Small area estimation. *Proceedings of the American Statistical Association, Section on Survey Research Methods, Vol. I,* 352–357.

Johnson, T. P., Hougland, J. G., Jr., & Clayton, R. R. (1989). Obtaining reports of sensitive behavior: A comparison of substance use reports from telephone and face-to-face interviews. *Social Science Quarterly, 70,* 174–183.

Johnson. T. P., Hougland, J. G., Jr., & Moore, R. W. (1991). Sex differences in reporting sensitive behavior: A comparison of interview methods. *Sex Roles, 24,* 669–680.

Johnson, T. P., Mitra, A., Newman, R., & Horm, J. (1993). Problems of definition in sampling special populations: The case of homeless persons. *Evaluation Practice, 14,* 119–126.

Johnson, T. P., O'Rourke, D., Chavez, N., Sudman, S., Warnecke, R., & Lacey, L. (1994). *Social cognition and responses to survey questions among culturally diverse populations.* Manuscript submitted for publication.

Jordan, L. A., Marcus, A. C., & Reeder, L. G. (1980). Response styles in telephone and household interviewing: A field experiment. *Public Opinion Quarterly, 44,* 210–222.

Jöreskog, K. G. (1993). *LISTREL 8 user's reference guide.* Chicago: Scientific Software International.

Jöreskog, K. G., & Sörbom, D. (1979). *Advances in factor analysis and structural equation models.* Cambridge, MA: Abt Books.

Joyce, C. (1988). This machine wants to help you. *Psychology Today, 22,* 44–50.

Judkins, D., Marker, D., & Waksberg, J. (1994). *National Health Interview Survey: Research for the 1995 redesign.* Rockville, MD: Westat.

Judkins, D., Massey, J., & Smith, V. (1992). Using surnames to oversample Hispanics from a list frame. *Proceedings of the American Statistical Association, Section on Survey Research Methods,* pp. 847–852.

Jylhä, M. (1994). Self-rated health revisited: Exploring survey interview episodes with elderly respondents. *Social Science and Medicine, 39,* 983–990.

Kahn, H. A., & Sempos, C. T. (1989). *Statistical methods in epidemiology.* New York: Oxford University Press.

Kahn, R. L., & Cannell, C. (1957). *The dynamics of interviewing: Theory, technique, and cases.* New York: Wiley.

Kalsbeek, W. D., Botman, S. L., Massey, J. T., & Liu, P.-W. (1994). Cost-efficiency and the number of allowable call attempts in the National Health Interview Survey. *Journal of Official Statistics, 10,* 133–152.

Kalton, G. (1983). *Introduction to survey sampling.* Thousand Oaks, CA: Sage.

Kalton, G. (1991). Sampling flows of mobile human populations. *Survey Methodology, 17,* 183–194.

Kalton, G., & Anderson, D. W. (1986). Sampling rare populations. *Journal of the Royal Statistical Society, 149,* 65–82.

Kalton, G., & Citro, C. F. (1993). Panel surveys: Adding the fourth dimension. *Survey Methodology, 19,* 205–215.

Kalton, G., Collins, M., & Brook, L. (1978). Experiments in wording opinion questions. *Journal of the Royal Statistical Society, 27* (Series C), 149–161.

Kalton G., & Kasprzyk, D. (1986). The treatment of missing survey data. *Survey Methodology, 12,* 1–16.

Kalton, G., & Schuman, H. (1982). The effect of the question on survey responses: A review. *Journal of the Royal Statistical Society, 145* (Series A, Part 1), 42–73.

Kaplan, R. M. (1989). Health outcome models for policy analysis. *Health Psychology, 8,* 723–735.

Kaplan, R. M., & Anderson, J. P. (1988). A general health policy model: Update and applications. *Health Services Research, 23,* 203–235.

Karweit, N., & Meyers, E. D., Jr. (1983). Computers in survey research. In P. H. Rossi, J. D. Wright, & A. B. Anderson (Eds.), *Handbook of survey research* (pp. 379–414). San Diego, CA: Academic Press.

Kasprzyk, D. (1988). Research issues in the Survey of Income and Program Participation. *Survey Methodology, 14,* 45–58.

Katz, S. (1987). The science of quality of life. *Journal of Chronic Diseases, 40,* 459–463.

Katz, S., Ford, A. B., Moskowitz, R. W., Jackson, B. A., & Jaffe, M. W. (1963). Studies of illness in the aged. The Index of ADL: A standardized measure of biological and psychosocial function. *Journal of the American Medical Association, 185,* 914–919.

Keeter, S. (1995). Estimating telephone noncoverage bias with a telephone survey. *Public Opinion Quarterly, 59,* 196–217.

Kehoe, R., Wu, S.-Y., Leske, M. C., & Chylack, L. T., Jr. (1994). Comparing self-reported and physician-reported medical history. *American Journal of Epidemiology, 139,* 813–818.

Keith, R. A. (1994). Functional status and health status. *Archives of Physical Medicine and Rehabilitation, 75,* 478–483.

Keller, D. M., Kovar, M. G., Jobe, J. B., & Branch, L. G. (1993). Problems eliciting elders' reports of functional status. *Journal of Aging and Health, 5,* 306–318

Kerwin, J. (1993a). *Questionnaire design research laboratory: Cognitive testing of the 1993 family resources supplement.* (Report No. 5, National Center for Health Statistics, Cognitive Methods Staff Working Paper Series). Hyattsville, MD: National Center for Health Statistics.

Kerwin, J. (1993b). *Questionnaire design research laboratory: Cognitive testing of the 1993 NHIS AIDS knowledge and attitudes supplement.* (Report No. 4, National Center for Health Statistics, Cognitive Methods Staff Working Paper Series). Hyattsville, MD: National Center for Health Statistics.

Khare, M., Little, R.J.A., Rubin, D. B., & Schafer, J. L. (1993). Multiple imputation of NHANES III. *Proceedings of the American Statistical Association, Section on Survey Research Methods, Vol. I,* 297–302.

Khurshid, A., & Sahai, H. (1993). Scales of measurements: An introduction and a selected bibliography. *Quality & Quantity, 27,* 303–324.

Kiecolt, K. J., & Nathan, L. E. (1985). *Secondary analysis of survey data.* Thousand Oaks, CA: Sage.

Kiesler, S., & Sproull, L. S. (1986). Response effects in the electronic survey. *Public Opinion Quarterly, 50,* 402–413.

Kim, J., & Mueller, C. W. (1978). *Introduction to factor analysis: What it is and how to do it.* Thousand Oaks, CA: Sage.

Kindel, K. K. (1991). Design and development of computer assisted survey information collection at the U.S. Census Bureau. *Proceedings of the American Statistical Association, Section on Social Statistics,* pp. 317–322.

Kirshner, B., & Guyatt, G. (1985). A methodological framework for assessing health indices. *Journal of Chronic Diseases, 38,* 27–36.

Kish, L. (1965). *Survey sampling.* New York: Wiley.

Kish, L. (1987). *Statistical design for research.* New York: Wiley.

Kish, L. (1990). Weighting: Why, when, and how? *Proceedings of the American Statistical Association, Section on Survey Research Methods,* pp. 121–130.

Kish, L. (1991). Taxonomy of elusive populations. *Journal of Official Statistics, 7,* 339–347.

Kitchens, L. J. (1987). *Exploring statistics: A modern introduction to data analysis and inference.* St. Paul, MN: West Publishing.

Klecka, W. R., & Tuchfarber, A. J. (1978). Random digit dialing: A comparison to personal surveys. *Public Opinion Quarterly, 42,* 105–114.

Kleinbaum, D. G., Kupper, L. L., & Morgenstern, H. (1982). *Epidemiologic research: Principles and quantitative methods.* Belmont, CA: Lifetime Learning.

Kohlmeier, L. (1994). Gaps in dietary assessment methodology: Meal- versus list-based methods. *American Journal of Clinical Nutrition, 59* (Suppl.), 175S–179S.

Kohn, R., & White, K. L. (Eds.). (1976). *Health care: An international study.* Oxford, England: Oxford University Press.

Korn, E. L., & Graubard, B. I. (1995). Analysis of large health surveys: Accounting for the sampling design. *Journal of the Royal Statistical Society, Series A—Statistics in Society, 158* (Part 2), 263–295.

Korn, E. L., & Graubard, B. I. (1991). Epidemiologic studies utilizing surveys: Accounting for the sampling design. *American Journal of Public Health, 81,* 1166–1173.

Kovar, M. G. (1990). Computer assisted personal interviewing: Lessons from experience. *Proceedings of the American Statistical Association, Section on Survey Research Methods,* pp. 378–381.

Kraemer, H. C., & Thiemann, S. (1987). *How many subjects? Statistical power analysis in research.* Thousand Oaks, CA: Sage.

Krause, N. M., & Jay, G. M. (1994). What do global self-rated health items measure? *Medical Care, 32,* 930–942.

Kreft, I.G.G. (Ed.). (1995). Hierarchical linear models: Problems and prospects. *Journal of Educational and Behavioral Statistics, 20* (2).

Kristal, A. R., White, E., Davis, J. R., Corycell, G., Raghunathan, T., Kinne, S., & Lin, T.-K. (1993). Effects of enhanced calling efforts on response rates, estimates of health behavior, and costs in a telephone health survey using random-digit dialing. *Public Health Reports, 108,* 372–379.

Kroeger, A. (1983). Health interview surveys in developing countries: A review of the methods and results. *International Journal of Epidemiology, 12,* 465–481.

Krosnick, J. A. (1991). Response strategies for coping with the cognitive demands of attitude measures in surveys. *Applied Cognitive Psychology, 5,* 213–236.

Krosnick, J. A., & Alwin, D. F. (1987). An evaluation of a cognitive theory of response-order effects in survey measurement. *Public Opinion Quarterly, 51,* 201–219.

Krueger, R. A. (1994). *Focus groups: A practical guide for applied research* (2nd ed.). Thousand Oaks, CA: Sage.

Krysan, M., Schuman, H., Scott, L. J., & Beatty, P. (1994). Response rates and response content in mail versus face-to-face surveys. *Public Opinion Quarterly, 58,* 381–399.

Kulka, R. A., Weeks, R. A., Lessler, J. T., & Whitmore, R. W. (1984). A comparison of the telephone and personal interview modes for conducting local household health surveys. In National Center for Health Services Research, *Health survey research methods: Proceedings of the fourth conference on health survey research methods.* (Report No. DHHS Publication No. [PHS] 84–3346, pp. 116–127). NCHSR Proceedings Series. Washington, DC: U.S. Government Printing Office.

Kviz, F. J. (1977). Toward a standard definition of response rate. *Public Opinion Quarterly, 41,* 265–267.

Lapham, R. J., & Westoff, C. F. (1986). Demographic and health surveys: Population and health information for the late 1980s. *Population Index, 52,* 28–34.

Larson, J. S. (1991). *The measurement of health: Concepts and indicators.* New York: Greenwood Press.

Last, J. M. (1988). *A dictionary of epidemiology* (2nd ed.). New York: Oxford University Press.

Laumann, E. O., Gagnon, J. H., Michael, R. T., & Michaels, S. (1994). *The social organization of sexuality: Sexual practices in the United States.* Chicago: University of Chicago Press.

Lavizzo-Mourey, R. J., Zinn, J., & Taylor, L. (1992). Ability of surrogates to represent satisfaction of nursing home residents with quality of care. *Journal of the American Geriatrics Society, 40,* 39–47.

Lavrakas, P. J. (1993). *Telephone survey methods: Sampling, selection, and supervision* (2nd ed.). Thousand Oaks, CA: Sage.

Lavrakas, P. J., Bauman, S. L., & Merkle, D. M. (1993). The last-birthday selection method & within-unit coverage problems. *Proceedings of the American Statistical Association, Section on Survey Research Methods, Vol. II,* 1107–1112.

Lazarsfeld, P., Pasanella, A., & Rosenberg, M. (Eds.). (1972). *Continuities in the language of social research.* New York: Free Press.

Lee, E. S., Forthofer, R. N., & Lorimor, R. J. (1986). Analysis of complex sample survey data: Problems and strategies. *Sociological Methods & Research, 15,* 69–100.

Lee, E. S., Forthofer, R. N., & Lorimor, R. J. (1989). *Analyzing complex survey data.* Thousand Oaks, CA: Sage.

Lee, R. M. (1993). *Doing research on sensitive topics.* Thousand Oaks: Sage.

Lee-Han, H., McGuire, V., & Boyd, N. F. (1989). A review of the methods used by studies of dietary measurement. *Journal of Clincial Epidemiology, 42,* 269–279.

Lemeshow, S., Hosmer, D. W., Jr., Klar, J., & Lwanga, S. K. (1990). *Adequacy of sample size in health studies.* New York: Wiley.

Lemeshow, S., & Robinson, D. (1985). Surveys to measure programme coverage and impact: A review of the methodology used by the Expanded Programme on Immunization. *World Health Statistics Quarterly, 38,* 65–75.

Lemeshow, S., & Stroh, G., Jr. (1989). Quality assurance sampling for evaluating health parameters in developing countries. *Survey Methodology, 15,* 71–81.

Lepkowski, J. M. (1988). Telephone sampling methods in the United States. In R. M. Groves, P. P. Biemer, L. E. Lyberg, J. T. Massey, W. L. Nicholls, II, & J. Waksberg (Eds.), *Telephone survey methodology* (pp. 73–98). New York: Wiley.

Lepkowski, J. M., Landis, J. R., & Stehouwer, S. A. (1987). Strategies for the analysis of imputed data from a sample survey. *Medical Care, 25,* 705–716.

Lessler, J. T. (1995). Choosing questions that people can understand and answer. *Medical Care, 33* (Suppl. 4), AS203–AS208.

Lessler, J. T., & Kalsbeek, W. D. (1992). *Nonsampling errors in surveys.* New York: Wiley.

Lessler, J. T., & Sirken, M. G. (1985). Laboratory-based research on the cognitive aspects of survey methodology: The goals and methods of the National Center for Health Statistics study. *Milbank Memorial Fund Quarterly: Health and Society, 63,* 565–581.

Letterie, G. S., Morgenstern, L. L., & Johnson, L. (1994). Graduate education: The role of an electronic mail system in the educational strategies of a residency in obstetrics and gynecology. *Obstetrics & Gynecology, 84,* 137–139.

Levy, P. S., & Lemeshow, S. (1980). *Sampling for health professionals.* Belmont, CA: Lifetime Learning.

Levy, P. S., & Lemeshow, S. (1991). *Sampling of populations: Methods and applications.* New York: Wiley.

Lewis, C. E., Freeman, H. E., & Corey, C. R. (1987). AIDS-related competence of California's primary care physicians. *American Journal of Public Health, 77,* 795–799.

Lewis, J. R. (1994). Patient views on quality care in general practice: Literature review. *Social Science and Medicine, 39,* 655–670.

Linder-Pelz, S. (1982). Toward a theory of patient satisfaction. *Social Science and Medicine, 16,* 577–582.

Lipkind, K. L. (1995). *National Hospital Ambulatory Medical Care Survey: 1993 outpatient department summary.* (Report No. DHHS Publication No. [PHS] 95–1250). Vital and Health Statistics Advance Data Series, No. 268. Washington, DC: U.S. Government Printing Office.

Lipsey, M. W. (1990). *Design sensitivity: Statistical power for experimental research.* Thousand Oaks, CA: Sage.

Little, R.J.A., & Rubin, D. B. (1989). The analysis of social science data with missing values. *Sociological Methods & Research, 18,* 292–326.

Locander, W. B., & Burton, J. P. (1976). The effect of question form on gathering income data by telephone. *Journal of Marketing Research, 13,* 189–192.

Loevy, S. S. (1984). Dual-frame sampling in the Community Hospital Program access evaluation. In National Center for Health Services Research, *Health survey research methods: Proceedings of the fourth conference on health survey research methods.* (Report No. DHHS Publication No. [PHS] 84–3346, pp. 264–271). NCHSR Proceedings Series. Washington, DC: U.S. Government Printing Office.

Loftus, E. F., Klinger, M. R., Smith, K. D., & Fiedler, J. (1990). A tale of two questions: Benefits of asking more than one question. *Public Opinion Quarterly, 54,* 330–345.

Lohr, K. N. (Ed.). (1989). Advances in health status assessment: Conference proceedings [Entire issue]. *Medical Care, 27* (Suppl. 3).

Lohr, K. N. (Ed.). (1992). Fostering the application of health status measures in clinical settings: Proceedings of a conference [Entire issue]. *Medical Care, 30* (Suppl. 5).

Lohr, K. N., & Ware, J. E., Jr. (Eds.). (1987). Proceedings of the advances in health assessment conference [Entire issue]. *Journal of Chronic Diseases, 40* (Suppl. 1).

Lwanga, S. K., & Lemeshow, S. (1991). *Sample size determination in health studies: A practical manual.* Geneva: World Health Organization.

MacKeigan, L. D., & Larson, L. N. (1989). Development and validation of an instrument to measure patient satisfaction with pharmacy services. *Medical Care, 27,* 522–536.

Madow, W. G., Nisselson, H., & Olkin, I. (Eds.) (1983). *Incomplete data in sample surveys.* San Diego, CA: Academic Press.

Madron, T. W., Tate, C. N., & Brookshire, R. G. (1985). *Using microcomputers in research.* Thousand Oaks, CA: Sage.

Magaziner, J., Simonsick, E. M., Kashner, T. M., & Hebel, J. R. (1988). Patient-proxy response comparability on measures of patient health and functional status. *Journal of Clinical Epidemiology, 41,* 1065–1074.

Maisel, R., & Persell, C. H. (1996). *How sampling works.* Thousand Oaks, CA: Pine Forge Press.

Makkai, T., & McAllister, I. (1992). Measuring social indicators in opinion surveys: A method to improve accuracy on sensitive questions. *Social Indicators Research, 27,* 169–186.

Makuc, D. M., & Feldman, J. J. (1993). Effect of recall period on measuring poverty and race differentials in physician utilization. *Proceedings of the American Statistical Association, Section on Social Statistics,* pp. 337–342.

Malec, D. (1995). Model-based state estimates from the National Health Interview Survey. In W. Schaible (Ed.), *Indirect estimators in U.S. federal programs* (pp. 145–167). New York: Springer.

Malec, D., & Sedransk, J. (1993). Bayesian predictive inference for units with small sample sizes: The case of binary random variables. *Medical Care, 31,* YS66–YS70.

Malec, D., Sedransk, J., & Tompkins, L. (1993). Bayesian predictive inference for small areas for binary variables in the National Health Interview Survey. In C. Gatsonis, J. S. Hodges, R. E. Kass, & N. D. Singpurwalla (Eds.), *Case studies in Bayesian statistics* (pp. 377–389). New York: Springer.

Mangione, T. W. (1995). *Mail surveys: Improving the quality.* Thousand Oaks, CA: Sage.

Mangione, T. W., Hingson, R., Barrett, J. (1982). Collecting sensitive data: A comparison of three survey strategies. *Sociological Methods & Research, 10,* 337–346.

Marcus, A. C., & Crane, L. A. (1986). Telephone surveys in public health research. *Medical Care, 24,* 97–112.

Marcus, A. C., & Telesky, C. W. (1984). Nonparticipation in telephone follow-up interviews. In National Center for Health Services Research, *Health survey research methods: Proceedings of the fourth conference on health survey methods.* (Report No. DHHS Publication No. [PHS] 84–3346, pp. 128–134). NCHSR Proceedings Series. Washington, DC: U.S. Government Printing Office.

Marin, G., & Marin, B. V. (1991). *Research with Hispanic populations.* Thousand Oaks, CA: Sage.

Marin, G., Vanoss, B., & Perez-Stable, E. J. (1990). Feasibility of a telephone survey to study a minority community: Hispanics in San Francisco. *American Journal of Public Health, 80,* 323–326.

Marker, D. A. (1993). Small area estimation for the U.S. National Health Interview Survey. *Proceedings of the American Statistical Association, Section on Survey Research Methods, Vol. I,* 11–20.

Marks, R. G. (1982). *Designing a research project: The basics of biomedical research methodology.* New York: Van Nostrand Reinhold.

Markus, H., & Zajonc, R. B. (1985). The cognitive perspective in social psychology. In G. Lindzey, & E. Aronson (Eds.) *The handbook of social psychology* (3rd ed., pp. 137–230). New York: Random House.

Marquis, K. H. (1978). *Record check validity of survey responses: A reassessment of bias in reports of hospitalizations.* Santa Monica, CA: RAND Corporation.

Marquis, K. H. (1984). Record checks for sample surveys. In T. B. Jabine, M. L. Straf, J. M. Tanur, & R. Tourangeau (Eds.), *Cognitive aspects of survey methodology: Building a bridge between disciplines* (pp. 130–147). Washington, DC: National Academy Press.

Marquis, K. H., Moore, J. C., & Bogen, K. (1993). Effects of a cognitive interviewing approach on response quality in a pretest for the SIPP. *Proceedings of the American Statistical Association, Section on Survey Research Methods, Vol. I,* 318–323.

Marquis, M. S., Davies, A. R., & Ware, J. E., Jr. (1983). Patient satisfaction and change in medical care provider: A longitudinal study. *Medical Care, 21,* 821–829.

Marshall, G. N., Hays, R. D., Sherbourne, C. D., & Wells, K. B. (1993). The structure of patient satisfaction with outpatient medical care. *Psychological Assessment, 5,* 477–483.

Martin, E., DeMaio, T. J., & Campanelli, P. C. (1990). Context effects for census measures of race and Hispanic origin. *Public Opinion Quarterly, 54,* 551–566.

Martin, J., Anderson, J., Romans, S., Mullen, P., & O'Shea, M. (1993). Asking about child sexual abuse: Methodological implications of a two-stage survey. *Child Abuse & Neglect, 17,* 383–392.

Martin, J., O'Muircheartaigh, C., & Curtice, J. (1993). The use of CAPI for attitude surveys: An experimental comparison with traditional methods. *Journal of Official Statistics, 9,* 641–661.

Mason, R., Carlson, J. E., & Tourangeau, R. (1994). Contrast effects and subtraction in part-whole questions. *Public Opinion Quarterly, 58,* 569–578.

Massey, M. M., Boyd, G., Mattson, M., & Feinleib, M. R. (1987). Inventory of surveys on smoking. *Public Health Reports, 102,* 430–438.

Mathiowetz, N. A. (1993). An assessment of alternative data replacement techniques. *Proceedings of the American Statistical Association, Section on Survey Research Methods, Vol. I,* 440–445.

Mathiowetz, N. A., & Groves, R. M. (1985). The effects of respondent rules on health survey reports. *American Journal of Public Health, 75,* 639–644.

Mays, V. M., & Jackson, J. S. (1991). AIDS survey methodology with black Americans. *Social Science and Medicine, 33,* 47–54.

McCall, L. A., & Rogers, P. L. (1992). Quality management approach to field procedures for the National Health Interview Survey. *Proceedings of the Annual Research Conference of the U.S. Bureau of the Census,* pp. 137–148.

McClendon, M. J. (1991). Acquiescence and recency response-order effects in interview surveys. *Sociological Methods & Research, 20,* 60–103.

McDaniel, C., & Nash, J. G. (1990). Compendium of instruments measuring patient satisfaction with nursing care. *Quality Review Bulletin, 60,* 182–188.

McDowell, I., & Newell, C. (1987). *Measuring health: A guide to rating scales and questionnaires.* New York: Oxford University Press.

McEwan, R. T., Harrington, B. E., Bhopal, R. S., Madhok, R., & McCallum, A. (1992). Social surveys in HIV/AIDS: Telling or writing? A comparison of interview and postal methods. *Health Education Research, 7,* 195–202.

McGraw, S. A., McKinlay, J. B., Crawford, S. A., Costa, L. A., & Cohen, D. L. (1992). Health survey methods with minority populations: Some lessons from recent experience. *Ethnicity & Disease, 2,* 273–287.

McHorney, C. A., Ware, J. E., Jr., Lu, J.F.R., & Sherbourne, C. D. (1994). The MOS 36-item short-form health survey (SF–36): III. Tests of data quality, scaling assumptions, and reliability across diverse patient groups. *Medical Care, 32,* 40–66.

McHorney, C. A., Ware, J. E., Jr., & Raczek, A. E. (1993). The MOS 36-item short-form health survey (SF–36): II. Psychometric and clinical tests of validity in measuring physical and mental health constructs. *Medical Care, 31,* 247–263.

McKillip, J. (1987). *Need analysis: Tools for the human services and education.* Thousand Oaks, CA: Sage.

Means, B., & Loftus, E. F. (1991). When personal history repeats itself: Decomposing memories for recurring events. *Applied Cognitive Psychology, 5,* 297–318.

Mechanic, D. (1989). Medical sociology: Some tensions among theory, method, and substance. *Journal of Health and Social Behavior, 30,* 147–160.

Medical Outcomes Trust, Scientific Advisory Committee. (1995). Instrument review criteria. *Medical Outcomes Trust Bulletin, 3* (4), I–IV.

Megivern, K., Halm, M. A., & Jones, G. (1992). Measuring patient satisfaction as an outcome of nursing care. *Journal of Nursing Care Quality, 6,* 9–24.

Menon, G., Bickart, B., Sudman, S., & Blair, J. (1995). How well do you know your partner? Strategies for formulating proxy-reports and their effects on convergence to self-reports. *Journal of Marketing Research, 32,* 75–84.

Merton, R. K., Fiske, M., & Kendall, P. L. (1990). *The focused interview: A manual of problems and procedures* (2nd ed.). New York: Free Press.

Meterko, M., Nelson, E. C., & Rubin, H. R. (Eds.). (1990). Patient judgments of hospital quality: Report of a pilot study. *Medical Care, 28* (Suppl.).

Milgrom, P., Fiset, L., Whitney, C., Conrad, D., Cullen, T., & O'Hara, D. (1994). Malpractice claims during 1988–1992: A national survey of dentists. *Journal of the American Dental Association, 125,* 462–469.

Milgrom, P., Whitney, C., Conrad, D., Fiset, L., & O'Hara, D. (1995). Tort reform and malpractice liability insurance. *Medical Care, 33,* 755–764.

Miller, D. C. (1991). *Handbook of research design and social measurement* (5th ed.). Thousand Oaks, CA: Sage.

Miller, P. V. (1984). A comparison of telephone and personal interviews in the Health Interview Survey. In National Center for Health Services Research, *Health survey research methods: Proceedings of the fourth conference on health survey research methods.* (Report No. DHHS Publication No. [PHS] 84–3346, pp. 135–145). NCHSR Proceedings Series. Washington, DC: U.S. Government Printing Office.

Mishler, E. G. (1986). *Research interviewing: Context and narrative.* Cambridge, MA: Harvard University Press.

Mishra, S. I., Dooley, D., Catalano, R., & Serxner, S. (1993). Telephone health surveys: Potential bias from noncompletion. *American Journal of Public Health, 83,* 94–99.

Mizes, J. S., Fleece, E. L., & Roos, C. (1984). Incentives for increasing return rates: Magnitude levels, response bias, and format. *Public Opinion Quarterly, 48,* 794–800.

Mohadjer, L. (1988). Stratification of prefix areas for sampling rare populations. In R. M. Groves, P. P. Biemer, L. E. Lyberg, J. T. Massey, W. L. Nicholls II, & J. Waksberg (Eds.), *Telephone survey methodology* (pp. 161–173). New York: Wiley.

Molenaar, N. J. (1991). Recent methodological studies on survey questioning. *Quality & Quantity, 25,* 167–187.

Mooney, L. A., & Gramling, R. (1991). Asking threatening questions and situational framing: The effects of decomposing survey items. *The Sociological Quarterly, 32,* 289–300.

Moore, J. C. (1988). Self/proxy response status and survey response quality: A review of the literature. *Journal of Official Statistics, 4,* 155–172.

Morgan, D. L. (Ed.). (1993). *Successful focus groups: Advancing the state of the art.* Thousand Oaks, CA: Sage.

Morrow, R. H., & Bryant, J. H. (1995). Health policy approaches to measuring and valuing human life: Conceptual and ethical issues. *American Journal of Public Health, 85,* 1356–1360.

Morton-Williams, J., & Sykes, W. (1984). The use of interaction coding and follow-up interviews to investigate comprehension of survey questions. *Journal of the Market Research Society, 26,* 109–127.

Mosely, R. R., II, & Wolinsky, F. D. (1986). The use of proxies in health surveys. *Medical Care, 24,* 496–510.

Moser, C. A., & Kalton, G. (1972). *Survey methods in social investigation* (2nd ed.) New York: Basic Books.

Mullen, P. D., Easling, I., Nixon, S. A., Koester, D. R., & Biddle, A. K. (1987). The cost-effectiveness of randomized incentive and follow-up contacts in a national mail survey of family physicians. *Evaluation & the Health Professions, 10,* 232–245.

Mulley, A. G., Jr. (1989). Assessing patients' utilities: Can the ends justify the means? *Medical Care, 27* (Suppl. 3), S269–S281.

Murray, D. M., McKinlay, S. M., Martin, D., Donner, A. P., Dwyer, J. H., Raudenbush, S. W., & Graubard, B. I. (1994). Design and analysis issues in community trials. *Evaluation Review, 18,* 493–514.

Myers, D. H., Leahy, A., Shoeb, H., & Ryder, J. (1990). The patients' view of life in a psychiatric hospital: A questionnaire study and associated methodological considerations. *British Journal of Psychiatry, 156,* 853–860.

Nachmias, C., & Nachmias, D. (1992). *Research methods in the social sciences* (4th ed.). New York: St. Martin's Press.

National Center for Health Services Research (1977a). *Advances in health survey methods: Proceedings of a national invitational conference.* (Report No. DHEW Publication no. [HRA] 77–3154). NCHSR Research Proceedings Series. Washington, DC: U.S. Government Printing Office.

National Center for Health Services Research. (1977b). Personal versus telephone interviews: The effects of telephone reinterviews on reporting of psychiatric symptomatology. In National Center for Health Services Research, *Experiments in interviewing techniques: Field experiments in health reporting.* (Report No. DHEW Publication No. [HRA] 78–3204). Washington, DC: U.S. Government Printing Office.

National Center for Health Services Research. (1978). *Experiments in interviewing techniques: Field experiments in health reporting 1971–1977.* (Report No. DHEW Publication No. [HRA] 78–3204). NCHSR Research Report Series. Washington, DC: U.S. Government Printing Office.

National Center for Health Services Research. (1979). *Health survey research methods: Second biennial conference.* (Report No. DHEW Publication No. [PHS] 79–3207). NCHSR Research Proceedings Series. Washington, DC: U.S. Government Printing Office.

National Center for Health Services Research (1981a). *Health survey research methods: Third biennial conference.* (Report No. DHHS Publication No. [PHS] 81–3268). NCHSR Research Proceedings Series. Washington, DC: U.S. Government Printing Office.

National Center for Health Services Research (1981b). *NMCES Household Interview Instruments: Instruments and Procedures 1.* Washington, DC: U.S. Government Printing Office.

National Center for Health Services Research. (1984). *Health survey research methods: Proceedings of the fourth conference on health survey research methods.* (Report No. DHHS Publication No. [PHS] 84–3346). NCHSR Research Proceedings Series. Washington, DC: U.S. Government Printing Office.

National Center for Health Services Research. (1987). *The 1987 National Medical Expenditure Survey: Its Design and Analytic Goals.* Rockville, MD: National Center for Health Services Research.

National Center for Health Statistics. (1977). *Synthetic estimation of state health characteristics based on the Health Interview Survey.* (Report No. DHEW Publication No. [PHS] 78–1349). Vital and Health Statistics Series 2, No. 75. Washington, DC: U.S. Government Printing Office.

National Center for Health Statistics. (1979). *Small area estimation: An empirical comparison of conventional and synthetic estimators for states.* (Report No. DHEW Publication No. [PHS] 80–1356). Vital and Health Statistics Series 2, No. 82. Washington DC: U.S. Government Printing Office.

National Center for Health Statistics. (1981a). *Basic data from wave I of the National Survey of Personal Health Practices and Consequences: United States, 1979.* (Report No. DHHS Publication No. [PHS] 81–1163). Vital and Health Statistics Series 5, No. 2. Washington, DC: U.S. Government Printing Office.

National Center for Health Statistics. (1981b). *Data systems of the National Center for Health Statistics.* (Report No. DHHS Publication No. [PHS] 82–1318). Vital and Health Statistics Series 1, No. 16. Washington, DC: U.S. Government Printing Office.

National Center for Health Statistics. (1981c). *Highlights from wave I of the National Survey of Personal Health Practices and Consequences: United States* (Report No. DHHS Publication No. [PHS] 81–1162). Vital and Health Statistics Series 5, No. 1. Washington, DC: U.S. Government Printing Office.

National Center for Health Statistics. (1983). *Procedures and questionnaires of the National Medical Care Utilization and Expenditure Survey.* Series A, Methodological Report No. 1. Washington, DC: U.S. Government Printing Office.

National Center for Health Statistics. (1984). *Health indicators for Hispanic, Black, and White Americans.* (Report No. DHHS Publication No. [PHS] 84–1576). Vital and Health Statistics Series 10, No. 148. Washington, DC: U.S. Government Printing Office.

National Center for Health Statistics. (1985a). *National Health Interview Survey 1985 Health Promotion and Disease Prevention Supplement: Sample Person Public Use File Codebook.* Hyattsville, MD: Author.

National Center for Health Statistics. (1985b). *Plan and operation of the Hispanic Health and Nutrition Examination Survey, 1982–84.* (Report No. DHHS Publication No. [PHS] 85–1321). Vital and Health Statistics Series 1, No. 19. Washington, DC: U.S. Government Printing Office.

National Center for Health Statistics. (1985c). *The National Health Interview Survey Design, 1973–84, and Procedures, 1975–83.* (Report No. DHHS Publication No. [PHS] 85–1320). Vital and Health Statistics Series 1, No. 18. Washington, DC: U.S. Government Printing Office.

National Center for Health Statistics. (1987a). *An experimental comparison of telephone and personal Health Interview Surveys.* (Report No. DHHS Publication No. [PHS] 87–1380). Vital and Health Statistics Series 2, No. 106. Washington, DC: U.S. Government Printing Office.

National Center for Health Statistics. (1987b). *The supplement on aging to the 1984 National Health Interview Survey.* (Report No. DHHS Publication No. [PHS] 87–1323). Vital and Health Statistics Series 1, No. 21. Washington, DC: U.S. Government Printing Office.

National Center for Health Statistics. (1987c). *Reporting chronic conditions in the National Health Interview Survey: A review of tendencies from evaluation studies and methodological test.* (Report No. DHHS Publication No. [PHS] 87–1379). Vital and Health Statistics Series 2, No. 105. Washington, DC: U.S. Government Printing Office.

National Center for Health Statistics. (1988a.). *Health promotion and disease prevention, United States, 1985.* (Report No. DHHS Publication No. [PHS] 88–1591). Vital and Health Statistics Series 10, No. 163. Washington, DC: U.S. Government Printing Office.

National Center for Health Statistics. (1988b). *Sample design, sampling variance, and estimation procedures for the National Ambulatory Medical Care Survey.* (Report No. DHHS Publication No. [PHS] 88–1382). Vital and Health Statistics Series 2, No. 108. Washington, DC: U.S. Government Printing Office.

National Center for Health Statistics. (1988c). *Use and interpretation of diagnostic statistics from selected data systems.* (Report No. DHHS Publication No. [PHS] 88–1381). Vital and Health Statistics Series 2, No. 107. Washington, DC: U.S. Government Printing Office.

National Center for Health Statistics. (1989a). *Autobiographical memory for health-related events.* (Report No. DHHS Publication No. [PHS] 89–1077). Vital and Health Statistics Series 6, No. 2. Washington, DC: U.S. Government Printing Office.

National Center for Health Statistics. (1989b). *Design and estimation for the National Health Interview Survey 1985–94.* (Report No. DHHS Publication No. [PHS] 89–1384). Vital and Health Statistics Series 2, No. 110. Washington, DC: U.S. Government Printing Office.

National Center for Health Statistics. (1989c). *Questionnaire design in the cognitive research laboratory.* (Report No. DHHS Publication No. [PHS] 89–1076). Vital and Health Statistics Series 6, No. 1. Washington, DC: U.S. Government Printing Office.

National Center For Health Statistics. (1989d). *Social cognition approach to reporting chronic conditions in health surveys.* (Report No. DHHS Publication No. [PHS] 89–1078). Vital and Health Statistics Series 6, No. 3. Washington, DC: U.S. Government Printing Office.

National Center for Health Statistics. (1990a). *Plan and operation of the NHANES I Epidemiologic Followup Study, 1986.* (Report No. DHHS Publication No. [PHS] 90–1307). Vital and Health Statistics Series 1, No. 25. Washington, DC: U.S. Government Printing Office.

National Center for Health Statistics. (1990b). *Questionnaires from the National Health Interview Survey, 1980–84.* (Report No. DHHS Publication No. [PHS] 90–1302). Vital and Health Statistics Series 1, No. 24. Washington DC: U.S. Government Printing Office.

National Center for Health Statistics. (1991a). *Cognitive processes in long-term dietary recall.* (Report No. DHHS Publication No. [PHS] 92–1079). Vital and Health Statistics Series 6, No. 4. Washington, DC: U.S. Government Printing Office.

National Center for Health Statistics. (1991b). *National Survey of Family Growth: Design, estimation, and inference.* (Report No. DHHS Publication No. [PHS] 91–1386). Vital and Health Statistics Series 2, No. 109. Washington, DC: U.S. Government Printing Office.

National Center for Health Statistics. (1992a). *Cognitive research on response error in survey questions on smoking.* (Report No. DHHS Publication No. [PHS] 92–1080). Vital and Health Statistics Series 6, No. 5. Washington, DC: U.S. Government Printing Office.

National Center for Health Statistics. (1992b). *Inventory of pain data from the National Center for Health Statistics.* (Report No. DHHS Publication No. [PHS] 92–1308). Vital and Health Statistics Series 1, No. 26. Washington, DC: U.S. Government Printing Office.

National Center for Health Statistics. (1992c). *Plan and operation of the NHANES I Epidemiologic Follow-Up Study, 1987.* (Report No. DHHS Publication No. [PHS] 92–1303). Vital and Health Statistics Series 1, No. 27. Washington, DC: U.S. Government Printing Office.

National Center for Health Statistics. (1992d). *Reporting chronic pain episodes on health surveys.* (Report No. DHHS Publication No. [PHS] 92–1081). Vital and Health Statistics Series 6, No. 6. Washington, DC: U.S. Government Printing Office.

National Center for Health Statistics. (1992e). *Sample design: Third National Health and Nutrition Examination Survey.* (Report No. DHHS Publication No. [PHS] 92–1387). Vital and Health Statistics Series 2, No. 113. Washington, DC: U.S. Government Printing Office.

National Center for Health Statistics. (1992f). *The longitudinal study of aging: 1984–90.* (Report No. DHHS Publication No. [PHS] 92–1304). Vital and Health Statistics Series 1, No. 28. Washington, DC: U.S. Government Printing Office.

National Center for Health Statistics. (1993a). *Development, methods, and response characteristics of the 1986 National Mortality Follow-Back Survey.* (Report No. DHHS Publication No. [PHS] 93–1305). Vital and Health Statistics Series 1, No. 29. Washington, DC: U.S. Government Printing Office.

National Center for Health Statistics. (1993b). *National Hospital Discharge Survey: Annual summary, 1991.* (Report No. DHHS Publication No. [PHS] 93–1775). Vital and Health Statistics Series 13, No. 114. Washington, DC: U.S. Government Printing Office.

National Center for Health Statistics. (1993c). *National Survey of Family Growth, cycle IV, evaluation of linked design.* (Report No. DHHS Publication No. [PHS] 93–1391). Vital and Health Statistics Series 2, No. 117. Washington, DC: U.S. Government Printing Office.

National Center for Health Statistics. (1993d). *Plan and operation: National Nursing Home Survey Follow-Up, 1987, 1988, 1990.* (Report No. DHHS Publication No. [PHS] 93–1306). Vital and Health Statistics Series 1, No. 30. Washington, DC: U.S. Government Printing Office.

National Center for Health Statistics. (1993c). *Questionnaires from the National Health Interview Survey, 1985–89.* (Report No. DHHS Publication No. [PHS] 93–1307). Vital and Health Statistics Series 1, No. 31. Washington, DC: U.S. Government Printing Office.

National Center for Health Statistics. (1994a). *Cognitive aspects of reporting cancer prevention examinations and tests.* (Report No. DHHS Publication No. [PHS] 94–1082). Vital and Health Statistics Series 6, No. 7. Washington, DC: U.S. Government Printing Office.

National Center for Health Statistics. (1994b). *Development of the National Home and Hospice Care Survey.* (Report No. DHHS Publication No. [PHS] 94–1309). Vital and Health Statistics Series 1, No. 33. Washington, DC: U.S. Government Printing Office.

National Center for Health Statistics. (1994c). *Evaluation of National Health Interview Survey diagnostic reporting.* (Report No. DHHS Publication No. [PHS] 94–1394). Vital and Health Statistics Series 2, No. 120. Washington DC: U.S. Government Printing Office.

National Center for Health Statistics. (1994d). *Fact sheet: SLICHS—State and Local Area Immunization Coverage and Health Survey.* Hyattsville, MD: Author.

National Center for Health Statistics. (1994e). *Plan and operation of the Third National Health and Nutrition Examination Survey, 1988–94.* (Report No. DHHS Publication No. [PHS] 94–1308). Vital and Health Statistics Series 1, No. 32. Washington, DC: U.S. Government Printing Office.

National Center for Health Statistics. (1995). *Health, United States, 1994.* (Report No. DHHS Publication No. [PHS] 95–1232). Washington, DC: U.S. Government Printing Office.

National Center for Health Statistics and U.S. Bureau of the Census. (1988). *Report of the 1987 automated National Health Interview Survey feasibility study: An investigation of computer-assisted personal interviews.* Hyattsville, MD: National Center for Health Statistics.

National Committee for Quality Assurance. (1993). *Healthplan employer data and information set and user's manual, version 2.0.* Washington, DC: Author.

National Committee for Quality Assurance. (1995a). *Annual Member Health Care Survey* (Version 1.0). Washington, DC: Author.

National Committee for Quality Assurance. (1995b). *Executive summary for report card pilot project.* Washington, DC: Author.

National Institute on Drug Abuse. (1991). *Drug abuse and drug abuse research: Third triennial report to Congress from the Secretary, Department of Health and Human Services.* (Report No. DHHS Publication No. ADM 91–1704). Washington, DC: U.S. Government Printing Office.

National Library of Medicine. (1992). *Health services: Sources of information for research.* (Report No. NLM PSD 92 01). Bethesda, MD: Author.

Nederhof, A. J. (1983). The effects of material incentives in mail surveys: Two studies. *Public Opinion Quarterly, 47,* 103–111.

Nelson, E. C., Hays, R. D., Larson, C., & Batalden, P. B. (1989). The patient judgment system: Reliability and validity. *Quality Review Bulletin, 15,* 185–191.

Nelson, E. C., & Larson, C. (1993). Patients' good and bad surprises: How do they relate to overall patient satisfaction? *Quality Review Bulletin, 19,* 89–94.

Nelson, E. C., Larson, C. O., Davies, A. R., Gustafson, D., Ferreira, P. L., & Ware, J. E., Jr. (1991). The patient comment card: A system to gather customer feedback. *Quality Review Bulletin, 17,* 278–286.

Nelson, E., Wasson, J., Kirk, J., Keller, A., Clark, D., Dietrich, A., Stewart, A., & Zubkoff, M. (1987). Assessment of function in routine clinical practice: Description of the COOP chart method and preliminary findings. *Journal of Chronic Diseases, 20* (Suppl. 1), 55S–63S.

Neter, J., Wasserman, W., & Kutner, M. H. (1990). *Applied linear statistical models: Regression, analysis of variance, and experimental designs* (3rd ed.). Homewood, IL: Irwin.

Nicholls, W. L., II. (1983). CATI research and development at the Census Bureau. *Sociological Methods & Research, 12,* 191–197.

Nicholls, W. L., II, & Groves, R. M. (1986). The status of computer-assisted telephone interviewing: Part I—Introduction and impact on cost and timeliness of survey data. *Journal of Official Statistics, 2,* 93–115.

Nicholls, W. L., II, & Kindel, K. K. (1993). Case management and communications for computer assisted personal interviewing. *Journal of Official Statistics, 9,* 623–639.

Norusis, M. J. (1990). *SPSS base system user's guide.* Chicago: SPSS [Statistical Package for the Social Sciences].

Norusis, M. J. (1992). *SPSS/PC+ base system user's guide, version 5.0.* Chicago: SPSS [Statistical Package for the Social Sciences].

Nunnally, J. C., & Bernstein, I. H. (1994). *Psychometric theory* (3rd ed.). New York: McGraw-Hill.

O'Brien, K. (1993). Using focus groups to develop health surveys: An example from research on social relationships and AIDS-preventive behavior. *Health Education Quarterly, 20,* 361–372.

O'Muircheartaigh, C. A., Gaskell, G. D., & Wright, D. B. (1993a). Evaluating numeric and verbal labels for response scales. *Proceedings of the American Statistical Association, Section on Survey Research Methods, Vol. II,* 1178–1182.

O'Muircheartaigh, C. A., Gaskell, G. D., & Wright, D. B. (1993b). Intensifiers in behavioral frequency questions. *Public Opinion Quarterly, 57,* 552–565.

O'Reilly, J. M., Hubbard, M. L., Lessler, J. T., Biemer, P. P., & Turner, C. F. (1994). Audio and video computer assisted self-interviewing: Preliminary tests of new technologies for data collection. *Journal of Official Statistics, 10,* 197–214.

O'Rourke, D., & Blair, J. (1983). Improving random respondent selection in telephone surveys. *Journal of Marketing Research, 20,* 428–432.

O'Rourke, D., & Lakner, E. (1989). Gender bias: Analysis of factors causing male underrepresentation in surveys. *International Journal of Public Opinion Research, 1,* 164–176.

Office of Management and Budget. (1994). *Standards for classification of Federal data on race and ethnicity.* (Report No. 59. Federal Register, 29831). Washington, DC: U.S. Government Printing Office.

Oksenberg, L., Cannell, C., & Kalton, G. (1991). New strategies for pretesting survey questions. *Journal of Official Statistics, 7,* 349–365.

Oksenberg, L., Coleman, L., & Cannell, C. (1986). Interviewers' voices and refusal rates in telephone surveys. *Public Opinion Quarterly, 50,* 97–111.

Oldendick, R. W. (1993). The effect of answering machines on the representativeness of samples in telephone surveys. *Journal of Official Statistics, 9,* 663–672.

Oldendick, R. W., & Link, M. W. (1994). The answering machine generation: Who are they and what problem do they pose for survey research? *Public Opinion Quarterly, 58,* 264–273.

Oppenheim, A. N. (1992). *Questionnaire design, interviewing and attitude measurement.* London: Pinter Publishers.

Orth-Gomer, K., & Unden, A. (1987). The measurement of social support in population surveys. *Social Science and Medicine, 24,* 83–94.

Orwin, R. G., & Boruch, R. F. (1982) RTT meets RDD: Statistical strategies for assuring response privacy in telephone surveys. *Public Opinion Quarterly, 46,* 560–571.

Palit, C., & Sharp, H. (1983). Microcomputer-assisted telephone interviewing. *Sociological Methods & Research, 12,* 169–189.

Parkerson, G. R., Jr., Broadhead, W. E., & Tse, C.-K. J. (1990). The Duke Health Profile: A 17-item measure of health and dysfunction. *Medical Care, 28,* 1056–1072.

Parkerson, G. R., Jr., Gehlbach, S. H., Wagner, E. H., James, S. A., Clapp, N. E., & Muhlbaier, L. H. (1981). The Duke-UNC Health Profile: An adult health status instrument for primary care. *Medical Care, 19,* 806–823.

Parsons, J. A., Johnson, T. P., Warnecke, R. B., & Kaluzny, A. (1993). The effect of interviewer characteristics on gatekeeper resistance in surveys of elite populations. *Evaluation Review, 17,* 131–143.

Parsons, J. A., Warnecke, R. B., Czaja, R. F., Barnsley, J., & Kaluzny, A. (1994). Factors associated with response rates in a national survey of primary care physicians. *Evaluation Review, 18,* 756–766.

Pascoe, G. C. (1983). Patient satisfaction in primary health care: A literature review and analysis. *Evaluation and Program Planning, 6,* 185–210.

Pascoe, G. C., Atkinson, C. C., & Roberts, R. E. (1983). Comparison of indirect and direct approaches to measuring patient satisfaction. *Evaluation and Program Planning, 6,* 359–371.

Passel, J. S., & Word, D. L. (1980, April). *Constructing the list of Spanish surnames for the 1980 Census: An application of Bayes' Theorem.* Paper presented at the annual meeting of the Population Association of America, Denver, CO.

Patrick, D. L., & Bergner, M. (1990). Measurement of health status in the 1990s. *Annual Review of Public Health, 11,* 165–183.

Patrick, D. L., Bush, J. W., & Chen, M. M. (1973). Toward an operational definition of health. *Journal of Health & Social Behavior, 14,* 6–23.

Patrick, D. L., & Deyo, R. A. (1989). Generic and disease-specific measures in assessing health status and quality of life. *Medical Care, 27* (Suppl. 3), S217–S232.

Patrick, D. L., & Erickson, P. (1993). *Health status and health policy: Quality of life in health care evaluation and resource allocation.* New York: Oxford University Press.

Paxson, M. C., Dillman, D. A., & Tarnai, J. (1995). Improving response to business mail surveys. In B. G. Cox, D. A. Binder, B. N. Chinnappa, A. Christianson, M. J. Colledge, & P. S. Kott (Eds.), *Business Survey Methods* (pp. 303–316). New York: Wiley.

Payne, S. L. (1951). *The art of asking questions.* Princeton, NJ: Princeton University Press.

Peck, J. K., & Dresch, S. P. (1981). Financial incentives, survey response, and sample representativeness: Does money matter? *Review of Public Data Use, 9,* 245–266.

Perkins, R. C. (1993). Evaluating the Passel-Word Spanish surname list. *Proceedings of the American Statistical Association, Section on Social Statistics,* pp. 65–70.

Perneger, T. V., Etter, J.-F., & Rougemont, A. (1993). Randomized trial of use of a monetary incentive and a reminder card to increase the response rate to a mailed health survey. *American Journal of Epidemiology, 138,* 714–722.

Perron, S., Berthelot, J.-M., & Blakeney, R. D. (1991). New technologies in data collection for business surveys. *Proceedings of the American Statistical Association, Section on Survey Research Methods,* pp. 707–712.

Peterson, R. A. (1984). Asking the age question: A research note. *Public Opinion Quarterly, 48,* 379–383.

Phipps, P. A., Robertson, K. W., & Keel, K. G. (1991). Does questionnaire color affect survey response rates? *Proceedings of the American Statistical Association, Section on Survey Research Methods,* pp. 484–489.

Phipps, P. A., & Tupek, A. R. (1991). Assessing measurement errors in a touchtone recognition survey. *Survey Methodology, 17,* 15–26.

Piazza, T. (1993). Meeting the challenge of answering machines. *Public Opinion Quarterly, 57,* 219–231.

Pierzchala, M. (1990). A review of the state of the art in automated data editing and imputation. *Journal of Official Statistics, 6,* 355–377.

Pierzchala, M. (1991). One agency's experience with the Blaise integrated survey processing system. *Proceedings of the American Statistical Association, Section on Survey Research Methods,* pp. 767–772.

Polissar, L., & Diehr, P. (1982). Regression analysis in health services research: The use of dummy variables. *Medical Care, 20,* 959–966.

Pope, G. C. (1988). Medical conditions, health status, and health services utilization. *Health Services Research, 22,* 857–877.

Potthoff, R. F. (1987). Some generalizations of the Mitofsky-Waksberg technique for random digit dialing. *Journal of the American Statistical Association, 82,* 409–418.

Presser, S., & Blair, J. (1994). Survey pretesting: Do different methods produce different results? *Sociological Methodology, 24,* 73–104.

Presser, S., & Schuman, H. (1980). The measurement of a middle position in attitude surveys. *Public Opinion Quarterly, 44,* 70–85.

Prohaska, T. R., Albrecht, G., Levy, J. A., Sugrue, N., & Kim, J. H. (1990). Determinants of self-perceived risk for AIDS. *Journal of Health and Social Behavior, 31,* 384–394.

Puska, P., Nissinen, A., Tuomilehto, J., Salonen, J. T., Koskela, K., McAlister, A., Kottke, T. E., Maccoby, N., & Farquhar, J. W. (1985). The community-based strategy to prevent coronary heart disease: Conclusions from the ten years of the North Karelia Project. *Annual Review of Public Health, 6,* 147–193.

Rabkin, J. G. (1986). Mental health needs assessment: A review of methods. *Medical Care, 24,* 1093–1109.

Rao, J.N.K., & Bellhouse, D. R. (1990). History and development of the theoretical foundations of survey based estimation and analysis. *Survey Methodology, 16,* 3–29.

Rasinski, K. A., Mingay, D., & Bradburn, N. M. (1994). Do respondents really "mark all that apply" on self-administered questionnaires? *Public Opinion Quarterly, 58,* 400–408.

Reese, S. D., Danielson, W. A., Shoemaker, P. J., Chang, T-K., & Hsu, H-L. (1986). Ethnicity-of-interviewer effects among Mexican-Americans and Anglos. *Public Opinion Quarterly, 50,* 563–572.

Regier, D. A., Myers, J. K., Kramer, M., Robins, L. N., Blazer, D. G., Hough, R. L., Eaton, W. W., & Locke, B. Z. (1984). The NIMH Epidemiologic Catchment Area Program. *Archives of General Psychiatry, 41,* 934–941.

Remington, P. L., Smith, M. Y., Williamson, D. F., Anda, R. F., Gentry, E. M., & Hogelin, G. C. (1988). Design, characteristics, and usefulness of state-based Behavioral Risk Factor Surveillance: 1981–87. *Public Health Reports, 103,* 366–375.

Revicki, D. A. (1992). Relationship between health utility and psychometric health status measures. *Medical Care, 30* (Suppl. 5), MS274–MS282.

Rhoads, M., Smith, J., Sperry, S., Shepherd, J., Dulaney, R., Hill, D., & Pennington, J. (1994, March). *CASIC Technologies Interchange: Demonstration of selected features from various Westat CAPI applications using Cheshire software.* Exhibit at the annual research conference of the U.S. Bureau of the Census, Arlington, VA.

Rhodes, P. J. (1994). Race-of-interviewer effects: A brief comment. *Sociology, 28,* 547–558.

Richardson, J. L., Lochner, T., McGuigan, K., & Levine, A. M. (1987). Physician attitudes and experience regarding the care of patients with Acquired Immunodeficiency Syndrome (AIDS) and Related Disorders (ARC). *Medical Care, 25,* 675–685.

Ricketts, T. (1992). Consumer satisfaction surveys in mental health. *British Journal of Nursing, 1,* 523–527.

Rizek, R. L., & Pao, E. M. (1990). Dietary intake methodology I. USDA surveys and supporting research. *Journal of Nutrition, 120* (Suppl. 11), 1525–1529.

Roberts, J. G., & Tugwell, P. (1987). Comparison of questionnaires determining patient satisfaction with medical care. *Health Services Research, 22,* 637–654.

Robert Wood Johnson Foundation. (1987). *Access to health care in the United States: Results of a 1986 survey.* Special Report. Princeton, NJ: Author.

Robine, J.-M., Mathers, C. D., & Bucquet, D. (1993). Distinguishing health expectancies and health-adjusted life expectancies from quality-adjusted life years. *American Journal of Public Health, 83,* 797–798.

Robins, L. N., & Regier, D. A. (Eds.). (1991). *Psychiatric disorders in America: The epidemiologic catchment area study.* New York: Free Press.

Rogers, T. F. (1976). Interviews by telephone and in person: Quality of responses and field performance. *Public Opinion Quarterly, 40,* 51–65.

Rosen, R. J., & Clayton, R. L. (1992). An operational test of fax for data collection. *Proceedings of the American Statistical Association, Section on Survey Research Methods,* pp. 602–607.

Rosen, R. J., Clayton, R. L., & Wolf, L. L. (1993). Long-term retention of sample members under automated self-response data collection. *Proceedings of the American Statistical Association, Section on Survey Research Methods, Vol. II,* 748–752.

Rosenberg, M. (1968). *The logic of survey analysis.* New York: Basic Books.

Rosner, B. (1994). *Fundamentals of biostatistics* (4th ed.). Belmont, CA: Wadsworth.

Ross, C. K., Steward, C. A., & Sinacore, J. M. (1995). A comparative study of seven measures of patient satisfaction. *Medical Care, 33,* 392–406.

Ross, D. A., & Vaughan, J. P. (1986). Health interview surveys in developing countries: A methodological review. *Studies in Family Planning, 17,* 78–94.

Rossi, P. H., & Freeman, H. E. (1993). *Evaluation: A systematic approach* (5th ed.). Thousand Oaks, CA: Sage.

Rowe, E. G., & Appel, M. V. (1993). Paperless fax image reporting system (PFIRS). *Proceedings of the American Statistical Association, Section on Survey Research Methods, Vol. I,* 168–172.

Rubin, D. B. (1987). *Multiple imputation for nonresponse in surveys.* New York: Wiley.

Rubin, H. J., & Rubin, I. S. (1995). *Qualitative interviewing: The art of hearing data.* Thousand Oaks, CA: Sage.

Rubin, H. R. (1990). Can patients evaluate the quality of hospital care? *Medical Care Review, 47,* 267–326.

Rubin, H. R., Gandek, B., Rogers, W. H., Kosinski, M., McHorney, C. A., & Ware, J. E., Jr. (1993). Patients' ratings of outpatient visits in different practice settings: Results from the medical outcomes study. *Journal of the American Medical Association, 270,* 835–840.

Rutten-van Mölken, M.P.M.H., Bakker, C. H., van Doorslaer, E.K.A., & van der Linden, S. (1995). Methodological issues of patient utility measurement: Experience from two clinical trials. *Medical Care, 33,* 922–937.

Saalfeld, A. (1993). Geographic information systems research at the Bureau of the Census. *Proceedings of the Annual Research Conference of the U.S. Bureau of the Census,* pp. 393–404.

Safran, D. G., Tarlov, A. R., & Rogers, W. H. (1994). Primary care performance in fee-for-service and prepaid health care systems: Results from the medical outcomes study. *Journal of the American Medical Association, 271,* 1579–1586.

Salant, P., & Dillman, D. A. (1994). *How to conduct your own survey.* New York: Wiley.

Salmon, C. T., & Nichols, J. S. (1983). The next-birthday method of respondent selection. *Public Opinion Quarterly, 47,* 270–276.

Salovey, P., Smith, A. F., Turk, D. C., Jobe, J. B., & Willis, G. B. (1993). The accuracy of memory for pain. *American Pain Society Journal, 2,* 184–191.

Saltzman, A. (1992). Improving response rates in disk-by-mail surveys. *Proceedings of the Sawtooth Software Conference* (pp. 27–38). Ketchum, ID.

Sanderson, M., Placek, P. J., & Keppel, K. G. (1991). The 1988 national maternal and infant health survey: Design, content, and data availability. *Birth, 18,* 26–32.

Saris, W. E. (1989). A technological revolution in data collection. *Quality & Quantity, 23,* 333–349.

Saris, W. E. (1991). *Computer-assisted interviewing.* Thousand Oaks, CA: Sage.

Sasao, T. (1994). Using surname-based telephone survey methodology in Asian-American communities: Practical issues and caveats. *Journal of Community Psychology, 22,* 283–295.

Scardina, S. A. (1994). SERVQUAL: A tool for evaluating patient satisfaction with nursing care. *Journal of Nursing Care Quality, 8,* 38–46.

Schaeffer, N. C. (1980). Evaluating race-of-interviewer effects in a national survey. *Sociological Methods & Research, 8,* 400–419.

Schaeffer, N. C. (1991). Hardly ever or constantly: Group comparisons using vague quantifiers. *Public Opinion Quarterly, 55,* 395–423.

Schafer, J. L., Khare, M., & Ezzati-Rice, T. M. (1993). Multiple imputation of missing data in NHANES III. *Proceedings of the Annual Research Conference of the U.S. Bureau of the Census,* pp. 459–480.

Scheaffer, R. L., Mendenhall, W., & Ott, L. (1990). *Elementary survey sampling* (4th ed.). Boston: PWS-KENT.

Schechter, S. (1993). *Investigations into the cognitive processes of answering self-assessed health status questions.* (Report No. 2, National Center for Health Statistics, Cognitive Methods Staff Working Papers Series). Hyattsville, MD: National Center for Health Statistics.

Schechter, S. (1994). *Proceedings of the 1993 NCHS Conference on the cognitive aspects of self-reported health status.* (Report No. 10, National Center for Health Statistics, Cognitive Methods Staff Working Paper Series). Hyattsville, MD: National Center for Health Statistics.

Schechter, S., & Beatty, P. (1994). *Conducting cognitive laboratory tests by telephone.* (Report No. 8, National Center for Health Statistics, Cognitive Methods Staff Working Paper Series). Hyattsville, MD: National Center for Health Statistics.

Schechter, S., Trunzo, D., & Parsons, P. E. (1993). Utilizing focus groups in the final stages of questionnaire design. *Proceedings of the American Statistical Association, Section on Survey Research Methods, Vol. II,* 1148–1153.

Schrodt, P. A. (1987). *Microcomputer methods for social scientists* (2nd ed.). Thousand Oaks, CA: Sage.

Schuman, H., & Kalton, G. (1985). Survey methods. In G. Lindzey & E. Aronson (Eds.), *The handbook of social psychology* (3rd ed.) (pp. 635–697). Reading, MA: Addison-Wesley.

Schuman, H., & Presser, S. (1981). *Questions and answers in attitude surveys: Experiments on question form, wording, and context.* San Diego, CA: Academic Press.

Schur, C. L., Bernstein, A. B., & Berk, M. L. (1987). The importance of distinguishing Hispanic subpopulations in the use of medical care. *Medical Care, 25,* 627–641.

Schwarz, N. (1990). What respondents learn from scales: The informative functions of response alternatives. *International Journal of Public Opinion Research, 2,* 274–285.

Schwarz, N., & Bienias, J. (1990). What mediates the impact of response alternatives on frequency reports of mundane behaviors? *Applied Cognitive Psychology, 4,* 61–72.

Schwarz, N., & Bless, H. (1992). Assimilation and contrast effects in attitude measurement: An inclusion/exclusion model. *Advances in Consumer Research, 19,* 72–77.

Schwarz, N., & Hippler, H.-J. (1991). The numeric values of rating scales: A comparison of their impact in mail surveys and telephone interviews. *International Journal of Public Opinion Research, 7,* 72–74.

Schwarz, N., & Hippler, H.-J. (1995). Subsequent questions may influence answers to preceding questions in mail surveys. *Public Opinion Quarterly, 59,* 93–97.

Schwarz, N., Knäuper, B., Hippler, H.-J., Noelle-Neumann, E., & Clark, L. (1991). Rating scales: Numeric values may change the meaning of scale labels. *Public Opinion Quarterly, 55,* 570–582.

Schwarz, N., Strack, F., Hippler, H.-J., & Bishop, G. (1991). The impact of administration mode on response effects in survey measurement. *Applied Cognitive Psychology, 5,* 193–212.

Schwarz, N., Strack, F., & Mai, H.-P. (1991). Assimilation and contrast effects in part-whole question sequences: A conversational logic analysis. *Public Opinion Quarterly, 55,* 3–23.

Schwarz, N., Strack, F., Müller, G., & Chassein, B. (1988). The range of response alternatives may determine the meaning of the question: Further evidence on informative functions of response alternatives. *Social Cognition, 6,* 107–117.

Schwarz, N., & Sudman, S. (Eds.). (1992). *Context effects in social and psychological research.* New York: Springer.

Schwarz, N., & Sudman, S. (Eds.). (1994). *Autobiographical memory and the validity of retrospective reports.* New York: Springer.

Schwarz, N., & Sudman, S. (Eds.). (1995). *Answering questions: Methodology for determining cognitive and communicative processes in survey research.* San Francisco: Jossey-Bass.

Shanks, J. M. (1983). The current status of computer-assisted telephone interviewing: Recent progress and future prospects. *Sociological Methods & Research, 12,* 119–142.

Sheatsley, P. B. (1983). Questionnaire construction and item writing. In P. Rossi, J. D. Wright, & A. B. Anderson (Eds.), *Handbook of survey research* (pp. 195–230). San Diego, CA: Academic Press.

Sheatsley, P. B., & Loft, J. D. (1981). On monetary incentives to respondents. *Public Opinion Quarterly, 45,* 571–572.

Sheps, C. G., Wagner, E. H., Schonfeld, W. H., DeFriese, G. H., Bachar, M., Brooks, E. F., Gillings, D. B., Guild, P. A., Konrad, T. R., McLaughlin, C. P., Ricketts, T. C., Seipp, C., & Stein, J. (1983). An evaluation of subsidized rural primary care programs: I. A typology of practice organizations. *American Journal of Public Health, 73,* 38–49.

Sherbourne, C. D., Hays, R. D., & Burton, T. (1995). Population-based surveys of access and consumer satisfaction with health care. In Agency for Health Care Policy and Research, *Consumer survey information in a reforming health care system* (Report No. AHCPR Publication No. 95–0083, pp. 37–56). Rockville, MD: Agency for Health Care Policy and Research.

Shiloh, S., Avdor, O., & Goodman, R. M. (1990). Satisfaction with genetic counseling: Dimensions and measurement. *American Journal of Medical Genetics, 37,* 522–529.

Shortell, S. M., & Richardson, W. C. (1978). *Health program evaluation.* St. Louis, MO: Mosby.

Shortell, S. M., Wickizer, T. M., & Wheeler, J. R. (1984). *Hospital-physician joint ventures.* Ann Arbor, MI: Health Administration Press.

Siemiatycki, J. (1979). A comparison of mail, telephone, and home interview strategies for household health surveys. *American Journal of Public Health, 69,* 238–245.

Simpson, G. (1993). Determining childhood disability and special needs children in the 1994–95 NHIS survey on disability. *Proceedings of the American Statistical Association, Section on Social Statistics,* pp. 396–400.

Simpson, G., Keer, D., & Cynamon, M. (1993). Plans for the 1993–94 National Health Interview Survey on Disability. *Disability Studies Quarterly,* 13, 21–24.

Singer, E. (1981). Telephone interviewing as a black box—Discussion: Response styles in telephone and household interviewing. In National Center for Health Services Research, *Health survey research methods: Third biennial conference.* (Report No. DHHS Publication No. [PHS] 81–3268, pp. 124–127). NCHSR Research Proceedings Series. Washington, D.C.: U.S. Government Printing Office.

Singer, E., Rogers, T. F., & Corcoran, M. (1987). The polls—A report: AIDS. *Public Opinion Quarterly, 51,* 580–595.

Smead, R. J., & Wilcox, J. (1980). Ring policy in telephone surveys. *Public Opinion Quarterly, 44,* 115–116.

Smith, A. F., Jobe, J. B., & Mingay, D. J. (1991a). Question-induced cognitive biases in reports of dietary intake by college men and women. *Health Psychology, 10,* 244–251.

Smith, A. F., Jobe, J. B., & Mingay, D. J. (1991b). Retrieval from memory of dietary information. *Applied Cognitive Psychology, 5,* 269–296.

Smith, G. S., & Olson, J. G. (1987). Rapid epidemiologic assessment: Evaluation of health problems and programs. *BOSTID Developments, 7,* 16–19.

Smith, J. E., & Vincent, C. (1990). Survey data quality improvement: Experience with computer-assisted methods in national surveys. *Proceedings of the Annual Research Conference of the U.S. Bureau of the Census,* pp. 703–712.

Smith, S. S. (1995). NCHS under full sail on the information highway. *Public Health Reports, 110,* 500–503.

Smith, S. S., & Lancashire, J. (1995). NCHS redesigns National Health Interview Survey. *Public Health Reports, 110,* 506–507.

Smith, T. W. (1987). The art of asking questions, 1938–1985. *Public Opinion Quarterly, 51,* S95–S108.

Smith, T. W. (1990). Phone home? An analysis of household telephone ownership. *International Journal of Public Opinion Research, 2,* 369–390.

Smith, T. W. (1992). Changing racial labels: From "colored" to "negro" to "black" to "African American." *Public Opinion Quarterly, 56,* 496–514.

Smith, T. W. (1993). An analysis of response patterns to the ten-point scalometer. *Proceedings of the American Statistical Association, Section on Survey Research Methods, Vol. II,* 1183–1188.

Snow, B. (1992). They stood up and were counted: Health surveys and public opinion polls on-line. *Database, 15,* 88–93.

Soeken, K. L., & Prescott, P. A. (1986). Issues in the use of Kappa to estimate reliability. *Medical Care, 24,* 733–741.

Spaeth, J. L., & O'Rourke, D. (1994). Designing and implementing the National Organizations Survey. *American Behavioral Scientist, 37,* 872–890.

Spaeth, M. A. (1987). CATI facilities at survey research organizations. *Survey Research, 18* (3–4), 19–22.

Spaeth, M. A. (1990). CATI facilities at academic survey research organizations. *Survey Research, 21* (2), 11–14.

Spector, P. E. (1992). *Summated rating scale construction: An introduction.* Thousand Oaks, CA: Sage.

Spilker, B., Molinek, F. R., Jr., Johnston, K. A., Simpson, R. L., Jr., & Tilson, H. H. (Eds.). (1990). Quality of life bibliography and indexes. *Medical Care, 28* (Suppl. 12).

Spitzer, W. O., Dobson, A. J., Hall, J., Chesterman, E., Levi, J., Shepherd, R., Battista, R. N., & Catchlove, B. R. (1981). Measuring the quality of life of cancer patients: A concise QL-Index for use by physicians. *Journal of Chronic Diseases, 34,* 585–597.

Stange, K. C., & Zyzanski, S. J. (1989). Integrating qualitative and quantitative research methods. *Family Medicine, 21,* 448–451.

Steckler, A., McLeroy, K. R., Goodman, R. M., Bird, S. T., & McCormick, L. (1992). Toward integrating qualitative and quantitative methods: An introduction. *Health Education Quarterly, 19,* 1–8.

Steinwachs, D. M., Wu, A. W., & Skinner, E. A. (1994). How will outcomes management work? *Health Affairs, 13* (4), 153–162.

Stephens, T., Jacobs, D. R., Jr., & White, C. C. (1985). A descriptive epidemiology of leisure-time physical activity. *Public Health Reports, 100,* 147–158.

Stewart, A. L., & Ware, J. E., Jr. (1992). *Measuring functioning and well-being: The medical outcomes study approach.* Durham: Duke University Press.

Stewart, D. W. (1984). *Secondary Research.* Thousand Oaks, CA: Sage.

Stewart, D. W., & Shamdasani, P. N. (1990). *Focus groups: Theory and practice.* Thousand Oaks, CA: Sage.

Stouthamer-Loeber, M., & van Kammen, W. B. (1995). *Data collection and management: A practical guide.* Thousand Oaks, CA: Sage.

Strasser, S., Aharony, L., & Greenberger, D. (1993). The patient satisfaction process: Moving toward a comprehensive model. *Medical Care Review, 50,* 219–248.

Streiner, D. L., & Norman, G. R. (1991). *Health measurement scales: A practical guide to their development and use.* Oxford: Oxford University Press.

Stussman, B. J. (1994). *Questionnaire design research laboratory: Cognitive laboratory testing of the 1993 Teenage Attitudes and Practices Survey II.* (Report No. 6, National Center for Health Statistics, Cognitive Methods Staff Working Paper Series). Hyattsville, MD: National Center for Health Statistics.

Stussman, B. J., Willis, G. B., & Allen, K. F. (1993). Collecting information from teenagers: Experiences from the cognitive lab. *Proceedings of the American Statistical Association, Section on Survey Research Methods, Vol. I,* 382–385.

Suchman, E. A. (1967). The survey method applied to public health and medicine. In C. Y. Glock (Ed.), *Survey Research in the Social Sciences* (pp. 425–517). New York: Russell Sage Foundation.

Suchman, L., & Jordan, B. (1990). Interactional troubles in face-to-face survey interviews. *Journal of the American Statistical Association, 85,* 232–241.

Sudman, S. (1989). Comment on "Medical sociology: Some tensions among theory, method, and substance." *Journal of Health and Social Behavior, 30,* 161–162.

Sudman, S. (1985). Mail surveys of reluctant professionals. *Evaluation Review, 9,* 349–360.

Sudman, S., & Bradburn, N. M. (1974). *Response effects in surveys.* Hawthorne, NY: Aldine.

Sudman, S., & Bradburn, N. M. (1982). *Asking questions: A practical guide to questionnaire design.* San Francisco: Jossey-Bass.

Sudman, S., Bradburn, N. M., & Schwarz, N. (1995). *Thinking about answers: The application of cognitive processes to survey methodology.* San Francisco: Jossey-Bass.

Sudman, S., Finn, A., & Lannom, L. (1984). The use of bounded recall procedures in single interviews. *Public Opinion Quarterly, 48,* 520–524.

Sudman, S., & Freeman, H. E. (1987, July). *Access to health care services in the U.S.A.: Results and methods.* Paper presented at International Symposium on Health Conduct and Health Care: Comparative Analyses in the United States and West Germany, Bad Homberg, Germany.

Sudman, S., & Freeman, H. E. (1988). The use of network sampling for locating the seriously ill. *Medical Care, 26,* 992–999.

Sudman, S., & Kalton, G. (1986). New developments in the sampling of special populations. *American Review of Sociology, 12,* 401–429.

Sudman, S., & Schwarz, N. (1989). Contributions of cognitive psychology to advertising research. *Journal of Advertising Research, 29* (3), 43–53.

Sudman, S., Sirken, M. G., & Cowan, C. D. (1988). Sampling rare and elusive populations. *Science, 240,* 991–996.

Sullivan, L. M., Dukes, K. A., Harris, L., Dittus, R. S., Greenfield, S., & Kaplan, S. H. (1995). A comparison of various methods of collecting self-reported health outcomes data among low-income and minority patients. *Medical Care, 33* (Suppl. 4), AS183–AS194.

The survey kit. (1995) (Vols. 1–9). Thousand Oaks, CA: Sage.

Survey Research Center, University of Michigan. (1990). *A report on the evaluation of three CATI systems.* Ann Arbor, MI: Author.

Survey Research Laboratory, University of Illinois. (1986). *Proposal: Survey of public knowledge, attitudes, perceptions, and behaviors concerning acquired immune deficiency syndrome (AIDS).* Chicago: Author.

Survey Research Laboratory, University of Illinois. (1987a). *Chicago Area General Population Survey on AIDS (SRL No. 606): Coding Manual.* Chicago: Author.

Survey Research Laboratory, University of Illinois. (1987b). *Chicago Area General Population Survey on AIDS (SRL No. 606): Interviewer Manual.* Chicago: Author.

Survey Research Laboratory, University of Illinois. (1988). *Sample report: Chicago area general population survey on AIDS.* Chicago: Author.

Survey Research Laboratory, University of Illinois. (1994a). *General training manual for face-to-face interviewers.* Chicago: Author.

Survey Research Laboratory, University of Illinois. (1994b). *General training manual for telephone interviewers.* Chicago: Author.

Survey Research Laboratory, University of Illinois. (1995). *Operations training manual.* Chicago: Author.

Susser, M. (1985). Epidemiology in the United States after World War II: The evolution of technique. *Epidemiologic Reviews, 7,* 147–177.

Swain, L. (1985). Basic principles of questionnaire design. *Survey Methodology, 11,* 161–170.

Sykes, W., & Morton-Williams, J. (1987). Evaluating survey questions. *Journal of Official Statistics, 3,* 191–207.

Tanur, J. M. (1982). Advances in methods for large-scale surveys and experiments. In R. M. Adams, N. J. Smelser, & D. J. Treiman (Eds.), *Behavioral and Social Research: A National Resource* (pp. 294–372). Washington, DC: National Academy Press.

Tanur, J. M. (1987). Some cognitive aspects of surveys. *Statistics Sweden, 3,* 465–475.

Tanur, J. M. (Ed.). (1992). *Questions about questions: Inquiries into the cognitive bases of surveys.* New York: Russell Sage Foundation.

Tedin, K. L., & Hofstetter, C. R. (1982). The effect of cost and importance factors on the return rate for single and multiple mailings. *Public Opinion Quarterly, 46,* 122–128.

Thornberry, O. T., & Massey, J. T. (1988). Trends in U.S. telephone coverage across time and subgroups. In R. M. Groves, P. P. Biemer, L. E. Lyberg, J. T. Massey, W. L. Nicholls, II, & J. Waksberg (Eds.), *Telephone survey methodology* (pp. 25–39). New York: Wiley.

Thornberry, O. T., Wilson, R. W., & Golden, P. M. (1986). The 1985 Health Promotion and Disease Prevention Survey. *Public Health Reports, 101,* 566–570.

Thran, S. L., & Gillis, K. D. (1992). A comparison of imputation techniques in a physician survey. *Proceedings of the American Statistical Association, Section on Survey Research Methods,* pp. 211–220.

Tillinghast, D. S. (1980). Direct magnitude estimation scales in public opinion surveys. *Public Opinion Quarterly, 44,* 377–383.

Torrance, G. W. (1986). Measurement of health state utilities for economic appraisal: A review. *Journal of Health Economics, 5,* 1–30.

Torrance, G. W. (1987). Utility approach to measuring health-related quality of life. *Journal of Chronic Diseases, 40,* 593–600.

Torrance, G. W., & Feeny, D. (1989). Utilities and quality-adjusted life years. *International Journal of Technology Assessment in Health Care, 5,* 559–575.

Tortora, R. D. (1985). CATI in an agricultural statistical agency. *Journal of Official Statistics, 1,* 301–314.

Tourangeau, R. (1984). Cognitive sciences and survey methods. In T. B. Jabine, M. L. Straf, J. M. Tanur, & R. Tourangeau (Eds.), *Cognitive aspects of survey methodology: Building a bridge between disciplines* (pp. 73–100). Washington, DC: National Academy Press.

Tourangeau, R., & Rasinski, K. A. (1988). Cognitive processes underlying context effects in attitude measurement. *Psychological Bulletin, 103,* 299–314.

Tourangeau, R., Rasinski, K. A., & Bradburn, N. (1991). Measuring happiness in surveys: A test of the subtraction hypothesis. *Public Opinion Quarterly, 55,* 255–266.

Tourangeau, R., Rasinski, K. A., Bradburn, N., & D'Andrade, R. (1989a). Belief accessibility and context effects in attitude measurement. *Journal of Experimental Social Psychology, 25,* 401–421.

Tourangeau, R., Rasinski, K. A., Bradburn, N., & D'Andrade, R. (1989b). Carryover effects in attitude surveys. *Public Opinion Quarterly, 53,* 495–524.

Tourangeau, R., Rasinski, K. A., & D'Andrade, R. (1991). Attitude structure and belief accessibility. *Journal of Experimental Social Psychology, 27,* 48–75.

Traub, R. E. (1994). *Reliability for the social sciences: Theory and applications.* Thousand Oaks, CA: Sage.

Trevino, F. M. (1982). Vital and health statistics for the U.S. Hispanic population. *American Journal of Public Health, 72,* 979–981.

Trevino, F. M. (1987). Standardized terminology for Hispanic populations. *American Journal of Public Health, 77,* 69–72.

Trevino, F. M. (1988). Uniform minimum data sets: In search of demographic comparability. *American Journal of Public Health, 78,* 126–127.

Trewin, D., & Lee, G. (1988). International comparisons of telephone coverage. In R. M. Groves, P. P. Biemer, L. E. Lyberg, J. T. Massey, W. L. Nicholls, II, & J. Waksberg (Eds.), *Telephone Survey Methodology* (pp. 9–24). New York: Wiley.

Trunzo, D., & Schechter, S. (1993). *Questionnaire design research laboratory: Focus groups on family health issues.* (Report No. 1, National Center for Health Statistics, Cognitive Methods Staff Working Paper Series). Hyattsville, MD: National Center for Health Statistics.

Tuckel, P. S., & Feinberg, B. M. (1991). The answering machine poses many questions for telephone survey researchers. *Public Opinion Quarterly, 55,* 200–217.

Tucker, C., Casady, R., & Lepkowski, J. (1992). Sample allocation for stratified telephone sample designs. *Proceedings of the American Statistical Association, Section on Survey Research Methods,* pp. 291–296.

Turner, C. F., & Martin, E. (Eds.). (1984). *Surveying subjective phenomena.* Vol. 1. New York: Russell Sage Foundation.

Turner, J. T., & Matthews, K. A. (1991). Measuring adolescent satisfaction with nursing care: In an ambulatory setting. *The Association of Black Nursing Faculty Journal, 1,* 48–52.

Twaddle, A. C., & Hessler, R. M. (1977). *A Sociology of Health.* St. Louis, MO: Mosby.

U.S. Bureau of the Census. (1994a). *Disability followback survey: Field representative's manual.* (Report No. DFS–100). Washington, DC: U. S. Government Printing Office.

U.S. Bureau of the Census. (1994b). *Disability followback survey: Guide for classroom training.* (Report No. DFS–300). Washington, DC: U.S. Government Printing Office.

U.S. Bureau of the Census. (1994c). *National health interview survey: Field representative's manual.* (Report No. HIS–100). Washington, DC: U.S. Government Printing Office.

Umesh, U. N., & Peterson, R. A. (1991). A critical evaluation of the randomized response method: Applications, validation, and research agenda. *Sociological Methods & Research, 20,* 104–138.

Verbrugge, L. M. (1980). Health diaries. *Medical Care, 18,* 73–95.

Verbrugge, L. M. (1994). *The disability supplement to the 1994–95 National Health Interview Survey (NHIS–Disability).* (Available from Lois M. Verbrugge, Institute of Gerontology, 300 North Ingalls, University of Michigan, Ann-Arbor, Michigan 48109–2007, (tel) 313–936–2103, (fax) 313–936–2116).

Vigderhous, G. (1981) Scheduling telephone interviews: A study of seasonal patterns. *Public Opinion Quarterly, 45,* 250–259.

Von Thurn, D. R., & Moore, J. C. (1993). The use of anthropological interviewing methods in survey research pretesting. *Proceedings of the American Statistical Association, Section on Survey Research Methods, Vol. I,* 571–576.

Voss, D. S., Gelman, A., & King, G. (1995). Preelection survey methodology: Details from eight polling organizations, 1988 and 1992. *Public Opinion Quarterly, 59,* 98–132.

Waksberg, J. (1978). Sampling methods for random digit dialing. *Journal of the American Statistical Association, 73,* 40–46.

Waksberg, J. (1983). A note on "Locating a special population using random digit dialing." *Public Opinion Quarterly, 47,* 576–579.

Waksberg, J., & Mohadjer, L. (1991). Automation of within-household sampling. *Proceedings of the American Statistical Association, Section on Survey Research Methods,* pp. 350–355.

Walker, J. T. (1994). Fax machines and social surveys: Teaching an old dog new tricks. *Journal of Quantitative Criminology, 10,* 181–188.

Wallace, R. B. (1994). Assessing the health of individuals and populations in surveys of the elderly: Some concepts and approaches. *The Gerontologist, 34,* 449–453.

Ware, J. E., Jr. (1978). Effects of acquiescent response set on patient satisfaction ratings. *Medical Care, 16,* 327–336.

Ware, J. E., Jr. (1986). The assessment of health status. In L. M. Aiken & D. Mechanic (Eds.), *Applications of Social Science to Clinical Medicine and Health Policy* (pp. 204–228). New Brunswick, NJ: Rutgers University Press.

Ware, J. E., Jr. (1987). Standards for validating health measures: Definition and content. *Journal of Chronic Diseases, 40,* 473–480.

Ware, J. E., Jr. (1995). The status of health assessment 1994. *Annual Review of Public Health, 16,* 327–354.

Ware, J. E., Jr., & Hays, R. D. (1988). Methods for measuring patient satisfaction with specific medical encounters. *Medical Care, 26,* 393–402.

Ware, J. E., Jr., Kosinski, M., Bayliss, M. S., McHorney, C. A., Rogers, W. H., & Raczek, A. (1995). Comparison of methods for the scoring and statistical analysis of SF-36 health profile and summary measures: Summary of results from the Medical Outcomes Study. *Medical Care, 33* (Suppl. 4), AS264–AS279.

Ware, J. E., Jr., Kosinski, M., & Keller, S. D. (1994). *SF–36 physical and mental health summary scales: A user's manual.* Boston: The Health Institute, New England Medical Center.

Ware, J. E., Jr., Kosinski, M., & Keller, S. D. (1995). *SF–12: How to score the SF–12 physical and mental health summary scales.* Boston: The Health Institute, New England Medical Center.

Ware, J. E., Jr., & Sherbourne, C. D. (1992). The MOS 36-item short-form health survey (SF–36): I. Conceptual framework and item selection. *Medical Care, 30,* 473–483.

Ware, J. E., Jr., Snow, K. K., Kosinski, M., & Gandek, B. (1993). *SF–36 health survey: Manual and interpretation guide.* Boston: The Health Institute, New England Medical Center.

Ware, J. E., Jr., & Snyder, M. K. (1975). Dimensions of patient attitudes regarding doctors and medical care services. *Medical Care, 13,* 669–682.

Ware, J. E., Jr., Snyder, M. K., Wright, W. R., & Davies, A. R. (1983). Defining and measuring patient satisfaction with medical care. *Evaluation and Program Planning, 6,* 247–263.

Ware, J. E., Jr., Wright, R., Snyder, M. K., & Chu, G. C. (1975). Consumer perceptions of health care services: Implications for academic medicine. *Journal of Medical Education, 50,* 839–848.

Warner, S. L. (1965). Randomized response: A survey technique for eliminating evasive answer bias. *Journal of the American Statistical Association, 60,* 63–69.

Wasson, J., Keller, A., Rubenstein, L., Hays, R., Nelson, E., Johnson, D., & the Dartmouth Primary Care COOP Project. (1992). Benefits and obstacles of health status assessment in ambulatory settings: The clinician's point of view. *Medical Care, 30* (Suppl. 5), MS42–MS49.

Weeks, M. F., Jones, B. L., Folsom, R. E., Jr., & Benrud, C. H. (1980). Optimal times to contact sample households. *Public Opinion Quarterly, 44,* 101–114.

Weeks, M. F., Kulka, R. A., Lessler, J. T., & Whitmore, R. W. (1983). Personal versus telephone surveys for collecting household health data at the local level. *American Journal of Public Health, 73,* 1389–1394.

Weeks, M. F., Kulka, R. A., & Pierson, S. A. (1987). Optimal call scheduling for a telephone survey. *Public Opinion Quarterly, 51,* 540–549.

Weeks, M. F., & Moore, R. P. (1981). Ethnicity-of-interviewer effects on ethnic respondents. *Public Opinion Quarterly, 45,* 245–249.

Weinberg, E. (1983). Data collection: Planning and management. In P. H. Rossi, J. D. Wright, & A. B. Anderson (Eds.), *Handbook of Survey Research* (pp. 329–358). San Diego, CA: Academic Press.

Weiss, B. D., & Senf, J. H. (1990). Patient satisfaction survey instrument for use in health maintenance organizations. *Medical Care, 28,* 434–445.

Westermeyer, J. (1988). Problems with surveillance methods for alcoholism: Differences in coding systems among federal, state, and private agencies. *American Journal of Public Health, 78,* 130–133.

White, A. A. (1983). Response rate calculation in RDD telephone health surveys: current practices. In *Proceedings of the American Statistical Association, Section on Survey Research Methods* (pp. 277–282). Washington, DC: American Statistical Association.

Wilensky, G. R. (1985). SIPP and health care issues. *Journal of Economic and Social Measurement, 13,* 295–298.

Wilkin, D., Hallam, L., & Doggett, M.-A. (1992). *Measures of need and outcome for primary health care.* New York: Oxford University Press.

Williams, B. (1994). Patient satisfaction: A valid concept? *Social Science and Medicine, 38,* 509–516.

Willimack, D. K., Schuman, H., Pennell, B.-E., & Lepkowski, J. M. (1995). Effects of a prepaid nonmonetary incentive on response rates and response quality in a face-to-face survey. *Public Opinion Quarterly, 59,* 78–92.

Willis, G. (1994a). *Cognitive interviewing and questionnaire design: A training manual.* (Report No. 7, National Center for Health Statistics, Cognitive Methods Staff Working Paper Series). Hyattsville, MD: National Center for Health Statistics.

Willis, G. B. (1994b). *The mini-pretest: Small-scale testing of a large-scale questionnaire.* (Report No. 15, National Center for Health Statistics, Cognitive Methods Staff Working Paper Series). Hyattsville, MD: National Center for Health Statistics.

Willis, G. B., Royston, P., & Bercini, D. (1991). The use of verbal report methods in the development and testing of survey questionnaires. *Applied Cognitive Psychology, 5,* 251–267.

Wilson, I. B., & Kaplan, S. (1995). Clinical practice and patients' health status: How are the two related? *Medical Care, 33* (Suppl. 1), AS209–AS214.

Wilson, R. W. (1981). Do health indicators indicate health? *American Journal of Public Health, 71,* 461–463.

Wilson, R. W., & Drury, T. F. (1984). Interpreting trends in illness and disability: Health statistics and health status. *Annual Review of Public Health, 5,* 83–106.

Wilson, R. W., & Elinson, J. (1981). National Survey of Personal Health Practices and Consequences: Background, conceptual issues, and selected findings. *Public Health Reports, 96,* 218–225.

Winglee, M., Ryaboy, L., & Judkins, D. (1993). Imputation for the income and assets module of the Medicare current beneficiaries survey (MCBS). *Proceedings of the American Statistical Association, Section on Survey Research Methods, Vol. I,* 463–467.

Winter, D.L.S., & Clayton, R. L. (1990). Speech data entry: Results of the first test of voice recognition for data collection. *Proceedings of the American Statistical Association, Section on Survey Research Methods,* pp. 387–392.

Witt, K., & Bernstein, S. (1992). Best practices in disk-by-mail surveys. *Proceedings of the Sawtooth Software Conference* (pp. 1–26). Ketchum, ID.

WONCA Classification Committee. (1990). *Functional status measurement in primary care.* New York: Springer.

Wood-Dauphinee, S., & Williams, J. I. (1987). Reintegration to normal living as a proxy to quality of life. *Journal of Chronic Diseases, 40,* 491–499.

World Health Organization. (1948). Constitution of the World Health Organization. In *Handbook of basic documents.* Geneva: Author.

Wright, R. A. (1991). Use of multiple entry diaries in panel studies of health care expenditure. *Proceedings of the American Statistical Association, Section on Survey Research Methods,* pp. 332–337.

Wunderlich, G. S. (Ed.). (1992). *Toward a national health care survey: A data system for the 21st century.* Washington, DC: National Academy Press.

Xu, M., Bates, B. J., & Schweitzer, J. C. (1993). The impact of messages on survey participation in answering machine households. *Public Opinion Quarterly, 57,* 232–237.

Yammarino, F. J., Skinner, S. J., & Childers, T. L. (1991). Understanding mail survey response behavior: A meta-analysis. *Public Opinion Quarterly, 55,* 613–639.

Yankauer, A. (1987). Hispanic-Latino: What's in a name? *American Journal of Public Health, 77,* 15–17.

Yu, E.S.H., & Liu, W. T. (1992). U.S. National Health Data on Asian Americans and Pacific Islanders: A research agenda for the 1990s. *American Journal of Public Health, 82,* 1645–1652.

Yu, J., & Cooper, H. (1983). A quantitative review of research design effects on response rates to questionnaires. *Journal of Marketing Research, 20,* 36–44.

Zeisel, H. (1968). *Say it with figures.* New York: HarperCollins.

Zyzanski, S. J., Hulka, B. S., & Cassel, J. C. (1974). Scale for the measurement of "satisfaction" with medical care: Modifications in content, format and scoring. *Medical Care, 12,* 611–620.

NAME INDEX

Aaronson, N. K., 210
Abramson, J. H., 43
Adair, E. G., 5, 186
Adams, M. M., 472, 478
Adams-Esquivel, H., 102
Adang, R. P., 95
Aday, L. A., 10, 14, 109, 137, 196, 198, 201, 218, 256, 307, 469, 472, 475, 478
Aharony, L., 257
Aiken, L. H., 469
Aitken, M. J., 109, 196, 307
Albrecht, G. L., 41, 72, 90, 104, 197, 348, 399, 479
Algina, J., 51, 67, 68, 72
Allen, H. M., Jr., 259
Allen, K. F., 197
Alonso, J., 220
Alwin, D. F., 50, 251, 252–253, 254
Ambergen, A. W., 95
Andersen, R. M., 10, 22, 106, 137, 181, 198, 218, 256, 467, 469, 472, 473, 474, 479
Anderson, A. B., 314
Anderson, D. W., 133
Anderson, J., 240
Anderson, J. P., 207
Andrews, F. M., 250, 253, 254, 276
Andrich, D., 71, 74
Aneshensel, C. S., 105, 110
Angel, R., 343
Anto, J. M., 220
Appel, M. V., 94–95
Aquilino, W. S., 105, 242
Armenian, H. K., 29
Armstrong, J. S., 286
Arnljot, H. A., 467, 474
Atkinson, C. C., 257
Austin, S. M., 31
Avdor, O., 257
Avila, R. A., 287
Axinn, W. G., 186
Ayidiya, S. A., 269

Babbie, E., 26, 30
Bachman, J. G., 250
Badia, X., 220
Bailar, B. A., 20
Bainbridge, W. S., 349
Bakker, C. H., 210
Balas, E. A., 31
Barbash, G. I., 287
Barer, M. L., 201
Barmes, D. E., 467, 474
Barnsley, J., 109
Barrett, J., 105
Basch, C. E., 185
Basilevsky, A., 314
Bastien, F., 259
Batalden, P. B., 259
Bates, B. J., 284
Bauman, L. J., 5, 186
Bauman, S. L., 132
Baumgartner, R., 286
Bayliss, M. S., 46, 68
Beatty, P., 102, 179, 186, 197
Beaufait, D. W., 207
Becerra, R. M., 110
Becker, M. H., 41
Beldt, S. F., 241
Bellhouse, D. R., 176
Belson, W., 180, 196
Benjamin, K. L., 202
Bennett, S., 124, 468
Benrud, C. H., 284
Benson, J., 471
Bercini, D., 186
Berglund, I., 260
Bergner, M., 207, 211, 214
Berk, M. L., 8, 226, 290, 291, 469
Berkanovic, E., 198
Berkman, L. F., 41, 472, 478
Bernstein, A. B., 226, 290, 291
Bernstein, I. H., 50, 51, 55, 56, 57, 58, 62, 67, 70, 260, 326
Bernstein, S., 95
Berry, S. H., 286

Berthelot, J. M., 94
Bethlehem, J. G., 93
Bhopal, R. S., 105
Bickart, B. A., 233, 288
Biddle, A. K., 286
Biemer, P. P., 22, 94, 105, 180, 183, 184, 196, 199, 304
Bienias, J., 232
Billiet, J., 295
Binson, D., 197, 198, 237
Bird, S. T., 5–6
Bishop, G. F., 105, 197, 247, 250, 253
Bittner, D., 106
Björkman, T., 260
Blair, E. A., 196, 232
Blair, J., 24, 129, 132, 133, 136, 139, 185, 197, 233, 288
Blakeney, R. D., 94
Blendon, R. J., 469, 471
Bless, H., 232, 255
Blixt, S., 185
Blyth, B., 94
Bobbitt, R. A., 207
Bogen, K., 182
Bohner, G., 232
Bohrnstedt, G. W., 349
Bolstein, R., 286
Borenstein, M., 144, 176
Boruch, R. F., 241
Botman, S. L., 284
Bourque, L. B., 304, 306, 312, 321
Bowling, A., 211, 221
Bowman, J. A., 233
Boyd, G., 471
Boyd, N. F., 233
Boyle, M. H., 207
Bradburn, N. M., 3, 6, 22, 24, 103, 180, 181, 182, 183, 197, 199, 224, 232, 236, 237, 238, 239, 240, 242, 244, 246, 247, 248, 249, 250, 251, 252, 253, 254, 255, 262, 263, 270, 272, 275, 277, 280, 303
Braden, J. J., 8

Branch, L. G., 197
Brandt, E. N., Jr., 467
Breslow, L., 41, 202, 472, 478
Brick, J. M., 127
Broadhead, W. E., 207
Brodie, M., 471
Brook, L., 253
Brook, R. H., 201, 207, 211, 259, 473, 478
Brookshire, R. G., 306
Brown, G. D., 31
Bryant, J. H., 208
Bucquet, D., 208
Burchell, B., 275
Burgess, M. J., 187
Buring, J. E., 26, 28, 30, 43, 60, 74, 90
Burnam, M. A., 97, 133
Burstein, L., 31
Burt, G., 108
Burt, V. L., 162
Burton, J. P., 228, 229
Burton, S., 196, 232
Burton, T., 257
Bush, J. W., 207
Buzzard, I. M., 233

Camburn, D., 94
Campanelli, P. C., 226
Campbell, B. A., 290
Campbell, D. T., 31, 42, 43, 63
Cannell, C., 100, 180, 187, 291, 295, 303–304
Cantor, J. C., 469
Caraballo, L. R., 197
Carlson, B. A., 468
Carlson, B. L., 162
Carlson, J. E., 255
Carmines, E. G., 51, 54n, 56, 57, 58, 63
Carter, W. B., 207
Cartwright, A., 10
Casady, R. J., 127, 136
Caspar, R., 22
Cassel, J. C., 70, 259, 471
Cassidy, C. M., 198
Catalano, R., 100
Catlin, G., 468, 474
Cella, D. F., 204, 210, 211
Chang, T. K., 290
Chapa, J., 226
Charlson, M., 216
Chassein, B., 232
Chen, M. M., 207
Chen, M. S., 218, 467, 474
Childers, T. L., 286
Chiu, G. Y., 198, 256
Chu, G. C., 259
Church, A. H., 286
Chylack, L. T., Jr., 60
Cialdini, R. B., 291, 304
Citro, C. F., 30
Clapp, N. E., 207
Clark, J. R., 263
Clark, L., 253
Clark, V. A., 105, 306, 312, 321
Clayton, R. L., 94
Clayton, R. R., 240

Cleary, P. D., 202, 256, 343
Cockburn, J., 257
Coffey, C. M., 110
Cohany, S. R., 471
Cohen, D. L., 302
Cohen, J., 144, 154, 155, 176, 290
Cohen, L. K., 265
Cohen, S. B., 8, 142, 162
Coleman, L., 291
Collier, C. M., 129
Collins, M., 253
Colombotos, J., 104
Connell, F. A., 8
Conover, W. J., 327
Conrad, D., 110
Converse, J. M., 24, 180, 182, 188
Cook, T. D., 42, 43
Cooper, H., 286
Corcoran, M., 245
Corey, C. R., 100, 102, 245, 469
Cornelius, L. J., 218
Cornelius, R. M., 468
Cornoni-Huntley, J., 469
Corrigan, J. M., 201
Costa, L. A., 302
Cotter, P. R., 290
Coulter, P. B., 290
Couper, M. P., 106, 108, 289, 291, 304
Cox, B. G., 8, 142, 162
Cowan, C. D., 133, 137
Crane, L. A., 100, 102, 103
Crawford, S. A., 302
Creswell, J. W., 43
Crocker, L., 51, 67, 68, 72
Cronbach, L. J., 51, 57
Cross, J., 95
Crowne, D. P., 252
Cummings, M. A., 202
Cummings, S. R., 26, 28, 30, 43
Currie, S., 126
Curtice, J., 108
Cynamon, M. L., 94, 221
Czaja, R., 24, 105, 109, 129, 133, 136, 139, 233

Daley, J., 15
Daly, M. B., 70, 259
D'Andrade, R., 255
Daniel, W. W., 241
Danielson, W. A., 290
Danis, C., 183, 236, 244
Darling, H., 259
David, M., 471
Davies, A. R., 257, 259
Davis, W. L., 233
Dawber, T. R., 473, 478
Dean, A. G., 144
DeFriese, G. H., 8
de Heer, W. F., 468
Delandshere, G., 31
Delbanco, T. L., 15
DeLeeuw, E. D., 286
Delgado, J. L., 226
DeLuise, T., 257
DeMaio, T. J., 180, 226, 233

Desvousges, W. H., 185
de Vaus, D. A., 43
DeVellis, R. F., 50, 51, 56, 57, 62, 67, 260, 326
Deyo, R. A., 211, 214, 216
Di, Z. X., 105
Dickinson, J. A., 233
DiClemente, R. J., 245
Diehr, P., 8, 319
Dielman, T. E., 108
Dijkstra, N., 187
Dillman, D. A., 95, 110, 111, 180, 199, 251, 262–263, 265, 266, 269, 270, 271, 272, 274, 275, 276, 280, 283, 284, 285, 286, 301, 302, 303, 304
Doggett, M. A., 211
Dooley, D., 100
Dornan, M. C., 257
Doyle, B. J., 259
Dresch, S. P., 286
Drew, J. D., 165
Drury, T. F., 31, 215
Duchan, K. L., 241
Dull, V. T., 110
Dykema, J., 185

Easling, I., 286
Eastman, E., 233
Edgell, S. E., 241
Edgman-Levitan, S., 15
Edwards, B., 30, 106, 471, 475
Edwards, S., 291, 294
Edwards, W. S., 30, 106, 471, 475
Elbeck, M., 260
Elinson, J., 211, 469
Epstein, A. M., 213, 257
Epstein, F. H., 473
Erickson, P., 14, 72, 204, 205n, 208, 210, 211, 221
Ericsson, K. A., 186
Estrada, L., 226
Etter, J. F., 286
Evans, R. G., 201
Ewigman, B. G., 31
Ezzati-Rice, T. M., 318

Fahimi, M., 318
Farquhar, J., 468
Fecso, R., 22
Fecteau, G., 260
Feeny, D. H., 207, 208
Feinberg, B. M., 101, 284
Feinleib, M. R., 471
Feinstein, A. R., 202, 203, 210
Feldman, J. J., 231
Fendrich, M., 242
Fern, E. F., 287
Ferreira, P. L., 259
Fiedler, J., 234
Fielder, E. P., 110, 304
Fienberg, S. E., 22, 24, 184, 186
Fink, A., 142, 343, 349
Fink, J. C., 93
Finn, A., 233–234
Fiset, L., 41, 72, 90, 110, 249, 345, 346, 348, 479

Fiske, D. W., 63
Fiske, M., 296
Fitzpatrick, R., 256
Fleece, E. L., 286
Fleming, G. V., 106, 469, 473, 475
Flendrig, J. A., 95
Foddy, W., 199
Folsom, R. E., Jr., 284
Fontana, A., 185
Ford, A. B., 215
Ford, K., 242
Forsman, G., 132
Forsyth, B. H., 186
Forthofer, R. N., 162, 327, 349
Fowler, J. J., Jr., 22, 95, 105, 187, 191,
    199, 202, 242, 280, 293, 295
Fox, J. A., 240, 241
Frankel, M. R., 22, 181
Freeman, H. E., 31, 43, 93, 100, 102,
    105, 109, 136, 245, 469
Freidenberg, J., 197
Frerichs, R. R., 105
Freund, D. A., 472
Frey, J. H., 185, 304
Fricke, T. E., 186
Froberg, D. G., 203, 208, 210
Fultz, N. H., 290
Furlong, W., 207
Furse, D. H., 286, 287

Gagnon, J. H., 472
Gandek, B., 46, 68, 207, 259
Ganesh, G. K., 232
Garcha, B. S., 241
Gardenier, J. S., 94, 110
Gaskell, G. D., 232
Geer, J. G., 195
Gelbach, S. H., 207
Gelman, A., 126
Gerteis, M., 15
Gibberd, R., 233
Gill, T. M., 210
Gillis, K. D., 318
Gilljam, M., 253–254
Gilson, B. S., 207
Gold, M., 257, 259n, 470
Goldberg, H. I., 202
Golden, P. M., 90, 470
Goldsmith, C. H., 207
Goodman, R. M., 5–6, 257
Gower, A. R., 184
Goyder, J., 100–101
Grady, K. E., 12
Grambling, R., 233
Granberg, D., 253–254
Graubard, B. I., 176
Gray, G. B., 165
Greenberger, D., 257
Greenfield, S., 201, 202
Grembowski, D., 37, 41, 72, 90, 249,
    345, 346, 348, 443, 479
Groves, R. M., 3, 20, 22, 95, 99, 102,
    103, 104, 106, 108, 111, 180, 182,
    183, 184, 196, 199, 287, 288, 289,
    290, 291, 303–304
Gunn, W. J., 286

Gustafson, D., 259
Guyatt, G. H., 214, 215, 216

Hadorn, D. C., 202
Hagan, D. E., 129
Hakim, C., 8
Haley, S. M., 71, 74
Hall, J. A., 213, 257
Hallam, L., 211
Halm, M. A., 260
Hambleton, R. K., 71, 74
Hanley, J. A., 343
Hansluwka, H. E., 211
Hansson, L., 260
Harrington, B. E., 105
Hart, L. G., 8
Hasman, A., 95
Hatcher, J., 207
Hay, D. A., 240
Hayes-Bautista, D. E., 226
Hays, R. D., 257, 259
Hebel, J. R., 288
Heberlein, T. A., 286
Hedges, L. V., 232
Hendershot, G. E., 16, 39, 221
Henry, G. T., 142
Herrmann, D., 231
Herzog, A. R., 100, 197
Hessler, R. M., 212
Hidiroglou, M. A., 165
Hild, T., 232
Hill, D., 257
Himmelfarb, S., 241
Hingson, R., 105
Hippler, G., 287
Hippler, H. J., 105, 184, 197, 248, 253,
    254, 278, 287
Hirschi, T., 76, 90
Hochstim, J. R., 104
Hofman, L.P.M.B., 93
Hofstetter, C. R., 286
Hollis, M., 31
Holte, J., 202
Horm, J., 133
Hornik, J., 287
Hosmer, D. W., Jr., 144, 152, 155, 161,
    176, 343
Hougland, J. G., Jr., 240
House, C. C., 108, 273
Hox, J. J., 286
Hsu, H. L., 290
Hubbard, M. L., 94, 105
Hubbard, R., 286
Hulka, B. S., 70, 257, 259
Hulley, S. B., 26, 28, 30, 43
Hum, D. P., 314
Hunt, S. D., 188
Hunt, S. M., 207
Hunter, P.B.V., 467
Hurley, R. E., 472
Huttenlocher, J., 232
Hyman, H., 76, 295

Irwig, L., 257
Israëls, A. Z., 468

Jabine, T. B., 183
Jackson, B. A., 215
Jackson, J. S., 241
Jacobs, D. R., Jr., 468, 471
Jacobs, M., 95
Jaffe, M. W., 215
James, J. M., 286
James, S. A., 207
Jay, G. M., 213
Jobe, J. B., 184, 186, 197, 221, 231, 232,
    233
Johnson, A. E., 8–9, 162
Johnson, L., 95
Johnson, T. P., 133, 197, 240, 291
Johnston, K. A., 204
Jones, B. L., 284
Jones, G., 260
Jones, G. K., 162
Jordan, B., 179, 295
Jordan, L. A., 104
Jöreskog, K. G., 67, 343
Joyce, C., 95
Judkins, D., 138, 226, 318
Jylhä, M., 202

Kahn, H. A., 349
Kahn, R. L., 95, 103, 104, 108, 180, 295
Kalsbeek, W. D., 22, 180, 199, 284
Kalton, G., 20, 22, 30, 121, 133, 137,
    142, 161, 180, 182, 187, 253, 292,
    314–315, 317
Kaluzny, A., 109, 291
Kane, R. L., 203, 208, 210
Kanouse, D. E., 286
Kaplan, R. M., 207
Kaplan, S., 213
Karweit, N., 310
Kashner, T. M., 288
Kasper, J., 22, 181
Kasprzyk, D., 314–315, 317, 471
Katz, S., 210, 214–215
Keel, K. G., 274
Keer, D., 198, 221, 237
Keeter, S., 101
Kehoe, R., 60
Keith, R. A., 211
Keller, D. M., 197
Keller, S. D., 46, 68, 207
Keller, W. J., 93
Kendall, P. L., 296
Keppel, K. G., 470, 477
Kerwin, J., 186
Khare, M., 318
Khurshid, A., 47
Kiecolt, K. J., 8, 100, 105
Kiesler, S., 95, 105
Kim, J., 62, 67
Kim, J. H., 41, 72, 90, 348
Kindel, K. K., 94, 107
King, G., 126
Kirshner, B., 214, 215, 216
Kish, L., 31, 120, 128, 137, 142, 169
Kitchens, L. J., 349
Klar, J., 144, 152, 155, 161, 176
Klecka, W. R., 104
Kleinbaum, D. G., 77, 90, 336, 349

Klinger, M. R., 234
Knäuper, B., 253
Knoke, D., 349
Koegel, P., 97, 133
Koester, D. R., 286
Kohlmeier, L., 233
Kohn, R., 467, 474
Korn, E. L., 176
Kosinski, M., 46, 68, 207, 257, 259
Kovar, M. G., 110, 197
Kraemer, H. C., 144, 155, 176
Krause, N. M., 213
Kreft, I.G.G., 176
Kremer, B., 137, 472, 478
Kressel, S., 207
Kristal, A. R., 100
Kroeger, A., 468
Krosnick, J. A., 247, 251, 252–253, 254
Krueger, R. A., 185
Krysan, M., 102
Kulka, R. A., 105, 108, 284
Kulp, D., 127
Kupper, L. L., 70, 77, 90, 259, 336, 349
Kutner, M. H., 343
Kvig, F. J., 165

Lakner, E., 132
Lancashire, J., 72
Landis, J. R., 318
Lang, D. A., 102
Lannom, L., 233–234
Lanphier, C. M., 20
Lapham, R. J., 468
Larson, C. O., 259
Larson, J. S., 211, 221
Larson, L. N., 260
Last, J. M., 28, 30
Laumann, E. O., 472
Lavizzo-Mourey, R. J., 255
Lavrakas, P. J., 132, 304
Lazarsfeld, P., 76, 90
Leahy, A., 260
Leclercq, M. H., 467, 474
Lee, E. S., 162, 327, 349
Lee, G., 97–98
Lee, R. M., 236, 242
Lee-Han, H., 233
Lemeshow, S., 124, 142, 144, 152, 155, 161, 176, 343, 468
Lepkowski, J. M., 126, 127, 286, 318
Leske, M. C., 60
Lessler, J. T., 22, 94, 105, 108, 180, 184, 185, 186, 199
Letterie, G. S., 95
Levine, A. M., 245
Levine, M. N., 216
Levy, J. A., 41, 72, 90, 348, 399, 479
Levy, P. S., 142
Lewis, C. E., 245
Lewis, J. R., 256
Li, L., 126
Linder-Pelz, S., 257
Link, M. W., 101, 284
Lipkind, K. L., 470, 476
Lipsey, M. W., 144, 154, 155, 159n, 176
Little, E. L., 286

Little, R.J.A., 315, 317, 318
Liu, P. W., 284
Liu, W. T., 226
Liyanage, W. M., 124, 468
Locander, W. B., 228, 229
Lochner, T., 245
Loevy, S. S., 137, 472, 478
Loft, J. D., 286
Loftus, E. F., 184, 186, 233, 234
Lohr, K. N., 211
Loosveldt, G., 295
Lorimor, R. J., 162, 327
LoSciuto, L. A., 242
Lu, J.F.R., 46, 56, 57, 68, 207
Lusk, E. J., 286
Lussier, R., 468, 474
Lwanga, S. K., 144, 152, 155, 161, 176
Lyberg, L. E., 22, 180, 183, 184, 196, 199, 304
Lyttle, C. S., 218, 467, 474

MacKeigan, L. D., 260
Madhok, R., 105
Madow, W. G., 315
Madron, T. W., 306
Magaziner, J., 202, 288
Magilavy, L. J., 287
Mai, H. P., 255
Maisel, R., 142
Makkai, T., 240
Makuc, D. M., 231
Malec, D., 9
Mangione, T. W., 105, 187, 293, 295, 304
Marcus, A. C., 100, 102, 103, 104
Marin, B. V., 197, 198
Marin, G., 110, 197, 198
Marker, D. A., 9, 138
Marks, R. G., 149, 151
Markus, H., 183
Marlowe, D., 252
Marmor, T. R., 201
Marquis, K. H., 182, 259
Marsh, C., 275
Marshall, G. N., 259
Martin, E., 181, 191, 226
Martin, J., 108, 240
Mason, R., 255
Massey, J. T., 98, 226, 284
Massey, M. M., 471
Mathers, C. D., 208
Mathiowetz, N. A., 22, 106, 180, 183, 184, 196, 199, 287–288, 304, 318
Matthews, K. A., 260
Mattson, M., 471
Mays, V. M., 241
McAllister, I., 240
McCall, L. A., 22
McCallum, A., 105
McClendon, M. J., 251, 269
McCormick, L., 5–6
McDaniel, C., 260
McDowell, I., 211, 213, 219, 221
McEwan, R. T., 105
McEwen, J., 207
McGinnis, J. M., 471

McGraw, S. A., 302
McGuigan, K., 245
McGuire, V., 233
McHorney, C. A., 46, 56, 57, 61, 62, 68, 71, 74, 207, 259
McKenna, S. P., 207
McKillip, J., 201
McKinlay, J. B., 302
McLeroy, K. R., 5–6
McNeil, B. J., 213, 256
McNeill, D. N., 259
Means, B., 233
Mechanic, D., 5
Megivern, K., 260
Mendenhall, W., 142
Menon, G., 288
Merkle, D. M., 132
Merton, R. K., 296
Meterko, M., 259
Meyers, E. D., Jr., 310
Michael, R. T., 472
Michaels, S., 472
Milburn, M. A., 257
Milgrom, P., 41, 72, 90, 110, 249, 345, 346, 348, 479
Miller, D. C., 43, 95
Miller, P. V., 106, 295, 304
Mingay, D. J., 184, 186, 197, 231, 232, 233, 272
Mishler, E. G., 179, 202, 295–296
Mishra, S. I., 100
Mitchell, A., 216
Mitchell, J. A., 31
Mitra, A., 133
Mizes, J. S., 286
Mohadjer, L., 126, 128, 135
Molenaar, N. J., 180
Molinek, F. R., Jr., 204
Monheit, A. C., 162
Monroe, K. B., 287
Mooney, L. A., 233
Moore, J. C., 182, 186, 197, 288
Moore, R. P., 290
Moore, R. W., 240
Moreno, C., 220
Morgan, D. L., 185
Morgenstern, H., 77, 90, 336, 349
Morgenstern, L. L., 95
Morgenstern, O., 203
Morris, J. R., 207
Morrow, R. H., 208
Morton-Williams, J., 187
Mosely, R. R., II, 287–288
Moser, C. A., 292
Moskowitz, R. W., 215
Mueller, C. W., 62, 67
Muhlbaier, L. H., 207
Mullen, P., 240
Mullen, P. D., 286
Müller, G., 232
Mulley, A. G., Jr., 210
Mullinex, C. F., 469
Mulvihill, M., 197
Murphy, P. A., 197, 198, 237
Murray, D. M., 31
Myers, D. H., 260

Nachmias, C., 349
Nachmias, D., 349
Nash, J. G., 260
Nathan, L. E., 8
Nederhof, A. J., 286
Nelson, E. C., 201, 202, 207, 259
Neter, J., 343
Newell, C., 211, 213, 219, 221
Newhouse, J. P., 259
Newman, R., 133
Nicholls, W. L., II, 94, 100, 105, 107, 108, 273
Nichols, J. S., 132
Nisselson, H., 315
Nixon, S. A., 286
Noelle-Neumann, E., 253
Norman, G. R., 62, 221
Norris, A., 242
Norusis, M. J., 56, 73, 74
Nunnally, J. C., 50, 51, 55, 56, 57, 58, 62, 67, 70, 260, 326

O'Brien, K., 185
O'Hara, D., 110
Oishi, S. M., 304
Oksenberg, L., 187, 291, 295, 304
Oldendick, R. W., 101, 247, 250, 284
Olkin, I., 315
Olson, J. G., 468
O'Malley, P. M., 250
O'Muircheartaigh, C. A., 108, 232, 253
Oppenheim, A. N., 260
O'Reilly, J. M., 94, 105
O'Rourke, D., 109, 132
Orth-Gomer, K., 211
Orwin, R. G., 241
O'Shea, M., 240
Ostrow, D. G., 41, 348, 479
Ott, L., 142

Palit, C., 93
Pao, E. M., 477
Papp, E., 207
Parkerson, G. R., Jr., 207
Parsons, J. A., 109, 291
Parsons, P. E., 185
Pasanella, A., 76, 90
Pascoe, G. C., 257
Passel, J. S., 226
Paton, D., 187
Patrick, D. L., 14, 72, 202, 204, 205n, 207, 208, 210, 211, 214, 221
Paul, J. E., 472
Paxson, M. C., 283
Payne, S. L., 180, 193, 194, 251
Peck, J. K., 286
Pennell, B. E., 286
Perez-Stable, E. J., 110
Perkins, R. C., 226
Perneger, T. V., 286
Perron, S., 94
Persell, C. H., 142
Peterson, J. R., 259
Peterson, R. A., 224, 241
Phipps, P. A., 94, 274
Piazza, T., 284

Pierson, S. A., 284
Pierzchala, M., 94, 312
Piper, H., 94
Placek, P. J., 470, 477
Polissar, L., 319
Polivka, A. E., 471
Pollard, W. E., 207
Pope, G. C., 213, 218
Potthoff, R. F., 127
Prescott, P. A., 55
Presser, S., 180, 182, 185, 188, 193, 196, 248, 249, 250, 251, 253, 255
Prohaska, T. R., 41, 72, 90, 348, 479
Puska, P., 468, 474

Rabkin, J. G., 211
Raczek, A. E., 46, 61, 62, 68, 207
Rados, D. L., 287
Rao, J. N. K., 176
Rasinski, K. A., 255, 272, 278
Redman, S., 233
Reeder, L. G., 104
Reese, S. D., 290
Regier, D. A., 473, 478
Remington, P. L., 472
Revicki, D. A., 204
Rhoads, M., 93
Rhodes, I. N., 286
Rhodes, P. J., 302
Richardson, J. L., 245
Richardson, W. C., 43, 63, 74
Ricketts, T., 260
Rips, L. J., 277
Rizek, R. L., 477
Roberts, J. G., 70
Roberts, R. E., 257
Robertson, K. W., 274
Robine, J. M., 208
Robins, L. N., 473, 478
Robinson, D., 468
Rodgers, W. L., 100, 197
Rogers, H. J., 71, 74
Rogers, P. L., 22
Rogers, T. F., 104, 245
Rogers, W. H., 259
Roman, A. M., 105
Romans, S., 240
Roos, C., 286
Rosen, R. J., 94
Rosenberg, M., 76, 90
Rosner, B., 339, 349
Ross, C. K., 257
Ross, D. A., 468
Rossi, P. H., 43
Rothgeb, J. M., 471
Rothman, M. L., 211, 214
Rougemont, A., 286
Rowe, E. G., 94–95
Royston, P. N., 136, 186
Rubin, D. B., 315, 317, 318
Rubin, H. J., 186
Rubin, H. R., 259
Rubin, I. S., 186
Rutten-van Mölken, M.P.M.H., 210
Ryaboy, L., 318
Ryder, J., 260

Saalfeld, A., 126
Safran, D. G., 259
Sahai, H., 47
Salant, P., 95, 110, 111, 199, 251, 262, 263, 269, 274, 280, 283, 284, 285, 286, 301, 303, 304
Salmon, C. T., 132
Salovey, P., 221
Saltzman, A., 95
Sanderson, M., 470, 477
Sangster, R. L., 111
Sanson-Fisher, R. W., 233
Saris, W. E., 92, 93, 94, 95, 106, 108, 111, 263, 273, 280, 302, 306, 321
Sasao, T., 133
Scardina, S. A., 260
Schaeffer, N. C., 242, 290
Schafer, J. L., 318
Scheaffer, R. L., 142
Schechter, S., 185, 197, 221
Schoen, F., 70, 259
Schofield, P., 257
Schrodt, P. A., 306
Schuler, R. H., 110
Schuman, H., 20, 22, 102, 180, 182, 193, 196, 248, 249, 250, 251, 253, 255, 286
Schur, C. L., 226, 469
Schwarz, N., 3, 6, 22, 105, 180, 184, 196, 197, 231, 232, 248, 253, 254, 255, 277, 278, 303
Schweitzer, J. C., 284
Scott, L. J., 102
Sebestik, J. P., 129
Sedransk, J., 9
Sellers, C., 10
Selvin, H., 76, 90
Sempos, C. T., 349
Senf, J. H., 68, 260
Serxner, S., 100
Shadmon, D., 287
Shamdasani, P. N., 185
Shanks, J. M., 93, 100, 105
Sharp, H., 93
Sheatsley, P. B., 180, 286
Sheps, C. G., 472
Sherbourne, C. D., 46, 49, 56, 57, 68, 207, 257, 259
Shevell, S. K., 277
Shiloh, S., 257
Ship, I. I., 467
Shoeb, H., 260
Shoemaker, P. J., 290
Shortell, S. M., 43, 63, 64, 74
Siegmann, A. E., 211
Siemiatycki, J., 104
Sievert, Y. A., 233
Simon, H. A., 186
Simonsick, E. M., 288
Simpson, G., 221
Simpson, R. L., Jr., 204
Sinacore, J. M., 257
Sinclair, M. D., 263
Singer, E., 104, 245
Sirken, M. G., 133, 137, 184
Sirotnik, K. A., 31

Skinner, E. A., 202
Skinner, S. J., 286
Smailes, E., 95
Smead, R. J., 284
Smith, A. F., 221, 231, 232, 233
Smith, D. L., 124, 468
Smith, G. S., 468
Smith, J. E., 22
Smith, K. D., 234
Smith, S. S., 72, 462
Smith, T. W., 100, 179, 226, 253, 295
Smith, V., 226
Snow, B., 460
Snow, K. K., 46, 68, 207
Snowden, C. B., 136
Snyder, M. K., 259
Soeken, K. L., 55
Sörbom, D., 343
Sorensen, J., 202
Spaeth, J. L., 109
Spaeth, M. A., 94
Sparkman, R. D., Jr., 188
Spector, P. E., 74
Sperry, S., 30, 106, 471, 475
Spilker, B. 204
Spitzer, W. O., 207
Sproull, L. S., 95, 105
Stange, K. C., 5
Stanley, J. C., 31, 42, 43
Starer, A., 127
Starfield, B., 41
Steckler, A., 5–6
Stehouwer, S. A., 318
Steinwachs, D. M., 202
Stephens, T., 471
Steward, C. A., 257
Stewart, A. L., 46, 49, 53, 58, 61, 63, 68,
     69, 201, 207, 211, 473, 479
Stewart, D. W., 8, 185, 286, 287
Stoddart, G. L., 201
Stouthamer-Loeber, M., 304
Strack, F., 105, 197, 232, 255
Straf, M. L., 183
Strasser, S., 257
Streiner, D. L., 62, 221
Stroh, G., Jr., 124
Stussman, B. J., 186, 197
Suchman, E. A., 10
Suchman, L., 179, 295
Sudman, S., 3, 6, 22, 24, 109, 133, 136,
     137, 180, 181, 183, 184, 196, 197,
     199, 224, 231, 233–234, 236, 237,
     238, 239, 240, 242, 244, 246, 247,
     248, 249, 250, 251, 252, 253, 254,
     255, 262, 263, 270, 275, 277, 278,
     280, 286, 288, 303, 304, 469
Sugrue, N. M., 41, 72, 90, 348, 399,
     479
Sullivan, L. M., 71
Susser, M., 26, 27
Swain, L., 180
Swaminathan, H., 71, 74
Sykes, W., 187

Taber, S., 343

Talmon, J. L., 95
Tanur, J. M., 20, 22, 24, 180, 183, 184,
     186
Tarlov, A. R., 259
Tarnai, J., 283
Tate, C. N., 306
Taylor, L., 255
Tedin, K. L., 286
Telesky, C. W., 100
Temoshok, L., 245
Thiemann, S., 144, 155, 176
Thompson, S. J., 259
Thornberry, O. T., 90, 98, 359, 470
Thornton, A., 186
Thran, S. L., 318
Tillinghast, D. S., 253
Tilson, H. H., 204
Tompkins, L., 9
Torrance, G. W., 205n, 207, 208, 209,
     210, 217
Tortora, R. D., 94
Tourangeau, R., 183, 230, 231, 232,
     236, 244, 255, 278
Tracy, P. E., 240, 241
Traub, R. E., 50
Trevino, F. M., 226
Trewin, D., 97–98
Trunzo, D. H., 136, 185
Tse, C.K.J., 207
Tuchfarber, A. J., 104, 247, 250
Tuckel, P. S., 101, 284
Tucker, C., 127
Tugwell, P., 70
Tupek, A. R., 94
Turk, D. C., 221
Turnbull, D., 257
Turner, C. F., 94, 105, 181, 191
Turner, J. T., 260
Twaddle, A. C., 212

Uebersax, J., 202
Umesh, U. N., 241
Unden, A., 211

van der Linden, S., 210
Van der Zouwen, J., 187
van Doorslaer, E.K.A., 210
van Kammen, W. B., 304
Vanoss, B., 110
Vaughan, J. P., 468
Vaughn, C. M., 242
Verbrugge, L. M., 16, 39, 221, 236
Vigderhous, G., 283
Vincent, C., 22
Vismans, F.J.F.E., 95
von Neumann, J., 203
Von Thurn, D. R., 186, 197
Voss, D. S., 126

Wagner, E. H., 207
Waksberg, J., 127, 128, 133, 138, 139
Walker, J. T., 95
Wall, D., 126
Wallace, R. B., 201
Wallston, B. S., 12

Ware, J. E., Jr., 46, 49, 53, 56, 57, 58,
     61, 62, 63, 68, 69, 71, 74, 201, 204,
     207, 211, 257, 259, 473, 479
Warnecke, R. B., 109, 291
Warner, S. L., 240
Wasserman, W., 343
Wasson, J., 202
Weeks, M. F., 105, 284, 290
Weeks, R. A., 105, 108
Wegener, D. H., 109, 196, 307
Weinberg, E., 289, 291, 292, 293, 296
Weiss, B. D., 68, 260
Wells, K. B., 259
Westermeyer, J., 226
Westoff, C. F., 468
Wheeler, J. R., 64
White, A. A., 167
White, C. C., 471
White, K. L., 467, 474
Whitmore, R. W., 105, 108
Whitney, C., 110
Wickizer, T. M., 64
Wilcox, J., 284
Wilcox, J. B., 188
Wilensky, G. R., 8, 471
Wilkin, D., 211
Williams, B., 256
Williams, J., 207
Willimack, D. K., 286
Willis, G. B., 186, 197, 221
Wilson, I. B., 213
Wilson, R. W., 31, 90, 215, 469, 470
Winglee, M., 318
Winter, D.L.S., 94
Witt, K., 95
Wolf, L. L., 94
Wolinsky, F. D., 287–288
Wood-Dauphinee, S., 207
Woods, T., 124, 468
Wooldridge, J., 257, 259n
Word, D. L., 226
Wright, D. B., 108, 232, 253
Wright, R. A., 236
Wright, W. R., 259
Wu, A. W., 202
Wu, S. Y., 60
Wunderlich, G. S., 470, 471

Xanthopoulos, J. A., 162
Xu, M., 284

Yammarino, F. J., 286
Yankauer, A., 226
Yokopenic, P. A., 105
Yu, E.S.H., 226
Yu, J., 286

Zaig, T., 287
Zajonc, R. B., 183
Zeisel, H., 76, 90
Zeller, R. A., 51, 54n, 56, 57, 58, 63
Zimmerman, R., 41, 197
Zinn, J., 255
Zorn, J., 245
Zyzanski, S. J., 5, 259

SUBJECT INDEX

Access Impact Evaluation Surveys, 472, 478

Accuracy, in sample design, 121

Advance notice, implementing, 282–283

Agency for Health Care Policy and Research: addresses for, 464, 465; conferences by, 22, 462, 465; funding by, 202; and large-scale surveys, 8, 235, 470–471, 473, 477; and satisfaction, 256. *See also* National Center for Health Services Research

Agency for International Development (AID), 468

Aided recall, for behavior questions, 234–235

AIDS Cost and Services Utilization Survey (ACSUS), 473

AIDS survey. *See* Chicago Area General Population Survey on AIDS

Alameda County Human Population Laboratory Study, 41, 472, 478

Alternative hypothesis (Ha): and data analysis, 327; and sample size, 152–154

American Hospital Association, 469, 474

American Medical Association, 469, 474

American Psychiatric Association, 61

American Psychological Association, 50, 58

American Statistical Association, 5, 8, 20, 462, 465

Americans with Disabilities Act of 1990, 16, 39

Analytical designs: characteristics of, 27, 29, 35; data analysis for, 334, 345; example of, 40–41; hypotheses for, 36, 38–39; and internal validity, 42; question for, 32–33, 34; sample size for, 147, 152–161

Annual Survey of Hospitals, 474

Anonymity: in data collection methods, 105; in future, 5; for threatening questions, 240–241

Area probability sample, procedures for, 123–126, 135, 138–139, 140–141

AT&T, computer-assisted interviewing for, 93

Attitude questions: aspects of, 247–256; and error issues, 260; examples of, 256–260; highlights on, 243–244; phrases in, 248–249; and population issues, 256; questionnaires for, 255, 277; responses to, 250–255; scales for strength of, 252–255; sentences for, 249–250; sources on, 260; words in, 248

Australia, software from, 301

Balance, in phrases, 193–194

Behavior coding, for question design, 187

Behavior questions: aspects of, 230–241; bounded recall for, 233–234; and cognitive psychology, 231–233; and error issues, 242; examples for, 242; highlights on, 222–223; memory aids for, 234–236; nonthreatening, 230–236; and overreporting and underreporting errors, 230–231; and population issues, 241–242; sources on, 242; threatening, 236–241

Behavioral Risk Factor Surveys, 472, 478

Bell Communications Research (BCR), BELLCORE of, 126, 127

Benefit versus harm, ethical issues of, 4–5

Bias errors: concept of, 22–23; of noncoverage and nonresponse, 101–102

Birthday method, last or next, 132–133

Bivariate statistics, for data analysis, 327, 333–339, 345–346

Boston, outcomes study in, 46

Bounded recall, for behavior questions, 233–234

Budget. *See* Costs

Burden, concept of, 71

California at Berkeley, University of, research organization at, 9, 110

California at Los Angeles, University of, and computer-assisted interviewing, 93

Canada: surveys in, 468, 474; telephone coverage in, 97

Canadian National Population Health Survey, 474

Capture-recapture method, for sampling mobile populations, 137

Case-control studies. *See* Group-comparison designs

Case studies, use of, 7

Category scaling methods, for health questions, 208

Center for Health Administration Studies, 235

Centers for Disease Control and Prevention (CDC): addresses for, 464, 465; and conferences, 462; and National Center for Health Statistics, 138, 359; and software, 162; studies by, 399, 470, 471, 472, 478

Central Bureau of Statistics, 301

Central tendency, measures of, 331–332

Chicago: Comprehensive AIDS Prevention/Education Program (CAPEP) in, 399; outcomes study in, 46

Chicago, University of: Center for Health Administration Studies at, 467, 469, 475; research organization at, 9, 466; researcher at, 303; total survey error framework at, 22

Chicago Area General Population Survey on AIDS: aspects of, 16–17, 479; attitude questions for, 248, 251; behavior questions for, 230, 235, 237–240, 242; data analysis for, 329–331, 336–337, 348; data collection methods for, 110; data preparation for, 321; demographic questions for, 225, 227–229; design of, 40–41;

implementation of, 285, 289, 293, 298–301, 302; knowledge questions for, 245–246; question design for, 198; questionnaire for, 263, 269, 270, 271, 272, 274, 276, 279, 399–441; questions for, 67, 72; sample design for, 132, 139–142; sample size for, 175

Chilton Research Services, 9, 93

Chunk sample, 116

Clarity, of words, 191, 193

Cleaning data, in data preparation, 313–314

Clinical practice assessment, 202

Clinometric norms, for health questions, 203

Closed-end questions, 195, 196, 306–307, 311

Cluster sample: procedures for, 120–121, 123; and sample size, 161–162

Coding, in data preparation, 306–310

Coefficient alpha reliability, 52, 55, 56–57

Cognitive Aspects of Survey Methodology (CASM), 182–183, 184

Cognitive psychology: and behavior questions, 231–233; in future, 3; and implementation, 288, 296; and knowledge and attitude questions, 243–244; and question design, 182–184; and questionnaire format, 277, 278

Cold-deck imputation, 315–316

Committee on National Statistics, 182

Commonwealth Fund, 257, 471

Community Hospital Program, 472, 478

Community needs assessment, 201

Complexity, in sample design, 121

Computer-assisted data collection (CADAC): and implementation, 285, 292, 301–302; and questionnaire format, 262, 263, 269, 275

Computer-assisted data entry (CADE), 308, 310, 312–313, 314

Computer-assisted personal interviews (CAPI), for data collection, 94, 103, 106, 110

Computer-assisted self-interviewing (CASI), for data collection, 94–95, 99, 104, 105

Computer Assisted Survey Methods, 301

Computer-assisted telephone interviews (CATI): for data collection, 93–94, 106–107, 109, 110; and follow-up contacts, 285

Computer interviewing by mail (CIM), 95

Computerized techniques: for data collection, 93–95, 103–107, 109–110; and data preparation, 305–308, 310–314, 321; in future, 3–4, 5; for implementation, 285, 292, 301–302; and questionnaires, 262, 263, 269, 275

Concurrent validity, in questions, 59, 60–61

Confidentiality, in future, 5

Confounding variables, 80–81

Connecticut, University of, Roper Center for Public Opinion Research at, 462, 466

Construct validity: for health questions, 210; in questions, 59, 61–63; and response effects, 182

Consumers, of survey results, 9–10

Content validity: for health questions, 210, 219; in questions, 58, 59, 62

Context: and question design, 184; for questionnaires, 278–279

Contingency checking, 313–314

Continuing Survey of Food Intake by Individuals, 477

Continuous Quality Improvement (CQI), 22

Control or test variables, 76, 89

Convergent validity, in questions, 59, 61–62

Corrected item-total reliability, 52, 55, 56

Costs: of data collection, 108–109; and implementation, 299–301; and pretesting, 190; and sample size, 164–165; and small budgets, 7–8

Coverage, and sampling, 97–99

Criterion validity: in questions, 59, 60–61, 62; and response effects, 181–182

Cross-sectional designs: characteristics of, 27, 28–29; data analysis for, 328; example of, 40–41; and external validity, 43; and health questions, 214; hypotheses for, 36; and internal validity, 42; question for, 33; sample size for, 146, 147–151; target population for, 114

Cumulative scales, 69

Current Employment Statistics Survey, 95

Current Population Surveys (CPS), 8, 224, 227, 471

Dartmouth Function Charts, 206–207

Data analysis: aspects of, 322–349; bivariate statistics for, 327, 333–339, 345–346; and data preparation, 319–320; descriptive or inferential, 326–327; and error issues, 348; examples of, 348; highlights on, 322–323; measurement matrix for, 323–326, 345; mock tables for, 347; multivariate statistics for, 327, 339–343; nonparametric, 327, 334–337, 339–341; parametric, 327, 337–339, 342–343; plan for, 343–346; and population issues, 347; preparing for, 107–108; procedures reviewed for, 326–329; in research report, 355, 358; sources on, 349; and turnaround speed, 108; univariate statistics for, 327, 329–333, 345

Data collection: aspects of methods for, 91–111; availability of methods for, 92–93; comparisons of, 95–109; computerized, 93–95; costs of, 108–109; criteria for, 92–93; and error issues, 111; examples of, 110; for health questions, 219; highlights on, 91–92; implementation of, 106–107, 281–304; and population issues, 109–110; pretesting, 189–190; questionnaires for, 105–106, 261–280; in research report, 354–355, 357; sampling for, 97–103; sources on, 111

Data preparation: aspects of, 305–321; cleaning in, 313–314; coding in, 306–310; and data analysis, 319–320; entering data for, 310–313; and error issues, 321; estimation for, 318; examples of, 321; highlights on, 305–306; and imputation, 314–318; and population issues, 320–321; pretesting, 190; and questionnaire format, 275; in research report, 355, 358; sources on, 321

Deductive imputation, 315

Demographic and Health Surveys (DHS), 468

Demographic questions: on age and sex, 224–225; aspects of, 223–229; on education, 227; on employment, 227–228; and error issues, 242; examples for, 242; format for, 272–273, 276–277; highlights on, 222–223; on household composition, 223–224; on income, 228–229; on marital status, 225; on occupation, 228; and population issues, 241–242; on race and ethnicity, 225–227; sources on, 242

Dentists. See Washington State Study of Dentists' Preferences. . .

Descriptive designs: characteristics of, 27, 35; data analysis for, 345; example of, 40; hypotheses for, 36, 38; question for, 32–33; sample size for, 144–152

Design: aspects of matching with objectives, 25–43; and error issues, 42–43; examples of, 39–41; health questions related to, 214–216; highlights on, 25–26; objectives and hypotheses stated for, 35–39; observational, 26–30; probability, 115–121; question stated for, 31–35; in research report, 354, 356; and sample size, 144; sources on, 43; types of, 26–31. See also Analytical; Cross-sectional; Descriptive; Experimental; Group-comparison; and Longitudinal designs

Design effects: on data collection, 102–103; formula for, 161; and sample size, 161–164

Diagnostic Interview Schedule, 61, 473

Diaries, for behavior questions, 235–236

Disability, concept of, 213

Dispersion measures, 332–333

Discriminant validity, in questions, 59, 61–62
Disproportionate sampling: for rare populations, 134, 135; weighting for, 169–170
Distance function matching, 317
Documentation: for coding, 308–310; of field procedures, 289
Donnelly Marketing Information Services, 126
Double-barreled questions, 194, 249
Dual-frame sampling, for rare populations, 134, 136–137
Duke Health Profile, 206–207
Dummy variables, 319–320

Economic norms, for health questions, 203, 204
Edge-coding, 310
Efficiency, in sample design, 121
Electronic mail, for data collection, 95
Eligibility proportions, and sample size, 164, 165–167
Entering data, for data preparation, 310–313
Environmental characteristics, 12
Epidemiological Catchment Area Surveys, 473, 478
Epidemiological Follow-Up Study, 469
Epidemiology: and designing surveys, 26, 28–31, 37, 41, 43; and health questions, 201–202; and testing hypotheses, 77
Equivalence, and reliability, 50
Errors: aspects of, 20–23; and attitude questions, 260; and behavior and demographic questions, 242; and data analysis, 348; and data collection, 111; and data preparation, 321; and design, 42–43; and health questions, 221; and implementation, 303–304; of overreporting and underreporting, 230–231; and question design, 179–182, 199; and questionnaires, 279–280; and questions, 73; in research report, 356–358; and response effects, 181; and sample design, 142; and sample size, 175–176; scale, 69; sources of, 179–182; and topics, 20–23; Type I and Type II, 153–154; types of, 21–23; and variables, 90. *See also* Standard error
Estimation, for data preparation, 318
Ethics: in experimental designs, 31; in future, 4–5
Ethnographic interviewing, for question design, 185–186
Euronut SENECA Investigators, 468, 477
European Quality of Life Index, 206–207
EuroQol Group, 207, 208
Expansion weights, 169–171
Expenditures, and population characteristics, 14–15

Experimental designs: characteristics of, 26, 27–28, 30–31, 35; data analysis for, 345; example of, 40–41; and external validity, 43; and health questions, 201, 215–216; hypotheses for, 36, 38; and internal validity, 42; question for, 33, 34; sample size for, 147, 152–161
Explanation, of variables, 79, 80–82
External validity, and design, 42–43
Extraneous variables, 80–81

FAX, 94, 95
Field procedures: documentation of, 289; for implementation, 282–289; supervising, 296–298
Finland, health surveys in, 468, 474
Flinn Foundation, 471
Florida, telephone interviews in, 105
Flowchart, for questionnaire order, 278
Focus groups, for question design, 185
Follow-up contacts, implementing, 284–286, 298
Foot-in-the-door technique, 287
Forced choice: in attitude questions, 250–251; for lists, 272
Format, for questionnaires, 262–275
Framingham Study, 473, 478
Frequencies, in data analysis, 329–331
Functioning and Well Being Profile (FWBP), 206–207

Gallup polls, 9, 462, 471
General Accounting Office (GAO), 12, 201
Generalizability, for questions, 72
GENESYS, 127
Geographic information systems (GIS), 126
Government Information Exchange, 464
Grammatik IV, 193
Group-comparison designs: characteristics of, 27–28, 29; data analysis for, 328, 333, 345; and external validity, 43; and health questions, 214–215; hypotheses for, 36; and internal validity, 42; question for, 33; sample size for, 146, 148, 151–152, 155–160; target population for, 114
Group Health Association of America (GHAA), 257, 258–259
Group interviews, for question design, 185
Guttman scale, for questions, 66, 67, 68–69

Hagan and Collier method, 129, 132
Handicap, concept of, 213
Harris polls, 462, 471
Health, concepts of, 13, 211–214
Health and Nutrition Examination Survey, 212
Health Belief Model, 41
Health Care Financing Administration, 30, 470, 471, 475
Health care system characteristics, 12–13

Health Care Technology Assessment, 443
Health Hazard Appraisal (HHA), 472
Health Insurance Experiment (HIE), 31, 201, 206–207, 473, 478
Health Plan Employer Data and Information System (HEDIS), 201
Health plan surveys, 201
Health questions: aspects of, 200–221; and conceptual issues, 211–214; criteria for, 202–204; data collection for, 219; design and objectives related to, 214–216; and error issues, 221; examples of, 221; highlights on, 200–202; number of, 217–218; phrasing, 220; and population issues, 220–221; reliability for, 210, 218; and sample design, 219–220; scales matched to, 216–218; sources on, 221; steps in creating, 210–220; utility-related scaling methods for, 204–210, 217; validity for, 210, 218–219
Health-related quality of life (HRQOL), and health questions, 201, 204, 208, 209
Health Risk Appraisal (HRA), 472
Health status, and population characteristics, 13–14
Health surveys: applications of, 201–202; computerized databases on, 461–462, 464; concept of, 1, 10; conferences on, 462, 465; data analysis for, 322–349; data archives on, 462, 465–466; data collection methods for, 91–111; data preparation for, 305–321; defining and clarifying variables for, 44–74; defining features of, 5–7; design for, 25–43; examples of, 15–17, 467–479; future, 2–5; implementation of, 106–107, 281–304; international, 458–468, 474; Internet sources on, 462, 464–465; journals on, 3, 9, 461, 463–464; large-scale, 8; map of, 18; national, 468–472, 474–477; question design for, 177–260; questionnaires for, 261–280; reasons for studying, 7–10; report on, 350–358; sample design for, 112–142; sample size for, 143–176; sources on, 461–466; by states and localities, 472–473, 478–479; steps in designing and conducting, 17–20; topics for, 1–24; variables related in, 75–90
Health Utilities Index (HUI), 206–207, 211
Hierarchical imputation, 317
Hispanic Health and Nutrition Examination Survey (HHANES), 469, 475
Hispanic subgroups, and demographic questions, 226
HIV Cost and Services Utilization Study (HCSUS), 473
Hot-deck imputation, 316–317
Hungary, telephone coverage in, 97

Hypotheses: alternative and null, 152–154, 327; concept of, 35, 37; examples of, 40; one- or two-tailed, 154, 159; stated, 35–39; and variables, 76–86

Illinois, University of, 303. *See also* Survey Research Laboratory
Impairment, concept of, 213
Implementation: aspects of, 281–304; and budget, 299–301; and computer-assisted data collection, 285, 292, 301–302; and error issues, 303–304; examples of, 302–303; field procedures for, 282–289; highlights on, 281–282; and interviewer hiring, 289–292; and interviewer training, 293–296; and management, 298–301; and population issues, 302; sources on, 304; and supervision, 296–298
Imputation of missing values: in data preparation, 314–318; need for, 107–108
Incentives, to respondents, 5, 286–287
Index of Independence in Activities of Daily Living, 214–215
Indexes, for questions, 64–65
Informed consent, in future, 4
Institute of Medicine, 41, 470
Instructions: criteria for, 196; formatting, 270–271; for threatening questions, 239
Interaction or effect modification, of variables, 84–85
Internal consistency reliability, 51, 52, 54, 55–58
Internal validity, and design, 42
International Collaborative Study of Medical Care Utilization, 467, 474
International Study of Dental Manpower Systems in Relation to Oral Health Status, 467, 474
Interpretability: concept of, 71; of variables, 79, 82–84
Inter-rater reliability, 51, 52, 54, 55
Inter-University Consortium for Political and Social Research, 465
Interval or ratio procedures: in data analysis, 337–338, 341; in questions, 48–50
Intervening variables, 82–83
Interviewers: field coding by, 308; and gender differences, 290; hiring, 289–292; observing, 297; physical characteristics of, 289–291; social, personal, and behavioral characteristics of, 291–292; supervising, 296–298; training, 293–296
Interviews: standardized, 295–296; validating, 297. *See also* Personal interviews; Telephone interviews
Iowa State University, Department of Statistics of, 162
Item response theory (IRT), and scales, 70–71, 74

Journals and publications, 3, 9, 461, 463–464

Kaiser Family Foundation, 471
Kish tables, 128–129, 130
Knowledge of AIDS Index, 72
Knowledge questions: aspects of, 244–247; highlights on, 243–244; phrasing, 245–246; and population issues, 256; questionnaire administration for, 246–247; responses to, 246

Laboratory and field experiments, for question design, 186–187
Likert scale, for questions, 66, 67–68
List-assisted frames, 126
List sample, procedures for, 127, 140, 142
Longitudinal designs: characteristics of, 27–28, 29–30; data analysis for, 328, 333–334, 345; example of, 39–40; and health questions, 215; hypotheses for, 36; and internal validity, 42; question for, 33, 34; sample size for, 146; target population for, 114
Longitudinal Study of Aging, 469
Los Angeles, outcomes study in, 46
Lottery procedure, for simple random sample, 118
Lou Harris Data Center, 465
Louis Harris and Associates, 9

Mail surveys: example of, 443–460; implementation of, 283, 284, 285–286, 288, 304. *See also* Self-administered questionnaires
Management, and implementation, 298–301
Marlowe-Crowne Social Desirability Scale, 251–252
Maryland, University of, 303
Mathematica Policy Research, 9
Mean, 332
Mean imputations, 316
Mean square error (MSE), formula for, 22–23
Measurement: of central tendencies, 331–332; of dispersion, 332–333; levels of, 47–50, 216–217; matrix for, 323–326, 345; in research report, 355, 357–358
Median, 331–332
Mediating variables, 82–83
Medical Care Satisfaction Questionnaire (MCSQ), 257, 258–259
Medical Outcomes Study (MOS): purpose of, 201, 473, 479; questions for, 46, 49; and reliability, 53, 56, 57–58; and satisfaction, 257; and scales, 68, 69, 71; and validity, 58, 61, 62, 63. *See also* Short-Form Health Survey
Medical Outcomes Trust, 71
Medicare Current Beneficiary Survey, 30, 471, 475
Memory aids, for behavior questions, 234–236

Mexico, telephone coverage in, 97
Michigan, University of: and implementation, 290, 295, 303; research organization at, 9, 465; and response rates, 100, 104, 180
Microtab Systems Pty Ltd., 301
Minnesota Heart Health Study, 468
Mixed procedures, in data analysis, 338–339, 341–343
Mock tables: for data analysis, 347; for variable analysis, 86–89
Mode, 331
Monetary incentives, 5, 286–287
Morbidity, concepts of, 212–213
Multiple frame sampling, 127
Multiple imputation, 317–318
Multiplicity sampling, 136
Multitrait multimethod approach (MTMM), 62, 63
Multivariate statistics, for data analysis, 327, 339–343

National Academy of Sciences, 181
National Ambulatory Medical Care Survey, 212, 470, 476
National Archives and Records Administration, 466
National Cancer Institute, 467
National Center for Health Services Research (NCHSR): and conferences, 22; and data collection, 97, 104; and implementation, 286, 295; and questions, 180; studies by, 443, 471, 477. *See also* Agency for Health Care Policy and Research
National Center for Health Statistics (NCHS): addresses for, 464, 466; and behavior questions, 233, 234, 235, 242; conferences by, 462; and data collection, 94, 98, 99, 100, 105, 110; and demographic questions, 226; and health questions, 212, 215, 217, 221; and implementation, 302; and knowledge and attitudes questions, 245; and large-scale surveys, 8, 13, 359, 469–470, 475–477; and question design, 184, 186, 187, 198; and secondary analyses, 9, 462. *See also* National Health Interview Survey
National Committee for Quality Assurance (NCQA), 12, 201, 257, 259, 473
National Employer Health Insurance Survey, 470
National Health and Nutrition Examination Survey (NHANES), 469, 475
National Health Care Survey (NHCS), 470, 476
National Health Interview Survey (NHIS): aspects of, 15–17; and behavior questions, 230–231, 233–234, 238, 239, 242; data analysis for, 348; data collection methods for, 97, 98, 100, 104, 105, 110; data preparation for, 308, 311, 313, 321; and demographic questions, 223–229; design

of, 30, 39–41; and health questions, 212, 215, 217–218, 221; implementation of, 282, 284, 287, 293–294, 302; and knowledge questions, 244–246; and question design, 183, 186, 198; questionnaire for, 272, 276, 277, 279, 359–398; questions for, 47, 50, 72; sample design for, 123, 135, 138–139, 140–141; sample size for, 174–175; uses of, 469, 470, 471, 475

National Health Promotion and Disease Prevention Survey, 470, 476

National Health Provider Inventory, 470

National Home and Hospice Care Survey, 470, 476

National Hospital Ambulatory Medical Care Survey, 470, 476

National Hospital Discharge Survey, 470, 476

National Household Survey Capability Programme, 468

National Immunization Survey, 470, 475

National Institute of Dental Research, 467

National Institute of Mental Health (NIMH), 471, 473, 478

National Institute on Drug Abuse, 471

National Institutes of Health, 464

National Library of Medicine, 461–462, 465

National Maternal and Infant Health Survey, 470, 477

National Medical Care Expenditure Survey (NMCES), 162, 233, 236, 290, 470, 471, 477

National Medical Care Utilization and Expenditure Survey, 470, 475

National Medical Expenditures Survey (NMES), 233, 236, 471, 477

National Mortality Followback Surveys, 470, 477

National Nursing Home Follow-Up Survey, 470

National Nursing Home Survey, 470, 476

National Opinion Research Center (NORC), 9, 466

National Science Foundation, 20, 182

National Survey of Ambulatory Surgery, 470, 476

National Survey of Family Growth, 470, 477

National Survey of Personal Health Practices and Consequences, 469, 475

National Technical Information Service, 466

Netherlands: public opinion polls in, 95; software from, 301

Network sampling, 134, 136

Neutral options, on attitude scales, 253–254

Nominal procedures: in data analysis, 334–336, 339; in questions, 47–49

Nonparametric data analysis, 327, 334–337, 339–341

Nonresponse or noncoverage: bias of, 101–102; weighting for, 172–173

North Carolina, University of, research organization at, 9, 465

North Karelia Project, 468, 474

Nottingham Health Profile (NHP), 206–207

Null hypothesis (Ho): and data analysis, 327; and sample size, 152–154, 155–161

Objectives: aspects of matching with design, 25–43; concept of study, 35; examples of, 40; health questions related to, 214–216

Objectives for Promoting Health and Preventing Disease, 469–470

Observation: of interviewers, 297; participant or nonparticipant, 6–7

Observational designs, characteristics of, 26–30

Odds ratio: in data analysis, 336; formula for, 77; and sample size, 160–161; and variables, 77–79, 81–82, 83, 85, 87

Office of Federal Statistical Policy and Standards, 225

Office of Management and Budget (OMB), 138, 190, 223, 225, 287, 462

One-group studies. See Cross-sectional designs

Open-ended questions, 103, 195–196, 307–308, 311

Operational definitions: for questions, 46–47; of target population, 114–115

Optical character recognition (OCR), 94, 312

Order, on questionnaires, 275–278

Ordinal procedures: in data analysis, 336–337, 339–341; in questions, 49–50

Organizations for research: choosing, 9; data archives from, 462, 465–466

Panel on Survey Measurement of Subjective Phenomena, 181

Panel surveys: bounded recall for, 233; characteristics of, 30

Paperwork Reduction Act of 1995, 287

Parametric data analysis, 327, 337–339, 341–343

Patient Comment Card (PCC), 257, 258–259

Patient Judgment system (PJS), 257, 258–259

Patient Outcomes Research Teams (PORTS), 202, 471

Patient Satisfaction Questionnaire (PSQ), 257, 258–259

Periodic Survey of Physicians, 469

Personal interviews: comparisons of, 96, 97, 99–100, 102–104, 106–110; computer-assisted, 94, 103, 106, 110; example of, 359–398; implementation of, 282, 284–285, 287–288, 290, 304; questionnaire formatting for, 262; rating scales for, 253; sample design for, 128–129

Phrases: in attitude questions, 248–249; criteria for, 193–194; in threatening questions, 237–238

Picker/Commonwealth Program for Patient-Centered Care, 257

Planning, for data analysis, 343–346

Populations: and attitude and knowledge questions, 256; and behavior and demographic questions, 241–242; characteristics of, 13–15; coverage of, 97–99; and data analysis, 347; and data collection, 109–110; and data preparation, 320–321; and design, 39; and health questions, 220–221; and implementation, 302; mobile, 137; and question design, 197–198; and questionnaires, 279; questions for, 71–72; rare, technologies for finding, 4; sample design for rare, 133–137; sample size weighting for, 168–174; target, 113–115; and variables, 89–90

Poststratification weighting, 173–174

Power analysis, 158–159

Pragmatic norms, for health questions, 203–204

Precision: formula for, 149, 150; in sample design, 121

Predictive validity, in questions, 59, 60–61

Pregnancy Risk Assessment Monitoring System (PRAMS), 472–478

Probability designs: and nonprobability designs, 115–116; types of, 116–121

Probability proportionate to size (PPS), 124–126

Proportional reduction in error (PRE), 336

Proportionate sampling, in stratified sample, 120

Proposal, and final report, 352–353

Prospective studies. See Longitudinal designs

Psychology. See Cognitive psychology

Psychometric issues, for health questions, 203, 204

Psychophysics, 203

Purposive samples, 116

Quality-adjusted life years (QALYS), 208

Quality of Life Index (QLI), 206–207

Quality of Well-Being Scale (QWB), 206–207

Quantitative measures, for reliability, 51

Question design: aspects of principles for, 177–199; and cognitive psychology, 182–184; criteria for, 191–197; on demographics and behavior, 222–242; and error issues, 199; error sources in, 179–182; examples of, 198; on health, 200–221; highlights on, 177–178; on knowledge and attitudes, 243–260; methods for, 185–187; and population issues, 197–198; pretesting, 187–190; in research report, 355; sources on, 199; steps in, 178–179

Questionnaire Design Research Laboratory (QDRL), 184, 186, 198
Questionnaires: administration of, 197, 240–241, 246–247, 255; appearance of, 274–275; aspects of, 261–280; for attitudes, 255, 277; context for, 278–279; criteria for, 197; for data collection, 105–106; and error issues, 279–280; examples of, 279; field editing, 297; format for, 262–275; highlights on, 261; for knowledge, 246–247; measurement matrix from, 323; order on, 275–278; and population issues, 279; precolumned, 311; pretesting, 189; sources on, 280; space on, 273–274; for threatening questions, 239–241; translating, 198, 220. *See also* Self-administered questionnaires
Questions: aspects of defining and clarifying, 44–74; closed-ended, 195, 196, 306–307, 311; concept of research, 35; criteria for, 191–194; and data collection methods, 92; for design, 31–35; dimensions of, 63–71; double-barreled, 194, 249; and error issues, 73; examples of, 40, 72; formulating, and data collection, 103–105; highlights on, 44–46; indexes for, 64–65; levels of measurement for, 47–50, 216–217; numbering, 263; open-ended, 103, 195–196, 307–308, 311; operational definitions for, 46–47; phrasing for, 271–272; and population issues, 71–72; pretesting, 188; reliability evaluation for, 50–58, 73; sample design related to, 113–116; and sample size, 144; scales for, 65–71; sources on, 73–74; threatening or sensitive, 104, 105, 236–241; typologies of, 64–65; validity evaluation for, 58–63, 73
Quota samples, 116

RAND Corporation, 9, 466, 479; Health Insurance Experiment of, 31, 201, 206–207, 473, 478
Random digit dialing (RDD): for data collection, 93, 99, 102; and informed consent, 4; procedures for, 126–127, 139–142
Random imputations, 316
Random numbers selection, 118
Random variation, and reliability, 45
Randomized responses, for threatening questions, 240–241
Randomized trials, characteristics of, 31
Range, in dispersion, 332–333
Range checking, 313, 314
Ranking and rating scales, on attitudes, 252–254
Ratio procedures, 48–50, 337–338, 341
Records: for behavior questions, 235; use of existing, 6
Reference person concept, 224
Regression imputation, 317

Relationships: bivariate statistics for, 333–339; existence or strength of, 328
Relative weights, 171–172
Reliability: evaluation of, 50–58, 73; for health questions, 210, 218; methods of computing, 54
Replication: and reports, 353; of variables, 79, 84, 86–87
Reports: aspects of, 350–358; audience for, 351; criteria for writing, 351–353; and error issues, 356–358; highlights on, 350; outline for, 352, 353–356; and replication, 353
Research Triangle Institute, 9, 105, 162
Respondent: procedures in selecting, 102, 128–133; proxy, 287–289
Response effects, and question design, 180–181, 197
Response rates: and data collection, 99–101; formula for, 165; and sample size, 164, 165–168; weighting for, 173
Responses: to attitude questions, 250–255; criteria for, 194–196; formats for, 263, 269, 270, 272–273; recoding, for 68; to knowledge questions, 246; randomized, 240–241; in threatening questions, 238, 240–241
Responsiveness, concept of, 71
Retrospective studies. *See* Group-comparison designs
Robert Wood Johnson Foundation, 98, 109, 469, 471
Roper Center User Services, 466
Roper polls, 462, 471

Sample design: aspects of, 112–142; combined methods for, 123–127; criteria for, 121–123; for data collection, 97–103; element in, 115; and error issues, 142; examples of, 137–142; frame for, 114–115; and health questions, 219–220; highlights on, 112–113; and population issues, 133–137; pretesting, 189; questions related to, 113–116; in research report, 354, 356–357; respondent selection procedures in, 128–133; sources on, 142; target population for, 113–114; types of, 115–121, 123–127
Sample size: adjustments in computing, 163–165; for analytical and experimental designs, 147, 152–161; aspects of, 143–176; and costs, 164–165; criteria for, 147; for cross-sectional designs, 146, 147–151; for descriptive designs, 144–152; and design, 144; and design effect, 161–164; and eligibility proportions, 164, 165–167; and error issues, 175–176; examples of, 174–175; formula for, 149, 150, 151, 152; for group-comparison designs, 146, 148, 151–152, 155–160; highlights on, 143; and response rates, 164,

165–168; sources on, 176; steps in estimating, 146–147, 163; weighting of, 168–174
Samples: independent or related, 328–329; normal distribution of, 145–146; univariate statistics to describe, 329–333
Satisfaction: attitude scales on, 256–260; and population characteristics, 15
Sawtooth Software, 301
Scales: for attitude questions, 252–255; construction of, 65–71; errors of, 69; for health questions, 204–210, 216–218; and reliability, 55–58; on satisfaction, 256–260
Schedule for contacts, implementing, 283–284, 298–299
Schemata: and behavior questions, 232; and question design, 183–184; and questionnaire format, 277
Screening, for rare populations, 133–135
Secondary analyses, conducting, 8–9
Self-administered questionnaires: comparisons of, 96, 98–99, 101, 103–110; computer-assisted, 94–95, 99, 104, 105; formatting, 262, 274, 276; on knowledge, 246–247. *See also* Mail surveys
SENECA Project, 468, 477
Sensitivity: and criterion validity, 60; cultural and language, 71
Sentences: for attitude questions, 249–250; criteria for, 194; in threatening questions, 238
Sequential imputation, 316–317
Service utilization, and population characteristics, 14
Short-Form Health Survey, 68, 71, 204, 206–207, 211
Sickness Impact Profile (SIP), 206–207
Simple random sample, procedures for, 117–118, 122
Sleepers, in knowledge questions, 247
Small area estimation procedures, 8
Social Security Administration, 471
Sociology: and designing surveys, 26, 29, 41, 43; and testing hypotheses, 76
Source data entry, 312–313
Specification, of variables, 79
Specificity, and criterion validity, 60
Split-half reliability, 52, 55, 56
Stability, and reliability, 50
Standard deviation, in dispersion, 333
Standard error: formula for, 149, 150; in sample size, 144–146; statistical procedures for, 162–163
Standard gamble approach, for health questions, 208–209
Stanford Three-Community Study, 468
Statistical imputation, 317
Statistical Package for the Social Sciences (SPSS), 56, 73, 171, 309, 313, 328–329
Statistics Canada, 184
Stratified sample: procedures for, 119–120, 123; and sample size, 161
Summative scales, 67–68

Supervision, of interviewers, 296–298
Survey of Income and Program Participation (SIPP), 471
Survey Research Center (California), 9
Survey Research Center (Michigan), 9, 100, 180, 302
Survey Research Laboratory: and cognitive psychology, 242; and data collection, 9, 110, 399; and implementation, 285, 289, 298–301, 302; and sampling, 139, 175; software from 321
Survey Sampling, Inc., 127
Surveys. *See* Health surveys
Sweden, telephone coverage in, 97
Switzerland, health surveys in, 468
Systematic departure, and validity, 45
Systematic random sample, procedures for, 118–119, 122–123, 137

Target population: operational definition of, 114–115; for sample design, 113–114
Techniques and technologies, in future, 2–4. *See* Computerized techniques
Telematch, 127
Telephone interviews: comparisons of, 96–106, 108–110; computer-assisted, 93–94, 106–107, 109, 110, 285; example of, 399–441; formatting, 262, 270; implementation of, 283, 284, 285, 288, 291, 298–301, 304; and informed consent, 4; rating scales for, 253; sample designs for, 126–127, 129, 132, 133, 139–142
Test or control variables, 76, 89
Test-retest reliability, 51, 52, 53, 54
Theoretic issues, for health questions, 202–203
Theory, concept of, 37
Think-aloud strategies: for behavior questions, 233; for question design, 186, 188
Thurstone Equal-Appearing Interval Scale, 66, 70, 217
Time trade-off method, for health questions, 209
Topics for surveys: aspects of, 1–24; classifying, 10–15; and defining features of surveys, 5–7; and errors, 20–23; examples of, 15–17; in future, 2; highlights on, 1–2; reasons for studying, 7–10; sources on, 24

Total Design Method: and implementation, 283, 285, 303; and questionnaire format, 262–263, 271, 274
Total Quality Management (TQM), 22
Total survey error framework. *See* Errors
Touchtone Data Entry (TDE), 94, 95
Training: in coding, 308, 309–310; of interviewers, 293–296
Transcriptive data entry, 310–311, 314
Transfer sheets, 310, 311
Translation of questionnaires, 198, 220
Trend studies, characteristics of, 30
Troldahl-Carter-Bryant (TCB) Tables, 129, 131

United Kingdom, health surveys in, 468
U.S. Bureau of Labor Statistics, 94, 95, 184, 471
U.S. Bureau of the Census: conferences by, 462; data collection by, 94, 110, 302; and data preparation, 308; and large-scale surveys, 8, 471; and question design, 184, 223, 224, 227, 228
U.S. Department of Agriculture, 94, 184, 477
U.S. Department of Commerce, 466
U.S. Department of Health and Human Services, 13, 39, 138, 359, 465
U.S. Department of Health Resources and Services Administration, 462
U.S. Public Health Service, 469–480
Univariate statistics, for data analysis, 327, 329–333, 345
Universe, for sample design, 113–114
Utility-related scaling methods, 204–210, 217

Validity: construct, 59, 61–63, 182, 210; content, 58, 59, 62, 210, 219; criterion, 59, 60–61, 62, 181–182; evaluation of, 58–63, 73; external, 42–43; for health questions, 210, 218–219; internal, 42; methods of computing, 62
Variable errors, concept of, 22–23
Variables: aspects of relationships between, 75–90; defining and clarifying, 44–74; dependent and independent, 38, 77–79; and error issues, 90; examples of, 90; explanation of, 79, 80–82; highlights on, 75; and hypotheses, 76–86; interpretation of, 79, 82–84; mock tables for,

86–89; and population issues, 89–90; replication of, 79, 84, 86–87; sources on, 90
Variance, in dispersion, 333
Veterans Administration, 471
Visit Satisfaction Questionnaire (VSQ), 257, 258–259
Voice Recognition Entry (VRE), 94, 95

Waksberg-Mitofsky procedure, 127, 133, 139–142
Washington, University of: and dentists' practice patterns, 41, 110; Department of Community Dentistry at, 443; Institutional Review Board of, 302–203
Washington Education Association (WEA), 40, 140, 142, 198, 348
Washington State Study of Dentists' Preferences in Prescribing Dental Therapy: aspects of, 16–17, 479; and attitude questions, 249, 252, 254; and behavior questions, 235; data analysis for, 323–326, 343–346, 348; data collection methods for, 110; data preparation for, 321; design of, 40–41; implementation of, 286, 288, 302–303; question design for, 198; questionnaire for, 263, 268, 270, 271, 272, 274, 443–460; questions for, 67, 72; sample design for, 140, 142; sample size for, 175
Washington State University, 303
Weighting, of sample, 168–174
Westat, 9, 162, 301
Wisconsin Survey Research Laboratory, 9
WONCA Classification Committee, 213
Words: in attitude questions, 248; criteria for, 191–193; in threatening questions, 237
World Fertility Survey (WFS), 467–468
World Health Organization (WHO): address of, 465; and concept of health, 13, 63, 211; Expanded Programme on Immunization (EPI) of, 124, 468; International Classification of Diseases by, 308; studies by, 467–468, 474

Yea-saying, avoiding, 250–252
Year 2000 Public Health Promotion and Disease Prevention Objectives for the Nation's Health, 16, 39, 224, 244